AF694122

Textbook of Pulmonary Rehabilitation

Enrico Clini • Anne E. Holland
Fabio Pitta • Thierry Troosters
Editors

Textbook of Pulmonary Rehabilitation

Springer

Editors

Enrico Clini
Department of Medical and Surgical Sciences
University of Modena
Azienda Ospedaliero Universitaria di Modena Policlinico
Modena, Italy

Fabio Pitta
State University of Londrina
Londrina, Paraná, Brazil

Anne E. Holland
Alfred Health and Institute for Breathing and Sleep, La Trobe University
Melbourne, Australia

Thierry Troosters
Department of Rehabilitation Sciences
KU Leuven, Respiratory Division and Rehabilitation
University Hospital Leuven
Leuven, Belgium

ISBN 978-3-319-65887-2 ISBN 978-3-319-65888-9 (eBook)
https://doi.org/10.1007/978-3-319-65888-9

Library of Congress Control Number: 2017962903

© Springer International Publishing AG 2018, corrected publication 2018
This work is subject to copyright. All rights are reserved by the Publisher, whether the whole or part of the material is concerned, specifically the rights of translation, reprinting, reuse of illustrations, recitation, broadcasting, reproduction on microfilms or in any other physical way, and transmission or information storage and retrieval, electronic adaptation, computer software, or by similar or dissimilar methodology now known or hereafter developed.
The use of general descriptive names, registered names, trademarks, service marks, etc. in this publication does not imply, even in the absence of a specific statement, that such names are exempt from the relevant protective laws and regulations and therefore free for general use.
The publisher, the authors and the editors are safe to assume that the advice and information in this book are believed to be true and accurate at the date of publication. Neither the publisher nor the authors or the editors give a warranty, express or implied, with respect to the material contained herein or for any errors or omissions that may have been made. The publisher remains neutral with regard to jurisdictional claims in published maps and institutional affiliations.

Printed on acid-free paper

This Springer imprint is published by Springer Nature
The registered company is Springer International Publishing AG
The registered company address is: Gewerbestrasse 11, 6330 Cham, Switzerland

Foreword

To borrow a phrase from Charles Dickens, for pulmonary rehabilitation this is the best of times and the worst of times. A strong scientific basis has been gathered which makes pulmonary rehabilitation arguably the most effective therapy we have to offer patients with pulmonary disease. Yet the lack of availability to the vast majority of patients lessens its impact. This is manifestly true for patients with chronic obstructive pulmonary disease (COPD), and even more so for patients with other chronic pulmonary conditions. This volume helps to clarify these issues and, hopefully, will provide a path forward.

Pulmonary rehabilitation is no longer a young discipline. Founded in the concepts of Alvan Barach, who more than 60 years ago posited that exercise was effective therapy for his emphysema patients. Made tangible by Tom Petty, who organized the first multidisciplinary team to deliver pulmonary rehabilitation almost 50 years ago. Nurtured by practitioners who understood the benefits, established programs and spread the word. Recognized by exercise scientists who established the scientific basis of the exercise programs that are the core of pulmonary rehabilitation, introducing concepts such as limb muscle dysfunction and dynamic hyperinflation, which have helped to rationalize new adjuncts to exercise programs. And then promoted as standard of care by every relevant professional organization in authoritative documents. The 2016 GOLD Guidelines concludes "…all COPD patients appear to benefit from rehabilitation and maintenance of physical activity, improving their exercise tolerance and experiencing decreased dyspnea and fatigue."

It is worth trying to discern why pulmonary rehabilitation is so little used despite its unequivocal benefits. Consider that there are three major therapies widely recognized as effective for COPD: bronchodilators, supplemental oxygen, and pulmonary rehabilitation. Although we have little in the way of head to head trials, it may be concluded that rehabilitation, in comparison to the other two, yields superior benefits in terms of enhancement of exercise tolerance, reduction of dyspnea, and improvement of health-related quality of life, all highly relevant patient-centered benefits. Yet uptake of these three therapies by COPD patients is quite the opposite. Bronchodilators, especially the long-acting variety, are almost universally used. Supplemental oxygen is widely available to those patients demonstrating clinically significant hypoxemia. In contrast, a 2013 survey (Desveaux et al., J. COPD) concludes: "the annual national capacity for pulmonary rehabilitation…consistently translated to ≤1.2% of the estimated COPD population" for the countries surveyed. In the United States, a recent Medicare database examination (Nishi et al. J Cardiopulm Rehabil, 2016) revealed that, among Medicare beneficiaries, pulmonary rehabilitation participation rate increased from 2.6% in 2003 to (only) 3.7% in 2012. As many COPD patients lack Medicare coverage, these percentages likely overestimate the participation in the overall COPD population in the United States. A 2015 American Thoracic Society/European Respiratory Society (ATS/ERS) Policy Statement (Rochester et al., Am J Respir Crit Care Med), dealing with strategies to enhance the implementation of pulmonary rehabilitation, concludes that "the ATS and ERS commit to undertake actions that will improve access to and delivery of PR services for suitable patients. They call on their members and other health professional societies, payers, patients, and patient advocacy groups to join in this commitment." But this call seems to be going largely unanswered.

This situation persists despite the fact that all three therapies have essentially universal support as standard of care for symptomatic COPD. Is this because of cost differentials? No, it can be seen that the annual cost of standard bronchodilator therapy, long-term oxygen therapy, and a program of pulmonary rehabilitation is roughly in the same range. In fact, analyses such as the one conducted by the British Thoracic Society (BTS Reports, 2012) conclude that pulmonary rehabilitation has a substantially lower cost per quality-adjusted life-year (QALY) than does bronchodilator therapy. It might be asked what pulmonary rehabilitation lacks that bronchodilator therapy and supplemental oxygen possess that explains the differential in uptake of these therapies. On reflection, bronchodilator therapy uptake is supported by an extensive marketing effort, both directly to patients and to medical providers. Oxygen therapy, on the other hand, is not marketed, but its provision is near mandatory because it is widely accepted that failure to provide long-term oxygen therapy to hypoxemic COPD patients is associated with substantially increased mortality. This conclusion is founded on two, relatively small, randomized clinical trials (total of about 300 patients) performed more than 35 years ago. Nevertheless, the perception that survival is enhanced by long-term oxygen therapy has made its provision (and funding) more or less mandatory for those meeting the criteria established in these clinical trials. Indeed, it may be asserted that *all* therapies that prolong survival have high priority.

It seems unlikely that pulmonary rehabilitation will ever be supported by an extensive marketing effort, but it might be asked whether rehabilitation reduces COPD mortality. It seems understandable that this information is not available. Large-scale multicenter investigations of pulmonary rehabilitation are almost nonexistent. Even if a substantial survival benefit is postulated, because, in stable COPD, the likelihood of dying in the short term is rather low, it would take a very large randomized clinical trial (many thousands of participants) to provide adequate resolution. A design that might be more feasible would be to study rehabilitation of patients shortly after a COPD hospitalization. Because post-hospitalization patients have a relatively high mortality, the number of participants to adequately investigate a given postulated reduction in mortality would be appreciably reduced.

As we look forward, it seems important to incorporate "next generation" features into our model of pulmonary rehabilitation. Formal behavior modification techniques can improve adherence and, especially, promote increases in physical activity in everyday life. Maintenance programs, perhaps incorporating telemedicine approaches, can help prolong benefit. Addition of these components might well increase the likelihood of the survival advantage whose establishment can be predicted to change the attitude of patients, providers, and payers alike, resulting in increased demand and better provision of pulmonary rehabilitation services.

Richard Casaburi, Ph.D., M.D.
UCLA School of Medicine, Rehabilitation Clinical Trials Center
Los Angeles Biomedical Research Institute,
Torrance, CA, USA

Contents

Part VII Specific Scenarios

Part I

Introductory Aspects

1 A Historical Perspective of Pulmonary Rehabilitation

Bartolome R. Celli and Roger S. Goldstein

1.1 Introduction

The association between a healthy body and a better functioning mind has been understood for a very long time. In his satires, the Roman poet Juvenal (English translation by Niall Rudd: http://books.google.ca/books?id=ngJemlYfB4MC&pg=PA86) condensed the concept into one of the most famous phrases in Western civilization "*Mens sana in corpore sano*," best translated as "A healthy mind lives within a healthy body." Indeed, all through antiquity and certainly in the Greco-Roman culture, a fit body was a sign of health and exercise became an integral part of their lives.

B.R. Celli, M.D., F.C.C.P., F.E.R.S. (✉)
Pulmonary and Critical Care Division,
Brigham and Women's Hospital,
Harvard Medical School,
Boston, MA, USA
e-mail: bcelli@partners.org

R.S. Goldstein, MB, ChB, FRCP(C), FCCP
National Sanitarium Chair in Respiratory Rehabilitation Research,
Program in Respiratory Rehabilitation,
West Park Healthcare Centre,
Medicine and Physical Therapy,
University of Toronto,
Toronto, ON, Canada
e-mail: rgoldste@westpark.org

1.2 Early Times

Unfortunately, loss of health was thought to be best treated with rest, which perhaps was beneficial for infectious diseases and trauma, which were the most frequent cause of death until our very recent past. Indeed, the development of "resting institutes" to care for the sick was first developed in the East, with the "Ayurvedic hospitals" of Sri Lanka representing the earliest example of actual physical places devoted to harboring the sick and helping them recover. Although the Greek culture also had its healing temples dedicated to their healer god Asclepius, it was the Romans who in the Western civilization first developed physical institutions called "*Valetudinaria*" to harbor and help the sick, primarily caring for sick slaves, gladiators, and soldiers (Medicine. An Illustrated History. Lyons A.S. and Petrucelli R.J. Aberdale Press, NY, 1987. pp. 175 and 205). This was needed to keep the empire functional and the health of the legions was central to this purpose. Bed rest as a therapy reached its highest acceptance in the nineteenth century when patients with many different illnesses were placed in absolute bed rest and were passively cared for by health assistants and nurses. This became particularly true for patients suffering from tuberculosis (Fig. 1.1), and the "*sanatoriums*" were built with the specific purpose of providing rest, good air, and nutrition for these patients [1]. Of note, what is known today

© Springer International Publishing AG 2018
E. Clini et al. (eds.), *Textbook of Pulmonary Rehabilitation*,
https://doi.org/10.1007/978-3-319-65888-9_1

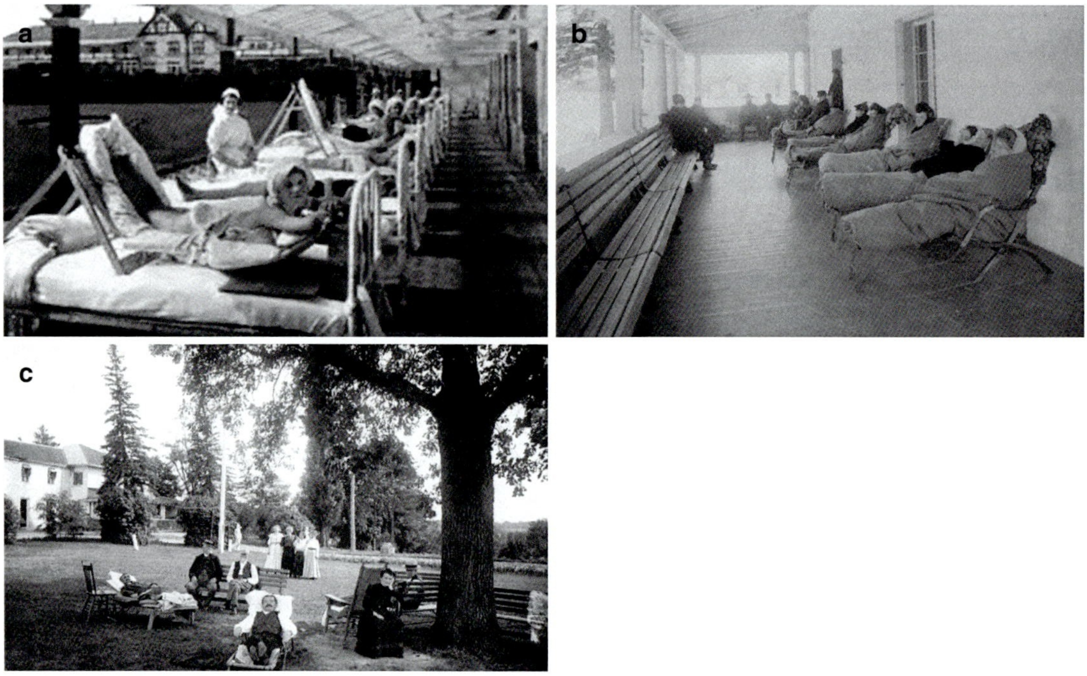

Fig. 1.1 (**a**) Patients with tuberculosis treated with bed rest, nutrition, and fresh air [1]. (**b**) Patients with tuberculosis taking the cure, midwinter 1905 [2]. (**c**) Patients with tuberculosis taking the cure under the oak tree, summer 1906 [2]

as "The American Thoracic Society (ATS)," an organization focused on improving care for pulmonary diseases, critical illnesses, and sleep-related breathing disorders, was established in 1905 as the American Sanatorium Association to assist with the care of patients with tuberculosis.

1.3 Pulmonary Rehabilitation Is Born

The belief was that a regimen of rest and good nutrition offered the best therapy to help individuals affected by tuberculosis to boost their own immune system to control the infection. In 1863, the first sanatorium opened in Europe (now Poland) for the treatment of tuberculosis. The accepted thought was that rest at high altitude, fresh air, and good nutrition could lead to resolution and control of the disease. Sanatoriums became quite popular and spread throughout the world, with the first one in the United States opening in 1885 in the Adirondack Region in Saranac Lake, New York, and the first one in Canada opening in Muskoka, Ontario, in 1897 (Fig. 1.1) [2]. The mountainous characteristics of these locations represented the perfect geography to develop these health resorts for patients with tuberculosis and many were built in these regions. It was the one in Denver, Colorado, that drew the attention of Dr. Charles Denison (1849–1909), a Vermont-born pulmonologist who was also a climatologist (Fig. 1.2). Having developed tuberculosis in Hartford, Connecticut, he moved to Texas for a short period and finally to Denver, where, after his recovery, he had a very successful career as a professor of medicine until his death. Dr. Denison had an inquisitive mind and noticed that he felt better after exercising rather than plain resting. Prompted by this observation, he wrote a book entitled *Exercise and Food for Pulmonary Invalids,* which constitutes the first written scientific testimony in the field of pulmonary rehabilitation (Fig. 1.2).

In his book, Dr. Denison wrote "Let it be understood that in recommending exercise for respiratory invalids, acute and inflammatory conditions of the lungs are excluded." Indeed, he recommended that the exercise become part of the "recuperative" period and that bed rest be limited

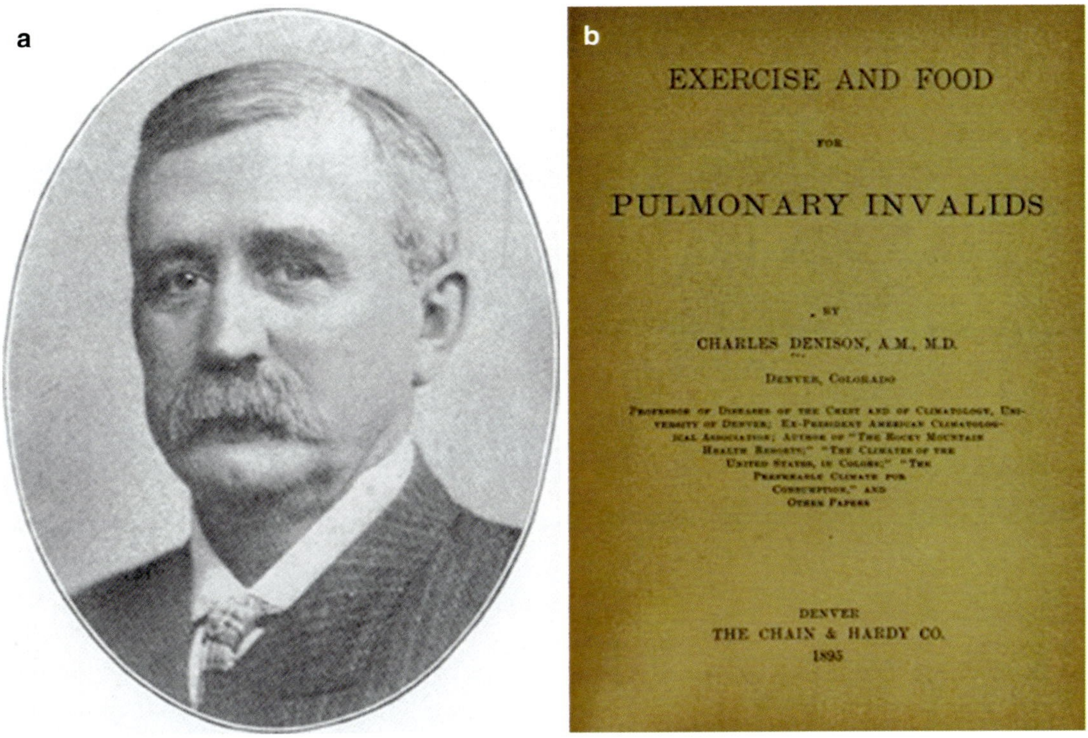

Fig. 1.2 (**a**) Photograph of Dr. Charles Denison, author of the first book on the use of exercise in respiratory invalids. (**b**) Exercise and food for pulmonary invalids. Charles Denison. The Chain and Hardy Co., Denver, Colorado, 1895

to the acute phases of the disease. Throughout the book, he expanded with excellent figures on breathing exercises, with particular emphasis of exercises of the upper extremities and expansion of the thorax. He also added that "walking, hill climbing, bicycling and rowing were excellent exercises that could help the patients." He went on to state "these forms of exercise are purposely graduated to enable the attending physician to know how far a given person should proceed a given time." In other words, he felt it would be wise to have some degree of supervision by a healthcare professional to determine the best program tailored to the individual patient. This was the insight that prompted the birth of pulmonary rehabilitation as we know it today. It was soon afterward, when at the early twentieth century, Dr. Alvan Barach in New York began to make observations and complete studies that constituted a first effort to consolidate the body of knowledge of pulmonary rehabilitation as a science. Barach was very interested in dyspnea as a cardinal symptom of respiratory disease. Indeed, he was the first to observe that the leaning forward position improved the sensation in patients with emphysema and wrote about a series of breathing exercise to improve this symptom in those patients [3, 4]. By expressing and writing his views on the topic, he raised some interest among certain groups, while his detractors discarded his ideas as being esoteric. However, the end result of his observations was an increase in the interest of the potential benefit of breathing exercises, and several clinical studies began to expand those observations to include whole-body exercise. His treatment manual for patients with emphysema published in 1969 (Fig. 1.3) highlighted the importance of exercise as part of comprehensive COPD management. At about this time, Dr. Albert Haas, also working in New York, expanded on the concepts of rehabilitation for patients with respiratory diseases. A native of Hungary, he received his MD from the University of Budapest in 1940. Of interest, like Denison, he also developed tuberculosis as a youngster, from which he recovered completely. He moved to

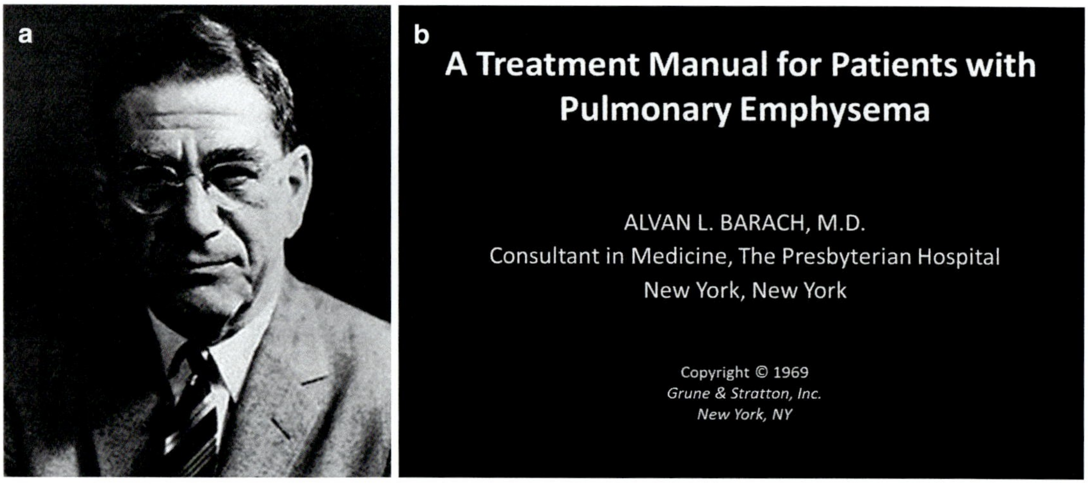

Fig. 1.3 (**a**) Photograph of Dr. Alvan L. Barach. (**b**) A treatment manual for patients with pulmonary emphysema. Alvan L. Barach, Grune & Stratton, New York, NY, 1969

France after the invasion of Hungary by the Nazis, and there, he joined the resistance. He was captured, made prisoner, and sent to the concentration camp in Dachau. Because of his medical training, but without being a surgeon, he was made to operate on sick individuals, which allowed him to acquire sufficient expertise in surgery to be of use in his career. He finally made his way to New York where he completed training in Bellevue and during his very academic and clinical career published a series of studies based on his own experience of exercise during his time with tuberculosis. Given this background, it came natural to him to study the value of breathing and whole-body exercise in patients with thoracoplasty and other thoracic surgical procedures [5–7]. The observational foundations laid by these pioneering scientists were followed by several important contributions by researchers who applied more modern methods to the explorations of questions related to the application of knowledge acquired from many different fields of medicine, primarily the new knowledge about mechanics of breathing, gas exchange, and cardiac as well as respiratory response to exercise [8, 9].

A second important event in this early period field of pulmonary rehabilitation was the novel idea that supplemental oxygen could be administered as a therapeutic agent to patients with respiratory ailments. Joseph Priestley in England, Carl Scheele in Sweden, and Antoine Lavoisier in France are all credited with the discovery of oxygen in the last quarter of the eighteenth century, but it took almost two centuries before Alvan Barach in the United States [10–12] and J. E. Cotes in England [13, 14] at almost the same time first reported the benefits of supplemental oxygen to patients with emphysema or respiratory insufficiency. These advances included the first references to portable oxygen in an attempt to improve the functional capacity of these patients [15].

1.4 Juvenile Years of the Field

By the midportion of the twentieth century, a group of pulmonary physicians attempted to integrate the experiences in the field into a comprehensive body of information. Of these attempts, the one that best relates to this historical review was the Eight Aspen Emphysema Conference that took place in Denver, Colorado. Instrumental in its organization and running was the then young Denver-born, attending Dr. Thomas Petty (Fig. 1.4), whose interest was centered in the clinical application of many of the concepts developed by the abovementioned pioneers with integration of pharmacotherapy and even potential surgical therapies, this being the conference where Otto C. Brantigan presented his

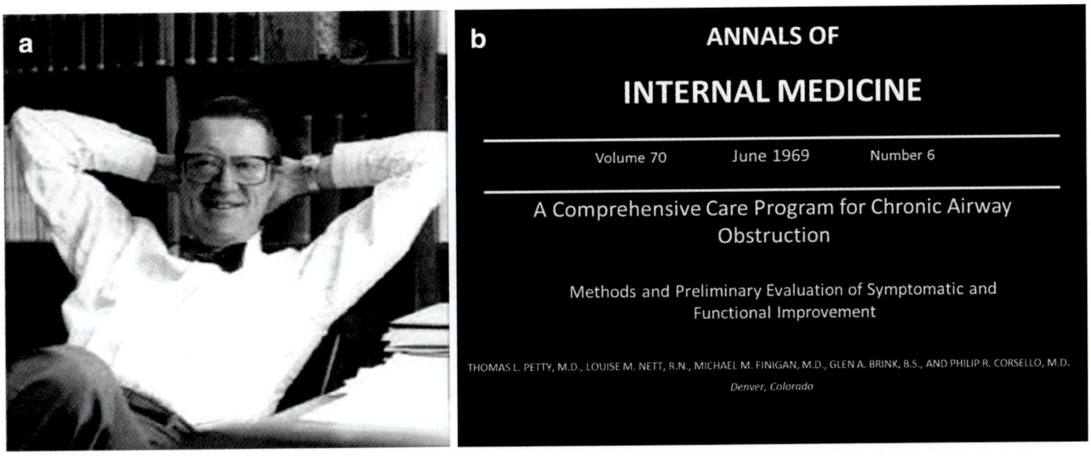

Fig. 1.4 (**a**) Photograph of Dr. Thomas Petty in his office at the University of Colorado. Dr. Petty coordinatored the Eighth Aspen Lung Conference, the first meeting where the concept of multidisciplinary treatment of patients with COPD was discussed. (**b**) One of the original rehabilitation studies "A comprehensive care program for chronic airway obstruction. Methods and preliminary evaluation of symptomatic and functional improvement." Thomas L. Petty [17]

results of operative techniques for advanced emphysema, with the attendance of Drs. William F. Miller from Dallas, who had already begun to publish results of trials of exercise in patients with emphysema [16], Ben V. Branscomb, Gordon L. Snider, and Reuben Cherniack. Most attendees discussed the interesting observation that the patients studied until then and reported significant improvement in their symptoms, but no objective evidence of lung function improvement, a problem that would puzzle many investigators in the field for decades. Indeed, the summary of that conference provided by Dr. Theodore Noehren centered on that difficult paradox that needed more research, and he even labeled that unknown factor as the Factor "R." As a consequence, Dr. Petty and coworkers applied and were granted a contract to develop and explore the scientific basis and benefits of a comprehensive pulmonary rehabilitation program funded by the Chronic Respiratory Disease Control Program of the Public Health Service. Actually two such demonstration projects were funded, the one in Denver and the other in Minneapolis. The description provided by Dr. Petty fully resembles the current components of modern-day pulmonary rehabilitation as it included patient and family education, pharmacological strategies, breathing retraining, physical reconditioning, and optimization of oxygen therapy. This program started in 1966 and had already collected over 180 patients by 1968, the findings of which were presented in the high-impact general medical journal the *Annals of Internal Medicine* in 1969 (Fig. 1.4) [17]. This breakthrough brought the field to a new level, as it began to be recognized as an important tool in the therapy of patients with chronic obstructive pulmonary diseases.

Another important push was added, when a specifically planned meeting took place in California, at the Human Interaction Research Institute, organized by Dr. Edward Glaser. The proceedings of this conference were published in the same year, and they may represent the first well-organized body of scientific information on pulmonary rehabilitation. Among other participants, there was another rising star, Dr. John Hodgkin from Loma Linda, California, who was tasked with the charge of organizing the proceeds and discussions into a coherent body of information. After receiving multiple versions, input, and thoughts from 29 authors, the summary was published in the *Journal of the American Medical Association* [18] and became the best source of comprehensive information in the field. Pulmonary rehabilitation had moved from an obscure form of therapy that had been considered the realm of charlatans to a concept that had enough evidence to have its principles published in the most prestigious journals in medicine. In the decade of the 1970s, the content of this workshop was expanded, and the American College of Chest Physicians published a book with a more comprehensive version of the topics. The growth and interest were not exclusive of the United States and pulmonary rehabilitation began to expand worldwide. The group in Nancy, France, and Spain led by Manuel Gimenez published studies on the beneficial use of breathing retraining in patients with chronic bronchitis [19, 20]. Simultaneously, an active interest in testing the potential benefit of oxygen therapy took the field to a new level. The results of two randomized clinical trials testing the effect of 12-h, 24-h, or no oxygen supplementation to hypoxemic patients with COPD, with mortality as the outcome, were undertaken in North America and in the United Kingdom [21, 22]. The results of these trials were revolutionary as both provided for the first time an agent capable of improving survival to patients with a chronic disease, for which there was consensus and there were no lifesaving options. Of interest, both trials were conducted on a background of comprehensive therapy, very similar to what would be considered pulmonary rehabilitation. These results elevated the field even more, by bringing into it the design of randomized trials to test the benefits and risks of any new intervention. The ground had been cleared for pulmonary rehabilitation to mature.

1.5 Pulmonary Rehabilitation Matures

The growth of pulmonary rehabilitation from anecdotal benefits of enthusiastic pioneers to it being accepted as the standard of care for chronic respiratory disease parallels a requirement for the establishment of many aspects of medical care, namely, scientific evidence. The four decades that span the period from the early 1980s until now have seen an explosion in the number and importance of studies related to pulmonary rehabilitation. This dramatic increase has been heralded by the development of valid, reproducible, interpretable, evaluative, outcome measures which enabled the transformation of clinical observations into science, thus setting the stage for randomized controlled trials. Key among these advances has been the introduction by Gordon Guyatt and colleagues of a disease-specific COPD questionnaire looking at domains of dyspnea, fatigue, emotional function, and mastery (Fig. 1.5) [23]. Other questionnaires such as

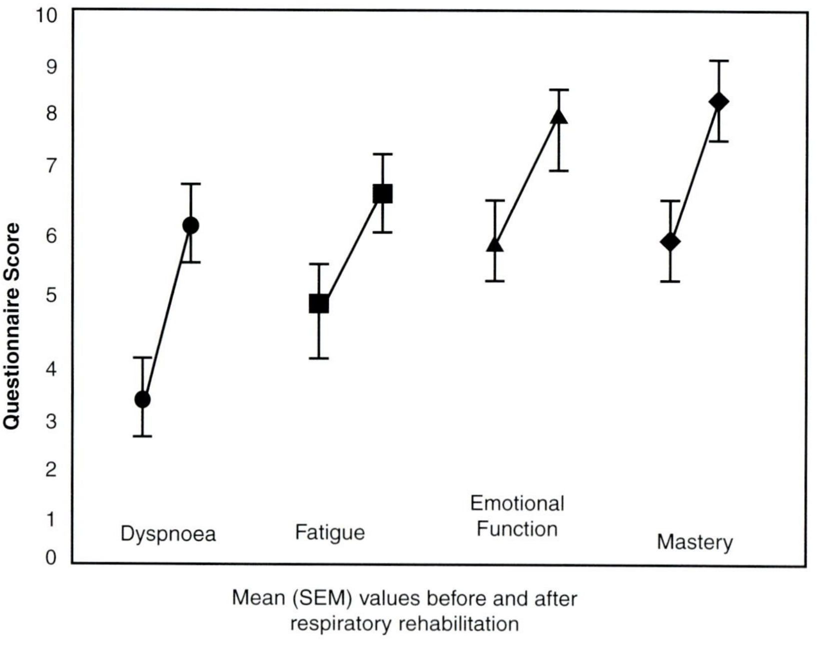

Fig. 1.5 A measure of quality of life for COPD. The Chronic Respiratory Disease Questionnaire (CRDQ) developed by Guyatt and colleagues [23]

the St. George's Respiratory Questionnaire (SGRQ) looking at symptom activity and impacts followed a few years later [24]. Today, there are at least 20 COPD disease-specific questionnaires, and the key is to know their psychometric properties and match the outcome selected to the clinical design for the question asked [25]. The other major outcome development was that of field exercise tests, recognizing that most PR patients could not be evaluated by a formal cardiopulmonary exercise test. The 6-min walk test came from the 12-min run (Fig. 1.6) [26–28] used to assess fitness in US military recruits and found to have similar results for maximum oxygen uptake to laboratory measures of incremental exercise. A few years later, the incremental and shuttle walk tests, originally used to test fitness among UK police applicants, were adapted for use in patients with COPD (Fig. 1.6) [29–31]. The concept of the minimum clinically important difference [32] enabled test interpretability to reach beyond statistical significance to clinical importance. Whereas 172 manuscripts were published in 1980, there were 1190 in the year 2016, a substantial increase not only in the number but in the quality of published papers. It is impossible to cite all of the important manuscripts and studies that have expanded the field. However, we shall make an attempt to reflect the most important developments. In 1980, Sahn and coworkers published the 10-year experience of the Denver cohort of patients [33]. In that study, a survival

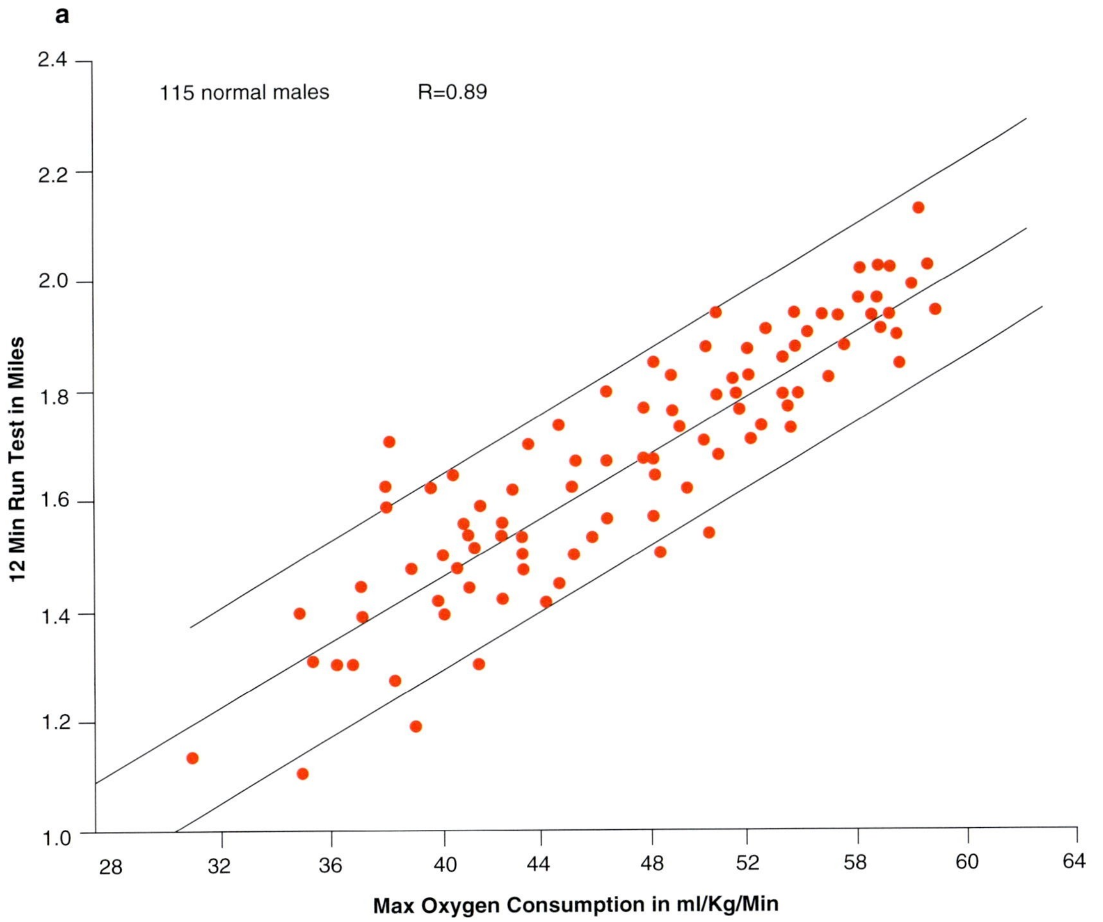

Fig. 1.6 (**a**) The 12-min run and maximal oxygen consumption. Taken from healthy males. Note the close association [26–28]. (**b**) The shuttle run and maximal oxygen consumption. Note the close association [29–31]

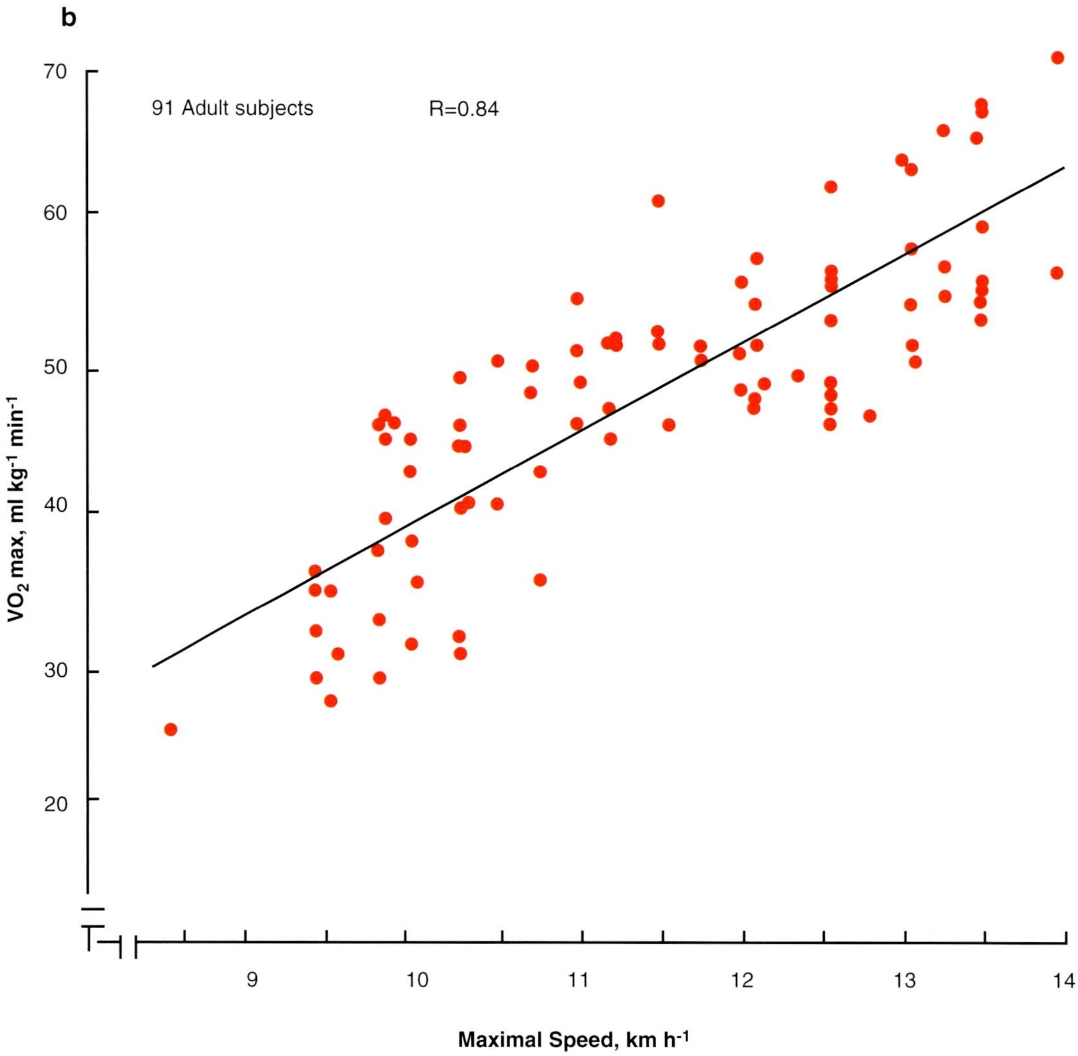

Fig. 1.6 (continued)

benefit was observed when compared to patients with the same degree of emphysema drawn from the Denver area. This provided even more impetus to scientists in the field to investigate the potential mechanism responsible for the reported and observed benefits of pulmonary rehabilitation. For the first time, the evidence, at least for patients with COPD, was acknowledged objectively by the American Thoracic Society [34], but the components, methods, and outcome measurements remained somewhat nebulous.

The content of comprehensive programs was placed in perspective by the publication of several books that have made an imprint on rehabilitation and have continued to do so. These books were edited by authorities who had helped develop the field and included *Pulmonary Rehabilitation: Guidelines to Success*. Under the leadership of Dr. John Hodgkin, this book was first edited in Boston by Butterworth in 1984, with the 4th edition published by Elsevier in 2009. Richard Casaburi and Thomas Petty edited the book entitled *Principles and Practice of Pulmonary Rehabilitation* in the United States, while several other books in different countries have followed, as the word on the benefit of these programs has expanded across the globe. In parallel to these developments, interest has grown in the review of evidence to grade recommendations. This concept has led to the development of guidelines aimed at providing help to healthcare deliverers and to improve overall health of afflicted patients. This also occurred in pulmonary rehabilitation. Independent international societies either on their own or in joint statements have published a flurry of guidelines addressing the large body of data that has accumulated on pulmonary rehabilitation. At an international level, collaborative consensus statements by international organizations such as the American Thoracic Society and European Respiratory Society have provided very detailed summaries of the evidence in support of pulmonary rehabilitation as well as the many unanswered questions [35–38]. The most important historical element is the high grade of evidence that supports many of the components that are recommended. The evidence is so strong that the Global Initiative for Obstructive Lung Disease (GOLD), in its most recent revision by Vogelmeier [39], includes pulmonary rehabilitation as one of the key therapeutic elements. They state "Pulmonary rehabilitation improves dyspnea, health status and exercise tolerance in stable patients (Evidence A). Pulmonary rehabilitation reduces hospitalizations in patients with recent exacerbation (≤4 weeks from prior hospitalization) (Evidence B)." Added to the statement on the benefits of oxygen therapy in hypoxemic patients (Evidence A), no other therapeutic package carries the same weight of evidence.

1.6 Major Recent Advances

Most medical advances occur by small increments, especially as the complexities of biology are deciphered at the molecular level and the gains are measured in microns. This is also true in the field of pulmonary rehabilitation. However, the last three decades have seen major developments. Let us review some of them.

Early randomized controlled trials of pulmonary rehabilitation [40–42] consistently reflected the improvements in dyspnea and quality of life associated with PR (Fig. 1.7) [43]. Whereas sensitization to dyspnea was thought to play a major role in the improved sensation of well-being after pulmonary rehabilitation in patients with COPD [44], studies documenting the increase in the oxidative enzyme content of the vastus lateralis muscle of COPD patients undergoing exercise training provided new insight into biological reasons for the increase in exercise endurance after rehabilitation [45]. These well-conducted physiological studies proved that patients with COPD could undergo intense training and derive important benefits in terms of improvements in lactic acid production, ventilatory requirements, and pattern of breathing that helped explained some of the increased tolerance to exercise and lower scores of dyspnea for the same work intensity (Fig. 1.8) [46]. The scales that allowed measurement of the sensation of dyspnea were further validated [47, 48], and with the advantage that extended to other domains [49, 50], the benefits on health status now became possible [23–25, 51–53]. Indices that reflect the multidimensional nature of COPD that respond to rehabilitation were also developed and tested [54, 55]. In the management of COPD, no therapy has matched the benefits seen in all of these scales after pulmonary rehabilitation. Together with the improvements in understanding the mechanisms responsible for the benefits of the programs, our knowledge about the type and duration of exercise to be recommended also improved [56–59]. Along with the improvement seen with leg exercise, evidence arose about the adverse effect of upper extremity exercise on breathing [60, 61] and the improvements seen when upper extremities are included in the training [62, 63]. When the norm was that patients were to be trained in well-supervised areas in hospital, several well-controlled studies have shown that benefits can be achieved in good home programs [64–66]. More recently evidence is accumulating that distance rehabilitation using tele-technology results in changes to quality of life and exercise similar to that reported from institutionally based outpatient programs [67].

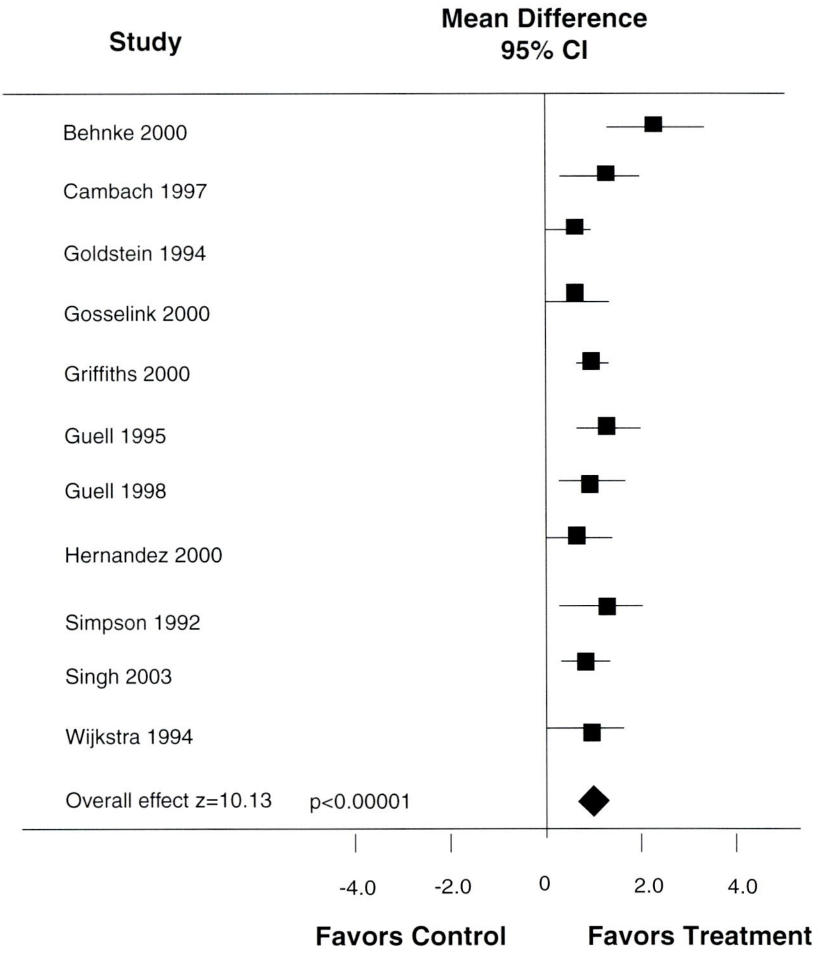

Fig. 1.7 Change in the dyspnea domain of chronic respiratory questionnaire following pulmonary rehabilitation [43]

This opens the way to more timely, less expensive, and equitable availability of PR for those in need. Different approaches to administering endurance exercise, such as interval training, are being explored [68]. Training has been augmented with electrical stimulation [69], ventilator support [70], hyperoxia [71], and by reducing the work of breathing using a mixture of helium and oxygen [72, 73]. Partitioned exercise using alternate single-leg training provides less of a central stimulus while maintaining a high muscle-specific training load. It has also been shown to increase maximum oxygen consumption, exercise capacity, and quality of life [74] as well as being a feasible addition to the exercise regimen of PR [75]. Randomized trials have been common in rehabilitation, all of them have shown improvement in patient-centered outcomes, and some have shown benefits in healthcare utilization of resources [76]. We now better appreciate the issue of reduced activity levels in COPD, even more so post exacerbation (Fig. 1.9) [77] as well as the relevance of activity as a predictor of morbidity and mortality [78, 79]. As a result, PR introduced early post exacerbation has shown promising improvements in function and quality of life with less powerful evidence in favor of reduced hospitalization [80, 81]. The challenge of diminution of the initial benefits over time from nonadherence has also been tackled using extended programs, repeat programs, cell phone encouragement, as well as by training community fitness instructors in the maintenance exercise for COPD [56, 82–84]. Another major step forward has been the realization that more

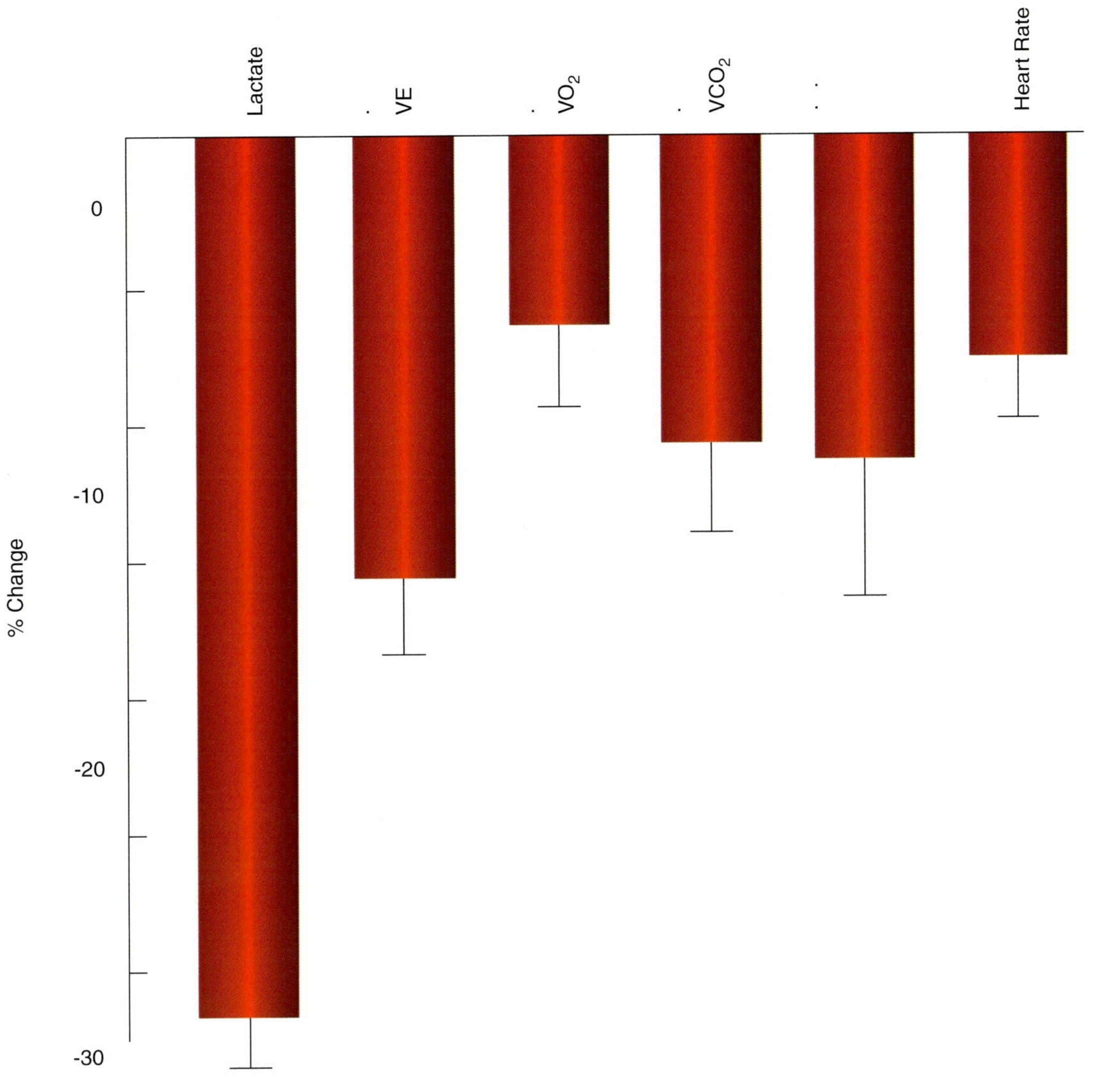

Fig. 1.8 Exercise responses to an identical work rate after exercise training in COPD. An original study by Casaburi and colleagues [46]

integrated care through case management (Fig. 1.10) [85–87] is associated in many reports with a diminution of hospitalization for exacerbations. Adding the benefits of PR within an integrated framework of case management holds great promise for the well-being of patients with COPD as well as for those responsible for diminishing healthcare resource utilization.

The benefits seen after pulmonary rehabilitation in patients with COPD have brought about its adoption as the standard of care for chronic respiratory conditions in the medical community as well as in the surgical community, where it is used in association with lung volume reduction as well as lung transplantation [88, 89]. Its effectiveness has generated an interest for the same techniques to be explored in diseases different from COPD. The results from studies in patients with cystic fibrosis, pulmonary artery hypertension, interstitial lung diseases, asthma, and lung cancer offer a testimony to the original observations of Dr. Denison in patients recovering from

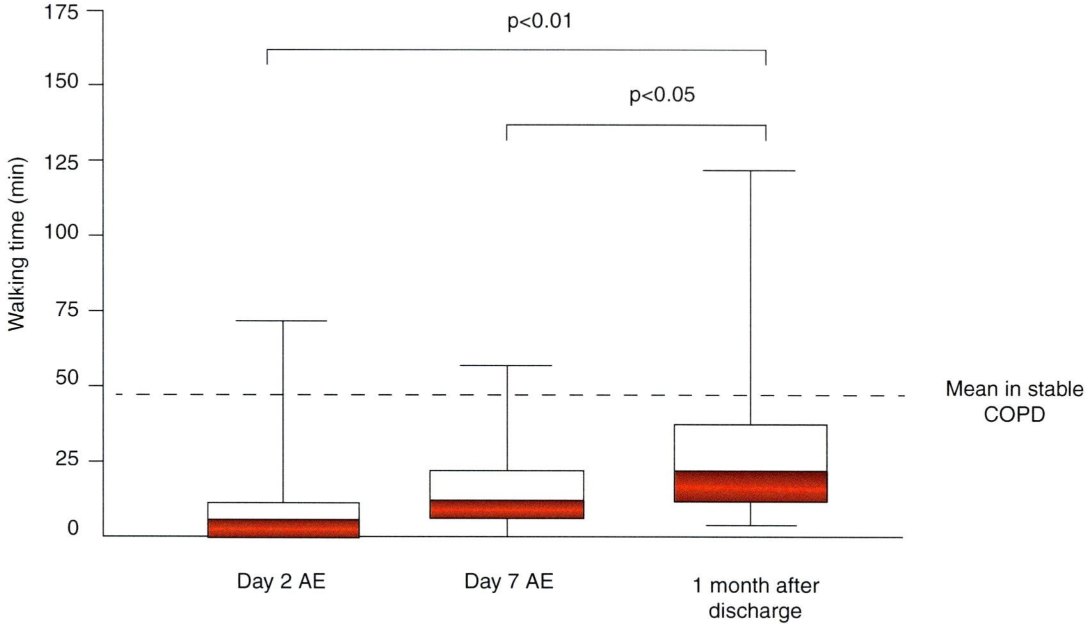

Fig. 1.9 Hospitalization and physical activity post AECOPD. Note the prolonged impact of low levels of activity following an acute exacerbation [77]

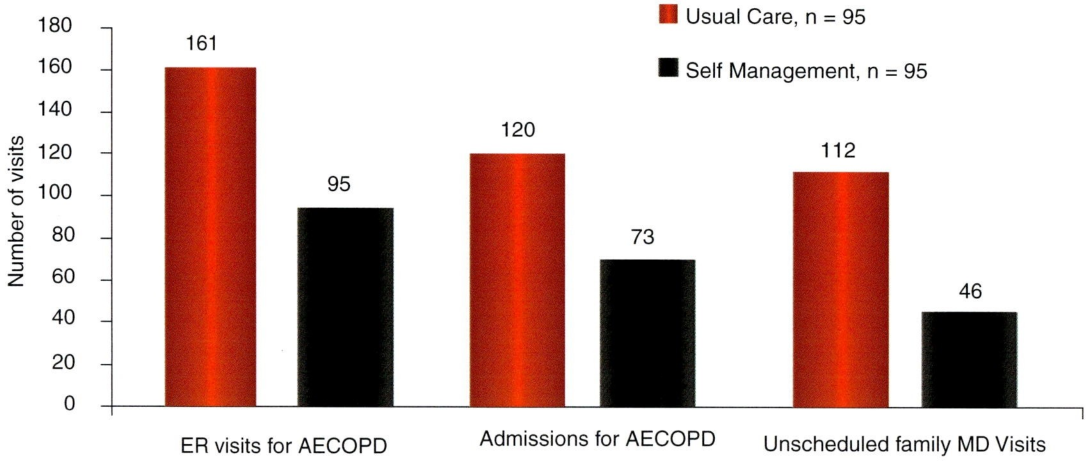

Fig. 1.10 Self-management education for COPD. Note the reduction in health resource utilization in the year following randomization [85]

tuberculosis. Most of these diseases are not only diseases of the lungs, and the consequences are systemic in nature and can be improved by improving the whole body. As a reflection of this paradigm, we might even consider changing the name of what we do from pulmonary rehabilitation to rehabilitation of the patient with pulmonary disease.

1.7 The Future

The history of pulmonary rehabilitation is interesting. What appeared to be a field with obscure benefits as late as five decades ago is now supported by evidence graded as "A" by grading experts. It has been a concerted effort by many, who having observed patients deteriorate over time have had the foresight to seek new avenues to improve their patient's lot. It is our hope that the years to come will provide even more exciting pathways. Perhaps the time to prevent aging and grow new tissue at earlier stages of all diseases will make "preventive rehabilitation" the futuristic version of our field. This book is proof of the existing interest and that young minds are at work to make this future possible.

References

1. DAVOS PLATZ: II. Sanatoriums and hotels. Br Med J. 1906;2:1407–10.
2. Baston A. Curing tuberculosis in Muskoka. Canada's First Sanatoria. Canada: Old Stone Books Limited; 2013.
3. Barach AL. Diaphragmatic breathing in pulmonary emphysema. J Chronic Dis. 1955;1:211–5.
4. Barach AL. Physiologic therapy of respiratory disease; with special reference to the management of pulmonary emphysema. N Y Med. 1946;2:21–6.
5. Dacso MM, Luczak AK, Haas A, Rusk HA. Bracing and rehabilitation training. Effect on the energy expenditure of the elderly hemiplegic; preliminary report. Postgrad Med. 1963;34:42–7.
6. Haas A, Rusk HA, Goodman WN. Rehabilitation in thoracic surgery. J Thorac Surg. 1952;24:304–22.
7. Haas A, Rusk HA, Zivan M. The results of a combined medical and rehabilitative program in tuberculosis; a preliminary report. Arch Phys Med Rehabil. 1954;35:77–86.
8. Mead J, Martin H. Principles of respiratory mechanics. Phys Ther. 1968;48:478–94.
9. Wasserman K. Breathing during exercise. N Engl J Med. 1978;298:780–5.
10. Barach AL. Physical exercise in breathless subjects with pulmonary emphysema, including a discussion of cigarette smoking. Dis Chest. 1964;45:113–28.
11. Barach AL. Ambulatory oxygen therapy: oxygen inhalation at home and out-of-doors. Dis Chest. 1959;35:229–41.
12. Barach AL. Increased effectiveness for oxygen therapy. Mod Hosp. 1946;67:90–2.
13. Cotes JE, Gilson JC. Improved portable oxygen apparatus with detachable cylinders for domiciliary use. Lancet. 1956;271:823.
14. Cotes JE, Gilson JC. Effect of oxygen on exercise ability in chronic respiratory insufficiency; use of portable apparatus. Lancet. 1956;270:872–6.
15. Barach AL. A Treatment Manual for Patients with Pulmonary Emphysema. New York, NY: Grune & Stratton, Inc.; 1969.
16. Miller WF. Physical therapeutic measures in the treatment of chronic bronchopulmonary disorders; methods for breathing training. Am J Med. 1958;24:929–40.
17. Petty TL, Nett LM, Finigan MM, Brink GA, Corsello PR. A comprehensive care program for chronic airway obstruction. Methods and preliminary evaluation of symptomatic and functional improvement. Ann Intern Med. 1969;70:1109–20.
18. Hodgkin JE, Balchum OJ, Kass I, Glaser EM, Miller WF, Haas A, Shaw DB, Kimbel P, Petty TL. Chronic obstructive airway diseases. Current concepts in diagnosis and comprehensive care. JAMA. 1975;232:1243–60.
19. Gimenez M. Physiotherapy of patients with severe chronic respiratory insufficiency. La Revue du Praticien. 1987;37:1017–22.
20. Gimenez M, Servera E, Vergara P, Bach JR, Polu JM. Endurance training in patients with chronic obstructive pulmonary disease: a comparison of high versus moderate intensity. Arch Phys Med Rehabil. 2000;81:102–9.
21. Continuous or nocturnal oxygen therapy in hypoxemic chronic obstructive lung disease: a clinical trial. Nocturnal Oxygen Therapy Trial Group. Ann Intern Med. 1980;93:391–8.
22. Long term domiciliary oxygen therapy in chronic hypoxic cor pulmonale complicating chronic bronchitis and emphysema. Report of the Medical Research Council Working Party. Lancet. 1981;1:681–6.
23. Guyatt GH, Berman LB, Townsend M, Pugsley SO, Chambers LW. A measure of quality of life for clinical trials in chronic lung disease. Thorax. 1987;42:773–8.
24. Jones PW, Quirk FH, Baveystock CM, Littlejohns P. A self-complete measure of health status for chronic airflow limitation. The St. George's Respiratory Questionnaire. Am Rev Respir Dis. 1992;145:1321–7.
25. Guyatt GH, King DR, Feeny DH, Stubbing D, Goldstein RS. Generic and specific measurement of health-related quality of life in a clinical trial of respiratory rehabilitation. J Clin Epidemiol. 1999;52:187–92.
26. Cooper KH. A means of assessing maximal oxygen intake. Correlation between field and treadmill testing. JAMA. 1968;203:201–4.
27. McGavin CR, Gupta SP, McHardy GJ. Twelve-minute walking test for assessing disability in chronic bronchitis. Br Med J. 1976;1:822–3.
28. Butland RJ, Pang J, Gross ER, Woodcock AA, Geddes DM. Two-, six-, and 12-minute walking tests in respiratory disease. Br Med J (Clin Res Ed). 1982;284:1607–8.
29. Leger LA, Lambert J. A maximal multistage 20-m shuttle run test to predict VO2 max. Eur J Appl Physiol Occup Physiol. 1982;49:1–12.
30. Singh SJ, Morgan MD, Scott S, Walters D, Hardman AE. Development of a shuttle walking test of disability in patients with chronic airways obstruction. Thorax. 1992;47:1019–24.
31. Revill SM, Morgan MD, Singh SJ, Williams J, Hardman AE. The endurance shuttle walk: a new field test for the assessment of endurance capacity in chronic obstructive pulmonary disease. Thorax. 1999;54:213–22.
32. Redelmeier DA, Guyatt GH, Goldstein RS. Assessing the minimal important difference in symptoms: a

comparison of two techniques. J Clin Epidemiol. 1996;49:1215–9.

33. Sahn SA, Nett LM, Petty TL. Ten year follow-up of a comprehensive rehabilitation program for severe COPD. Chest. 1980;77:311–4.
34. Hodgkin JE, Farrell MJ, Gibson SR, Kanner RE, Kass I, Lampton LM, Nield M, Petty TL. American thoracic society. Medical section of the American lung association. Pulmonary rehabilitation. Am Rev Respir Dis. 1981;124:663–6.
35. Pulmonary rehabilitation: joint ACCP/AACVPR evidence-based guidelines. ACCP/AACVPR Pulmonary Rehabilitation Guidelines Panel. American College of Chest Physicians. American Association of Cardiovascular and Pulmonary Rehabilitation. Chest. 1997;112:1363–96.
36. Nici L, Donner C, Wouters E, Zuwallack R, Ambrosino N, Bourbeau J, Carone M, Celli B, Engelen M, Fahy B, Garvey C, Goldstein R, Gosselink R, Lareau S, MacIntyre N, Maltais F, Morgan M, O'Donnell D, Prefault C, Reardon J, Rochester C, Schols A, Singh S, Troosters T. American Thoracic Society/European Respiratory Society statement on pulmonary rehabilitation. Am J Respir Crit Care Med. 2006;173:1390–413.
37. Spruit MA, Singh SJ, Garvey C, ZuWallack R, Nici L, Rochester C, Hill K, Holland AE, Lareau SC, Man WD, Pitta F, Sewell L, Raskin J, Bourbeau J, Crouch R, Franssen FM, Casaburi R, Vercoulen JH, Vogiatzis I, Gosselink R, Clini EM, Effing TW, Maltais F, van der Palen J, Troosters T, Janssen DJ, Collins E, Garcia-Aymerich J, Brooks D, Fahy BF, Puhan MA, Hoogendoorn M, Garrod R, Schols AM, Carlin B, Benzo R, Meek P, Morgan M, Rutten-van Molken MP, Ries AL, Make B, Goldstein RS, Dowson CA, Brozek JL, Donner CF, Wouters EF, Rehabilitation AETFP. An official American Thoracic Society/European Respiratory Society statement: key concepts and advances in pulmonary rehabilitation. Am J Respir Crit Care Med. 2013;188:e13–64.
38. Rochester CL, Vogiatzis I, Holland AE, Lareau SC, Marciniuk DD, Puhan MA, Spruit MA, Masefield S, Casaburi R, Clini EM, Crouch R, Garcia-Aymerich J, Garvey C, Goldstein RS, Hill K, Morgan M, Nici L, Pitta F, Ries AL, Singh SJ, Troosters T, Wijkstra PJ, Yawn BP, ZuWallack RL, Rehabilitation AETFPP. An Official American Thoracic Society/European Respiratory Society Policy Statement: enhancing implementation, use, and delivery of pulmonary rehabilitation. Am J Respir Crit Care Med. 2015;192:1373–86.
39. Vogelmeier CF, Criner GJ, Martinez FJ, Anzueto A, Barnes PJ, Bourbeau J, Celli BR, Chen R, Decramer M, Fabbri LM, Frith P, Halpin DM, Victorina Lopez Varela M, Nishimura M, Roche N, Rodriguez-Roisin R, Sin DD, Singh D, Stockley R, Vestbo J, Wedzicha JA, Agusti A. Global strategy for the diagnosis, management, and prevention of chronic obstructive lung disease 2017 report. GOLD executive summary. Am J Respir Crit Care Med. 2017;195(5):557–82.
40. Goldstein RS, Gort EH, Stubbing D, Avendano MA, Guyatt GH. Randomised controlled trial of respiratory rehabilitation. Lancet. 1994;344:1394–7.
41. Wijkstra PJ, Van Altena R, Kraan J, Otten V, Postma DS, Koeter GH. Quality of life in patients with chronic obstructive pulmonary disease improves after rehabilitation at home. Eur Respir J. 1994;7:269–73.
42. Ries AL, Kaplan RM, Limberg TM, Prewitt LM. Effects of pulmonary rehabilitation on physiologic and psychosocial outcomes in patients with chronic obstructive pulmonary disease. Ann Intern Med. 1995;122:823–32.
43. Lacasse Y, Goldstein R, Lasserson TJ, Martin S. Pulmonary rehabilitation for chronic obstructive pulmonary disease. Cochrane Database Syst Rev. 2006;2:CD003793.
44. Belman MJ, Kendregan BA. Exercise training fails to increase skeletal muscle enzymes in patients with chronic obstructive pulmonary disease. Am Rev Respir Dis. 1981;123:256–61.
45. Maltais F, LeBlanc P, Simard C, Jobin J, Berube C, Bruneau J, Carrier L, Belleau R. Skeletal muscle adaptation to endurance training in patients with chronic obstructive pulmonary disease. Am J Respir Crit Care Med. 1996;154:442–7.
46. Casaburi R, Patessio A, Ioli F, Zanaboni S, Donner CF, Wasserman K. Reductions in exercise lactic acidosis and ventilation as a result of exercise training in patients with obstructive lung disease. Am Rev Respir Dis. 1991;143:9–18.
47. Mahler DA, Waterman LA, Ward J, McCusker C, ZuWallack R, Baird JC. Validity and responsiveness of the self-administered computerized versions of the baseline and transition dyspnea indexes. Chest. 2007;132:1283–90.
48. Nishimura K, Izumi T, Tsukino M, Oga T. Dyspnea is a better predictor of 5-year survival than airway obstruction in patients with COPD. Chest. 2002;121:1434–40.
49. Aldred MA, Comhair SA, Varella-Garcia M, Asosingh K, Xu W, Noon GP, Thistlethwaite PA, Tuder RM, Erzurum SC, Geraci MW, Coldren CD. Somatic chromosome abnormalities in the lungs of patients with pulmonary arterial hypertension. Am J Respir Crit Care Med. 2010;182:1153–60.
50. Singh SJ, Puhan MA, Andrianopoulos V, Hernandes NA, Mitchell KE, Hill CJ, Lee AL, Camillo CA, Troosters T, Spruit MA, Carlin BW, Wanger J, Pepin V, Saey D, Pitta F, Kaminsky DA, McCormack MC, MacIntyre N, Culver BH, Sciurba FC, Revill SM, Delafosse V, Holland AE. An official systematic review of the European Respiratory Society/American Thoracic Society: measurement properties of field walking tests in chronic respiratory disease. Eur Respir J. 2014;44:1447–78.
51. Roflumilast: APTA 2217, B9302-107, BY 217, BYK 20869. Drugs R&D. 2004;5:176–81.

52. Jones PW, Harding G, Berry P, Wiklund I, Chen WH, Kline Leidy N. Development and first validation of the COPD assessment test. Eur Respir J. 2009;34:648–54.
53. Guyatt GH, Townsend M, Keller J, Singer J, Nogradi S. Measuring functional status in chronic lung disease: conclusions from a randomized control trial. Respir Med. 1989;83:293–7.
54. Celli BR, Cote CG, Marin JM, Casanova C, Montes de Oca M, Mendez RA, Pinto Plata V, Cabral HJ. The body-mass index, airflow obstruction, dyspnea, and exercise capacity index in chronic obstructive pulmonary disease. N Engl J Med. 2004;350:1005–12.
55. Cote CG, Celli BR. Pulmonary rehabilitation and the BODE index in COPD. Eur Respir J. 2005;26:630–6.
56. Guell MR, Cejudo P, Ortega F, Puy MC, Rodriguez-Trigo G, Pijoan JI, Martinez-Indart L, Gorostiza A, Bdeir K, Celli B, Galdiz JB. Benefits of long-term pulmonary rehabilitation maintenance program in severe COPD patients: 3 year follow-up. Am J Respir Crit Care Med. 2017;195(5):622–9.
57. Guell R, Casan P, Belda J, Sangenis M, Morante F, Guyatt GH, Sanchis J. Long-term effects of outpatient rehabilitation of COPD: a randomized trial. Chest. 2000;117:976–83.
58. Griffiths TL, Burr ML, Campbell IA, Lewis-Jenkins V, Mullins J, Shiels K, Turner-Lawlor PJ, Payne N, Newcombe RG, Ionescu AA, Thomas J, Tunbridge J. Results at 1 year of outpatient multidisciplinary pulmonary rehabilitation: a randomised controlled trial. Lancet. 2000;355:362–8.
59. Troosters T, Gosselink R, Decramer M. Short- and long-term effects of outpatient rehabilitation in patients with chronic obstructive pulmonary disease: a randomized trial. Am J Med. 2000;109:207–12.
60. Celli BR, Rassulo J, Make BJ. Dyssynchronous breathing during arm but not leg exercise in patients with chronic airflow obstruction. N Engl J Med. 1986;314:1485–90.
61. Velloso M, do Nascimento NH, Gazzotti MR, Jardim JR. Evaluation of effects of shoulder girdle training on strength and performance of activities of daily living in patients with chronic obstructive pulmonary disease. Int J Chron Obstruct Pulmon Dis. 2013;8:187–92.
62. Martinez FJ, Vogel PD, Dupont DN, Stanopoulos I, Gray A, Beamis JF. Supported arm exercise vs unsupported arm exercise in the rehabilitation of patients with severe chronic airflow obstruction. Chest. 1993;103:1397–402.
63. Costi S, Crisafulli E, Antoni FD, Beneventi C, Fabbri LM, Clini EM. Effects of unsupported upper extremity exercise training in patients with COPD: a randomized clinical trial. Chest. 2009;136:387–95.
64. Effing T, Zielhuis G, Kerstjens H, van der Valk P, van der Palen J. Community based physiotherapeutic exercise in COPD self-management: a randomised controlled trial. Respir Med. 2011;105:418–26.
65. Maltais F, Bourbeau J, Shapiro S, Lacasse Y, Perrault H, Baltzan M, Hernandez P, Rouleau M, Julien M, Parenteau S, Paradis B, Levy RD, Camp P, Lecours R, Audet R, Hutton B, Penrod JR, Picard D, Bernard S. Effects of home-based pulmonary rehabilitation in patients with chronic obstructive pulmonary disease: a randomized trial. Ann Intern Med. 2008;149:869–78.
66. Strijbos JH, Postma DS, van Altena R, Gimeno F, Koeter GH. A comparison between an outpatient hospital-based pulmonary rehabilitation program and a home-care pulmonary rehabilitation program in patients with COPD. A follow-up of 18 months. Chest. 1996;109:366–72.
67. Stickland M, Jourdain T, Wong EY, Rodgers WM, Jendzjowsky NG, Macdonald GF. Using Telehealth technology to deliver pulmonary rehabilitation in chronic obstructive pulmonary disease patients. Can Respir J. 2011;18:216–20.
68. Beauchamp MK, Nonoyama M, Goldstein RS, Hill K, Dolmage TE, Mathur S, Brooks D. Interval versus continuous training in individuals with chronic obstructive pulmonary disease—a systematic review. Thorax. 2010;65:157–64.
69. Maddocks M, Nolan CM, Man WD, Polkey MI, Hart N, Gao W, Rafferty GF, Moxham J, Higginson IJ. Neuromuscular electrical stimulation to improve exercise capacity in patients with severe COPD: a randomised double-blind, placebo-controlled trial. Lancet Respir Med. 2016;4:27–36.
70. Dolmage TE, Goldstein RS. Proportional assist ventilation and exercise tolerance in subjects with COPD. Chest. 1997;111:948–54.
71. O'Donnell DE, D'Arsigny C, Webb KA. Effects of hyperoxia on ventilatory limitation during exercise in advanced chronic obstructive pulmonary disease. Am J Respir Crit Care Med. 2001;163:892–8.
72. Eves ND, Sandmeyer LC, Wong EY, Jones LW, MacDonald GF, Ford GT, Petersen SR, Bibeau MD, Jones RL. Helium-hyperoxia: a novel intervention to improve the benefits of pulmonary rehabilitation for patients with COPD. Chest. 2009;135:609–18.
73. Dolmage TE, Evans RA, Brooks D, Goldstein RS. Breathing helium-hyperoxia and tolerance of partitioned exercise in patients with COPD. J Cardiopulm Rehabil Prev. 2014;34:69–74.
74. Dolmage TE, Goldstein RS. Effects of One-Legged Exercise Training of Patients With COPD. Chest. 2008;133:370–6.
75. Evans RA, Hill K, Dolmage TE, Blouin M, O'Hoski S, Brooks D, Goldstein RS. Properties of self-paced walking in chronic respiratory disease: a patient goal-oriented assessment. Chest. 2011;140:737–43.
76. Griffiths TL, Phillips CJ, Davies S, Burr ML, Campbell IA. Cost effectiveness of an outpatient multidisciplinary pulmonary rehabilitation programme. Thorax. 2001;56:779–84.
77. Pitta F, Troosters T, Probst VS, Spruit MA, Decramer M, Gosselink R. Physical activity and hospitalization for exacerbation of COPD. Chest. 2006;129:536–44.
78. Garcia-Aymerich J, Hernandez C, Alonso A, Casas A, Rodriguez-Roisin R, Anto JM, Roca J. Effects of an

integrated care intervention on risk factors of COPD readmission. Respir Med. 2007;101:1462–9.
79. Waschki B, Kirsten A, Holz O, Muller KC, Meyer T, Watz H, Magnussen H. Physical activity is the strongest predictor of all-cause mortality in patients with COPD: a prospective cohort study. Chest. 2011;140:331–42.
80. Man WD, Polkey MI, Donaldson N, Gray BJ, Moxham J. Community pulmonary rehabilitation after hospitalisation for acute exacerbations of chronic obstructive pulmonary disease: randomised controlled study. BMJ. 2004;329:1209.
81. Puhan MA, Gimeno-Santos E, Cates CJ, Troosters T. Pulmonary rehabilitation following exacerbations of chronic obstructive pulmonary disease. Cochrane Database Syst Rev. 2016;12:CD005305.
82. Beauchamp MK, Francella S, Romano JM, Goldstein RS, Brooks D. A novel approach to long-term respiratory care: results of a community-based post-rehabilitation maintenance program in COPD. Respir Med. 2013;107:1210–6.
83. Hill K, Bansal V, Brooks D, Goldstein RS. Repeat pulmonary rehabilitation programs confer similar increases in functional exercise capacity to initial programs. J Cardiopulm Rehabil Prev. 2008;28:410–4.
84. Foglio K, Bianchi L, Ambrosino NI. it really useful to repeat outpatient pulmonary rehabilitation programs in patients with chronic airway obstruction? A 2-year controlled study. Chest. 2001;119:1696–704.
85. Bourbeau J, Julien M, Maltais F, Rouleau M, Beaupre A, Begin R, Renzi P, Nault D, Borycki E, Schwartzman K, Singh R, Collet JP. Chronic Obstructive Pulmonary Disease axis of the Respiratory Network Fonds de la Recherche en Sante du Q. Reduction of hospital utilization in patients with chronic obstructive pulmonary disease: a disease-specific self-management intervention. Arch Intern Med. 2003;163:585–91.
86. Casas A, Troosters T, Garcia-Aymerich J, Roca J, Hernandez C, Alonso A, del Pozo F, de Toledo P, Anto JM, Rodriguez-Roisin R, Decramer M. members of the CP. Integrated care prevents hospitalisations for exacerbations in COPD patients. Eur Respir J. 2006;28:123–30.
87. Rice KL, Dewan N, Bloomfield HE, Grill J, Schult TM, Nelson DB, Kumari S, Thomas M, Geist LJ, Beaner C, Caldwell M, Niewoehner DE. Disease management program for chronic obstructive pulmonary disease: a randomized controlled trial. Am J Respir Crit Care Med. 2010;182:890–6.
88. Ries AL, Make BJ, Lee SM, Krasna MJ, Bartels M, Crouch R, Fishman AP, National Emphysema Treatment Trial Research G. The effects of pulmonary rehabilitation in the national emphysema treatment trial. Chest. 2005;128:3799–809.
89. Langer D, Gosselink R, Pitta F, Burtin C, Verleden G, Dupont L, Decramer M, Troosters T. Physical activity in daily life 1 year after lung transplantation. J Heart Lung Transplant. 2009;28:572–8.

Current Concepts and Definitions

2

Martijn Spruit and Linda Nici

The individual components of pulmonary rehabilitation have been provided as part of standard medical care for patients with chronic respiratory diseases for a very long time. Beginning in the 1960s, clinicians began to recognize that organizing these components into a comprehensive program could lead to substantial benefits for their patients [1]. These bundled interventions (typically walking exercises, supplemental oxygen therapy, bronchial hygiene techniques, and breathing retraining) were officially given the label of pulmonary rehabilitation by the American College of Chest Physicians in 1974, and in 1981 the American Thoracic Society published its first statement on pulmonary rehabilitation [2]. In the ensuing 35 years, numerous scientific advances both in our understanding of the systemic effects of chronic respiratory disease and the changes induced by the process of pulmonary rehabilitation have led to a broader application of this treatment modality in a wide range of settings leading to significant benefits for both the individual and society.

The most recent American Thoracic Society/European Respiratory Society Statement on Pulmonary Rehabilitation defines pulmonary rehabilitation as follows: "A comprehensive intervention based on a thorough patient assessment followed by patient-tailored therapies which include, but are not limited to, exercise training, education and behavior change, designed to improve the physical and emotional condition of people with chronic respiratory disease and to promote the long-term adherence to health-enhancing behaviors" [3].

Pulmonary rehabilitation is defined by its multidisciplinary, multifaceted approach which provides individualized, goal-directed care. The overarching principles of pulmonary rehabilitation are to minimize symptom burden and enhance exercise capacity, thereby maximizing the patient's independence and functioning within the community. Although pulmonary rehabilitation has multiple components (exercise training, self-management education, nutritional and psychosocial support), it is an entity on its own. Each component has benefits for the patient, but when bundled and delivered by professionals with expertise and experience in this area, pulmonary rehabilitation exceeds the sum of its parts. This requires a dedicated interdisciplinary team which may include physicians, nurses, nurse practitioners, physiotherapists, exercise physiologists, respiratory therapists, occupational therapists, psychologists, social workers, and nutritionists.

Pulmonary rehabilitation leads to substantial benefits in dyspnea, exercise capacity, health-related quality of life, and healthcare utilization [3]. These benefits, which are often of greater magni-

M. Spruit
CIRO, Maastricht University & Hasselt University, The Netherlands
e-mail: martijnspruit@ciro-horn.nl

L. Nici (✉)
Providence VA Medical Center, Rhode Island, USA
e-mail: linda_nici@brown.edu

© Springer International Publishing AG 2018
E. Clini et al. (eds.), *Textbook of Pulmonary Rehabilitation*,
https://doi.org/10.1007/978-3-319-65888-9_2

tude than that seen with other medical therapies such as bronchodilators, are achieved without discernible improvements in traditional measures of physiological impairment, such as the FEV1. This apparent paradox is explained by the fact that this intervention addresses the systemic effects of chronic respiratory disease, including peripheral muscle dysfunction, physical inactivity leading to deconditioning, anxiety and depression, and maladaptive behaviors such as a sedentary lifestyle and poor adherence to prescribed therapies.

A thorough patient assessment is essential to identify and treat the often complex and unique comorbidities of the individual with chronic respiratory disease [4]. For instance, exercise limitation may result from multiple factors including ventilatory constraints, pulmonary gas exchange abnormalities, peripheral muscle dysfunction, cardiac dysfunction, anxiety, depression, poor motivation, or any combination of the above. Identification of the distinctive set of factors at play in each patient allows for targeted, efficient, and effective therapy. The explanation for the beneficial effects of exercise training in this setting is likewise complex. For example, exercise training results in an increase in oxidative enzymes in ambulatory muscles, leading to less lactate production and less ventilatory requirement at any given workload. This, in turn, allows for a slower respiratory rate at that particular workload, and this longer expiratory time facilitates greater emptying of the lung, thereby reducing dynamic hyperinflation. The adaptive muscle changes and reduction in dynamic hyperinflation, coupled with greater self-efficacy and less anxiety associated with dyspnea-producing activity, result in less exertional dyspnea and improved health-related quality of life. Although exercise training directly targets exercise limitation, it would be naive to think that 6–12 weeks of exercise training would have substantial long-term effects on fitness. This underscores the need to couple exercise training with efforts aimed at promoting self-management skills and positive health behavior change in order to maintain long-term benefits.

Pulmonary rehabilitation can be delivered at multiple points in the disease trajectory of any individual patient, though its focus and components will vary depending on the patient's goals and functional impairments, as well as the stage of disease. Historically, pulmonary rehabilitation has been provided to stable patients with moderate-to-severe COPD, typically in an outpatient setting. However, a growing body of scientific evidence has challenged this narrow application and supports the role for pulmonary rehabilitation in nontraditional settings. For example, patients with mild to moderate airflow obstruction appear to benefit to a similar degree to those with more advanced disease. This appears to be at least partially due to the presence of lower limb muscle weakness and low levels of daily physical activity [5–7]. Pulmonary rehabilitation provided to the COPD patient in the peri-exacerbation period reduces hospital days, readmissions and, perhaps, even mortality [8]. Evidence now supports the effectiveness and often equivalent benefits of pulmonary rehabilitation in the non-COPD respiratory patient, likely due to similarities in the disablement processes across chronic respiratory diseases [9]. Finally, home-based pulmonary rehabilitation, when carefully structured, can result in similar benefits to traditional center-based programs [10].

Despite advances in our understanding of the complex systemic effects of chronic respiratory disease and the mechanisms of benefit from pulmonary rehabilitation, challenges still remain in further defining its effectiveness and improving its accessibility. Although pulmonary rehabilitation provides substantial beneficial effects in dyspnea, exercise performance, and health-related quality of life, these gains tend to diminish in the months to years following the formal intervention. This decline is likely due to several factors, including disease progression (with intervening exacerbations), the acute nature of the pulmonary rehabilitation intervention, and suboptimal behavior change. More research is needed to determine which modifications to the pulmonary rehabilitation approach would lead to longer-term benefits, including prolonging programs, maintenance programs, and successful behavior change. More information is needed to better understand the learning styles of our patients and ways to adapt educational and behavioral techniques to foster self-efficacy.

Lower levels of daily physical activity predict poor outcome in patients with COPD, independent of other measures of disease severity. While the higher levels of exercise capacity that are achieved during pulmonary rehabilitation are necessary to allow for increased physical activity in the home setting, other factors such as motivation, self-efficacy for walking, and cultural issues undoubtedly play a role in modulating baseline physical activity. We must focus more effort on fostering physical activity during pulmonary rehabilitation and standardized ways to evaluate this important outcome.

A significant barrier to the effective utilization of pulmonary rehabilitation in the community is the lack of patient referrals, likely due to a lack of awareness among many healthcare providers of the nature and benefits of this intervention. Education of primary care physicians, hospitalists, and other health professionals, including nurses, nurse practitioners, physical therapists, occupational therapists, and respiratory therapists, is needed to increase utilization of pulmonary rehabilitation. Newer data demonstrating reductions in healthcare utilization after pulmonary rehabilitation should aid in promoting awareness of this intervention.

Optimal treatment of the often complex patient with chronic respiratory disease requires a high degree of coordination and collaboration across the healthcare system. This is the concept of integrated care, which can be defined as, "The continuum of patient centered services organized as a care delivery value chain for patients with chronic conditions with the goal of achieving the optimal daily functioning and health status for the individual patient and to achieve and maintain the individual's independence and functioning in the community" [11]. The essence of this integrated care approach is to provide the right treatment to the right patient at the right time, which requires a seamless transition of care across settings (hospital, rehabilitation, community) and disciplines (primary care, subspecialty, home services) throughout the trajectory of disease [12]. Since pulmonary rehabilitation is an integrated, interdisciplinary approach to the management of the individual with chronic respiratory disease, it fits perfectly into the concept of integrated care. Pulmonary rehabilitation may include providing smoking cessation therapy when necessary, promoting regular exercise and physical activity in the home and community settings, fostering collaborative self-management strategies, optimizing pharmacotherapy and medication adherence, and—when needed—offering palliative care and hospice services. This requires partnering, communication, and coordination among healthcare providers, patients, and their families.

References

1. Petty TL, Nett LM, Finigan MM, et al. A comprehensive care program for chronic airway obstruction. Methods and preliminary evaluation of symptomatic and functional improvement. Ann Intern Med. 1969;70:1109–20.
2. Casaburi R. A brief history of pulmonary rehabilitation. Respir Care. 2008;53:1185–9.
3. Spruit MA, Singh SJ, Garvey C, et al. An official American Thoracic Society/European Respiratory Society statement: key concepts and advances in pulmonary rehabilitation. Am J Respir Crit Care Med. 2013;188:e13–64.
4. Evans RA, Morgan MDL. The systemic nature of chronic lung disease. Clin Chest Med. 2014;35:283–03.
5. Seymour JM, Spruit MA, Hopkinson NS, Natanek SA, Man WD, Jackson A, Gosker HR, Schols AM, Moxham J, Polkey MI, Wouters EF. The prevalence of quadriceps weakness in copd and the relationship with disease severity. Eur Respir J. 2010;36:81–8.
6. Ofir D, Laveneziana P, Webb KA, Lam YM, O'Donnell DE. Mechanisms of dyspnea during cycle exercise in symptomatic patients with gold stage I chronic obstructive pulmonary disease. Am J Respir Crit Care Med. 2008;177:622–9.
7. Berry MJ, Rejeski WJ, Adair NE, Zaccaro D. Exercise rehabilitation and chronic obstructive pulmonary disease stage. Am J Respir Crit Care Med. 1999;160:1248–53.
8. Puhan MA, Gimeno-Santos E, Scharplatz M, Troosters T, Walters EH, Steurer J. Pulmonary rehabilitation following exacerbations of chronic obstructive pulmonary disease. Cochrane Database Syst Rev. 2011;10:CD005305.

9. Rochester CL, Fairburn C, Crouch RH. Pulmonary rehabilitation for respiratory disorders other than chronic obstructive pulmonary disease. Clin Chest Med. 2014;35:369–89.
10. Holland AE, Mahal A, Hill CJ, et al. Benefits and costs of home-based pulmonary rehabilitation in chronic obstructive pulmonary disease- a multi-center randomized controlled equivalence trial. BMC Pulm Med. 2013;13:57.
11. Nici L, ZuWallack R. An official American Thoracic Society workshop report: the integrated care of the COPD patient. Proc Am Thorac Soc. 2012;9:9–18.
12. Grone O, Garcia-Barbero M. Integrated care. A position paper of the WHO European office for integrated healthcare services. Int J Integr Care. 2001;1:1–15.

Part II

Participants

3 Identifying Candidates for Pulmonary Rehabilitation

Thierry Troosters

3.1 Introduction

Pulmonary rehabilitation is an evidence-based treatment option for patients with respiratory disorders. The numbers needed to treat in order to have one successful participant on a particular outcome are estimated to be around three. Such low numbers are surely speaking for themselves in terms of the overall effectiveness of rehabilitation, but still a number of patients do not benefit from pulmonary rehabilitation, never start the program, or drop out. In this chapter, we will summarize the current state of the art in terms of patient selection for rehabilitation.

Pulmonary rehabilitation is a patient-centered intervention which can contain different components tailored to the individual patient, based on a thorough and multidisciplinary assessment. Hence—in principle—all patients are potential candidates for some form of rehabilitation, provided the program is tailored to their needs. In clinical practice, however, programs do not have unlimited flexibility, and patients are selected based on clear clinical needs in terms of lack of physical fitness, symptoms, or—more recently—lack of physical activity.

Key to the selection process is therefore the identification of the problems in an individual patient that can be targeted by rehabilitation interventions. Subsequently, the program will need to be adapted to tackle the identified problems. As pulmonary rehabilitation will typically contain exercise training, the selection of patients that might be responsible to exercise interventions has received most attention in the literature. However, other problems can be identified and solved with rehabilitation programs. Furthermore, the question can be asked which candidates eligible for rehabilitation are more likely to accept the offer for rehabilitation and what efforts can be taken to modify the program such that more patients become good candidates or are likely to accept the offer for rehabilitation.

Guidelines are generally relatively liberal in their criteria for rehabilitation. Interestingly, most of the recommendations take only disease severity into account as assessed by symptoms (often only of breathlessness) and lung function impairment. Recommendations are also made regarding referral of patients after acute exacerbations. Table 3.1 provides a selection of guidelines and what they quote on the issue of "patient selection criteria." At a local or regional level, local policy may also determine which patient (if any) is eligible to receive rehabilitation. In Belgium, for example, patients who meet the

T. Troosters, P.T., Ph.D.
Department of Rehabilitation Sciences, KU Leuven,
Respiratory Division and Rehabilitation,
University Hospital Leuven, Leuven, Belgium
e-mail: thierry.troosters@kuleuven.be

© Springer International Publishing AG 2018
E. Clini et al. (eds.), *Textbook of Pulmonary Rehabilitation*,
https://doi.org/10.1007/978-3-319-65888-9_3

Table 3.1 A selection of guidelines that address pulmonary rehabilitation and the selection of candidates

Available documents recommending rehabilitation as a treatment strategy
2007 ACCP/AACVPR [2]: A program of exercise training of the muscles of ambulation is recommended as a mandatory component of pulmonary rehabilitation *for patients with COPD*. Grade of Recommendation: 1A
2010 Canadian Thoracic Society Clinical Practice Guideline [3]: Pulmonary rehabilitation is standard of care for individuals with COPD who remain symptomatic despite bronchodilator therapies. It is strongly recommended that patients with moderate, severe, and very severe COPD participate in PR (grade 1C); there are insufficient data to make a recommendation regarding mild COPD. It is strongly recommended that patients undergo PR following an acute exacerbation of COPD
GOLD 2017 [4]: Rehabilitation is appropriate for most patients with COPD; improved functional exercise capacity and health-related quality of life have been demonstrated across all grades of COPD severity, although the evidence is especially strong in moderate to severe disease. Even patients with hypercapnic failure show benefit. Patients with high symptom burden and risk of exacerbations (groups B, C, D) should be encouraged to take part in a full rehabilitation program
NICE 2016 [5]: Make pulmonary rehabilitation available to all appropriate people with COPD, including those who have had a recent hospital admission for an acute exacerbation (updated recommendation). Offer pulmonary rehabilitation to all patients who consider themselves functionally disabled by COPD. Pulmonary rehabilitation is not suitable for patients who are unable to walk, have unstable angina, or had a recent myocardial infarction
British Thoracic Society guidelines on PR [6]: Patients with a Medical Research Council (MRC) dyspnea scale of 3–5 who are functionally limited by breathlessness should be referred for outpatient pulmonary rehabilitation. Grade A, patients with a MRC dyspnea scale of 2 who are functionally limited by breathlessness should be referred for pulmonary rehabilitation. Grade D, patients with a MRC dyspnea score of 5 who are housebound should not routinely be offered supervised pulmonary rehabilitation within their home. Grade B, flexible and pragmatic approaches should be considered to facilitate exercise training in patients who have less severe COPD and who are less breathless

following criteria are eligible for outpatient pulmonary rehabilitation in highly specialized programs, FEV1 and/or diffusion capacity <50% of the predicted normal value, and at least two of the following five criteria: (1) respiratory or (2) peripheral muscle strength less than 70% of the predicted value, (3) 6-min walking distance less than 70% of the predicted normal value, (4) peak work rate less than 90 W, or (5) a score on the Chronic Respiratory Disease Questionnaire less than 100 for the total score or 20 for dyspnea. Patients with less advanced disease are allowed rehabilitation in somewhat less complex programs (FEV1 < 60% or significant desaturation during exercise). These selection criteria were put forward by the Federal Ministry of Health in an attempt to direct rehabilitation to those patients with COPD that were deemed to have the largest needs and with a perspective of cost containment. There is no evidence base however to support these criteria as "the best selection criteria."

Several clinical practice documents advise pulmonary rehabilitation for patients with lung diseases. Generally, these documents only scratch the surface as to who might be a candidate for pulmonary rehabilitation. Typically, this guidance is poorly evidence based and rather broad. In addition, the guidelines lump all "pulmonary rehabilitation" programs together. In clinical reality, one should perhaps try to make a match between a program offered and the possible candidate. Such efforts were made in the clinical practice guidance from the Dutch physiotherapist society (KNGF, Fig. 3.1). These practice guidelines direct less complex patients toward simpler—first-line or community-based—programs, whereas more complex patients are directed to multidisciplinary programs [1].

3.2 What Are the Problems Amenable to Rehabilitation

The definition of pulmonary rehabilitation provided by the European Respiratory Society and American Thoracic Society in 2013 is rather vague on the precise outcomes to expect from pulmonary rehabilitation [7]. The definition states that pulmonary rehabilitation is "designed to improve the physical and psychological condition of people

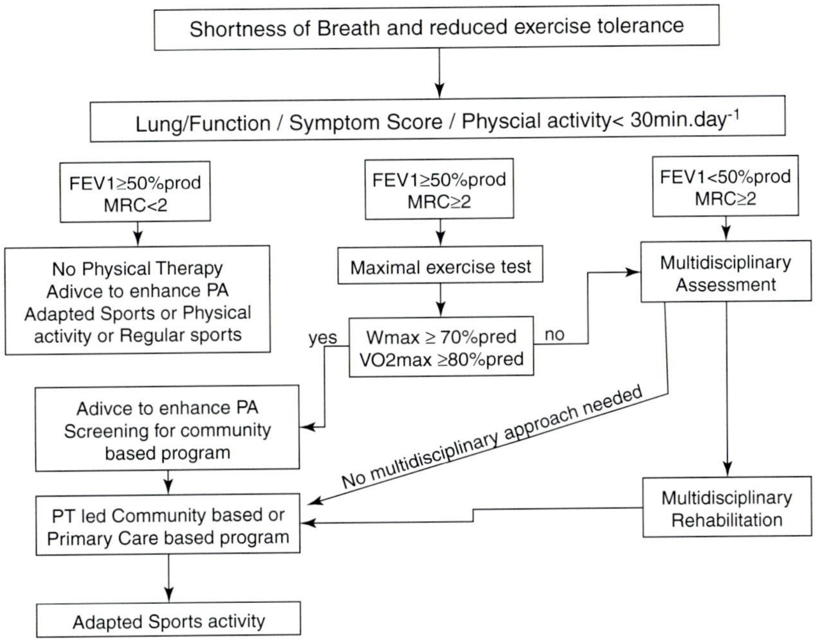

Fig. 3.1 Flowchart presented in Dutch practice guidelines for referral of patients to different programs (Adapted from Dutch practice guideline for treatment of COPD)

with chronic respiratory disease and to promote the long term adherence to health enhancing behaviors." Hence, patients with physical or psychological dysfunction as well as those with suboptimal adherence to health-enhancing behaviors are candidates for rehabilitation. Clearly such problems should be residual when reasonable pharmacological interventions (e.g., bronchodilator therapy) have been implemented, and pulmonary rehabilitation should be seen as an integrated part of the care program offered to a patient. Comorbidity is a typical feature of COPD. It is rather seldom that a patient with COPD that is considered for rehabilitation has no comorbidities. Comorbidities typically do not impose a contraindication for rehabilitation, but it should be clear that rehabilitation programs for patients with respiratory disease have to take recommendations for rehabilitation for the comorbidity into account. Relevant guidelines exist, for example, for rehabilitation in patients with cardiovascular disease [8, 9], osteoporosis [10], diabetes [11], obese people [12], joint disease, cognitive dysfunction, and depression [13]. In particular, around pharmacological treatments and self-management components of these comorbidities, important steps should be taken. Interestingly, exercise training is advised for many—if not all—of these conditions. For patients with poor nutritional status and/or deranged body composition, specific guidance is provided that can be readily integrated into pulmonary rehabilitation programs [14].

Table 3.2 attempts to provide operational definitions of the concepts above that can be used to evaluate in clinical practice whether a patient has an indication for pulmonary rehabilitation. Such assessment can be made in virtually all settings (indicated with A) or in more specific settings (indicated with B), allowing for an initial and more thorough screening, if needed. It follows that a comprehensive assessment of a candidate will need to be conducted prior to enrolment in a pulmonary rehabilitation program. Lung function is generally not considered to be a good selection criterion. Patients with mild lung function impairments can benefit from rehabilitation, and also very severe patients benefit from rehabilitation. Clearly, the program content will be different for these subgroups, and also the focus and targeted end points or goals for rehabilitation may differ.

Events may mark the patients' referral for pulmonary rehabilitation. Given the impressive effect of pulmonary rehabilitation programs that are started after a hospital admission for COPD [15],

Table 3.2 Issues to be addressed in the intake (concept) and items to be assessed with examples of tests that can be performed

Concept	Type of test	Complexity	Examples of assessment tools
Physical condition	Exercise tolerance	A	6-min walking test
		B	Peak oxygen consumption
		B	Whole-body endurance
	Occupational performance	B	Pulmonary functional status and dyspnea scale
	Skeletal muscle dysfunction	B	Early lactic acidosis
		B	Quadriceps force
		B	Respiratory muscle force
	Nutritional status	A	Body mass index
		B	Fat-free mass index
	Symptoms	A	Disabling dyspnea (mMRC, CDRQ)
		B	Disabling fatigue (CRDQ)
	High utilization of health-care resources	A	Hospital admission
		A	Frequent exacerbations
Psychological condition	Coping skills	B	Interview
	Depressive symptoms	B	Hospital anxiety and depression scale
	Anxiety (for dyspnea)	B	Breathlessness belief questionnaire
	Poor self-efficacy	B	Self-efficacy for walking scale
Health-enhancing behavior	Adherence	B	Interview around adherence to medication and agreed health behaviors
	Low physical activity	B	Accelerometry for >4 days
	Self-management skills	B	Interview
	Active smoking	B	Interview

Easy tests that can be used as screening in virtually all health-care settings are indicated with "A," and more specific tests are identified with "B"

it is of utmost importance that all patients that have been admitted for an exacerbation of COPD are considered as candidates for exacerbations. Similarly, listing for lung transplantation and volume reduction surgery prompt for rehabilitation prior to undergoing such interventions is typically advised, and also after volume reduction surgery or transplantation, pulmonary rehabilitation is advised to ensure a swift recovery of exercise tolerance and physical activity [16].

3.3 What Patients Are Typically Recruited for Rehabilitation (And Therefore Become "Candidates")

In order to become a candidate for pulmonary rehabilitation, patients need to be referred and subsequently accept the offer of pulmonary rehabilitation. Referral is an important first step and remains a bottleneck [17]. Efforts should be made to inform clinicians across the lines of health care about the pathways for referral and the effects of rehabilitation programs.

Inevitably, clinical study reports on pulmonary rehabilitation are biased by their recruitment. Few studies have investigated which patients declined the offer of rehabilitation. A systematic review investigated factors related to uptake (taking up the offer for pulmonary rehabilitation) and completion [18]. Only five studies (mainly qualitative studies) investigated why patients did not take up the offer to start rehabilitation. The disruption of daily routines or inconvenient timing of rehabilitation, travel, and location as well as the lack of seeing convincing arguments from a doctor they were unfamiliar with or their own practitioner or the belief that the program would not yield important benefits was most reported. Other factors identified were social factors (i.e., patients that were divorced or widowed) and being a current smoker. A large study investigating characteristics of >700 patients who were invited to take part in PR showed that 69% of patients took up the offer, but nearly 30% of patients were nonadherent to a rehabilitation program [19]. Being a current smoker and lack of social support were again identified as predictors of nonattendance. Travel distance was also larger in those not attending the rehabilitation program. No physiological measurements were identified as being linked to poor uptake, although uptake in studies that investigated rehabilitation after exacerbations was notably low [20]. A more recent systematic review [21] confirmed that environmental context and resources were the most studied factors associated to barriers and facilitators for being referral to, starting of, and completion of rehabilitation. System factors may also need to be considered as a recent study in the UK concluded that people from more deprived areas in the UK were less likely to complete pulmonary rehabilitation [22]. This social inequality, seen across health-care services, would suggest that particular actions toward these populations might be required to attract people from these areas into rehabilitation programs. Further claims on which patients have larger effects from pulmonary rehabilitation need to take into account that many patients never started the program.

A question to be addressed is whether flexibility in program delivery may make programs more appealing to a broader range of patients without losing effectiveness. In addition, in cardiac rehabilitation, specific interventions have been designed to increase uptake. These include structured nurse or therapist-led contacts to motivate patients for participation, early appointments after discharge, motivational letters, gender-specific programs, and intermediate-phase programs for older patients [23].

A particular group of patients in whom pulmonary rehabilitation is essential in achieving significant improvements are patients after exacerbations. In these frail patients, uptake is even lower than in stable patients, whereas the potential benefits are striking in those that take part [15]. Recent qualitative research in 19 patients identified four themes why these patients declined PR: declining related to chronic obstructive pulmonary disease and comorbidity or multi-morbidity, declining related also to lack of relevance (I'm too good or too bad), declining related to bad timing and other priorities, and declining related to the referral process [24]. It was of interest to see that patients sometimes just did not remember the offer for pulmonary rehabilitation which was made at discharge from their hospital stay. So a repeated request could perhaps improve recruitment. This idea was recently conformed in another study where repeated asking to enter rehabilitation also attracted more patients to rehabilitation after an acute exacerbation as time progressed [25].

It remains a working point for pulmonary rehabilitation to increase uptake and adherence to programs. Regardless of the exact percentage of patients included in pulmonary rehabilitation, it is clear that only a fraction of patients that could potentially benefit from such an intervention are effectively recruited into programs. Part of this gap has to do with the unavailability of programs; however, part of the problem is also the lack of success in recruiting patients into programs even when they would theoretically be able to take part in a program.

It seems therefore reasonable to conclude that patients can become a candidate for pulmonary rehabilitation if they can be properly advised on the expected results of the program, and a program is available within a reasonable travel distance. More attention should be given to active smokers and patients with poor (practical) social support as these patients are likely to decline the offer for rehabilitation.

In order to be more successful in the future, the policy statement of the European Respiratory Society and the American Thoracic Society [17] proposed a comprehensive action plan which involves (a) increasing awareness around PR by all health-care providers across lines of health care, (b) enhancing payers' buy-in to rehabilitation and providing incentives when the offer for PR is taken up, (c) increasing patient awareness through lay public campaigns, and (d) improving access to rehabilitation by having sufficient programs available around patients. Ideally the offer for pulmonary rehab should be made repeatedly by all health-care actors around the patient, including the general practitioner, a nurse, and specialists. The offer should preferably be endorsed by the loved ones around the patient for it to be successful. When patients remain symptomatic of experienced problems in daily life, the possibility for pulmonary rehabilitation should be brought to the table, when stable or (and especially) after an exacerbation in each health-care contact.

3.4 What Patients Should Not Be Referred to Pulmonary Rehabilitation

There are very few contraindications to refer a patient to a rehabilitation program [7]. Only when exercise training would place the patient at increased risk for adverse events patients should not be referred to rehabilitation programs. Such patients, however, can still benefit from other components of a multidisciplinary program. Patients may benefit from adaptations in their daily life offered by an occupational therapist or from disease management skills offered in the self-management component of rehabilitation. Similarly, clinicians may be more restricted in sending patients who are in a palliative track to a conventional rehabilitation program. Where it can be argued that programs should be able to deal with patients in a palliative care track, it is best verified upfront whether the program is able to take such patients under their care. When prognosis is limited, the burden of attending rehabilitation should be carefully balanced with eventual benefits. In many countries, dedicated palliative care teams are available, and although they typically use components of rehabilitation, these teams are better equipped to deal with end-of-life issues comprehensively. That said, it is important that advanced care planning has a place in all rehabilitation programs as it offers patients and their families comfort and security regarding life-threatening situations. An excellent review on the topic was recently provided by Janssen and colleagues [26].

3.5 What Is the Best Candidate for Exercise Training

3.5.1 Candidates for Conventional Exercise Training

Exercise training improves skeletal muscle function, exercise tolerance, and exercise-induced symptoms. These effects have been convincingly demonstrated at the histological and molecular biological level of skeletal muscle function (fiber cross-sectional area, oxidative enzyme capacity), as well as on the macroscopic level (enhanced skeletal muscle strength and endurance, reduced ventilatory requirements for identical work rate and oxygen consumption, and generally improved exercise tolerance). Despite the overwhelming evidence for exercise training [27], it is also widely recognized that not all patients benefit equally from an exercise training program. While some patients experience very large benefits, others do not improve their exercise tolerance, despite attending the training sessions (see Fig. 3.2).

Genetic factors: In healthy subject, variability in training response is also well accepted, and training response in a particular outcome (typically peak VO_2 or skeletal muscle strength after resistance exercise training) is to some extent explained by the genotype of the subjects [28]. Similar suggestions were made in 850 patients that followed cardiac rehabilitation [29]. In patients with respiratory diseases, no studies showed so far candidate genes that would predispose patients to more or less effects of training. Perhaps in the future, (epi-) genetic screening may offer additional insight in the adaptation potential with specific training regimes. More research focused on the physiological determinants of exercise training success.

Skeletal muscle dysfunction: Since exercise training programs aim at restoring cardiovascular but also skeletal muscle function, it has become clear that patients with more abnormal muscle function at baseline are better candidates for an exercise training program. Some years ago, we investigated the predictors of exercise training response, and indeed skeletal muscle weakness

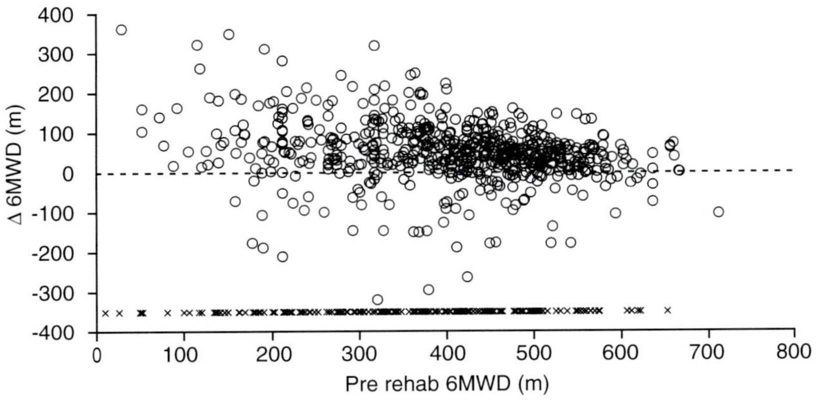

Fig. 3.2 Variability in pulmonary rehabilitation response. Change in pulmonary rehabilitation in the 6-min walking distance as a function of the baseline 6-min walking distance. Average effect of the program was 47 ± 81 m with 63% of 616 COPD patients reassessed reached the MID of 30 m in this outcome. Patients with low 6MWD can obtain significant benefits of exercise training programs. Patients who dropped out from the program are identified as "*x*." Patients with a poor (<350 m) baseline 6MWD were more likely to drop out from the program than patients with better preserved 6MWD at baseline (see text for explanation)

was an important predictor of success of a training intervention [30, 31]. Later, two studies investigated what skeletal muscle characteristic was most linked to improvements after exercise training. Patients with fatigable quadriceps muscle upon a training session or exhaustive exercise were more likely to have significant training effects [32, 33]. Importantly, patients that were more responsive to bronchodilators were those with an "opposite" phenotype: patients with less profound muscular fatigue after a single exercise bout [34]. These observations may help to select patients for either exercise training interventions (when fatigue) or more emphasis on improving lung function, when no fatigue is observed.

Other factors: Clearly baseline deconditioning is a factor that can be associated to better training outcomes. If patients can make their way through the training program, typically those with more impaired exercise capacity benefit more from a training program [35]. Figure 3.2 highlights the fact that many patients with an initially low 6MWD are very good candidates for exercise training. It deserves to be mentioned, however, that patients with poorer exercise tolerance (arbitrarily determined to be a 6MWD < 350 m) had higher likelihood of dropping out from our program (37%) compared to patients with better exercise tolerance (20% dropout, $p < 0.001$). A similar trend was observed in another large cohort of patients [36]. The poor 6MWD might be a surrogate measure of frailty, and other groups have also identified twice as much dropout rates in patients who were formally identified as frail [37]. This indicates that in these more frail patients, perhaps more attention should be given to signs of intolerance to the program, and closer monitoring might be required when patients miss a session (often because of intermittent exacerbations).

The exercise limitation has been put forward as a factor that is associated with response to exercise training. Patients with more overt ventilatory limitations were suggested to have less response to conventional exercise training. While this may be true, when the training program is not adapted to the exercise limitation of the patient (see below), it is possible to train patients with ventilator limitations using training modalities that are less challenging for the ventilatory system.

More recently, a study in Barcelona identified patients with non-anemic iron deficiency (defined as ferritin levels < 1000 μg/mL) as patients with less response to a training program as assessed by the changes in peak VO_2. This subgroup of patients included 48% of all patients recruited in that study [38]. Data would need further confirmation, and it is unknown whether treatment of the abnormality with iron supplements would yield better training outcomes.

Several factors were shown not to be related to exercise training outcomes. Gender, age, lung function impairment, comorbidities, and hypoxia are not or at best poorly associated with the outcome of an exercise training program in COPD.

3.5.2 What Is the Best Candidate for Comprehensive Rehabilitation

When patients suffer from non-respiratory consequences of their lung disease, or when they have insufficient knowledge or self-management skills to cope with their disease, they are candidates for multidisciplinary rehabilitation. Non-respiratory problems that impact on the patients' burden of the disease may be in the symptom control of the patient and coping with the disease; knowledge and self-management of the lung disease; psychologic problems (e.g., depression); social problems (poor social support or poor social conditions); nutritional problems (e.g., over- or underweight, difficulties with calorie uptake or unhealthy nutritional habits); speech problems; problems with activities of daily living; and the organization thereof in terms of pacing or maladapted living conditions. If any of the above occur, patients should be referred to multidisciplinary rehabilitation. The different team members available in well-equipped rehabilitation teams can tackle these problems with individualized therapies tailored to the patient. These therapies are discussed in much detail in Part IV of this handbook.

3.6 Improving Acceptability for Programs: Factors Related to the Program

3.6.1 Organizing the Program to the Patient's Preference

One of the challenges of patient selection and referral is to ensure that there is a good fit between patients and programs. As outlined in Part V of this handbook, programs can differ in terms of their content, duration, location, and supervision. While some patients may be difficult to manage in a specific setting, they may be excellent candidates for other types of programs. A severe patient with multi-morbidity may be difficult to manage in a community-based program, while that same patient may do very well in a hospital-based third-line program. To the best of our knowledge, no studies have formally investigated whether triage of patients has beneficial effects, but clearly such an approach makes clinical sense. In such a system, the complexity of the patient, the rehabilitation center's expertise, the reimbursement options, and the preference of the patient need to be considered. Figure 3.3 provides an overview of different options for rehabilitation that can be considered and discussed with patients [39]. While no firm advice can be provided, our center and others have created networks of centers and options for different types of patients. We actively engage in postgraduate formation in order to ensure standards of care across settings. The "network consists" of a third-line rehabilitation facility, second-line centers in neighboring cities, primary care physiotherapy practices, fitness centers, and a self-care group largely managed where a maintenance exercise is organized in a local sports club. Patients that are screened can be placed in the most optimal and preferred location. Patients can also move from one program to another, for example, to ensure an appropriate maintenance program after an outpatient-centered-based program.

More accessible variants of rehabilitation have been described. Exercise training offered in the home of the patient, for example, can resolve issues of accessibility, while adequate monitoring through telemedicine application can be ensured [40]. Such variants have not yet proven to work effectively when a high throughput of patients is required, as usually in clinical care. More real-world effectiveness studies are needed to confirm the benefits of these novel variants. So far, small-scale studies are showing very encouraging results.

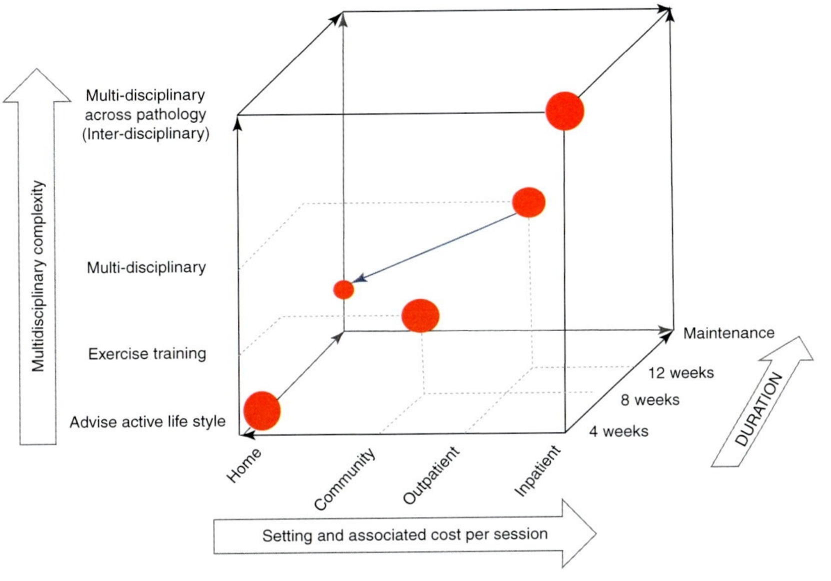

Fig. 3.3 Possible forms of rehabilitation, organized in terms of duration of the program, complexity, and setting. Different rehabilitation program options, in terms of setting and its associated cost per session, the involvement of a multidisciplinary team, and the duration of the program. Redrawn from [38]

3.6.2 Adapting the Program

For severe or frail patients, "classic" programs can be difficult to cope with. Several strategies can be applied to make the training program more feasible for patients with extreme ventilatory limitation, muscle weakness, or gas exchange abnormalities. Training modalities that are very suitable for patients with limited ventilatory capacity and are relatively easy to implement include interval training, single-leg training, resistance training, or eccentric work (e.g., downhill walking [41] or eccentric cycling [42]). Patients with overt muscle weakness may be good candidates for resistance training or neuromuscular electrical stimulation. The latter intervention was successfully used in patients that were too frail to participate in regular rehabilitation but were able to receive this intervention in the home setting [43]. For patients with gas exchange problems, supplemental oxygen can be offered to reduce the ventilatory burden during the training and improve oxygen saturation.

By altering the training modality better to the patient's possibilities, exercise training becomes more feasible and within reach for patients. Studies showed that patients have less unexpected breaks and less symptoms, while training effects were guaranteed as well as with conventional training, but with higher completion rates [44–47]. Proper assessment of the patient providing insight in the exercise limitation can help determining what training modality is best selected for a patient.

3.6.3 Adapting Other Aspects of Pulmonary Rehabilitation

While exercise training is typically conducted in groups of patients, other disciplines typically offer their interventions to individual patients. These interventions are therefore by definition individualized. Nevertheless, conventional approaches need to be adapted when patients suffer from other lung diseases than COPD or when there are important comorbidities that need to be taken into account and may sometimes hinder a patient more than the respiratory disease. For example, educational packages geared to COPD should not be offered to patients with other lung diseases. Self-management techniques may also be different.

3.7 In Summary

While no evidence-based guidance exists around which patients should be identified as candidates for pulmonary rehabilitation, there is general consensus that those patients who have remaining symptoms or have insufficient physical activity despite optimal pharmacological treatment or those patients who suffered from an exacerbation should be referred for PR. Unfortunately, few of the candidates eventually receive and complete this highly effective intervention. More efforts are needed to repeatedly and consistently propose rehabilitation as a treatment option by all health professionals. This requires that the whole health-care system is made aware of the benefits of rehabilitation, sufficient options for rehabilitation can be offered, and patients are made aware of the importance of this treatment option.

Multidisciplinary rehabilitation including exercise training can also be modified and should also be individualized so that patients find the program acceptable while remaining effective in tackling physiological and other problems of patients with respiratory disease. This requires an adaptation of the exercise training program and an individualized multidisciplinary approach.

References

1. Langer D, Hendriks E, Burtin C, Probst V, van der Schans C, Paterson W, Verhoef-de WM, Straver R, Klaassen M, Troosters T, et al. A clinical practice guideline for physiotherapists treating patients with chronic obstructive pulmonary disease based on a systematic review of available evidence. Clin Rehabil. 2009;23:445–62.
2. Ries AL, Bauldoff GS, Carlin BW, Casaburi R, Emery CF, Mahler DA, Make B, Rochester CL, ZuWallack R, Herrerias C. Pulmonary rehabilitation: joint ACCP/AACVPR evidence-based clinical practice guidelines. *Chest*. 2007;131:4S–42S.
3. Marciniuk DD, Brooks D, Butcher S, Debigare R, Dechman G, Ford G, Pepin V, Reid D, Sheel AW, Stickland MK, et al. Optimizing pulmonary rehabilitation in chronic obstructive pulmonary disease—practical issues: a Canadian Thoracic Society Clinical Practice Guideline. Can Respir J. 2010;17:159–68.
4. Vogelmeier CF, Criner GJ, Martinez FJ, Anzueto A, Barnes PJ, Bourbeau J, Celli BR, Chen R, Decramer M, Fabbri LM, et al. Global strategy for the diagnosis, management, and prevention of chronic obstructive lung disease 2017 report: gold executive summary. Eur Respir J. 2017;49(3):1700214.
5. National institute for Health and Care Excellence (NICE). Chronic obstructive pulmonary disease in adults. 2016. Ref Type: Online Source.
6. Bolton CE, Bevan-Smith EF, Blakey JD, Crowe P, Elkin SL, Garrod R, Greening NJ, Heslop K, Hull JH, Man WD, et al. British thoracic society guideline on pulmonary rehabilitation in adults. Thorax. 2013;68(Suppl 2):ii1–30.
7. Spruit MA, Singh SJ, Garvey C, ZuWallack R, Nici L, Rochester C, Hill K, Holland AE, Lareau SC, Man WD, et al. An official American Thoracic Society/European Respiratory Society statement: key concepts and advances in pulmonary rehabilitation. Am J Respir Crit Care Med. 2013;188:e13–64.
8. Piepoli MF, Conraads V, Corra U, Dickstein K, Francis DP, Jaarsma T, McMurray J, Pieske B, Piotrowicz E, Schmid JP, et al. Exercise training in heart failure: from theory to practice. A consensus document of the Heart Failure Association and the European Association for Cardiovascular Prevention and Rehabilitation. Eur J Heart Fail. 2011;13:347–57.
9. Piepoli MF, Corra U, Adamopoulos S, Benzer W, Bjarnason-Wehrens B, Cupples M, Dendale P, Doherty P, Gaita D, Hofer S, et al. Secondary prevention in the clinical management of patients with cardiovascular diseases. Core components, standards and outcome measures for referral and delivery: a policy statement from the cardiac rehabilitation section of the European Association for Cardiovascular Prevention & Rehabilitation. Endorsed by the Committee for Practice Guidelines of the European Society of Cardiology. Eur J Prev Cardiol. 2014;21:664–81.
10. Giangregorio LM, Papaioannou A, Macintyre NJ, Ashe MC, Heinonen A, Shipp K, Wark J, McGill S, Keller H, Jain R, et al. Too fit to fracture: exercise recommendations for individuals with osteoporosis or osteoporotic vertebral fracture. Osteoporos Int. 2014;25:821–35.
11. Colberg SR, Sigal RJ, Fernhall B, Regensteiner JG, Rubin RR, Chasan-Taber L, Albright AL, Broun B, American College of Sports Medicine; American Diabetes Association. Exercise and type 2 diabetes: the American College of Sports Medicine and the American Diabetes Association: Joint Position Statement. Diabetes Care. 2010;33:e147–67.
12. Executive Summary: Guidelines. For the management of overweight and obesity in adults: a report of the American College of Cardiology/American Heart Association Task Force on Practice Guidelines and the Obesity Society published by the Obesity Society

and American College of Cardiology/American Heart Association Task Force on Practice Guidelines. Based on a systematic review from the obesity expert panel, 2013. Obesity (Silver Spring). 2013;22(Suppl 2):S5–39.
13. Qaseem A, Barry MJ, Kansagara D. Nonpharmacologic versus pharmacologic treatment of adult patients with major depressive disorder: a clinical practice guideline from the American college of physicians. Ann Intern Med. 2016;164:350–9.
14. Schols AM, Ferreira IM, Franssen FM, Gosker HR, Janssens W, Muscaritoli M, Pison C, Rutten-van MM, Slinde F, Steiner MC, et al. Nutritional assessment and therapy in COPD: a European Respiratory Society statement. Eur Respir J. 2014;44:1504–20.
15. Puhan MA, Gimeno-Santos E, Cates CJ, Troosters T. Pulmonary rehabilitation following exacerbations of chronic obstructive pulmonary disease. Cochrane Database Syst Rev. 2016;12:CD005305.
16. Langer D, Burtin C, Schepers L, Ivanova A, Verleden G, Decramer M, Troosters T, Gosselink R. Exercise training after lung transplantation improves participation in daily activity: a randomized controlled trial. Am J Transplant. 2012;12:1584–92.
17. Rochester CL, Vogiatzis I, Holland AE, Lareau SC, Marciniuk DD, Puhan MA, Spruit MA, Masefield S, Casaburi R, Clini EM, et al. An official American Thoracic Society/European respiratory society policy statement: enhancing implementation, use, and delivery of pulmonary rehabilitation. Am J Respir Crit Care Med. 2015;192:1373–86.
18. Keating A, Lee A, Holland AE. What prevents people with chronic obstructive pulmonary disease from attending pulmonary rehabilitation? A systematic review. Chron Respir Dis. 2011;8:89–99.
19. Hayton C, Clark A, Olive S, Browne P, Galey P, Knights E, Staunton L, Jones A, Coombes E, Wilson AM. Barriers to pulmonary rehabilitation: characteristics that predict patient attendance and adherence. Respir Med. 2013;107:401–7.
20. Jones SE, Green SA, Clark AL, Dickson MJ, Nolan AM, Moloney C, Kon SS, Kamal F, Godden J, Howe C, et al. Pulmonary rehabilitation following hospitalisation for acute exacerbation of COPD: referrals, uptake and adherence. Thorax. 2014;69:181–2.
21. Cox NS, Oliveira CC, Lahham A, Holland AE. Pulmonary rehabilitation referral and participation are commonly influenced by environment, knowledge, and beliefs about consequences: a systematic review using the theoretical domains framework. J Physiother. 2017;63:84–93.
22. Steiner MC, Lowe D, Beckford K, Blakey J, Bolton CE, Elkin S, Man WD, Roberts CM, Sewell L, Walker P, et al. Socioeconomic deprivation and the outcome of pulmonary rehabilitation in England and Wales. Thorax. 2017;72:530–7.
23. Karmali KN, Davies P, Taylor F, Beswick A, Martin N, Ebrahim S. Promoting patient uptake and adherence in cardiac rehabilitation. Cochrane Database Syst Rev. 2014;6:CD007131.
24. Mathar H, Fastholm P, Lange P, Larsen NS. Why do patients decline participation in offered pulmonary rehabilitation? A qualitative study. Clin Rehabil. 2017:269215517708821.
25. Ko FW, Cheung NK, Rainer TH, Lum C, Wong I, Hui DS. Comprehensive care programme for patients with chronic obstructive pulmonary disease: a randomised controlled trial. Thorax. 2016;72(2):107–8.
26. Janssen DJ, McCormick JR. Palliative care and pulmonary rehabilitation. Clin Chest Med. 2014;35:411–21.
27. McCarthy B, Casey D, Devane D, Murphy K, Murphy E, Lacasse Y. Pulmonary rehabilitation for chronic obstructive pulmonary disease. Cochrane Database Syst Rev. 2015;2:CD003793.
28. Bouchard C. Genomic predictors of trainability. Exp Physiol. 2012;97:347–52.
29. Thomaes T, Thomis M, Onkelinx S, Fagard R, Matthijs G, Buys R, Schepers D, Cornelissen V, Vanhees L. A genetic predisposition score for muscular endophenotypes predicts the increase in aerobic power after training: the CAREGENE study. BMC Genet. 2011;12:84.
30. Troosters T, Gosselink R, Decramer M. Exercise training in COPD: how to distinguish responders from nonresponders. J Cardpulm Rehabil. 2001;21:10–7.
31. Walsh JR, Morris NR, McKeough ZJ, Yerkovich ST, Paratz JD. A simple clinical measure of quadriceps muscle strength identifies responders to pulmonary rehabilitation. Pulm Med. 2014;2014:782702.
32. Burtin C, Saey D, Saglam M, Langer D, Gosselink R, Janssens W, Decramer M, Maltais F, Troosters T. Effectiveness of exercise training in patients with COPD: the role of muscle fatigue. Eur Respir J. 2012;40:338–44.
33. Mador MJ, Mogri M, Patel A. Contractile fatigue of the quadriceps muscle predicts improvement in exercise performance after pulmonary rehabilitation. J Cardiopulm Rehabil Prev. 2014;34:54–61.
34. Saey D, Debigare R, LeBlanc P, Mador MJ, Cote CH, Jobin J, Maltais F. Contractile leg fatigue after cycle exercise: a factor limiting exercise in patients with chronic obstructive pulmonary disease. Am J Respir Crit Care Med. 2003;168:425–30.
35. Vagaggini B, Costa F, Antonelli S, De SC, De CG, Martino F, Santerini S, Paggiaro P. Clinical predictors of the efficacy of a pulmonary rehabilitation programme in patients with COPD. Respir Med. 2009;103:1224–30.
36. Selzler AM, Simmonds L, Rodgers WM, Wong EY, Stickland MK. Pulmonary rehabilitation in chronic obstructive pulmonary disease: predictors of program completion and success. COPD. 2012;9:538–45.
37. Maddocks M, Kon SS, Canavan JL, Jones SE, Nolan CM, Labey A, Polkey MI, Man WD. Physical frailty and pulmonary rehabilitation in COPD: a prospective cohort study. Thorax. 2016;71:988–95.
38. Barberan-Garcia A, Rodriguez DA, Blanco I, Gea J, Torralba Y, Arbillaga-Etxarri A, Barbera JA, Vilaro J, Roca J, Orozco-Levi M. Non-anaemic iron deficiency impairs response to pulmonary rehabilitation in COPD. Respirology. 2015;20:1089–95.

39. Troosters T, Demeyer H, Hornikx M, Camillo CA, Janssens W. Pulmonary rehabilitation. Clin Chest Med. 2014;35:241–9.
40. Paneroni M, Colombo F, Papalia A, Colitta A, Borghi G, Saleri M, Cabiaglia A, Azzalini E, Vitacca M. Is telerehabilitation a safe and viable option for patients with COPD? A feasibility study. COPD. 2015;12:217–25.
41. Camillo CA, Burtin C, Hornikx M, Demeyer H, De BK, van RH, Osadnik CR, Janssens W, Troosters T. Physiological responses during downhill walking: a new exercise modality for subjects with chronic obstructive pulmonary disease? Chron Respir Dis. 2015;12:155–64.
42. MacMillan NJ, Kapchinsky S, Konokhova Y, Gouspillou G, de Sousa SR, Jagoe RT, Baril J, Carver TE, Andersen RE, Richard R, et al. Eccentric ergometer training promotes locomotor muscle strength but not mitochondrial adaptation in patients with severe chronic obstructive pulmonary disease. Front Physiol. 2017;8:114.
43. Neder JA, Sword D, Ward SA, Mackay E, Cochrane LM, Clark CJ. Home based neuromuscular electrical stimulation as a new rehabilitative strategy for severely disabled patients with chronic obstructive pulmonary disease (COPD). Thorax. 2002;57:333–7.
44. Puhan MA, Busching G, Schunemann HJ, van Oort E, Zaugg C, Frey M. Interval versus continuous high-intensity exercise in chronic obstructive pulmonary disease: a randomized trial. Ann Intern Med. 2006;145:816–25.
45. Puhan MA, Schunemann HJ, Buesching G, van Oort E, Spaar A, Frey M. COPD patients' ability to follow exercise influences short-term outcomes of rehabilitation. Eur Respir J. 2008;31:304–10.
46. Vogiatzis I, Nanas S, Roussos C. Interval training as an alternative modality to continuous exercise in patients with COPD. Eur Respir J. 2002;20:12–9.
47. Vogiatzis I, Terzis G, Nanas S, Stratakos G, Simoes DC, Georgiadou O, Zakynthinos S, Roussos C. Skeletal muscle adaptations to interval training in patients with advanced COPD. Chest. 2005;128:3838–45.

The Complexity of a Respiratory Patient

4

Lowie E.G.W. Vanfleteren

Although chronic obstructive pulmonary disease (COPD) is defined by the presence of chronic airflow limitation, it is considered a complex, heterogeneous, and multicomponent disease. The heterogeneity and complexity is seen in the pulmonary expression of the disease, ranging from chronic bronchitis without emphysema to emphysema without bronchitis, in the presence or absence of exacerbations, in the differential diagnosis with asthma, but also in comorbidities and extrapulmonary manifestations, which have important contributions to disease expression, disease burden, and survival.

4.1 Heterogeneity

Most guidelines on diagnosis and treatment of COPD relate to the document published by the Global Initiative for Chronic Obstructive Lung Disease (GOLD). GOLD was initiated in 1997 to increase the attention worldwide for COPD as an emerging problem and improve prevention and management [1]. By consensus, COPD was defined based on the unidimensional pulmonary physiological parameter, namely, the forced expiratory volume in 1 s, less than 70% of the forced vital capacity of the same patient (FEV1/FVC < 0.7). The severity of the disease was further defined according to the impairment of FEV1 related to reference values. In the past decades, it came increasingly clear that FEV1 has important shortcomings in the evaluation of the disease severity of the individual patient. More details were needed to estimate the real burden of disease of patients with COPD. In the course of the years, multiple combined indices were proposed that provided a better prediction of prognosis, than only lung function or FEV1. A well-known example is the BODE index that also considered low body weight, degree of dyspnea, and exercise impairment, next to the impairment in pulmonary function [2]. For the first time, an extrapulmonary manifestation of the disease, namely, body weight, was taken in the balance to predict prognosis. Ten years after the first GOLD document, in 2007 a first revision was published, and the revised definition of COPD recognized that extrapulmonary effects could contribute to the disease severity of the individual patient [3]. Moreover, it was emphasized that FEV1 need to be considered for spirometric classification of the degree of airflow limitation, but not to establish disease severity.

The heterogeneity of COPD was also well shown within the Evaluation of COPD Longitudinally to Identify Predictive Surrogate End-points (ECLIPSE) study. The distribution of the degree of breathlessness, health status, pres-

Lowie E.G.W. Vanfleteren
CIRO, A Centre of Expertise for Chronic Organ Failure, Horn, The Netherlands

Respiratory Department, Maastricht University Medical Centre, Maastricht, The Netherlands
e-mail: lowievanfleteren@ciro-horn.nl

© Springer International Publishing AG 2018
E. Clini et al. (eds.), *Textbook of Pulmonary Rehabilitation*,
https://doi.org/10.1007/978-3-319-65888-9_4

ence of comorbidity, exercise capacity, and number of exacerbations reported in the year before the study was wide within each GOLD stage [1]. This heterogeneity is also well illustrated in Fig. 4.1. For a given FEV1, exercise capacity or health-related quality of life is unpredictable.

In the update of the GOLD document in 2013, additional characteristics were put forward to assess and treat COPD [2]. Next to the severity of airflow limitation, also exacerbation frequency and subjective well-being/amount of symptoms (measured with validated COPD-specific questionnaires) were included. These multiple dimensions resulted in four quadrants (A–B–C–D). The combination of the quadrants with the degree of airflow limitation was further refined in the 2017 GOLD update [3].

4.2 Heterogeneity and Complexity, Toward a Phenotype of Disease

The recognition of the heterogeneity of COPD led to the stratification of patients with similar characteristics. This so-called stratified medicine

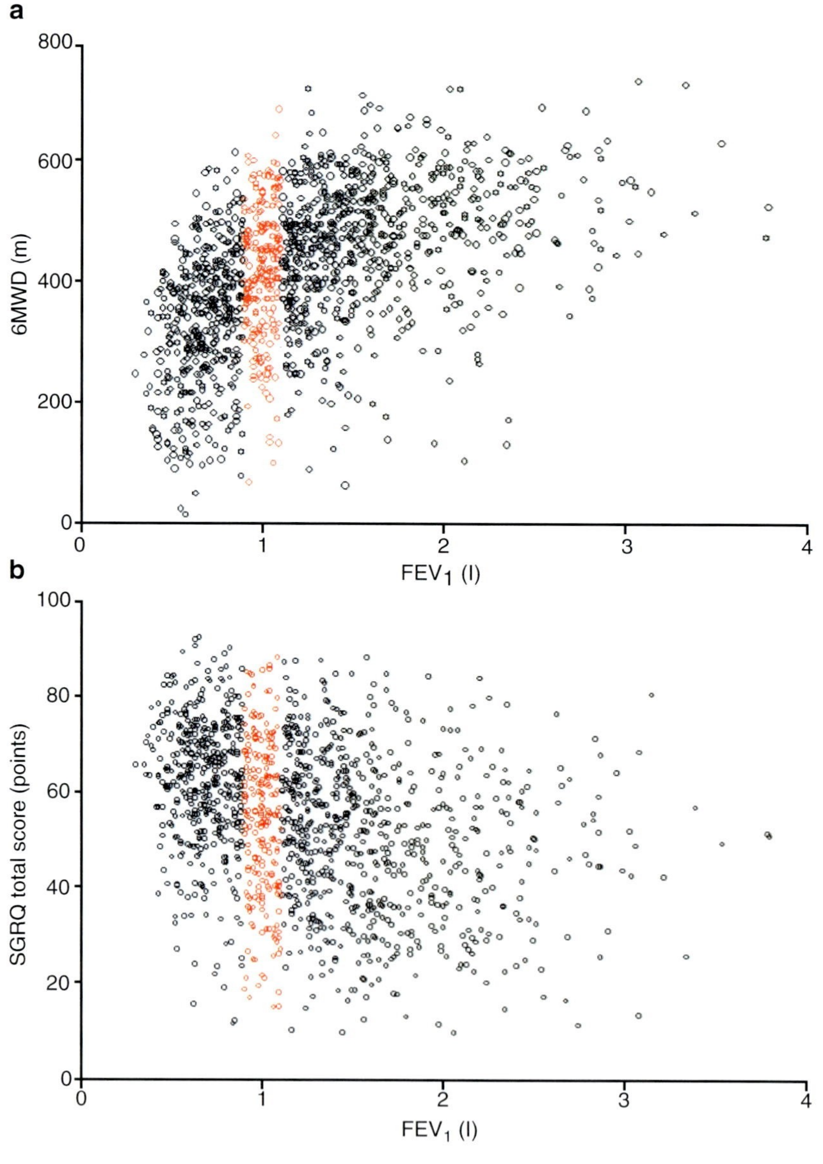

Fig. 4.1 1326 patients with COPD from the CIRO® dataset. (**a**) Correlation between forced expiratory volume in the first second: FEV1 and 6-min walking distance. (**b**) Correlation between FEV1 and SGRQ: St. George Respiratory Questionnaire (Courtesy of Dr. Martijn Spruit)

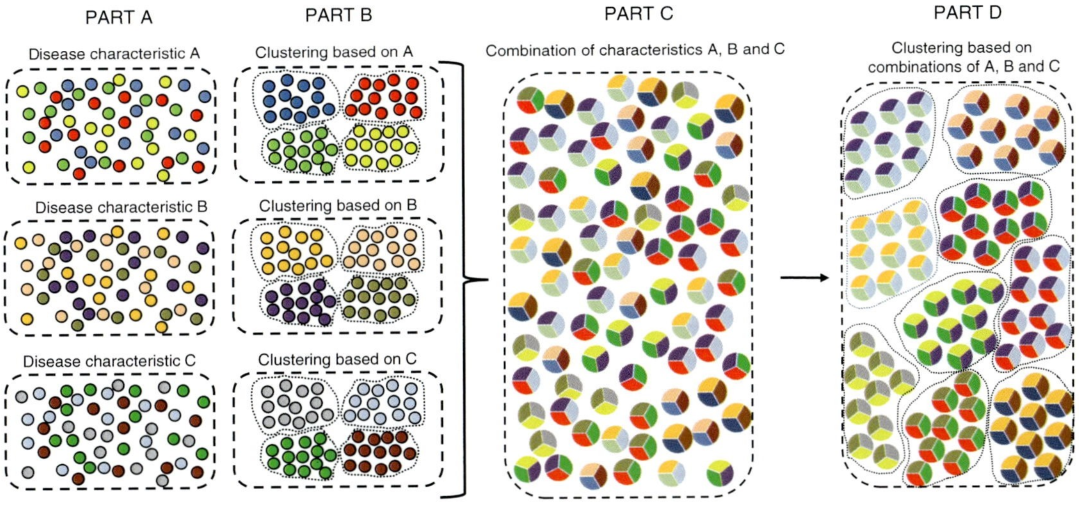

Fig. 4.2 Heterogeneity and complexity of COPD. *Part A*: As an example, three disease (treatable or non-treatable) characteristics (*A*, *B*, and *C*) are presented. *Part A*: Disease characteristic can be absent or expressed in different ways. *Part B*: Patients can be grouped based on the evaluation of the single disease characteristics. *Part C*: All characteristics are less or more expressed in every single patient. *Part D*: Patients can therefore be grouped, based on the expression of different disease characteristics

resulted from the insights that patients with COPD might respond differently to treatments or may have different outcomes or prognosis. A group of researchers defined the identification of different groups of patients based on characteristics related to prognosis, outcome, and response to therapy as "clinical phenotypes" [4]. Agusti rightfully mentioned that although the stratified medicine is helpful for research and to identify groups of patients that respond to therapy, an individual patient with COPD is also complex, and multiple "clinical phenotypes" might be recognized within one patient [5].

Figure 4.2 provides a graphical representation of heterogeneity and complexity of COPD. Each color represents one clinical characteristic. Multiple treatable and non-treatable characteristics of individual patients with COPD result in specific clinical phenotypes; and patients with COPD with comparable "clinical phenotypes" or "treatable traits" can be clustered, and hence result is a distinctive phenotype. So, an in-depth characterization seems the basis of a personalized treatment in patients with COPD.

4.3 Pulmonary Heterogeneity

COPD is an umbrella term that covers in many clinical subtypes of patients with chronic airflow limitation. As described above, the unidimensional (patho)physiological description of airflow limitation is insufficient to describe the complexity of a respiratory patient. Within the broader epidemiological context of COPD, we need to consider that subjects with persistent airflow limitation may have clearly different clinical disease expressions and underlying pathology that underlies that airflow limitation. Also a clinical disease entity like chronic bronchitis or emphysema may exist without airflow limitation. In addition, a clear different disease like uncontrolled severe allergic asthma may also be associated with persistent airflow limitation, but is objectionable called COPD. Hence, we need to consider this pulmonary heterogeneity and complexity in the approach of our patient with COPD. Here below, I discuss some of the pulmonary disease expressions related to COPD, with associated specific treatment options (Fig. 4.3).

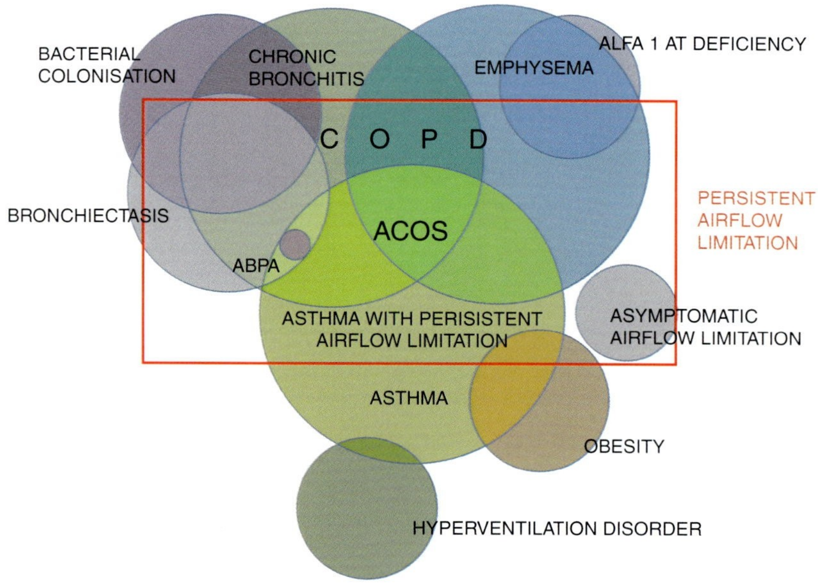

Fig. 4.3 Persistent airflow limitation in view of pulmonary disease entities

4.3.1 Chronic Bronchitis, Bronchiectasis, Bacterial Colonization

Chronic bronchitis or the presence of cough and sputum production for at least 3 months in each of two consecutive years has often been used to clinically describe COPD. However, it is important to recognize that chronic cough and sputum production (chronic bronchitis) is an independent disease entity that may precede or follow the development of airflow limitation. Chronic bronchitis also exists in patients with normal spirometry. Patients with COPD and chronic bronchitis, producing large volumes of sputum, may have underlying bronchiectasis, which increases the risk of bacterial infection and colonization, and exacerbations. Subjects with frequent exacerbations and chronic bronchitis have a higher likelihood to respond to roflumilast in terms of a reduced exacerbation frequency [6]. Also, neomacrolide is a treatment option for frequent bronchitic exacerbators [7], certainly when bronchiectasis or bacterial colonization is present [8].

4.3.2 Emphysema

Emphysema is a destructive process of the lung parenchyma characterized by the permanent enlargement of air spaces distal to the terminal bronchioles, due to inhalation of noxious substances. It is considered a distinct disease entity and may also exist in the absence of airflow limitation. The pathological process leads to lung hyperinflation, which may exaggerate during exercise (dynamic hyperinflation) and is importantly related to dyspnea. Bronchodilation therapy has only limited success in these patients. Specific treatments for patients with severe emphysema and hyperinflation exist of both surgical and endobronchial lung volume reduction strategies. The National Emphysema Treatment Trial (NETT) identified patients with upper lobe-predominant emphysema with low baseline exercise capacity as responders for lung volume reduction surgery, but at the cost of a relatively high morbidity and mortality [9]. Innovative endobronchial therapeutic strategies that induce lung volume reduction have been developed in the past decade and indicate that precise emphysema phenotyping is necessary and that it provides personalized therapies for patients with emphysema [10].

4.3.3 Asthma: COPD Overlap Syndrome

COPD and asthma are regarded as two distinct disease entities. But both conditions are now recognized as heterogeneous and often overlapping conditions. The term "asthma—COPD overlap syndrome" (ACOS) has been applied to the condition in which a person has clinical features of both asthma and COPD [11]. In most cases the differential diagnosis between asthma and COPD is easy, but in more advanced age categories, and certainly if there is an amount of exposure to noxious substances, the clinical presentation might be very similar. Indeed, irreversible airway obstruction might develop over time in patients with asthma owing to airway remodeling. On the other hand, patients with COPD often show bronchodilator reversibility that meets criteria for asthma. Bronchial hyperreactivity, a key characteristic of asthma, is also often seen in COPD [11]. Eosinophilic airway inflammation, which has been traditionally associated with asthma, has recently become a biomarker for response to inhaled corticosteroids in COPD [12]. Recently, the Global Initiative for Asthma (GINA) and GOLD issued a joint document that describes ACOS as a clinical entity and proposes that clinicians should assemble the features for asthma and for COPD that best describe the patient and compare the number of features in favor of each diagnosis [13].

4.4 Comorbidities and Extrapulmonary Manifestations of COPD

Multiple recent studies illustrated the importance and high frequency of extrapulmonary manifestations and/or comorbidities in patients with COPD as these comorbidities contribute to the heterogeneity of COPD [14]. Most probably there is a multifactorial explanation for the excess comorbidity frequency in patients with COPD. It seems that different chronic conditions develop at different speed on an individual susceptible genetic background, in response to common risk factors, as smoking, alcohol, nutrition, exposition to air pollution, physical inactivity, etc. [15] (Fig. 4.4). The theory that inflammatory activity from the lungs spills over into the systemic blood circulation and causes pathology in other organ systems is increasingly abandoned [16]. Systemic inflammation is found in patients with COPD [17], but is heterogeneous [18], often not persistent [19], and in a stable condition, it is often not pulmonary originated, given the lack of correlation between inflammatory cytokines in the airways and the blood [20].

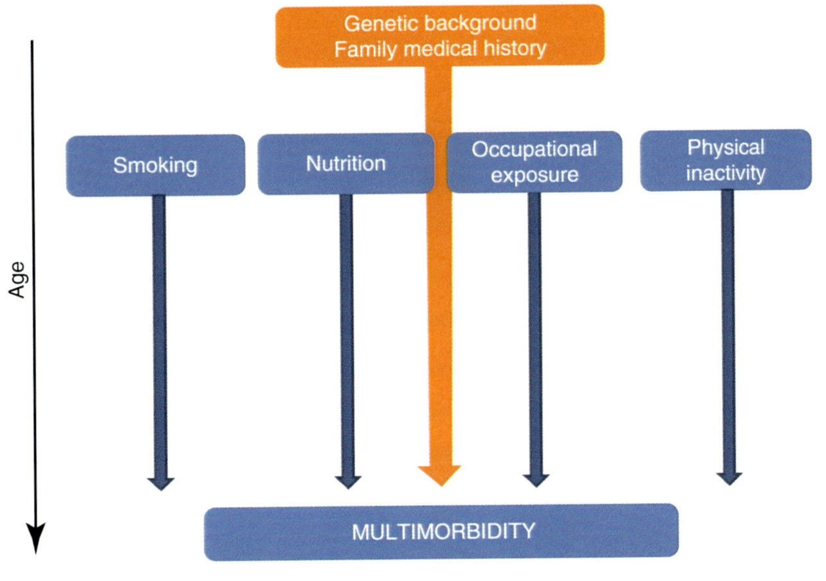

Fig. 4.4 Comorbidities develop at different speed in a susceptible subject as a consequence of common risk factors

The inflammation is commonly not specific to the presence of COPD and related to smoking, older age, and an increased fat mass [19, 21].

Anyhow, comorbidities have an important impact on health status and well-being, the amount of hospitalizations, and survival of the patient with COPD [22–24]. Given this high prevalence and impact of comorbidities in COPD, the GOLD committee recognized its importance and included the role of comorbidities in the definition of COPD in the second revision in 2011 [2]. In the most recent 2017 revision, comorbidities are no longer included in the definition, but its importance is still emphasized [3].

Comorbidities are currently not included in the COPD classification system. The presence of comorbidities has been shown to be highest in the former category B, the category that was defined by a high symptom burden, but less severe airflow limitation [25, 26]. Hence, symptoms are also determined by the presence of comorbidity. It remains a point of discussion whether and to which extent other conditions can weigh on the evaluation of the severity of the disease COPD and on how comorbidities could be incorporated in a disease-evaluation diagram [27].

The recognition of the important impact of these comorbidities on the disease burden of the individual patient by the GOLD committee by including in the definition of COPD is an important step forward [2]. It has direct consequences, as the care for COPD patients is not limited to the prescription of bronchodilators, and therapy to prevent exacerbations, but is a comprehensive and holistic approach, in which accurate diagnosis and management of COPD-related systemic manifestations and comorbidities, both pharmacologically and non-pharmacologically, need to be considered [28].

4.5 Frailty and Multimorbidity

COPD is entangled in a network of other chronic conditions which may additionally impact on the patient and the healthcare system. Not only the single conditions but also the treatment burden and the burden of healthcare appointments, unscheduled visits, hospitalizations, etc. may impact on the well-being and quality of life of the patient. Patients with COPD often fulfill criteria of frailty [29]. Pharmacological and non-pharmacological treatment need to be carefully considered, balanced, and discussed with the patient. The treatment of patients with COPD is generally not limited to inhaler therapy. In fact, multimorbidity clusters were identified in COPD [14], and treatments for these multiple conditions may interfere with each other and may increase the risk of adverse events [30]. Adherence to guidelines for individual chronic diseases might lead to complex medication regimes in multimorbid patients with potential cumulative side effects, interactions, and poor compliance [30, 31]. Polypharmacy in people with multimorbidity is not only due to drugs meant to reduce daily symptoms but often also driven by multiple drugs intended to prevent future morbidity and mortality. The case for using such drugs weakens as life expectancy shortens. The recently published NICE guideline on the management of multimorbidity notes that clinicians should not blindly follow single condition guidelines recommendations for all patients because treatment decisions should always be made in the context of an individual's circumstances. Accurate assessment of often not diagnosed relevant comorbidities is needed, but then again judgment of treatment strategies in the context of the individual patient needs to be done.

Conclusions

COPD consists of heterogeneous and complex group of patients which can be stratified according to treatable and untreatable characteristics. Not only the pulmonary clinical stratification is very diverse but also different groups of patients with different health status can be identified on the basis of their comorbidity profile. The presence of co-occurring chronic noncommunicable diseases and other physical and psychological manifestations needs to be recognized in our approach to characterize and manage individual patients with COPD. Systemic manifestations and comorbidities of COPD also contribute to different clinical phenotypes and warrant an individualized approach as part of integrated disease management.

References

1. Agusti A, et al. Characterisation of COPD heterogeneity in the ECLIPSE cohort. Respir Res. 2010;11:122.
2. Vestbo J, et al. Global strategy for the diagnosis, management, and prevention of chronic obstructive pulmonary disease: GOLD executive summary. Am J Respir Crit Care Med. 2013;187(4):347–65.
3. From the global strategy for the diagnosis, management and prevention of COPD, global initiative for chronic obstructive lung disease (GOLD) 2017. http://goldcopd.org.
4. Han MK, et al. Chronic obstructive pulmonary disease phenotypes: the future of COPD. Am J Respir Crit Care Med. 2010;182(5):598–604.
5. Agusti A. The path to personalised medicine in COPD. Thorax. 2014;69(9):857–64.
6. Martinez FJ, et al. Effect of roflumilast on exacerbations in patients with severe chronic obstructive pulmonary disease uncontrolled by combination therapy (REACT): a multicentre randomised controlled trial. Lancet. 2015;385(9971):857–66.
7. Uzun S, et al. Azithromycin maintenance treatment in patients with frequent exacerbations of chronic obstructive pulmonary disease (COLUMBUS): a randomised, double-blind, placebo-controlled trial. Lancet Respir Med. 2014;2(5):361–8.
8. Miravitlles M, et al. Pharmacological strategies to reduce exacerbation risk in COPD: a narrative review. Respir Res. 2016;17(1):112.
9. Fishman A, et al. A randomized trial comparing lung-volume-reduction surgery with medical therapy for severe emphysema. N Engl J Med. 2003;348(21):2059–73.
10. Shah PL, et al. Lung volume reduction for emphysema. Lancet Respir Med. 2016;
11. Postma DS, Rabe KF. The asthma-COPD overlap syndrome. N Engl J Med. 2015;373(13):1241–9.
12. Pascoe S, et al. Blood eosinophil counts, exacerbations, and response to the addition of inhaled fluticasone furoate to vilanterol in patients with chronic obstructive pulmonary disease: a secondary analysis of data from two parallel randomised controlled trials. Lancet Respir Med. 2015;3(6):435–42.
13. http://ginasthma.org/asthma-copd-and-asthma-copd-overlap-syndrome-acos.
14. Vanfleteren LE, et al. Clusters of comorbidities based on validated objective measurements and systemic inflammation in patients with chronic obstructive pulmonary disease. Am J Respir Crit Care Med. 2013;187(7):728–35.
15. Clini EM, Beghe B, Fabbri LM. Chronic obstructive pulmonary disease is just one component of the complex multimorbidities in patients with COPD. Am J Respir Crit Care Med. 2013;187(7):668–71.
16. Fabbri LM, Rabe KF. From COPD to chronic systemic inflammatory syndrome? Lancet. 2007;370(9589):797–9.
17. Gan WQ, et al. Association between chronic obstructive pulmonary disease and systemic inflammation: a systematic review and a meta-analysis. Thorax. 2004;59(7):574–80.
18. Vanfleteren LE, et al. Arterial stiffness in patients with COPD: the role of systemic inflammation and the effects of pulmonary rehabilitation. Eur Respir J. 2014;43(5):1306–15.
19. Agusti A, et al. Persistent systemic inflammation is associated with poor clinical outcomes in COPD: a novel phenotype. PLoS One. 2012;7(5):e37483.
20. Sinden NJ, Stockley RA. Systemic inflammation and comorbidity in COPD: a result of 'overspill' of inflammatory mediators from the lungs? Review of the evidence. Thorax. 2010;65(10):930–6.
21. Breyer MK, et al. Highly elevated C-reactive protein levels in obese patients with COPD: a fat chance? Clin Nutr. 2009;28(6):642–7.
22. Mannino DM, et al. Prevalence and outcomes of diabetes, hypertension and cardiovascular disease in COPD. Eur Respir J. 2008;32(4):962–9.
23. Divo M, et al. Comorbidities and risk of mortality in patients with COPD. Am J Respir Crit Care Med. 2012;186(2):155–61.
24. Vanfleteren LE, et al. Frequency and relevance of ischemic electrocardiographic findings in patients with chronic obstructive pulmonary disease. Am J Cardiol. 2011;108(11):1669–74.
25. Lange P, et al. Prediction of the clinical course of chronic obstructive pulmonary disease, using the new GOLD classification: a study of the general population. Am J Respir Crit Care Med. 2012;186(10):975–81.
26. Agusti A, et al. Characteristics, stability and outcomes of the 2011 GOLD COPD groups in the ECLIPSE cohort. Eur Respir J. 2013;42(3):636–46.
27. Agusti A, et al. FAQs about the GOLD 2011 assessment proposal of COPD: a comparative analysis of four different cohorts. Eur Respir J. 2013;42(5):1391–401.
28. Wouters EF. COPD: a chronic and overlooked pulmonary disease. Lancet. 2007;370(9589):715–6.
29. Maddocks M, et al. Physical frailty and pulmonary rehabilitation in COPD: a prospective cohort study. Thorax. 2016;
30. Boyd CM, et al. Clinical practice guidelines and quality of care for older patients with multiple comorbid diseases: implications for pay for performance. JAMA. 2005;294(6):716–24.
31. Doos L, et al. Multi-drug therapy in chronic condition multimorbidity: a systematic review. Fam Pract. 2014;31(6):654–63.

Part III

Assessment

5 Assessment of Exercise Capacity

Ioannis Vogiatzis, Paolo Palange,
and Pierantonio Laveneziana

5.1 Factors Limiting Exercise Capacity

Exercise intolerance is a condition where the patient is unable to undertake physical exercise at the level and/or for the duration that would be expected of someone in his or her age and general physical condition. When this inability is triggered by impaired function of one or more of the physiological systems (i.e. central haemodynamic, respiratory, peripheral muscles), the result is the intensification of the perceptions of dyspnoea, often in conjunction with peripheral muscle discomfort that is often triggered by peripheral muscle fatigue [1].

Dyspnoea is typically perceived as the distressing sensation of unsatisfied inspiration (i.e. neuromechanical coupling) [2]. The mechanisms that exacerbate dyspnoea sensations are relevant to an imbalance between the central respiratory efferent drive and the response of the respiratory muscles. In patients with chronic lung diseases, dyspnoea is exaggerated during exercise secondary to the reduced breathing efficiency that results from the deteriorating ventilatory mechanics in one hand and the increased ventilatory requirement on the other hand.

Peripheral muscle contractile fatigue, associated with the subjective feeling of leg discomfort, is manifested by a decrease in muscle force output, and it is due to a limitation in oxygen supply to, and/or utilization of oxygen by, the mitochondria [3]. This suggestion is supported by the finding that the degree of exercise-induced quadriceps muscle fatigue in COPD negatively correlates with peak oxygen utilization [4]. According to this scenario, cellular oxygen demand either exceeds the normal maximal oxygen transfer capacity of the oxygen transport chain (i.e. when maximal oxygen consumption has been truly achieved) or stresses an impaired physiological system or mechanism preventing the achieve-

I. Vogiatzis
Faculty of Physical Education and Sports Sciences, National and Kapodistrian University of Athens, Athens, Greece
e-mail: ioannis.vogiatzis@northumbria.ac.uk

Faculty of Health and Life Sciences, Department of Sport, Exercise and Rehabilitation, Northumbria University, Newcastle Upon Tyne, UK

P. Palange
Department of Public Health and Infectious Diseases, Sapienza University of Rome, Rome, Italy
e-mail: paolo.palange@uniroma1.it

P. Laveneziana (✉)
Sorbonne Universités, UPMC Université Paris 06, INSERM, UMRS_1158 Neurophysiologie Respiratoire Expérimentale et Clinique, Paris, France
e-mail: pierantonio.laveneziana@aphp.fr

Assistance Publique-Hôpitaux de Paris (AP-HP), Groupe Hospitalier Pitié-Salpêtrière Charles Foix, Service des Explorations Fonctionnelles de la Respiration, de l'Exercice et de la Dyspnée (Département "R3S", Pôle PRAGUES), Paris, France
e-mail: pierantonio.laveneziana@aphp.fr

© Springer International Publishing AG 2018
E. Clini et al. (eds.), *Textbook of Pulmonary Rehabilitation*,
https://doi.org/10.1007/978-3-319-65888-9_5

ment of a true maximal oxygen consumption (i.e. achieving, as in COPD, peak but not normal maximal oxygen consumption) [5]. In the latter case, a series of malfunctions at the level of respiratory and cardiovascular systems may impair the normal peripheral muscle oxygen delivery and conductance capabilities [3, 6]. Hence, the factors that limit exercise tolerance in healthy individuals (the former case) are different to that constraining exercise capacity in patients with cardiorespiratory diseases (the latter case).

5.1.1 Exercise Testing in Lung Diseases

To evaluate exercise intolerance, cardiopulmonary exercise testing (CPET) is considered the gold standard as it allows simultaneous assessment of objective (i.e. cardiopulmonary responses, operational lung volumes, etc.) and subjective variables (intensity of dyspnoea and leg discomfort sensations). There are two types of exercise protocols taking place either on the treadmill or the cycle ergometer that are commonly implemented: the maximal incremental test and the constant work-rate test.

The maximal incremental test provides to the subject a smooth gradational stress of all the physiological systems involved in the exercise response as the intensity of exercise is progressively increased to volitional termination. The incremental test not only allows determination of a variety of physiological responses at the limit of tolerance (i.e. peak oxygen uptake) but also enables the evaluation of trending phenomena as the severity of exercise progresses from submaximal to maximal tolerable levels. Such trends may, for example, refer to the response of minute ventilation relative to oxygen uptake ($\dot{V}O_2$) or to carbon dioxide production ($\dot{V}CO_2$), reflecting "ventilatory efficiency". Also, the rate of change in $\dot{V}CO_2$ relative to the change in $\dot{V}O_2$ is commonly used to non-invasively identify the "anaerobic threshold". Similarly, when the test is performed on the bicycle ergometer, the rate of change in $\dot{V}O_2$ relative to work rate is taken to reflect "aerobic work efficiency" (Fig. 5.1) [7].

During the constant work-rate test, the work rate is set at a constant fraction of the predetermined maximal or peak work rate (usually 50–80%), and individuals are asked to exercise for as long as they can tolerate the imposed load. The time to exercise limitation is measured. During these tests, a steady-state response (where the energy demands of the working muscles are met by the energy supply mechanisms) may or may not be achieved depending on the work intensity and the disability level of the individual. Nevertheless, even if a steady state in the cardiorespiratory response is to be achieved, this will not occur instantaneously, but it will happen over a period of time. Hence, the period of dynamic adjustment in cardiorespiratory and metabolic responses provides valuable information of

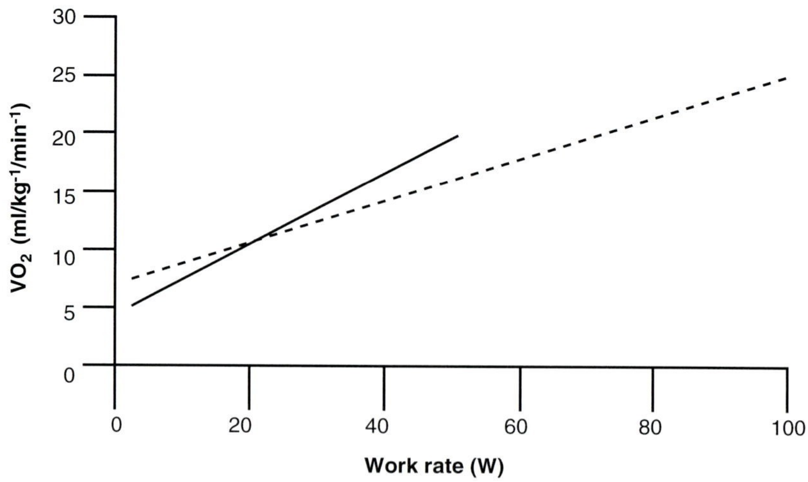

Fig. 5.1 Change of the oxygen uptake in relation to work rate on a cycle ergometer in a healthy individual (*dotted line*) and in a patient with COPD (*solid line*)

the dynamic behaviour of the respiratory and cardiorespiratory function as well as of the capacity of the body to reach a steady state of oxygen utilization [1, 5].

Besides cardiopulmonary exercise testing that provides plethora of information on physiological responses, there are exercise tests that yield less physiological information but still provide a measure of exercise limitation. These are the 6-min walking test [8] and the incremental and endurance shuttle walking tests [9, 10], which provide information in regard to the magnitude of exercise intolerance, the intensity of symptoms and the degree of reduction in arterial oxygen saturation. The 6-min walking test has been shown to be of submaximal intensity and is often used to evaluate the effects of interventions on patients' endurance capacity [11, 12]. Patients are allowed to walk at own pace and encouraged to go around a set of cones positioned on the floor as many times as possible. One study [11] demonstrated that the 6-min walking test generates a high but sustainable oxygen uptake, thereby emphasizing the high prognostic value of the 6-min walking test.

The incremental shuttle walk test [9] is a test where the walking speed is continuously increased until the patient reaches the level of his/her tolerance. As such, the incremental shuttle walk test is considered as equivalent to the maximal incremental test performed on the treadmill. The intensity of the endurance walking test corresponds to a fraction of the patient's maximum exercise performance assessed by the incremental shuttle walking tests. Although the sustained intensity is submaximal (i.e. 75 and 85% of intensity) [10], patients often reach their level of tolerance.

5.1.2 Factors Determining Exercise Tolerance in Healthy Young Individuals

In healthy subjects exercise tolerance refers to the capacity of an individual to achieve the maximum attainable amount of work during an exercise protocol where the intensity increases progressively until maximum capacity is reached. In this case, exercise tolerance is assessed by the maximum capacity of the individual's body to transport and utilize oxygen (i.e. $\dot{V}O_2$ max). In turn the achieved $\dot{V}O_2$ max depends on the convective and conductive oxygen delivery and muscle oxygen utilization [3].

Over the past few decades, a number of studies have been conducted with the aim to investigate the limiting factors for achieving $\dot{V}O_{2max}$ in healthy subjects [13–15]. A fundamental approach to establish the limiting factors is to compare the physiological responses recorded from sedentary and well-trained individuals during incremental exercise. Such studies have clearly shown that in healthy sedentary subjects compared to highly trained athletes, the main variable that limits $\dot{V}O_{2max}$ is cardiac output [16–19]. In fact, the implemented experimental procedures demonstrated a linear relationship between $\dot{V}O_{2max}$ and maximal cardiac output showing that an average of 5.0 L/min–6.0 L/min of cardiac output is needed per litre of $\dot{V}O_2$ in sedentary subjects, whereas in highly trained subjects, cardiac output often reaches 6.0–7.0 L/min per litre of $\dot{V}O_2$. This difference in maximal cardiac output and $\dot{V}O_2$ between sedentary and well-trained subjects was mainly attributed to the lower stroke volume in untrained compared to trained individuals [15]. Additionally, the lower haemoglobin concentration exhibited by the sedentary individuals has been considered as another contributor to the difference in $\dot{V}O_{2max}$ [16–19] as this impacts on the arterial oxygen content. Experimental reduction in maximal cardiac output and in arterial oxygen content (either through the reduction in blood volume or haemoglobin concentration alone) has led to a reduction in systemic oxygen delivery [20–24].

Besides systemic oxygen delivery, skeletal muscle oxygen extraction as well as mitochondrial rate of oxygen consumption has also been shown to differentiate a sedentary from a well-trained individual in terms of the potential to achieve a high value for $\dot{V}O_{2max.}$ Specifically, skeletal muscle oxygen extraction limitation could be due to (1) limited diffusive conductance for oxygen between the red blood cells and the mitochondria, (2) non-uniformity of perfusion in relation to metabolic rate and/or (3) shunting of blood between arterioles and venules, bypassing muscle fibres [1]. The limited diffusive conductance for oxygen appears to be the major contributor in limiting oxygen transport by limiting oxygen extraction [1, 3].

As a final point, $\dot{V}O_{2max}$ can be affected also by factors as alveolar ventilation/pulmonary perfusion ($\dot{V}_A/Q$) inequality [25] and post-pulmonary shunts [26] which are playing a small but demonstrable role in reducing arterial oxygenation [27]. Accordingly, in healthy subjects a limitation primarily in oxygen transport and also in the capacity of oxygen utilization by the working muscles constitutes important factors determining exercise capacity. Defects in the mechanism of oxygen transport and utilization also determine the magnitude of exercise intolerance in patients with chronic lung diseases.

5.1.3 Factors Determining Exercise Tolerance in Healthy Elderly Individuals

The response of the cardiovascular and respiratory systems during exercise is attenuated to various degrees in the elderly. Importantly, there are considerable changes in the connective tissue matrix of the lung that may reduce the elastic recoil pressure and hence the airway radial traction, thus predisposing to expiratory flow limitation and air trapping [28]. This is the reason why it is common practice in clinical research to compare the responses recorded by patients with lung disease with those of healthy age-matched individuals. Accordingly, it is important to separately consider the limiting factors to exercise capacity in healthy elderly individuals.

Age-associated changes in cardiovascular structure and function [29, 30] as well as in mitochondrial content and quality [31] indicate that the ability of the older adult to increase convective oxygen delivery and muscle oxygen utilization is impaired. These two factors may contribute to a slowed adaptation of muscle oxygen consumption and early metabolic acidosis in the older compared to the young individual [32, 33]. In addition, ageing is associated with a reduced maximal heart rate [34], reduced left ventricular function [30], increased total peripheral resistance [29], reduced capillary density [35], endothelial dysfunction and altered capillary haemodynamics [36], all of which are expected to compromise the convective oxygen transport to working muscles during exercise. In addition, with ageing there is an increase in pulmonary vascular stiffness, resistance and pressures along with increased heterogeneity of alveolar ventilation and pulmonary perfusion as well as decreased pulmonary capillary blood volume and membrane diffusing capacity that is consistent with a reduction in alveolar-capillary surface area [37].

Studies have shown that besides the aforementioned changes in pulmonary haemodynamics, ageing is associated with numerous structural and functional alterations, related to reductions in the elastic recoil of the lung, in chest wall compliance and in respiratory muscle performance [38–40]. As the compliance of the lung increases and that of the chest wall decreases at a higher extent than that of the lung, thoracic expansion becomes limited, and an old subject would have to do ~20% more elastic work at a given level of ventilation than a 40-year younger fellow [38]. As a result, the respiratory muscles of the old subjects would be expected to work harder since they are acting on a stiffer chest wall [41–43]. This would most likely require an increased share of cardiac output, thus potentially limiting blood flow to the lower limbs [43, 44].

Based on such evidence, chest wall volume regulation would be expected to differ among old and healthy individuals. The normal response of operational chest wall volume regulation during exercise has been previously and extensively described in healthy young adults. Although a similar pattern to that described for healthy young adults [45, 46] has been observed in healthy older subjects in terms of reducing end-expiratory chest wall volume during incremental exercise [47], at peak exercise the end-inspiratory chest wall volume in older subjects often reaches ~80% of the chest wall volume at total lung capacity (TLC), whilst in healthy young subjects, the ratio of end-inspiratory lung volume to TLC does not exceed 70% [43, 46]. This difference exists because young subjects are capable of reducing end-expiratory chest wall volume by expiratory muscle recruitment, thus allowing tidal volume to expand by encroachment into both the inspiratory and expiratory reserve volume. In elderly, due to flow limitation, end-expiratory chest wall volume only slightly decreases, so expansion of tidal volume takes place primarily by encroachment on the inspiratory reserve volume (288), thereby end-inspiratory lung volume reaches close to TLC with consequent increasing of the elastic work associated with breathing near to TLC [47]. In the setting of significant restrictive mechanical constraints on tidal volume expansion, an increase in ventilatory demand during exercise intensifies exertional breathlessness to a greater degree in older individuals than in healthy young individuals [41, 42].

5.1.4 Factors Impairing Exercise Tolerance in Chronic Lung Diseases

Exercise intolerance in patients with chronic lung diseases is multifactorial, involving ventilatory, gas exchange, cardiovascular and peripheral muscle abnormalities.

5.1.4.1 Ventilatory Constraints

During exercise of progressively increasing intensity, healthy elderly individuals can increase their breathing frequency and their tidal volume to provide up to a 10–15 fold increase in minute ventilation that is essential to clear the carbon dioxide production and meet the increased oxygen demand [41–43, 48]. Under such circumstances, ventilatory function is often not the limiting factor, at least for a wide range of submaximal exercise levels, as minute ventilation ($\dot{V}_E$) is maintained well below the maximum ventilatory capacity (MVC) [49]. Ventilatory limitation, however, may occur in healthy elderly individuals, particularly women [50] during maximal exercise, as the ratio of $\dot{V}_E$ to MVC ($\dot{V}_E$/MVC) approaches or even exceeds 85% [33, 51].

In the majority of respiratory disorders, the $\dot{V}_E$/MVC ratio often exceeds 85% even during moderate levels of exercise, commonly reflecting reduced ventilatory capacity [48, 52]. In fact, in patients with chronic lung diseases, a disparity is developed between the decreased ventilatory capacity, which is manifested by diminished maximum and sustainable voluntary capacity and eventually by the inability to sufficiently increase minute ventilation during exercise, and the increased ventilatory requirement and workload. This disparity leads to intense dyspnoea sensation that is the symptom limiting exercise in a large fraction of patients with chronic lung diseases [53, 54]. The factors contributing to decreased ventilatory capacity or increased ventilatory requirement/workload are in brief described below.

Reduced ventilatory capacity during exercise is due to the abnormal respiratory system mechanics and the dysfunction of the respiratory muscles. In patients with chronic lung diseases, the high inspiratory (and expiratory) airway resistance and/or reduced compliance can substantially increase the pressure requirement for airflow and thus increase the work to breathe [54–56]. Respiratory muscles are frequently weakened and unable to endure adequately due to the presence of hyperinflation and/or intrinsic muscle dysfunction/hypoperfusion.

Ventilatory demand is increased during exercise owing to gas exchange abnormalities (i.e. worsening of $\dot{V}_E/Q$ mismatch and increased dead space ventilation) which lead to hypoxemia and hypercapnia [51]. The ventilatory demand of exercise is regulated not only by the metabolic rate but also by the arterial carbon dioxide tension and the physiological dead space fraction of breath [7]. Metabolic acidosis also increases the ventilatory requirement of exercise [57]. Therefore in chronic lung diseases, for a given rate of CO_2 output ($\dot{V}CO_2$) and $PaCO_2$, $\dot{V}_E$ is usually increased because of higher dead space ventilation [1]. Moreover, *ventilatory workload is increased* during exercise because of abnormal dynamic ventilatory mechanics.

5.1.4.2 Gas Exchange Limitations

Age-related changes in pulmonary circulation would be expected to make elderly individuals more susceptible to gas exchange abnormalities during exercise. However, despite the deterioration in ventilatory reserve with ageing, healthy older adults appear able to maintain alveolar ventilation at a level that allows maintenance of arterial blood gases within normal limits, even during heavy exercise [49, 51, 58, 59]. Accordingly, the ventilation-perfusion ratio ($\dot{V}_A / Q$) remains near unity as both ventilation and perfusion increase severalfold with increasing exercise intensity. Moreover, alveolar-capillary diffusion also remains intact, and consequently PaO_2 remains normal, even at high exercise intensities [48, 49, 51]. Furthermore, in healthy elderly individuals, exercise-induced tidal volume (V_T) increase occurs in the setting of relatively fixed anatomic dead space (V_D), so the V_D/V_T ratio decreases such that effective alveolar ventilation increases as a proportion of the increased minute ventilation.

In contrast, gas exchange regulation is impaired in chronic lung diseases that involve the airways, the pulmonary vasculature and the alveolar-capillary interface to varying degrees thus producing varying degrees of abnormal $\dot{V}_A / Q$ inequalities, diffusion impairment and hypoxemia at rest and during exercise [13, 28, 54, 60]. In fact, many patients with severe lung disease experience arterial oxygen desaturation during exercise. Furthermore, in chronic lung diseases that affect the pulmonary vasculature, arterial PCO_2 may be higher than in healthy subjects as V_D is increased owing to reduced $\dot{V}_A$ [61–63].

5.1.4.3 Central and Peripheral Haemodynamic Factors

Cardiac output in healthy elderly subjects can increase severalfold in response to exercise [29, 30, 49, 51, 58]. In the majority of healthy elderly subjects, cardiac output is often the "rate-limiting step" to exercise, and normal maximal exercise is usually accompanied by a heart rate that often approaches the maximal predicted. In contrast in chronic lung diseases, the following mechanisms that involve oxygen transport are frequently impaired resulting in reduction of cardiovascular function. Firstly, coexisting right or left ventricular dysfunction can impair exercise function simply because of poor cardiac-output capability, which often leads to impaired oxygen delivery and early development of metabolic acidosis. Similarly, functionally important arrhythmias may also impair the normal increase in cardiac output as a function of an increase in work rate [49, 51, 58, 64]. Secondly, in chronic lung diseases, especially in the presence of pulmonary vascular abnormalities, pulmonary hypertension and right ventricular dysfunction may develop [65]. The impaired right ventricle may thus contribute to a limited increase in cardiac output. These phenomena may worsen in the presence of hypoxemia. Hypoxemia can in turn elevate pulmonary vascular resistance and create pulmonary arterial hypertension with consequent right heart failure [60, 65–71]. The resulting restrained increase in cardiac output, coupled with the low oxygen content, reduces systemic oxygen delivery to all organs of the body, including skeletal muscles. Interestingly, because the work of breathing is often substantially increased in chronic lung diseases, there might also exist a respiratory muscle "steal" of blood flow away from the locomotor muscles, which further compromises peripheral muscle function [44, 72].

5.1.4.4 Skeletal Muscle Abnormalities

Respiratory insufficiency may lead to inactivity, chronic under loading of the locomotor muscles and weakness, which is associated with less muscle mass and altered muscle fibre distribution in particular with reference to the proportion of type-I (slow-twitch oxidative) fibres [73–79]. Reduction in the proportion of oxidative fibres reduces the oxidative potential of the muscles and would make them more prone to fatigue during high-intensity exercise. There is also less capillary density that reduces regional blood flow and oxygen/nutrient delivery. Such structural and metabolic abnormalities of the limb muscles may lead to early lactic acidosis and task failure with exercise [73–77].

5.2 Cardiopulmonary Exercise Testing (CPET)

Cardiopulmonary exercise testing is often applied in clinical practice to investigate the mechanisms responsible for the limitation of exercise capacity and the extent of their contribution (Table 5.1).

Table 5.1 Mechanisms limiting exercise capacity in chronic respiratory diseases

1	Expiratory flow limitation
2	Exercise-induced dynamic hyperinflation
3	Increased work of breathing
4	Disturbance between alveolar ventilation/perfusion ratio
5	Impaired cardiac performance
6	Peripheral muscle dysfunction

Table 5.2 Diagnostic uses of exercise testing

1	Myocardial ischemia
2	Peripheral vascular disease
3	Exercise-induced asthma
4	Unfitness
5	Psychogenic dyspnoea
6	Muscle phosphorylase deficiency

This test allows the concurrent study of the function of three organ systems: cardiovascular, respiratory and metabolic of muscle cells in well-controlled laboratory conditions during exercise [80]. At the same time, cardiopulmonary exercise testing (CPET) allows recordings of subjective factors such as dyspnoea and muscle discomfort in conditions where symptoms are apparent or become more pronounced. CPET test indicated in patients with limited exercise capacity, when the causes of exercise limitation have not been sufficiently clarified following a thorough respiratory or central haemodynamic evaluation [64, 81]. Applications of CPET are presented in Table 5.2.

The most widely used types of exercise testing that are applied in the clinical evaluation of patients are the incremental exercise test to the limit of tolerance and the constant-load exercise test sustained at a fraction of peak exercise capacity. More often these tests are conducted on an electromagnetically braked cycle ergometer [82].

5.2.1 Types of Cardiopulmonary Exercise Testing

5.2.1.1 Incremental Exercise

This test subjects the patient to a gradually increase of load upon all physiological systems responding during exercise. The intensity gradually increases until symptoms of dyspnoea and/or muscle discomfort limit further increase of the imposed work. This test allows determination of biological responses of transport and utilization of oxygen up to the limit of exercise tolerance (i.e. the peak oxygen uptake (VO_2 peak). Furthermore when the test is performed on a cycle ergometer, the rate of change of oxygen uptake (VO_2) in relation to the work rate (WR) reflects the sufficiency of the operating physiological systems involved in the transport to and utilization of oxygen by the operating organs during conditions of increasing external load [7, 80, 81] (Fig. 5.1).

5.2.1.2 Constant-Load Exercise

During constant-load exercise testing, the patient is asked to perform work that corresponds to a certain fraction of his/her peak exercise capacity (which typically ranges between 50 and 75%) to the limit of tolerance caused by intense dyspnoea and/or muscle discomfort symptoms (Fig. 5.2). The period of dynamic adaptation until stabilisation of cardiorespiratory and metabolic responses provides valuable information about the operation and response of the capacity of the respiratory, cardiovascular and metabolic systems to sufficiently respond to a given load [82, 83]. Table 5.3 shows the effect of different types of interventions during constant-load exercise in patients with COPD [7].

Besides the two aforementioned tests, there are tests that provide less information concerning the physiological responses, but even like this they allow the determination of the exercise capacity to some extent. The most widely used test is the 6-min walk test, which is submaximal and is often applied to evaluate the efficacy of pharmaceutical or non-pharmaceutical interventions [7].

5.2.2 Recorded Variables During Cardiopulmonary Exercise Testing

Peak oxygen uptake (VO_2 peak): The classic criterion for the determination of exercise capacity and cardiorespiratory efficiency is provided by

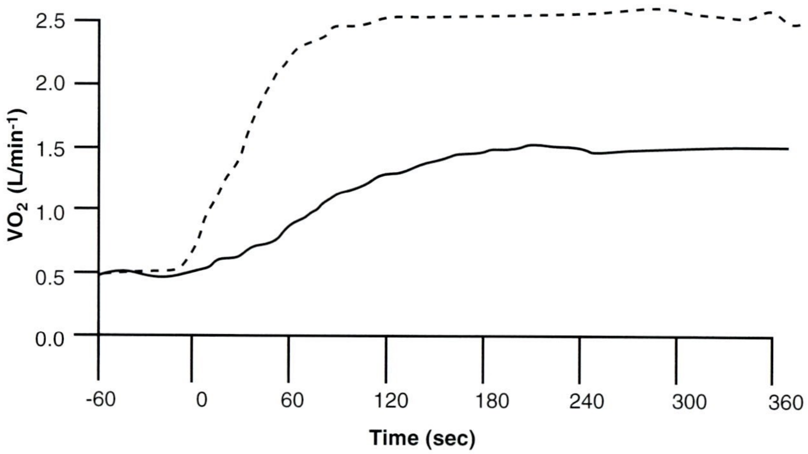

Fig. 5.2 Changes in oxygen uptake during the transition from unloading exercise to constant-load exercise in a healthy man (*dotted line*) and in a patient with COPD (*solid line*)

Table 5.3 Effect of different types of interventions during constant-load exercise in patients with COPD

Type of intervention	Medication (tiotropium)	Oxygen supplementation 50%	Helium (79%) and oxygen (21%) supplementation	Rehabilitation
Exercise intensity (%) predicted	75	75	80	75
Change in exercise tolerance time (%)	+21	+145	+115	+224
Change in inspiratory capacity (%)	+12	+24	+12	+15
Change in dyspnoea sensation (%)	−14	−40	−25	−30

recording peak oxygen uptake. In a well-executed incremental test, the peak oxygen uptake reflects the maximum aerobic capacity. This parameter reflects the oxygen-binding capacity of haemoglobin molecules in alveolar level, the transfer to the periphery through the mediation of the cardiovascular system and its utilization by mitochondria in skeletal muscle to produce external work. Values lower than 80% predicted are considered abnormal, and values below 50% predicted indicate serious dysfunction of the above physiological systems (Table 5.4) [7, 81].

Anaerobic threshold: The anaerobic threshold (AT) is often considered as an index for the initiation of metabolic acidosis, which is the result of the increase of lactic acid in arterial blood during exercise [83]. Normal values when detecting the anaerobic threshold represent at least 45–50% of peak oxygen uptake (Table 5.4).

Oxygen pulse: It reflects the amount of oxygen extracted from the peripheral muscles within each heartbeat. According to the modified equation of Fick, the oxygenic pulse is numerically equal to the product of stroke volume (SV) and arteriovenous oxygen difference ($C(a\text{-}v)O_2$), i.e. $VO_2/HR = SV \times C(a\text{-}v)O_2$ and is commonly used as an index of stroke volume during exercise [7].

Breathing reserve: The degree of ventilatory limitation profoundly contributes to the impaired exercise capacity, and can be evaluated from the respiratory reserve, which reflects the relationship of respiratory requirement in relation to respiratory capacity. For most healthy adults, the maximum pulmonary ventilation (V_E) during exercise does not exceed 70% of maximum voluntary ventilation (MVV), although this fraction may increase (V_E/MVV > 0.75) indicating limited respiratory reserve in chronic cardiorespiratory diseases [7, 80, 81].

Table 5.4 Values of physiological responses in a patient with COPD during incremental exercise testing, expressed as a fraction of the expected values in healthy individuals

Variable	Predicted	Measured	Presentence of predicted (%)
Peak oxygen uptake, VO_2 peak (L/min)	1.67	0.90	54
Peak heart rate			
(beats/min)	151	136	90
Peak work rate (W)	60	30	50
Peak oxygen pulse			
(mL/beats)	11.1	6.6	60
Change in oxygen uptake/change in work rate $\Delta VO_2/\Delta WR$ (mL/min/W)	10.3	8.9	–
Anaerobic threshold (L/min of VO_2)	1.0	0.5	50
Peak ventilation V_E (L/min)	90	40	45

5.2.3 Pathophysiological Manifestations

5.2.3.1 Chronic Obstructive Pulmonary Disease (COPD)

Reduced exercise capacity in patients with COPD is usually manifested by reduced peak oxygen uptake (Fig. 5.3a), and early onset of the anaerobic threshold, which reflects early metabolic acidosis. The premature termination of exercise testing is accompanied by additional low value of peak pulmonary ventilation (V_E) (Fig. 5.3b) and by breathlessness (Fig. 5.3c) and muscle discomfort [80].

It is well documented that exercise tolerance during constant-load testing on a cycle ergometer largely depends on the imposing load, as the time to the limit of tolerance in patients with COPD decreases proportionally to increasing power output. Studies have shown that the rate of change in oxygen uptake during the transitional phase from unloading cycling to constant-load exercise is faster in healthy individuals (approximately 35 s) compared to patients with COPD (approximately 75 s) [83] (Fig. 5.2). The slower kinetic response of oxygen uptake is considered to lead to an early and greater reliance on anaerobic metabolism causing the accumulation of by-products of metabolism accelerating the onset of muscle fatigue [83].

5.2.3.2 Interstitial Lung Disease

During cardiopulmonary exercise testing, the peak values of work rate and oxygen uptake (Fig. 5.3a), the oxygen tension in the arterial blood (Fig. 5.3d) and the respiratory reserve are all reduced in patients with interstitial lung disease, compared to healthy individuals. For given oxygen consumption, the rate of increase of pulmonary ventilation (V_E) is disproportionately increased compared to healthy age-matched individuals (Fig. 5.3b). At peak exercise tolerance, a significant heart rate reserve is observed as peak heart rate is reduced.

During constant-load exercise, patients with interstitial lung disease have increased pulmonary ventilation (V_E), for a given load or a given oxygen consumption, and increased values of the produced carbon dioxide output (VCO_2) due to increased dead space ventilation. In these patients, the ratio between minute ventilation to oxygen uptake (VO_2) and the produced carbon dioxide (VCO_2) is abnormally high. The occurrence of arterial hypoxemia during cardiopulmonary exercise testing is commonly associated with an unusually broad arteriovenous oxygen difference and reduced tissue oxygenation. These factors play an important role in the early onset of metabolic acidosis during submaximal exercise. Thus, limitation of exercise tolerance is often due to symptoms of both dyspnoea and discomfort of the lower limbs [7, 80, 81].

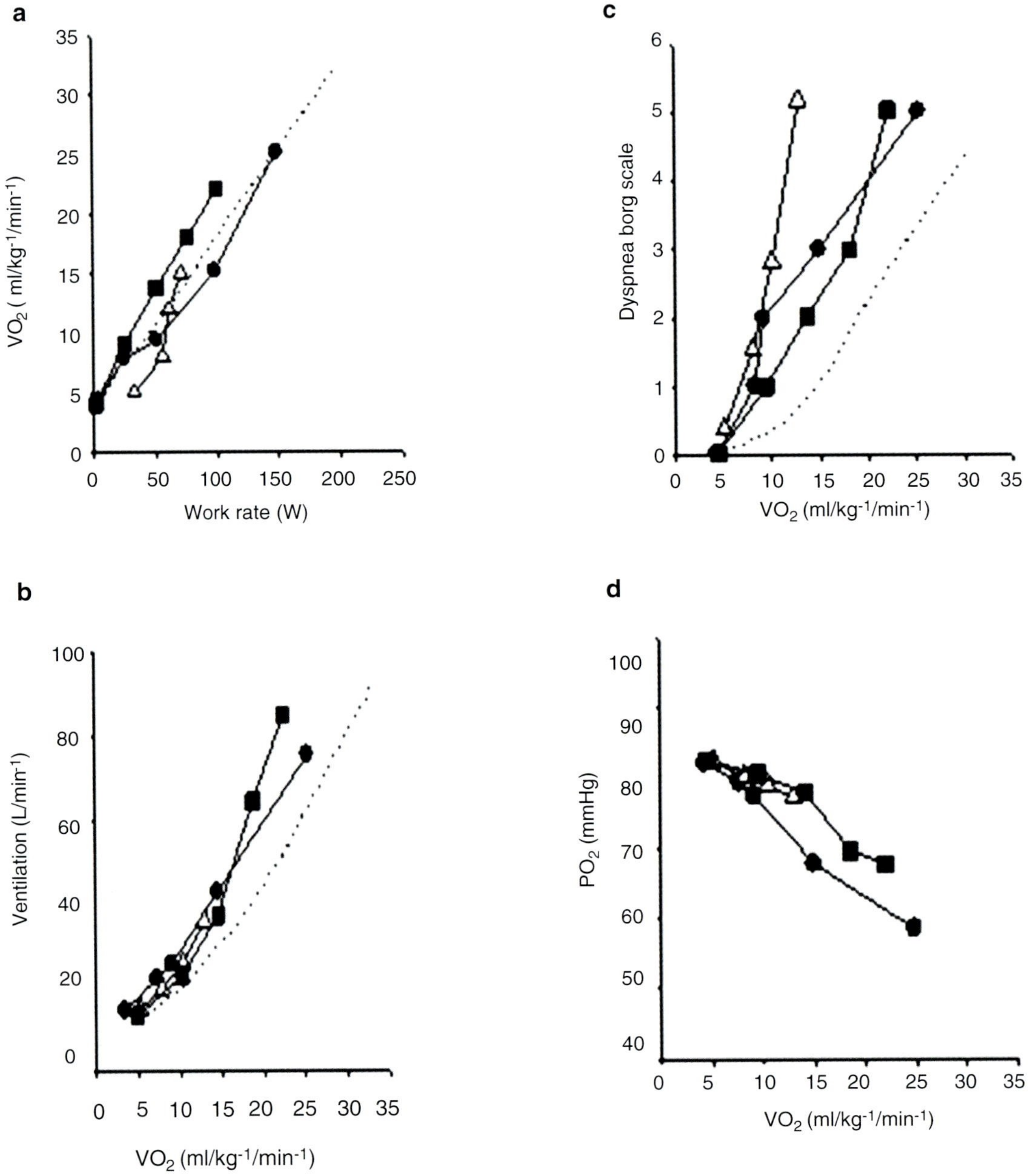

Fig. 5.3 Responses of (**a**) oxygen uptake, (**b**) pulmonary ventilation, (**c**) dyspnoea sensations and (**d**) oxygen tension in the arterial blood during cardiopulmonary exercise testing in patients with COPD (*triangles*), with pulmonary hypertension (*squares*) and with interstitial lung diseases (*circles*) compared with healthy age-matched individuals (*dotted lines*) [80]

5.2.3.3 Pulmonary Hypertension

During cardiopulmonary exercise testing, peak values of oxygen uptake (VO_2) (Fig. 5.3a) and of work rate are reduced in patients with pulmonary hypertension compared to healthy age matched. However, the slope of the relationship of the oxygen uptake over the work rate is normal (Fig. 5.3a). At peak exercise tolerance, heart rate reaches the maximum predicted value, whilst pulmonary ventilation exceeds 85% of maximum voluntary ventilation (Fig. 5.3b), thus exercise in these patients is often limited by both cardiovascular and respiratory factors [7, 80].

During submaximal exercise these patients exhibit tachycardia due to increased pulmonary vascular resistance and the consequent increase in the afterload of the right ventricle, which limits the increase in stroke volume. On the other hand, excessive enlargement of arteriovenous oxygen tension and an unusually high ratio between pulmonary ventilation and carbon dioxide output imply an increase of dead space ventilation due to the high heterogeneity between alveolar ventilation and blood flow (V_A/Q) causing severe hypoxemia (Fig. 5.3d). Such a model of cardiopulmonary disorder promotes early onset of metabolic acidosis and limits the quantity of readily available oxygen to peripheral muscles, thereby causing premature occurrence of peripheral muscle fatigue [7, 80, 81].

5.3 CPET: A Tool for Predicting Mortality

Cardiopulmonary exercise testing emerges as a useful tool for the prognosis of mortality in patients with lung diseases. Peak oxygen intake is the most important predictor of mortality rate at a depth of 5 years in patients with chronic obstructive pulmonary disease and is a significant predictor of survival in patients with pulmonary hypertension [7, 81]. In patients with interstitial lung disease, cardiopulmonary exercise testing has proved particularly useful in predicting the prognosis of the disease. The peak oxygen consumption, oxygen consumption corresponding to the anaerobic threshold and the slope of change in pulmonary ventilation over carbon dioxide output are useful predictors of patient survival with chronic respiratory diseases; however, a wider range of factors are also playing an important role in the survival of these patients, and thus they should be taken into account [7, 64, 82].

5.4 CPET: A Tool for Evaluating Exertional Dyspnoea

Is dyspnoea worth documenting and accurately assessing? The answer is "Undoubtedly YES", for at least the following reasons: (1) activity-related dyspnoea is usually the earliest and most troublesome complaint for which patients with cardiopulmonary diseases seek medical attention; (2) this symptom progresses relentlessly as the underlying disease advances leading invariably to avoidance of activity with consequent skeletal muscle deconditioning and an impoverished quality of life; (3) it is estimated that up to a quarter of the general population and half of severely ill patients are affected by it; and (4) dyspnoea is also an important predictor of quality of life, exercise tolerance and mortality in various conditions. In patients with chronic obstructive pulmonary disease (COPD), it has been shown to be a better predictor of mortality than forced expiratory volume in 1 s (FEV1). In patients with heart disease referred for clinical exercise testing, it is a better predictor of mortality than angina; (5) dyspnoea is also associated with decreased functional status and worse psychological health in older individuals living at home; (6) it is also a factor in the low adherence to exercise training programmes in sedentary adults and in patients with COPD; (7) the effective management of exertional dyspnoea remains a major challenge for caregivers, and modern treatment strategies that are based on attempts to reverse the underlying chronic condition are only partially successful [83–89].

The perception of dyspnoea involves the integration of afferent and efferent inputs at cortical level and is modulated by affective/emotional/behavioural components. The recent statements of the American Thoracic Society [90] and European Respiratory Society [83] have underlined the multidimensional nature of dyspnoea which comprises three major dimensions: (1) the sensory-perceptual domain, (2) the affective distress and (3) the symptom impact or burden.

Dyspnoea is a complex, multifaceted and highly personalised sensory experience, the source and mechanisms of which are incompletely understood: there is no unique central or peripheral source of this symptom. The definition given by the latest ATS statement (*a subjective experience of breathing discomfort that consists of qualitatively distinct sensations that vary in intensity*) highlights the importance of the different qualities (descriptors) covered by the term dyspnoea, the cortical integration of multiple sources of neural inputs about breathing and the physiological affective and behavioural consequences [90]. More specifically, it is believed that dyspnoea arises when there is a conscious awareness of dissociation between what the brain expects (through the "corollary discharge", i.e. copy of the descending motor activity to perceptual areas) and what it receives in terms of neural inputs from the respiratory system, respiratory muscles, peripheral chemoreceptors and locomotor muscles [90]. Of course, not all conscious breathing sensations are labelled as "dyspnoea" because the brain is able to "filter" all the respiratory sensations and let only some of them reach the conscious level [83]. This sensory gating process hinders the brain from being constantly overloaded by irrelevant sensory information. Human beings have the voluntary capacity to bring "breathing" into awareness at any moment. On the other hand, breathing may come to conscious awareness automatically if it needs to be attended to (gate-in). This "gating process" is instrumental in monitoring essential biological and physiological functions and adopting appropriate behaviour. It has been proposed that respiratory sensations are the result of neural gating into the cerebral cortex of respiratory afferent input eliciting a somatosensory cognitive awareness of breathing and an affective response [83].

It can be summarised in a very simplistic yet pedagogic way that dyspnoea may result from two processes: (1) a discriminative one which identifies relevant afferent information on respiratory disruption/abnormalities and brings them to consciousness (sensory components: intensity and quality) and (2) an affective one which labels the now conscious sensation as unpleasant or threatening, i.e. dyspnoea (Fig. 5.4).

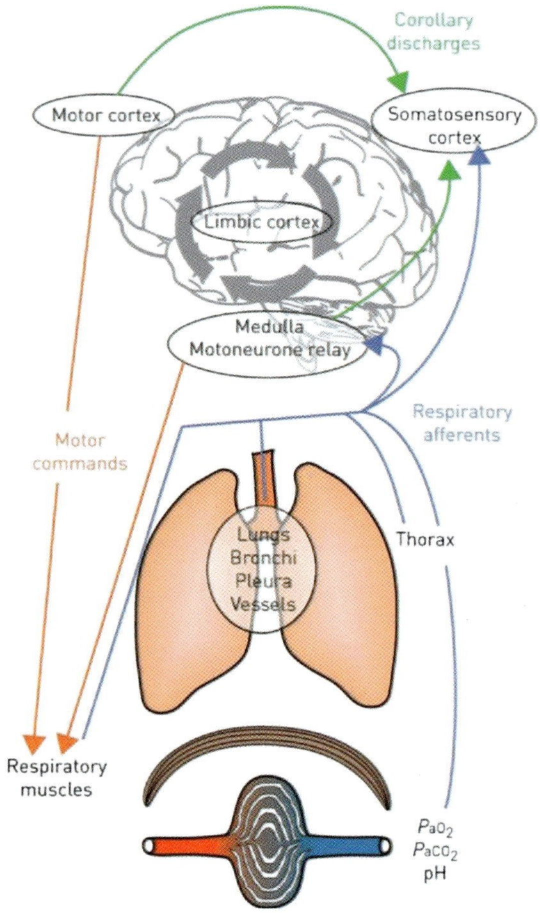

Fig. 5.4 Integrative mechanisms at the origin of dyspnoea. Respiratory command derives from inputs from both the motor cortex and the medulla. These commands are integrated at the spinal level and transmitted to the muscular effectors of the respiratory system. The subsequent activation of the respiratory muscles will generate afferent inputs that are fed back to the respiratory command centres and the somatosensory cortex. The comparison of the corollary discharge and the ensuing afferent feedback may present a mismatch, and dyspnoea will occur when a negative affective sensation is attributed to this mismatch by the limbic cortex, which will also be influenced and modulated by memory and the prevailing environment. Adapted from reference: Laviolette L, Laveneziana P. Eur Respir J. 2014;43(6):1750–1762, with permission [83]

Dyspnoea is not a single sensation, and our brain is able to distinguish among different afferent information and give each of them a distinct cognitive sensation, notably: (1) *work/effort* ("breathing requires work or effort"), (2) *tightness* ("chest is constricted, chest feels tight") and (3) *air hunger* ("unsatisfied inspiration, starved for air, urge to breathe, like breath holding"). It is generally accepted that these sensations do not share the same physiological mechanisms [83, 90]. Some of these sensations, such as *work/effort* and *air hunger* may exist and vary independently in the same subject or experimental condition. Notwithstanding, whether there are multiple types of dyspnoea, whether they are subjective expressions of different neurophysiological mechanisms or whether the same neurophysiological mechanisms may be expressed differently in relation to language, psychological, cultural and/or social context is at the moment unclear and required additional research.

Dyspnoea can also be quantified ("intensity"). Exertional dyspnoea can be easily defined as "the perception of respiratory discomfort that occurs for an activity level that does not normally lead to breathing discomfort". It follows that the intensity of dyspnoea can be determined by assessing the activity level required to produce dyspnoea (i.e. dyspnoea at rest is more severe than dyspnoea when climbing stairs) [83].

Dyspnoea can be therefore evaluated during a physical task, such as cardiopulmonary exercise testing (CPET) [83, 90]. For this purpose, the 10-point Borg scale can be used to rate a specific respiratory sensation (e.g. inspiratory difficulty, breathing effort, expiratory difficulty, air hunger, etc.) or a more general one (e.g. breathing difficulty, breathlessness). The magnitude of respiratory sensation should be anchored at both extremes of the scale such that a rating of "0" represents no breathing discomfort and "10" represents the maximal breathlessness that the subject had ever experienced or could imagine experiencing. Though somewhat less popular, the visual analogue scale (VAS) is another dyspnoea measuring instrument with proven construct validity used during CPET. Both the VAS and Borg scale have been shown to provide similar scores during CPET and to be reliable and reproducible over time in healthy subjects and in patients with chronic respiratory diseases undergoing CPET [82]. The advantage of using the Borg or VAS scales in individual patients is the possibility of reliably comparing "intensity of exertional dyspnoea" at the same level of exercise activity (*standardised* work rate or oxygen consumption or ventilation during CPET) between subjects and before and after a pharmacological and/or non-pharmacological treatment [82]. Studies in cardiopulmonary diseases have shown that during CPET there is a close correlation between the magnitude (and duration) of respiratory effort (measured by tidal oesophageal pressure relative to maximum) and the intensity of dyspnoea (measured by the Borg scale) and that pharmacological manipulations able to reduce the magnitude (and duration) of respiratory effort are clearly and consistently associated with reduced dyspnoea intensity [82, 83].

Quality and quantity of dyspnoea can also be measured together during CPET. Few studies have shown that moderate-to-severe chronic obstructive pulmonary disease (COPD) and even mild stable asthmatics are able to "perceive" dynamic changes in their mechanics of breathing during exercise: once a critical inspiratory reserve volume (IRV) is attained (0.3–0.5 L from total lung capacity), tidal volume expansion is critically constrained, dyspnoea intensity rises abruptly and there is a transition in the dominant qualitative descriptor choice from *work/effort* to *difficult/unsatisfied inspiration* [83]. The clinical relevance of these findings is that by asking the quality of dyspnoea at the end of an exercise bout, one can ascertain whether a critical IRV (*difficult/unsatisfied inspiration*) or not (*work/effort*) has been reached, i.e. the likelihood of developing exercise-related critical volume constraints [83].

Things are, however, somehow different in chronic heart failure. Indeed heart failure patients may report dyspnoea alone or in variable combination with leg discomfort as the exercise-limiting symptoms. In heart failure no haemodynamic and respiratory variables, either at rest or during exercise, seems to be able to discriminate between heart failure patients who complain of dyspnoea as the predominant exercise-limiting symptom from those who report leg discomfort. Clearly the issue is still unsolved, and more studies are needed [83].

Cardiopulmonary exercise testing (CPET) is therefore well suited for understanding mechanisms underlying dyspnoea during exercise ("exertional dyspnoea") both in research and clinical settings. CPET may also help clinicians identify additional mechanisms underpinning the greater dyspnoea intensity which could be "independent of" or "not directly related to" the main/obvious pathophysiological determinant of the disease under consideration.

We hope we have convinced the readers about the importance of assessing dyspnoea on exertion. This "chapter" will therefore focus on the "clinical use of CPET" to explore and unmask the mechanisms underlying dyspnoea during exercise in an abroad spectrum of cardiorespiratory disorders.

5.4.1 Dyspnoea Can Be Perceived as a Sense of Respiratory Effort

During voluntary increase in ventilation, the motor cortex increases the outgoing motor signal to respiratory muscles and conveys a copy (central corollary discharge) through cortical interneurons to the sensory/association cortex, which is informed of the voluntary effort to increase ventilation. It is also likely that the sense of the respiratory effort arises from the simultaneous activation of the sensory cortex and muscle contraction: a variety of muscle receptors provides feedback to the central nervous system about force and tension, and information from these receptors may conceivably underlie the sense of effort. For clinical purposes, the perceived magnitude of respiratory effort is expressed by the ratio of the tidal oesophageal pressure (P_{oes}) to the maximal pressure generation capacity of the respiratory muscles ($P_{I,max}$). In healthy subjects, volitional respiratory effort is matched with lung/chest wall displacement (i.e. change in tidal volume (V_T) as percentage of vital capacity (VC)) via concurrent afferent proprioceptive information, transmitted via vagal, glossopharyngeal, spinal and phrenic nerves that monitor displacement and are processed and integrated in the sensory cortex. The result is a harmonious neuromechanical coupling with avoidance of respiratory discomfort or distress [83, 90].

5.4.2 Dyspnoea Can Be Perceived as a Sense of Air Hunger

Under some clinical and experimental circumstances, the relationship between dyspnoea and effort is less apparent. If normal subjects suppress their ventilation to a level below that dictated by chemical drive (CO_2), dyspnoea increases without corresponding increases in indices of respiratory effort [83, 90]. Likewise, in experimental and clinical conditions where peripheral stretch receptors are inhibited, the sensory cortex is not informed of the ventilatory response. In these circumstances, dyspnoea is perceived as a sensation of air hunger whose intensity depends on the mismatch between the level of chemical-stimulated drive and the ongoing inhibition from pulmonary mechanosensors signalling the current level of ventilation [83, 90]. In turn, dyspnoea arises and may qualitatively change when peripheral afferent feedback is altered and inspiratory motor output either increases or stabilises [83, 90].

5.4.3 Dyspnoea on Exertion in Healthy, Nonathletic Subjects

During exercise, breathing is tightly coupled to muscular and cardiovascular demands. In healthy, nonathletic subjects, exercise is more of a challenge to the cardiovascular and locomotor muscle systems than the respiratory system. Healthy subjects therefore usually report limb muscle fatigue as the primary cause for exercise cessation, although high-level athletes may encounter respiratory limitation to exercise performance [83]. Dyspnoea in healthy humans increases in proportion to increasing ventilation and respiratory contractile effort; the later measured as the ratio of tidal oesophageal pressure swing relative to maximal pressure (*see above*). Healthy young adults at the symptom-limited peak of exercise generally rate dyspnoea intensity as "moderate" or "severe" (Fig. 5.5) and describe a heightened sense of effort, "work" or "heaviness" of breathing [83].

Such sensations are not usually perceived as threatening in this population because they represent, based on learning and experience, the anticipated ventilatory response to heavy exercise [83]. The current accepted theory is that dyspnoea results from a conscious awareness of

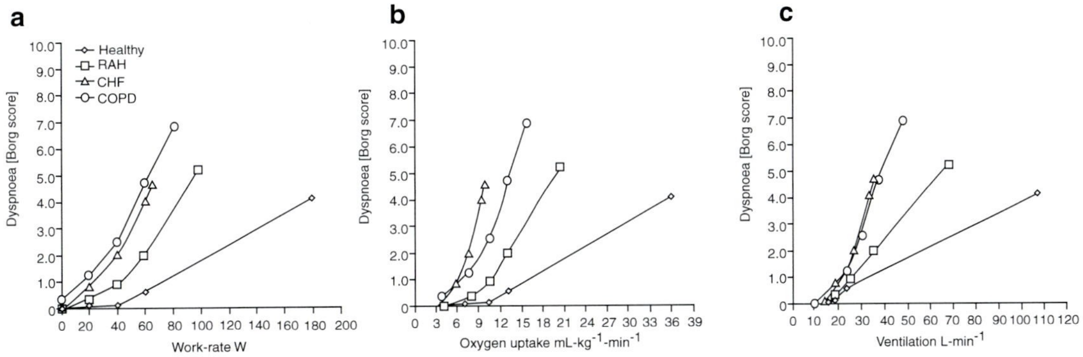

Fig. 5.5 Dyspnoea on exertion (rated using the Borg scale) with increasing work rate (**a**), oxygen uptake (**b**) and minute ventilation (**c**) in health, COPD, chronic heart failure and pulmonary arterial hypertension. Data from the authors' laboratory in Paris, France. Adapted from reference: Laviolette L, Laveneziana P. Eur Respir J. 2014;43(6):1750–1762, with permission [83]

the dissociation between what the brain expects and what it receives in terms of afferent information from receptors in the respiratory muscles, lungs, airways and chest wall. This feedback from peripheral sensory afferents may enable the brain to assess the effectiveness of the motor output to the respiratory muscles. When the mechanical/muscular response of the respiratory system is appropriate for the prevailing level of central respiratory motor drive, then dyspnoea intensity increases in direct proportion to the level of drive and is described as a heightened sense of effort, work or heaviness of breathing [83, 90].

5.4.4 Dyspnoea in Cardiorespiratory Disorders

In patients with respiratory and cardiovascular diseases, respiratory limitation during exercise is often encountered, although limb muscle fatigue may also play an important role in exercise limitation. Whether the respective role of dyspnoea and limb muscle fatigue may be influenced by the testing modality is still debated. When compared to aged-matched controls, dyspnoea in patients with cardiorespiratory diseases is significantly increased for a given level of work rate, oxygen uptake and minute ventilation (Fig. 5.5). In the next chapters we will explore its underlying mechanisms.

5.4.5 COPD

Two qualitative descriptor clusters of dyspnoea are commonly selected by patients with COPD during physical activity [2, 91–93]. The descriptor cluster that alludes to *increased respiratory work/effort* ("breathing requires more effort or work") is commonly selected by patients with COPD. Increased sense of *work/effort* is related to the increased motor drive to the respiratory muscles and increased central neural drive (due to chemo-stimulation) as a consequence of progressive metabolic and ventilation/perfusion disruptions during exercise. Therefore, increased perceived *work/effort* during physical activity in part reflects the greater ventilatory demand for a given task compared with health. In addition, contractile muscle effort is increased for any given ventilation because of (1) the acutely increased intrinsic mechanical (elastic/threshold) loading and (2) functional respiratory muscle weakness. These respiratory mechanical/muscular abnormalities are, in part, related to resting and dynamic hyperinflation during exercise and may be leading to either a decrease in $P_{I,max}$ or a further increase in P_{oes} as percentage $P_{I,max}$. Because of these effects, greater neural drive or electrical activation of the respiratory muscle is required to generate a given force. Furthermore, because of the limbic system activation, the corollary discharge may be sensed as abnormal, thus evoking a sensation of distress.

The other descriptor cluster alludes to *unsatisfied inspiration*. Structural abnormalities (chronic bronchitis and emphysema), via their physiological negative consequences, i.e. expiratory flow limitation and dynamic hyperinflation, result in dyspnoea [94]. Breathing at a high-lung volume has serious mechanical and sensory consequences. Dynamic lung hyperinflation forces tidal volume (V_T) to be accommodated only within the inspiratory reserve volume, which becomes progressively reduced (i.e. close to total lung capacity (TLC)) and the upper non-linear reaches of the respiratory system pressure-volume relationship. The elastic loading of inspiratory muscles can be substantial under this situation. As lung hyperinflation develops, the inspiratory muscles must overcome the combined inward recoil of the lung and chest wall at the onset of inspiration, before the inspiratory flow commences. Dynamic lung hyperinflation shortens the operating length of the inspiratory muscles, thereby affecting their ability to generate pressure. The combination of excessive elastic, threshold and resistive loading results in functional muscle weakness, and the inspiratory muscles are forced to use a large fraction of their maximal force-generating capacity during tidal breathing. The net consequence is that the ratio of oesophageal pressure (expressed as percentage of maximal inspiratory pressure) to V_T response (expressed as percentage of TLC or vital capacity (VC)) increases considerably. A mechanical consequence of lung hyperinflation is that V_T expansion becomes severely constrained: thoracic displacement is greatly reduced (the V_T response relative to TLC or VC diminishes or even reaches a discernable plateau) despite the patient being able to generate a near-maximal inspiratory motor output (the oesophageal pressure relative to maximal inspiratory pressure goes up). This neuromechanical or neuroventilatory dissociation induced by dynamic hyperinflation is an important contributor to dyspnoea intensity and quality in COPD [2, 83, 91–95].

A patient's physical activity is indeed characterised by a growing mismatch between increase in central neural output to the respiratory muscles and the blunted respiratory mechanical/muscular response (lung/chest wall displacement). This mismatch, which we called above neuroventilatory dissociation, has been proposed to be, at least in part, the neurophysiological basis of the perceived *unsatisfied inspiration*. In a clinical setting, the slope that defines neuroventilatory dissociation (i.e. effort versus displacement) is steeper and shifted upwards in patients compared with healthy subjects. At any respiratory workload, a steeper slope will therefore result in a greater intensity of dyspnoea. In particular, patients experience intolerable dyspnoea during exercise because V_T expansion is constrained "from below" (by the effects of dynamic lung hyperinflation or the already critically reduced resting inspiratory capacity) [94]. As mentioned, this so-called dyspnoea threshold seems to be at the level at which the inspiratory reserve volume (IRV) critically approaches 0.5 L [93]. Once this critical IRV is achieved, further expansion in V_T is greatly impaired, the effort-volume displacement ratio ($P_{oes}/P_{I,max}$: V_T/VC) increases sharply and dyspnoea intensity rises steeply to intolerable levels [2, 91–93], regardless of the exercise testing protocol (incremental or constant work rate) [91]. In addition, the attainment of critical constraints on V_T expansion marked also the point where there is a transition in the dominant qualitative descriptor choice from "work and effort" to "unsatisfied inspiration" [91] (Fig. 5.6).

Intensity and quality of dyspnoea evolve separately and are strongly influenced by mechanical constraints on V_T expansion during exercise in COPD [91, 92]. These data support the central importance of mechanical restriction in causing dyspnoea in COPD patients [95].

5.4.6 Neuromuscular Disorders (NMD)

Patients with NMD exhibit heightened neuromotor output, which is sensed as increased respiratory muscle effort and as such is likely to be the principal mechanism of dyspnoea in NMD [96]. Nonetheless, a significant positive relationship between increased dyspnoea per unit increase in ventilation and dynamic elastance affects the coupling between respiratory effort and displacement [96].

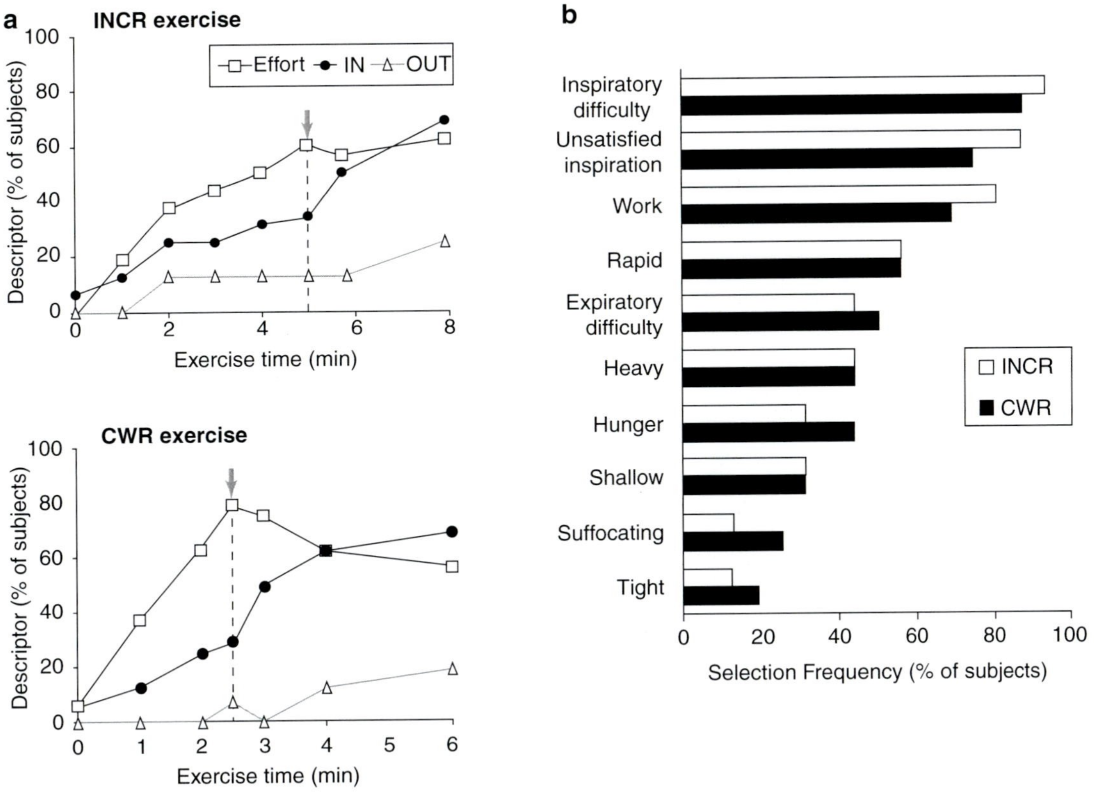

Fig. 5.6 (**a**) Choice of descriptor for dyspnoea evaluated during incremental (*INCR*) and constant work rate (*CWR*) exercise: increased work and effort (*Effort*), unsatisfied inspiration (*IN*) and unsatisfied expiration (*OUT*). The *grey arrow* represents the onset of the inflection point of the relationship between tidal volume and minute ventilation. (**b**) Choice of descriptor for dyspnoea evaluated at the end of the exercise test. Adapted from reference: Laveneziana P et al. Am J Respir Crit Care Med. 2011;184:1367–1373, with permission [91]

5.4.7 Interstitial Lung Disease (ILD)

As in COPD, restrictive dynamic respiratory mechanics limit the ability of patients with ILD to increase ventilation in response to increased metabolic demands of physical tasks [97]. One of the characteristic features of ILD is a reduction in lung compliance and lung volumes. This has two major consequences: (1) greater pressure generation is required by the inspiratory muscles for a given V_T and (2) the resting TLC and IRV are often diminished compared with health. Therefore V_T expansion is constrained early in exercise "from above" (reflecting the reduced TLC and IRV), which results in greater reliance on increasing breathing frequency to increase ventilation. Differences in dynamic ventilatory mechanics, including possible expiratory flow limitation in some patients, account for distinct qualitative perception in ILD patients, namely *inspiratory difficulty/unsatisfied inspiration* and rapid shallow breathing [97]. Because of increase in both dynamic elastance and efferent respiratory drive, *inspiratory difficulty/unsatisfied inspiration* may have its neurophysiological basis in the conscious awareness of a dissociation between the increased drive to breathe (and concurrent increased respiratory effort, i.e. $P_{oes}/P_{I,max}$) and the restricted mechanical response of the respiratory system (i.e. V_T/VC), i.e. the inability to expand V_T appropriately in the face of an increased drive to breathe [97]. In turn, the possibility has also been put forwards that the intensity of exertional dyspnoea in ILD is more closely linked to mechanical constraints on volume expansion than to indexes of inspiratory effort per se [97].

5.4.8 Chronic Heart Failure (HF)

The key message that has emerged from therapeutic intervention studies in patients with HF is that exertional dyspnoea alleviation is consistently associated with reduced excessive ventilatory demand (secondary to reduced central neural drive), improved respiratory mechanics and muscle function and, consequently, enhanced neuromechanical coupling of the respiratory system during exercise. Pressure support has been reported to reduce the tidal inspiratory pleural pressure-time slope without affecting submaximal dyspnoea ratings but allowed patients to exercise for additional minutes without experiencing any significant rise in dyspnoea [98]. New insights into mechanisms of exertional dyspnoea in patients with advanced CHF have emerged as a result of a study that used biventricular pacing to increase cardiac output during cardiopulmonary exercise testing [99]. Laveneziana et al. showed that biventricular pacing was associated with improved dyspnoea intensity at a given V_E and oxygen consumption (VO_2). The dyspnoea/V_E slopes were consistently reduced by ~50% during exercise in response to active cardiac pacing [99]. Improved dyspnoea during active pacing (compared with inactive pacing modality) was associated with (1) a reduced ventilatory requirement likely due to (a) delayed onset of metabolic acidosis secondary to improved oxygen delivery or utilization or both (as suggested by a consistent increase in the anaerobic threshold) and (b) improved ventilation-perfusion relations as a result of an improved ability to reduce a higher physiological dead space during exercise due to improved pulmonary perfusion (as suggested by the improved V_E/VCO_2 slope and ratios) and (2) improved dynamic operating lung volumes [due to either reduced dynamic hyperinflation (as reflected by the increased inspiratory capacity on exertion), improved respiratory muscle function or both] and an increased ability to expand V_T during exercise [99]. The available data suggest that increased ventilatory demand, abnormal dynamic ventilatory mechanics and respiratory muscle dysfunction are instrumental in causing exertional dyspnoea in patients with severe cardiac impairment [98, 99].

5.4.9 Pulmonary Arterial Hypertension (PAH)

Exertional dyspnoea is by far the dominant symptom in patients with pulmonary arterial hypertension (PAH) [100–102]. Recent advances in PAH have clearly demonstrated that some PAH patients (up to 60%) may exhibit reduced expiratory flows in tidal operating range, which could promote exercise-induced dynamic lung hyperinflation (Fig. 5.7) [100]. Laveneziana and collaborators were the first to examine the impact of potential dynamic lung hyperinflation-induced critical mechanical constraints on the intensity of dyspnoea in young non-smoking patients with idiopathic and heritable PAH undergoing symptom-limited incremental CPET [100]. They showed that reduced expiratory flows at low lung volumes at spirometry exist in a large proportion of idiopathic and heritable PAH patients (60%) despite a preserved FEV_1/VC ratio. When increased ventilation/perfusion mismatching was superimposed on pre-existing abnormal airway function, greater troublesome exertional symptoms ensued. Although dyspnoea in these patients was likely multifactorial, their results clearly indicate that increased ventilatory demand and abnormal dynamic ventilatory mechanics should be considered in PAH patients [100], in the absence of respiratory muscle dysfunction [102] or TLC changes [100].

5.4.10 Obesity

An increase in respiratory neural drive is thought to be the reason for the similar increase in dyspnoea in obese and lean subjects [103]. However, different underlying mechanisms may affect dyspnoea in obese subjects. Exercise performance is impaired compared with healthy normal-weight subjects when corrected for the increased lean body mass [104] but normal when expressed as a percentage of predicted for ideal body weight in subjects who hyperinflate to the same extent as those obese subjects who "deflate", with both groups reaching similar dyspnoea scores [105]. In "hyperinflators", dynamic hyperinflation along

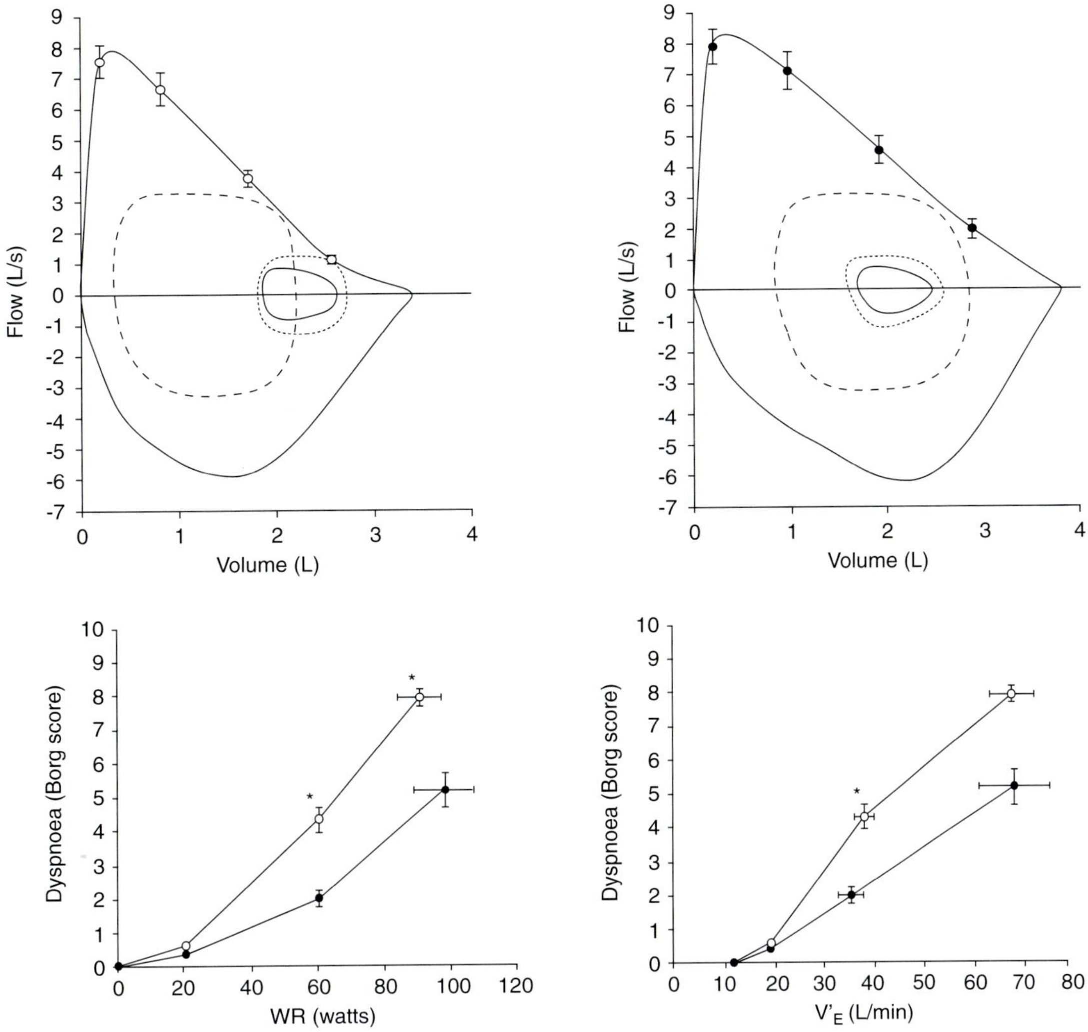

Fig. 5.7 *Upper panels*: maximal and tidal flow-volume loops (*full lines*) in patients with pulmonary arterial hypertension (*PAH*) with exercise-induced hyperinflation (*PAH–H*; $n = 15$, age 40 ± 11 years; *upper left panel*) and without hyperinflation (PAH–NH; $n = 10$, age 35 ± 13 years; *upper right panel*). Flow-volume loops are shown for early exercise (*small dotted line*) and at peak exercise (*dashed line*). In the *left panel*, a decrease in inspiratory capacity is observable, confirming dynamic hyperinflation. *Lower panels*: Dyspnoea on exertion (rated using the Borg scale) with increasing work rate (*left panel*), (WR; *lower left panel*) and minute ventilation (V'_E; *lower right panel*) during incremental cycle exercise in patients with PAH–H (*open circles*) and in PAH–NH patients (*filled circles*). Data show values at rest, 20, 60 W and peak exercise. *$p < 0.05$, PAH–H versus PAH–NH. Adapted and modified from reference: Laveneziana P et al. Eur Respir J. 2013;41(3):578–587, with permission [100]

with a decrease in inspiratory reserve volume increases respiratory muscle loading, respiratory drive and perception of respiratory discomfort [105]. In contrast, "deflators" exhibit a negative relationship between resting end-expiratory lung volume (EELV) and perceptual respiratory response during exercise: the lower the EELV, the greater the Borg score [105]. A low resting EELV has three important and related consequences during exercise: (1) a decrease in expiratory reserve volume, (2) dynamic airway compression and (3) changes in transmural airway pressure resulting in airway dynamic compression. Thus, an alteration in the central drive to the respiratory muscles in response to afferent activity from upper airway mechanoreceptors may also contribute to the unpleasant respiratory sensation in obese subjects.

5.4.11 Asthma

Three dominant qualitative descriptors of dyspnoea emerge in patients with asthma under different conditions ranging from induced bronchoconstriction to physical exercise: (1) chest tightness, (2) increased work/effort ("breathing requires more work or effort"), and (3) unsatisfied/unrewarded inspiration ("can't get enough air in") [106–108]. Recent studies have examined sensory-mechanical relations during the methacholine provocation test [108–110] thus allowing us to evaluate intensity [107, 111, 112] and quality [107, 109, 113] of the sensation over a broad range of physiological perturbations ranging from minor bronchoconstriction to severe lung hyperinflation [107, 108]. Mechanical factors, including loading and activity of the ventilatory muscles associated with lung hyperinflation [108, 114], have been proposed to influence the perception of dyspnoea during acute bronchoconstriction in asthma [108, 115]. Moreover, the effect of lung hyperinflation on the intensity and quality of dyspnoea has recently been evaluated in patients with asthma undergoing cycling exercise [106]. The language of dyspnoea has also proven to be a useful supplement to overall ratings of dyspnoea intensity whilst monitoring the response to bronchodilator therapy in patients with acute asthma [116].

The many descriptors that characterise bronchial asthma indicate that different pathophysiological mechanisms are potentially in action, suggesting the possibility of distinguishing among them by utilizing symptom discrimination [113]. Based on the contrasting effects of airway obstruction and dynamic lung hyperinflation on the language of dyspnoea during methacholine challenge test [108, 109], and on previous findings that in short exercise sessions an increase in lung volumes does not appear to be a crucial contributor to exercise limitation and dyspnoea intensity in severe asthma [117], Laveneziana and collaborators [107] have hypothesized that regardless of the global score of intensity of dyspnoea, different descriptors may be selected by asthmatic patients during short cycle exercise sessions and methacholine challenge test (Fig. 5.8). Airway obstruction and dynamic lung hyperinflation, as measured by the decrease in IC, correlated best with dyspnoea during methacholine challenge test [107]. *Chest tightness* was the highest reported descriptor (68%) during methacholine inhalation [107]. During short cycle exercise, V_E was the best predictor of dyspnoea, and *work/effort* was the highest reported descriptor (72%) [107]. IC decreased

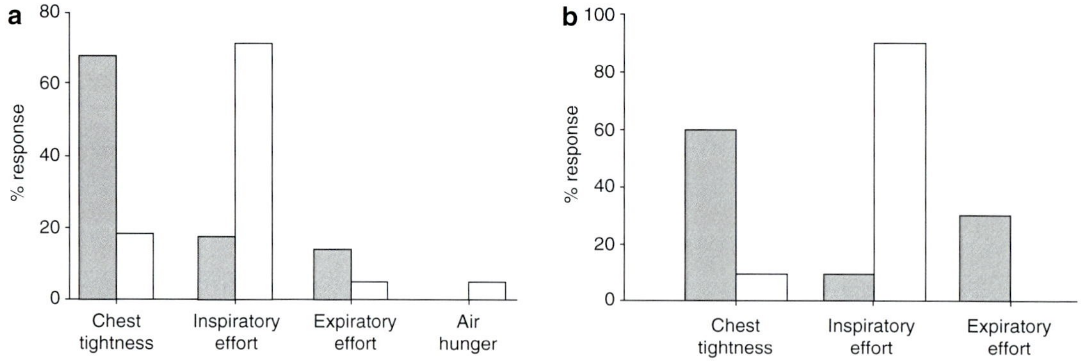

Fig. 5.8 Choice of descriptor for dyspnoea after methacholine challenge (*grey columns*) and cardiopulmonary exercise test (*white columns*) (panel **a**). Panel **b** displays the same information, limited to the subjects that had a similar degree of hyperinflation at the end of the tests. Adapted from reference: Laveneziana P et al. Eur Respir J. 2006;27:742–747, with permission [107]

in eight patients during exercise. Of interest, these eight patients showed a similar degree of hyperinflation during methacholine challenge test, but their description of dyspnoea was different between the two tests: during methacholine challenge test, 60% of the responses were *chest tightness*, 10% were *inspiratory effort* and 30% were *expiratory effort*; during exercise, 90% were *inspiratory effort* and 10% were *chest tightness* (Fig. 5.8) [107].

More recently, Laveneziana and co-workers [106] have argued that the presence of expiratory flow limitation at rest and during exercise may have explained the significant decrease in IC (i.e. dynamic lung hyperinflation) observed in a subgroup of patients with stable mild asthma undergoing high-intensity constant work-rate cycle exercise. A strong correlation was found between the extent of expiratory flow limitation and the reduction in IC (expressed as % of predicted TLC) during exercise ($r = -0.82$, $p = 0.04$) [106]. However, the lack of oesophageal pressure-derived measurements did not allow the authors to rule out the contribution of other mechanical factors in dynamic lung hyperinflation causation.

In the same study, the quantitative and qualitative aspects of dyspnoea in patients with asthma ($n = 16$) were evaluated [106]. The investigators showed that even mild stable asthmatics were able to perceive critical mechanical constraints on V_T expansion during exercise [106]. They demonstrated that V_T expansion became constrained due to dynamic lung hyperinflation at a critically reduced inspiratory reserve volume (IRV) only in 37.5% of subjects, and it marked the point where dyspnoea intensity rose abruptly and there was a transition in the dominant qualitative descriptor choice from *work/effort* to *difficult/unsatisfied inspiration* [106]. In contrast, V_T expansion flattened at a preserved IRV in 62.5% of subjects, and it did not mark a mechanical event with important sensory consequences [106]. The corollary of this is that therapeutic interventions that effectively delay the appearance of the V_T constraints at a critically reduced IRV should theoretically reduce the attendant dyspnoea during physical activity even in patients with mild stable asthma. The clinical relevance of these findings is that, pending confirmation in larger samples, by asking the quality of dyspnoea at the end of an exercise bout, one can ascertain whether a critical IRV (*difficult/unsatisfied inspiration*) or not (*work/effort*) has been reached, i.e. the likelihood of developing exercise-related critical volume constraints in asthmatics [106].

5.4.12 Effects of Interventions on Dyspnoea

Effective improvement in exertional dyspnoea represents one of the most challenging targets of management in patients with cardiopulmonary disease. Traditionally, the approach to improving exertional dyspnoea in all of the major cardiopulmonary diseases involves interventions that (1) reduce ventilatory demand (by reducing the drive to breathe), (2) improve ventilatory capacity, (3) improve respiratory mechanics (by reducing the mechanical load), (4) increase the functional strength of weakened or ineffective ventilatory muscles, (5) address the affective dimension of dyspnoea and (6) any combination of the above. It is of note that these interventions should be selected based on the underlying pathophysiological background of the specific disease under examination and may differ from one disease to another. However, multiple interventions are generally required and appear to have additive or synergistic effects.

Some of these interventions include bronchodilators, oxygen, heliox, exercise training, biventricular pacing (specific for HF patients), respiratory muscle training, biofeedback techniques, non-invasive ventilation, lung volume reduction surgery and related endoscopic techniques and various combinations of these. All of the above strategies have proven to provide beneficial sensory consequences in a variety of patients with cardiopulmonary diseases. In selected patients, interventions such as opiates (oral and inhaled) reduce respiratory drive and alter affective components of dyspnoea. Recently, it has been shown that inhaled furosemide may modulate respiratory sensation by altering afferent inputs from vagal receptors within the lungs.

Psychological counselling, cognitive/behavioural modification and anxiolytics can have favourable influences on the affective dimension of chronic dyspnoea.

5.4.13 Summary

Dyspnoea is a multifaceted symptom, involving the interaction between various physiological, psychological and environmental factors. Its understanding may only derive from a multidisciplinary and multidimensional approach. Although mechanical factors are important contributors to dyspnoea, the precise mechanisms of dyspnoea remain obscure. One approach to the study of this symptom is to identify the major qualitative dimensions of the symptom in an attempt to uncover different underlying neurophysiological mechanisms. The remarkable similarity in choices of qualitative descriptors (work/effort, inspiratory difficulty/unsatisfied inspiration, air hunger, rapid breathing) for exertional dyspnoea in patients with restrictive and obstructive syndromes raises the intriguing possibility that they share some common underlying mechanisms.

Conclusions

Functional measurements at rest do not always provide an accurate diagnosis and a proper stratification of severity in patients with chronic respiratory diseases. Cardiopulmonary exercise testing complimentary applied to functional tests at rest, provides useful information on exercise capacity and a comprehensive evaluation of the biological mechanisms that limit exercise tolerance.

References

1. Whipp BJ, Wagner PD, Agusti A. Determinants of the physiological systems responses to muscular exercise in healthy subjects. In: European respiratory monograph. United Kingdom: European Respiratory Society; 2007. p. 30–4.
2. O'Donnell DE, et al. Qualitative aspects of exertional breathlessness in chronic airflow limitation: pathophysiologic mechanisms. Am J Respir Crit Care Med. 1997;155(1):109–15.
3. Wagner PD. Determinants of maximal oxygen transport and utilization. Annu Rev Physiol. 1996;58:21–50.
4. Mador MJ, Kufel TJ, Pineda L. Quadriceps fatigue after cycle exercise in patients with chronic obstructive pulmonary disease. Am J Respir Crit Care Med. 2000;161(2 Pt 1):447–53.
5. Roca J, et al. Guidelines for interpretation. In: Roca J, Whipp BJ, editors. European respiratory monograph. United Knigdom: European Respiratory Society; 1997. p. 88–114.
6. Killian KJ. Limitation to muscular activity in chronic obstructive pulmonary disease. Eur Respir J. 2004;24(1):6–7.
7. Palange P, et al. Recommendation on the use of exercise testing in clinical practice. Eur Respir J. 2007;29:185–209.
8. ATS Committee on Proficiency Standards for Clinical Pulmonary Function Laboratories. ATS statement: guidelines for the six-minute walk test. Am J Respir Crit Care Med. 2002;**166**(1):111–7.
9. Singh SJ, et al. Development of a shuttle walking test of disability in patients with chronic airways obstruction. Thorax. 1992;47(12):1019–24.
10. Revill SM, et al. The endurance shuttle walk: a new field test for the assessment of endurance capacity in chronic obstructive pulmonary disease. Thorax. 1999;54(3):213–22.
11. Troosters T, et al. Physiological responses to the 6-min walk test in patients with chronic obstructive pulmonary disease. Eur Respir J. 2002;20(3):564–9.
12. Onorati P, et al. Non-invasive evaluation of gas exchange during a shuttle walking test vs. a 6-min walking test to assess exercise tolerance in COPD patients. Eur J Appl Physiol. 2003;89(3–4):331–6.
13. Rice AJ, et al. Pulmonary gas exchange during exercise in highly trained cyclists with arterial hypoxemia. J Appl Physiol. 1999;87(5):1802–12.
14. Richardson RS, et al. Determinants of maximal exercise VO2 during single leg knee-extensor exercise in humans. Am J Phys. 1995;268(4 Pt 2):H1453–61.
15. Saltin B, Calbet JA, Wagner PD. Point: in health and in a normoxic environment, VO2 max is limited primarily by cardiac output and locomotor muscle blood flow. J Appl Physiol. 2006;100:744–8.
16. Ekblom B, Hermansen L. Cardiac output in athletes. J Appl Physiol. 1968;25(5):619–25.
17. Grimby G, Nilsson NJ, Saltin B. Cardiac output during submaximal and maximal exercise in active middle-aged athletes. J Appl Physiol. 1966;21(4):1150–6.
18. Mitchell JH, Sproule BJ, Chapman CB. The physiological meaning of the maximal oxygen intake test. J Clin Invest. 1958;37(4):538–47.
19. Saltin B. Circulatory response to submaximal and maximal exercise after thermal dehydration. J Appl Physiol. 1964;19:1125–32.
20. Koskolou MD, et al. Cardiovascular responses to dynamic exercise with acute anemia in humans. Am J Phys. 1997;273(4 Pt 2):H1787–93.

21. Stenberg J, Ekblom B, Messin R. Hemodynamic response to work at simulated altitude, 4,000 m. J Appl Physiol. 1966;21(5):1589–94.
22. Roach RC, et al. Arterial O2 content and tension in regulation of cardiac output and leg blood flow during exercise in humans. Am J Phys. 1999;276(2 Pt 2):H438–45.
23. Ekblom B, Wilson G, Astrand PO. Central circulation during exercise after venesection and reinfusion of red blood cells. J Appl Physiol. 1976;40(3):379–83.
24. Krip B, et al. Effect of alterations in blood volume on cardiac function during maximal exercise. Med Sci Sports Exerc. 1997;29(11):1469–76.
25. Torre-Bueno JR, et al. Diffusion limitation in normal humans during exercise at sea level and simulated altitude. J Appl Physiol. 1985;58(3):989–95.
26. Gledhill N, Froese AB, Dempsey JA. Ventilation to perfusion distribution during exercise in health. In: Dempsey JA, Reed CE, editors. Muscular exercise and the lung. Wisconsin: University of Wisconsin; 1977. p. 325–44.
27. Powers SK, et al. Effects of incomplete pulmonary gas exchange on VO2 max. J Appl Physiol. 1989;66(6):2491–5.
28. O'Donnell DE, Ofir D, Laveneziana P. Patterns of cardiopulmonary response to exercise in lung diseases. In: European respiratory monograph. United Kingdom: European Respiratory Society; 2007. p. 69–92.
29. Lakatta EG, Levy D. Arterial and cardiac aging: major shareholders in cardiovascular disease enterprises: Part I: aging arteries: a "set up" for vascular disease. Circulation. 2003a;107(1):139–46.
30. Lakatta EG, Levy D. Arterial and cardiac aging: major shareholders in cardiovascular disease enterprises: Part II: the aging heart in health: links to heart disease. Circulation. 2003b;107(2):346–54.
31. Marcinek DJ, et al. Reduced mitochondrial coupling in vivo alters cellular energetics in aged mouse skeletal muscle. J Physiol. 2005;569(Pt 2):467–73.
32. DeLorey DS, Paterson DH, Kowalchuk JM. Effects of ageing on muscle O2 utilization and muscle oxygenation during the transition to moderate-intensity exercise. Appl Physiol Nutr Metab. 2007;32(6):1251–62.
33. DeLorey DS, Babb TG. Progressive mechanical ventilatory constraints with aging. Am J Respir Crit Care Med. 1999;160(1):169–77.
34. Stathokostas L, et al. Longitudinal changes in aerobic power in older men and women. J Appl Physiol. 2004;97(2):781–9.
35. Coggan AR, et al. Histochemical and enzymatic comparison of the gastrocnemius muscle of young and elderly men and women. J Gerontol. 1992;47(3):B71–6.
36. Russell JA, et al. Effects of aging on capillary geometry and hemodynamics in rat spinotrapezius muscle. Am J Physiol Heart Circ Physiol. 2003;285(1):H251–8.
37. Taylor BJ, Johnson BD. The pulmonary circulation and exercise responses in the elderly. Semin Respir Crit Care Med. 2010;31(5):528–38.
38. Turner JM, Mead J, Wohl ME. Elasticity of human lungs in relation to age. J Appl Physiol. 1968;25(6): 664–71.
39. Walsh J, et al. Structural change of the thorax in chronic obstructive pulmonary disease. J Appl Physiol. 1992;72:1270–8.
40. Tolep K, et al. Comparison of diaphragm strength between healthy adult elderly and young men. Am J Respir Crit Care Med. 1995;152(2):677–82.
41. Johnson BD, Badr MS, Dempsey JA. Impact of the aging pulmonary system on the response to exercise. Clin Chest Med. 1994;15(2):229–46.
42. Johnson BD, et al. Flow limitation and regulation of functional residual capacity during exercise in a physically active aging population. Am Rev Respir Dis. 1991;143(5 Pt 1):960–7.
43. Johnson BD, et al. Mechanical constraints on exercise hyperpnea in a fit aging population. Am Rev Respir Dis. 1991;143(5 Pt 1):968–77.
44. Harms CA, et al. Respiratory muscle work compromises leg blood flow during maximal exercise. J Appl Physiol. 1997;82(5):1573–83.
45. Aliverti A, et al. Human respiratory muscle actions and control during exercise. J Appl Physiol. 1997;83(4):1256–69.
46. Vogiatzis I, et al. Respiratory kinematics by optoelectronic plethysmography during exercise in men and women. Eur J Appl Physiol. 2005;93(5–6):581–7.
47. Vogiatzis I, et al. Chest wall volume regulation during exercise in COPD patients with GOLD stages II to IV. Eur Respir J. 2008;32(1):42–52.
48. Gallagher C. Exercise limitation and clinical exercise testing in chronic obstructive pulmonary disease. Clin Chest Med. 1994;15(2):305–26.
49. American Thoracic Society; American College of Chest Physicians. ATS/ACCP Statement on cardiopulmonary exercise testing. Am J Respir Crit Care Med. 2003;167(2):211–77.
50. Harms CA. Does gender affect pulmonary function and exercise capacity? Respir Physiol Neurobiol. 2006;151(2–3):124–31.
51. Wasserman K, et al. Exercise testing and interpretation: an overview. In: Weinberg WR, editor. Principles of exercise testing and interpretation. Baltimore, PA: Lippincott Williams & Wilkins; 2005. p. 1–9.
52. Dillard TA, Piantadosi S, Rajagopal KR. Prediction of ventilation at maximal exercise in chronic airflow obstruction. Am Rev Respir Dis. 1985;132: 230–5.
53. Laveneziana P, Parker CM, O'Donnell DE. Ventilatory constraints and dyspnea during exercise in chronic obstructive pulmonary disease. Appl Physiol Nutr Metab. 2007;32(6):1225–38.
54. MacIntyre NR. Mechanisms of functional loss in patients with chronic lung disease. Respir Care. 2008;53(9):1177–84.
55. Levison H, Cherniack RM. Ventilatory cost of exercise in chronic obstructive pulmonary disease. J Appl Physiol. 1968;25(1):21–7.

56. MacIntyre NR, Leatherman NE. Mechanical loads on the ventilatory muscles. A theoretical analysis. Am Rev Respir Dis. 1989;139(4):968–73.
57. Casaburi R, et al. Reductions in exercise lactic acidosis and ventilation as a result of exercise training in patients with obstructive lung disease. Am Rev Respir Dis. 1991;143(1):9–18.
58. O'Donnell DE. Exercise limitation and clinical exercise testing in chronic obstructive pulmonary disease. In: Weisman I, Zeballos R, editors. Progress in respiratory research. Basel: Karger; 2002. p. 138–58.
59. West JB. State of the art: ventilation-perfusion relationships. Am Rev Respir Dis. 1977;116(5):919–43.
60. Agusti A, Cotes J, Wagner P. Responses to exercise in lung diseases. In: European respiratory monograph. UK: ERS Journals; 1997. p. 32–50.
61. Hyatt RE. Expiratory flow limitation. J Appl Physiol. 1983;55(1 Pt 1):1–7.
62. Martinez FJ, et al. Lung-volume reduction improves dyspnea, dynamic hyperinflation, and respiratory muscle function. Am J Respir Crit Care Med. 1997;155(6):1984–90.
63. O'Donnell DE, Revill S, Webb K. Dynamic hyperinflation and exercise intolerance in COPD. Am J Respir Crit Care Med. 2001;164:770–7.
64. Ferrazza A, et al. Cardiopulmonary exercise testing in the functional and prognostic evaluation of patients with pulmonary diseases. Respiration. 2009;77:3–17.
65. Naeije R. Pulmonary hypertension and right heart failure in chronic obstructive pulmonary disease. Proc Am Thorac Soc. 2005;2(1):20–2.
66. Agusti AG, et al. Hypoxic pulmonary vasoconstriction and gas exchange during exercise in chronic obstructive pulmonary disease. Chest. 1990;97(2):268–75.
67. Agusti AG, et al. Mechanisms of gas-exchange impairment in idiopathic pulmonary fibrosis. Am Rev Respir Dis. 1991;143(2):219–25.
68. D'Alonzo GE, et al. Comparison of progressive exercise performance of normal subjects and patients with primary pulmonary hypertension. Chest. 1987;92(1):57–62.
69. Dantzker DR, D'Alonzo GE. The effect of exercise on pulmonary gas exchange in patients with severe chronic obstructive pulmonary disease. Am Rev Respir Dis. 1986;134(6):1135–9.
70. Dantzker DR, et al. Pulmonary gas exchange during exercise in patients with chronic obliterative pulmonary hypertension. Am Rev Respir Dis. 1984;130(3):412–6.
71. Janicki JS. Influence of the pericardium and ventricular interdependence on left ventricular diastolic and systolic function in patients with heart failure. Circulation. 1990;81(2 Suppl):III15–20.
72. Dempsey JA, Harms CA, Ainsworth DM. Respiratory muscle perfusion and energetics during exercise. Med Sci Sports Exerc. 1996;28(9):1123–8.
73. Gosselink R, Troosters T, Decramer M. Peripheral muscle weakness contributes to exercise limitation in COPD. Am J Respir Crit Care Med Sci Sports Exerc. 1996;153(3):976–80.
74. Hamilton AL, et al. Muscle strength, symptom intensity, and exercise capacity in patients with cardiorespiratory disorders. Am J Respir Crit Care Med. 1995;152(6 Pt 1):2021–31.
75. Bernard S, et al. Peripheral muscle weakness in patients with chronic obstructive pulmonary disease. Am J Respir Crit Care Med. 1998;158(2):629–34.
76. Serres I, et al. Impaired skeletal muscle endurance related to physical inactivity and altered lung function in COPD patients. Chest. 1998;113(4):900–5.
77. Booth F, Gollnick P. Effects of disease on the structure and function of skeletal muscle. Med Sci Sports Exerc. 1983;15(5):415–20.
78. Coyle EF, et al. Effects of detraining on responses to submaximal exercise. J Appl Physiol. 1985; 59(3):853–9.
79. Mainguy V, et al. Peripheral muscle dysfunction in idiopathic pulmonary arterial hypertension. Thorax. 2010;65(2):113–7.
80. Vogiatzis I, Zakynthinos S. Factors limiting exercise tolerance in chronic lung diseases. Compr Physiol. 2012;2(3):1779–817.
81. Johnson B. ATS/ACCP Statement on cardiopulmonary exercise testing. Am J Respir Crit Care Med. 2003;167(2):211–77.
82. Puente-Maestu L, et al. Use of exercise testing in the evaluation of interventional efficacy: an official ERS statement. Eur Respir J. 2016;47(2):429–60.
83. Laviolette L, Laveneziana P. Dyspnoea: a multidimensional and multidisciplinary approach. Eur Respir J. 2014;43(6):1750–62.
84. Banzett RB, O'Donnell CR. Should we measure dyspnoea in everyone? Eur Respir J. 2014;43(6):1547–50.
85. Gronseth R, et al. Predictors of dyspnoea prevalence: results from the BOLD study. Eur Respir J. 2014;43(6):1610–20.
86. Nishimura K, et al. Dyspnea is a better predictor of 5-year survival than airway obstruction in patients with COPD. Chest. 2002;121(5):1434–40.
87. Abidov A, et al. Prognostic significance of dyspnea in patients referred for cardiac stress testing. N Engl J Med. 2005;353(18):1889–98.
88. Ho SF, et al. Dyspnoea and quality of life in older people at home. Age Ageing. 2001;30(2):155–9.
89. Hayton C, et al. Barriers to pulmonary rehabilitation: characteristics that predict patient attendance and adherence. Respir Med. 2013;107(3):401–7.
90. Parshall MB, et al. An official American Thoracic Society statement: update on the mechanisms, assessment, and management of dyspnea. Am J Respir Crit Care Med. 2012;185(4):435–52.
91. Laveneziana P, et al. Evolution of dyspnea during exercise in chronic obstructive pulmonary disease: impact of critical volume constraints. Am J Respir Crit Care Med. 2011;184(12):1367–73.
92. Laveneziana P, et al. Does expiratory muscle activity influence dynamic hyperinflation and exertional

dyspnea in COPD? Respir Physiol Neurobiol. 2014;199:24–33.
93. O'Donnell DE, Hamilton AL, Webb KA. Sensory-mechanical relationships during high-intensity, constant-work-rate exercise in COPD. J Appl Physiol. 2006;101(4):1025–35.
94. Guenette JA, Webb KA, O'Donnell DE. Does dynamic hyperinflation contribute to dyspnoea during exercise in patients with COPD? Eur Respir J. 2012;40(2):322–9.
95. Hudson AL, Laveneziana P. Do we "drive" dyspnoea? Eur Respir J. 2015;45(2):301–4.
96. Lanini B, et al. Perception of dyspnea in patients with neuromuscular disease. Chest. 2001;120(2):402–8.
97. O'Donnell DE, Chau LK, Webb KA. Qualitative aspects of exertional dyspnea in patients with interstitial lung disease. J Appl Physiol. 1998;84(6): 2000–9.
98. O'Donnell DE, et al. Ventilatory assistance improves exercise endurance in stable congestive heart failure. Am J Respir Crit Care Med. 1999;160(6):1804–11.
99. Laveneziana P, et al. Effect of biventricular pacing on ventilatory and perceptual responses to exercise in patients with stable chronic heart failure. J Appl Physiol. 2009;106(5):1574–83.
100. Laveneziana P, et al. Dynamic respiratory mechanics and exertional dyspnoea in pulmonary arterial hypertension. Eur Respir J. 2013;41(3):578–87.
101. Laveneziana P, et al. Mechanisms of exertional dyspnoea in pulmonary veno-occlusive disease with EIF2AK4 mutations. Eur Respir J. 2014;44(4):1069–72.
102. Laveneziana P, et al. Inspiratory muscle function, dynamic hyperinflation and exertional dyspnoea in pulmonary arterial hypertension. Eur Respir J. 2015;45(5):1495–8.
103. DeLorey DS, Wyrick BL, Babb TG. Mild-to-moderate obesity: implications for respiratory mechanics at rest and during exercise in young men. Int J Obes. 2005;29(9):1039–47.
104. Ofir D, et al. Ventilatory and perceptual responses to cycle exercise in obese women. J Appl Physiol. 2007;102(6):2217–26.
105. Romagnoli I, et al. Role of hyperinflation vs. deflation on dyspnoea in severely to extremely obese subjects. Acta Physiol (Oxford). 2008;193(4):393–402.
106. Laveneziana P, et al. Tidal volume inflection and its sensory consequences during exercise in patients with stable asthma. Respir Physiol Neurobiol. 2012;185(2):374–9.
107. Laveneziana P, et al. Mechanisms of dyspnoea and its language in patients with asthma. Eur Respir J. 2006;27(4):742–7.
108. Lougheed MD, Fisher T, O'Donnell DE. Dynamic hyperinflation during bronchoconstriction in asthma: implications for symptom perception. Chest. 2006;130(4):1072–81.
109. Moy ML, et al. Quality of dyspnea in bronchoconstriction differs from external resistive loads. Am J Respir Crit Care Med. 2000;162(2 Pt 1):451–5.
110. Lougheed MD, et al. Breathlessness during acute bronchoconstriction in asthma. Pathophysiologic mechanisms. Am Rev Respir Dis. 1993;148(6 Pt 1):1452–9.
111. Ottanelli R, et al. Do inhaled corticosteroids affect perception of dyspnea during bronchoconstriction in asthma? Chest. 2001;120(3):770–7.
112. Ottanelli R, et al. Perception of bronchoconstriction and bronchial hyper-responsiveness in asthma. Clin Sci (Lond). 2000;98(6):681–7.
113. Killian KJ, et al. Symptom perception during acute bronchoconstriction. Am J Respir Crit Care Med. 2000;162(2 Pt 1):490–6.
114. Gorini M, et al. Chest wall hyperinflation during acute bronchoconstriction in asthma. Am J Respir Crit Care Med. 1999;160(3):808–16.
115. Filippelli M, et al. Overall contribution of chest wall hyperinflation to breathlessness in asthma. Chest. 2003;124(6):2164–70.
116. Moy ML, et al. Language of dyspnea in assessment of patients with acute asthma treated with nebulized albuterol. Am J Respir Crit Care Med. 1998;158(3):749–53.
117. Barreiro E, et al. Dyspnoea at rest and at the end of different exercises in patients with near-fatal asthma. Eur Respir J. 2004;24(2):219–25.

Assessment of Limb Muscle Function

6

Roberto A. Rabinovich, Kim-Ly Bui, André Nyberg, Didier Saey, and François Maltais

6.1 Limb Muscle Dysfunction in Patients with COPD: A Clinically Relevant Problem

Limb muscle dysfunction is frequent in COPD and contributes to its morbidity and mortality. Limb muscle dysfunction encompasses several manifestations including muscle atrophy and weakness, susceptibility to muscle fatigue and reduced oxidative capacity and mitochondrial function. Depending on the criteria used, up to a third of patients with COPD expresses some form of muscle dysfunction, including atrophy and weakness [1]. Although the extent of muscle atrophy and weakness is greater in more advanced disease, it is important to recognize that muscle dysfunction may also occur in early disease [1, 2]. The typical patients with COPD entering a pulmonary rehabilitation program have already lost about 30% of muscle mass and strength [3]. One important aspect of limb muscle dysfunction is that it is amenable to therapy, the most effective for this problem being exercise training [4–7]. Arguably, the most perverse consequence of muscle dysfunction is its negative effect on life expectancy. Parameters such as reduced mid-thigh cross-sectional area [8], fat-free mass [9], lower quadriceps strength [10] and *vastus lateralis* fibre-type shift [11] are predictors of mortality in subjects with COPD. Beyond its negative impact on survival, limb muscle dysfunction also contributes to exercise intolerance in COPD and poor quality of life in this disease. For example, quadriceps strength is a strong determinant of exercise capacity [12]. Premature leg fatigue reduces the ability of bronchodilators to enhance exercise tolerance [13, 14]. The links that exist between limb muscle function and relevant clinical outcomes in COPD stress out the importance for clinicians to carefully monitor body composition and muscle function when evaluating a patient with COPD, particularly before pulmonary rehabilitation where one goal of the intervention is to improve limb muscle function.

6.2 Evaluation of Muscle Mass and Body Composition

Body weight loss is present in 17–35% of COPD patients depending on the studied population [15–19] and has been related to mortality in

R.A. Rabinovich
ELEGI Colt Laboratory, Centre for Inflammation Research, The Queen's Medical Research Institute, University of Edinburgh, 47 Little France Crescent, Edinburgh EH16 4TJ, Scotland, UK
e-mail: roberto.rabinovich@ed.ac.uk

K.-L. Bui • A. Nyberg • D. Saey • F. Maltais (✉)
Institut Universitaire de Cardiologie et de Pneumologie de Québec, Université Laval, 2725 Chemin Ste-Foy, Québec G1V 4G5, Canada
e-mail: kim-ly.bui@criucpq.ulaval.ca; andre.nyberg@criucpq.ulaval.ca; Didier.Saey@rea.ulaval.ca; Francois.Maltais@fmed.ulaval.ca

© Springer International Publishing AG 2018
E. Clini et al. (eds.), *Textbook of Pulmonary Rehabilitation*,
https://doi.org/10.1007/978-3-319-65888-9_6

chronic respiratory conditions such as COPD [8, 20]. However, assessing only body weight or even body mass index (BMI) is insufficient to quantify the different body compartments in these population and does not provide information on body composition shifts or fat distribution [9]. Muscle mass loss is the main cause of weight loss in this population [16] and relates to muscle strength [3, 21, 22] and exercise tolerance [16, 23, 24], independent of the degree of airway obstruction [25]. Hence, muscle wasting is a better predictor of health-related quality of life [26] and survival [8] than body weight or BMI [23].

A two-compartment model of body composition provides a more accurate approach to assess the impact of chronic conditions such as COPD on the different body compartments, particularly on muscle mass. This model divides the body mass into fat-free mass (FFM) and fat mass (FM). In turn, FFM can be divided in an intracellular compartment (including muscle mass, bone mineral mass and other metabolizing tissues) and an extracellular fluid compartment. In clinically stable patients, FFM has been commonly used as a surrogate for muscle mass. FFM loss is present in 18–36% of these patients and can be evident in 6–21% of patients with normal weight [15–17]. A FFM index (FFMI) below 16 kg/m^2 (male) or 15 kg/m^2 (female) associates with approximately a twofold increase in mortality in COPD [9, 27, 28]. Other cut-offs have also been established for COPD (Table 6.1).

There are numerous techniques to estimate body composition. None of the methods actually measure FM; the only direct way to truly measure it would be to dissect and chemically analyse tissues in the body. Therefore, the techniques to estimate FM (and therefore FFM) are by definition indirect and based on the relationship between FM and other factors that can be accurately measured (Table 6.2). Deuterium oxide or oxygen-18-labelled water dilution techniques are considered by many to be the current gold standard. These methods estimate total body water (TBW) and require sampling a biologic fluid (blood, saliva or urine), before and after the administration of the isotope. FFM is calculated from the equation TBW/0.73. One limitation of these dilution techniques is that their use is restricted to highly specialized laboratories.

Table 6.1 Commonly used FFMI cut-offs in COPD

Study	Rationale	Men (kg/m^2)	Women (kg/m^2)
Schols et al. [16]	FFM corresponding to a weight of <90% of ideal body weight according to Metropolitan Health Insurance Tables	<16	<15
Vestbo et al. [143]	10th percentile of FFM in Copenhagen City Heart Study	<17.1	<14.6
Coin et al. [144]	10th percentile of FFM in the age range 60–69 year	<17.8	<14.6

Definition of abbreviations: *FFM* fat-free mass. Modified with permission from [35]

Table 6.2 Commonly used methods to assess body composition (FM/FFM) and muscle mass

Deuterium dilution
Skinfolds
Hydrostatic weighing
Air displacement plethysmography
Bioelectrical impedance analysis
Dual-energy X-ray absorptiometry
Computed tomography
Magnetic resonance
Ultrasound

On the other spectrum of tests, measuring skinfold thickness is one of the most frequently performed tests to estimate percentage of FM. The method is simple, non-invasive and inexpensive; however, it typically overestimates FFM compared with other methods [29, 30]. The method is based in the assumption that skinfold thickness is proportional to the gain in adipose tissue. The accurate assessment of skinfold thickness is dependent upon the identification of the appropriate skinfold site, measuring the skinfold with a calliper and selecting the adequate equation to convert the measurements into proportion of fat tissue.

Two common methods to estimate body composition based on densitometry are the hydrostatic weighing (or underwater weighing) and air displacement plethysmography (i.e. BodPod). These methods are by far more accurate than measuring the skinfold thickness and were long considered the gold standard for the estimation of FM and body composition. Therefore, they were used as a criterion method for validation of other body composition methods. However, more recent findings from studies using anatomical and chemical models have emphasized the limitations of densitometry. The density of an object is defined as the ratio of its weight to its volume (weight/volume = density). These methods measure the volume of the body by assessing the displacement of water (based on Archimedes principle) or air (relying on the physics of Boyle's law) and subsequently calculate body density. The density of fat tissue is far less than that of the muscle density (or bone) and is assumed to be 0.9 kg/L. Different equations are used to convert fat density into percentage of fat/fat-free tissue [31].

So far, the methods that have been described require special equipment and specialized laboratories to be conducted. Two reasonable compromises are bioelectrical impedance analysis (BIA) and dual-energy X-ray absorptiometry (DEXA) scan. BIA is based on the higher conductivity of an electric current through FFM than FM [32]. By measuring a voltage drop between two electrodes, it determines the electrical impedance (or opposition to the flow of an electric current through body tissue) to estimate TBW. When longitudinal assessments are needed, it is recommended to perform BIA measurements under the same fluid balance conditions, at the same time of the day. Although multi-frequency analysers exist, most BIA equipment use a single-frequency current of 50 kHz. BIA is low cost, non-invasive and quick and does not require patient's collaboration. BIA has been validated against total body water assessed by deuterium dilution in COPD [33]. FFM obtained with BIA has shown to be lower than FFM obtained with DEXA in patients with COPD especially in the male population [29, 30, 34]. When estimating FFM from BIA impedance, it is important to use equations that have been validated in the population studied and to be cautious with built-in equations provided by manufacturers [29, 34].

In turn, DEXA scan is based on the comparison of X-ray attenuations of two different energies measuring total body composition and fat content. Similar to BIA, this method does not require the patient collaboration and is considered a valid, reliable, safe and non-invasive technique for assessment of FFM in COPD [30, 35]. The method is, however, more expensive and less accessible than BIA. DEXA provides systematically higher values for FFM compared with other techniques such as deuterium dilution [36]. It is important to be aware that DEXA results may differ between different commercial devices. This is particularly important when longitudinal assessments are made.

Lower extremities play a major role in locomotion and account for a large proportion of muscle tissue in the body. Measurement of the thigh circumference is a simple and cheap approach, but it may not reflect accurately local muscle mass [8]. Direct estimation of regional muscle mass can be achieved by imaging techniques such as computed tomography (CT scan), magnetic resonance imaging (MRI) and ultrasound (US) [8, 37, 38] (Table 6.2) that have all been used in patients with COPD. The quantification of muscle mass using these techniques has been related to relevant outcomes such as strength and survival [8, 38]. CT scan and MRI techniques may provide additional information such as muscle fat infiltration which may have implications for muscle performance [39–41]. Moreover, as correlations between regional and whole-body muscle mass are poor, direct estimation of thigh muscle mass may constitute a more relevant measurement and may be more responsive to changes associated to therapeutic interventions such as exercise training [38].

6.3 Evaluation of Muscle Strength

Limb muscle strength, defined as the force-generating capacity of the muscle, is reduced in patients with COPD when compared with age-matched controls [1] and is most often assessed with maximum voluntary contractions. Effort-dependent muscle strength assessment of muscle strength can be done by portable devices (e.g. strain gauge, hand-held dynamometer), more complex systems (e.g. computerized dynamometers) or weight machines [42]. Electrical or magnetic stimulation of the muscle or its motor nerve is another way of measuring muscle strength, independently from the patient's effort [43].

Velocity of shortening, type of contraction, joint angle position and length of the muscle are important determinants of muscle strength [35]. Muscle strength assessment protocols, techniques (static or dynamic) and devices must be chosen based on their advantages and limitations as well as on the desired information [44, 45]. Static testing ensures that muscle length and joint angle remain identical throughout the contraction and is thus called "isometric". Some daily life activities rely on isometric strength, such as carrying grocery bags. Muscle function is, however, only assessed at the specific angle used for testing which limits its applicability in other functional activities. Isokinetic (fixed speed of movement) and isotonic (fixed resistance applied to the muscle during the movement) testing are dynamic techniques that may better reflect functional activities by describing muscle function throughout the full range of motion and/or at different speeds. Table 6.3 presents different static and dynamic strategies commonly used to assess limb muscle strength in patients with COPD.

Muscle strength assessment values can be expressed in percentage of reference values established for healthy subjects, based on sex, gender and weight. Such normal values are available (even though not yet widely accepted) for isometric muscle strength measurement with strain gauges [46], hand-held dynamometers [47], computerized dynamometers [48] and for isotonic measures [49]. Familiarization sessions with the device and/or protocol used before the first evaluation should be conducted to obtain accurate and reliable results and avoid any underestimation or one's accurate maximal strength [50] or any learning effect that could overestimate the effects of a strength training program [51]. Another important element to be considered is whether or not visual and/or verbal feedback should be provided. The use of one or both forms of feedback significantly increases peak torques deployed among various populations, with different contraction types (concentric, eccentric, isometric) [52–58]. If provided, feedback should be consistent in frequency and intensity while performing longitudinal assessment of muscle strength.

Supramaximal electrical or magnetic stimulation of a peripheral nerve has been used to assess muscle strength in non-effort-dependent manner [59]. Quadriceps twitch force is reduced in patients with COPD and normal values are available (though only reported for a small healthy subject sample) [38]. Magnetic stimulation is relatively non-invasive, results in higher peak torques and is less painful (with a mean of about five points less on a visual analog scale) than electrical stimulation since it avoids stimulation of skin nociceptors [60]. Stimulation output needs to slowly increase until the attained twitch force reaches its peak before diminishing [35] in order to ensure supra-maximality and thus a reliable measure [61] with less day-to-day variability than maximal voluntary contractions [62]. Stimulation can be applied on a rested muscle (unpotentiated twitch) or a few seconds after a maximal voluntary contraction (potentiated twitch). The latter however still requires patient's full cooperation, while the first requires a 20-min complete relaxation of the tested muscle in order to achieve depotentiation, which might be difficult for some patients [35].

6.3.1 Manual Testing

Manual strength testing was first described by Wright et al. in 1912 [63]. It allows a quick and tool-free qualitative assessment of muscle strength from "no contraction at all" to "normal". The Medical Research Council scale is mostly used in critically ill settings (with the sum of 12 muscle group score [64, 65]) and ranges strength on a five-point scale, from no visible or palpable contraction (zero) to normal muscle contraction against full resistance (five), and a score of three means that a limb can be moved in the full range of motion with no resistance added other than gravity. This type of testing however depends on a subjective examiner rating, and interobserver reliability is thus questionable [66]. It was also shown to be less accurate and responsive in ambulant patients with muscle weakness when compared with hand-held dynamometer measures [67].

Table 6.3 Strategies used to assess limb muscle strength, endurance and fatigability in patients with COPD

Measuring equipment	1. Strain gauge or hand-held systems	2. Computerized dynamometers	3. Repetition maximum	4. Handgrip gauges	5. Non-volitional (electrical or magnetic nerve stimulation)
Type of contraction	Isometric	Isometric and isokinetic	Isotonic	Isometric	Isometric
Picture of measurement/device	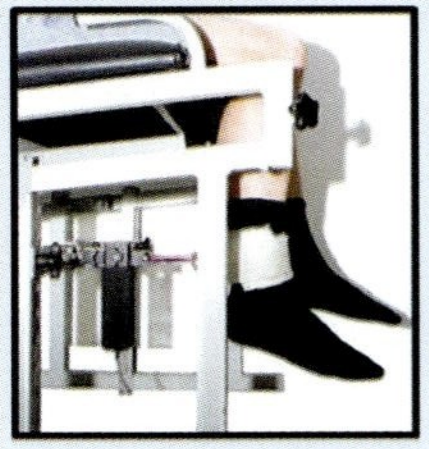	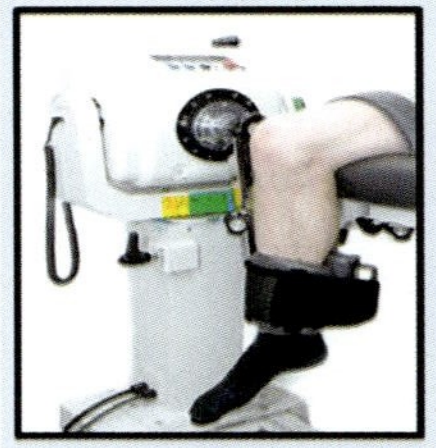	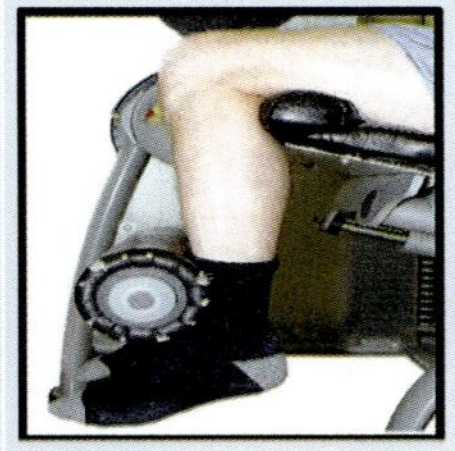	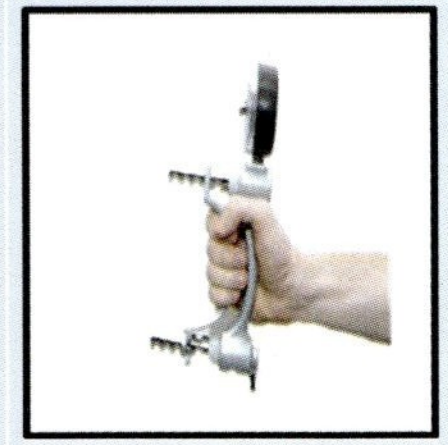	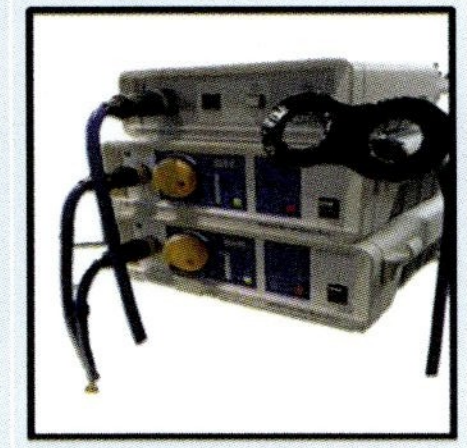
Positioning of tested limbs in COPD studies [42, 77, 145]	Knee and hip flexed at 90°, elbow and/or shoulder flexed at 90°	**Isometric**: elbow flexed at 90°, knee flexed 60°–120° **Isokinetic**: knee flexed at 90° to full knee extension	Not well described in COPD studies	Elbow flexed at 90° with arm unsupported	Knee and hip flexed at 90°
Measurements of **muscle strength** in COPD studies [42, 72]	Perform 3 MVC, each lasting 3–5 s with at least 30-s rest between attempts. Highest value used as measurement of strength	Perform 3–5 MVC (*isometric: hold each contraction for 3 s*) and 1–2-min rest between attempts. Highest value used as measurement of strength	Not well described in COPD studies. Follow ACSM recommendations + use metronome and control start and stop positions	Perform 3 MVC with each lasting at least 3-s and 30-s rest between attempts. Highest value used as measurement of strength	Three stimulations at 100% stimulator output in a relaxed muscle. Highest value used as measurement of strength
Measurements of **muscle endurance** in COPD studies [49, 77, 96, 97]	Measure the time during which a contraction at 60–80% of MVC can be maintained in one set (only performed using strain gauges in COPD studies)	**Isometric**: has not previously been used in COPD. **Isokinetic**: measure the total amount of work performed from 1 set of 30 MVC at 60° or 90°/s	Number of repetitions performed. One set of dynamic contractions at 30–40% of MVC until exhaustion. Contraction cycle of 6–12 contractions	Has not previously been done in COPD. Strain gauge procedure might be feasible	One set of repeated magnetic stimulations using a train of impulsions at 20–30% of MVC until a 70–80% reduction in force is seen

(continued)

Table 6.3 (continued)

Measuring equipment	1. Strain gauge or hand-held systems	2. Computerized dynamometers	3. Repetition maximum	4. Handgrip gauges	5. Non-volitional (electrical or magnetic nerve stimulation)
Type of contraction	Isometric	Isometric and isokinetic	Isotonic	Isometric	Isometric
Measurements of **muscle fatigue** in COPD studies [77, 93, 146]	Calculates and measures the change in EMG median frequency and/or root mean square over time. Measure muscle strength before and after a specific activity	**Isokinetic**: measures the slope of the fall in force over time from one set of 30 MVC at 60° or 90°/s	Calculates and measures the change in EMG median frequency and/or root mean square over time. Measure muscle strength before and after a specific activity	Has not previously been done in COPD	Measures twitch muscle force before and after specific muscle activity
Advantages [62, 69, 72, 147–149]	Results are valid, reliable and reproducible. Easy to use, portable, time efficient and inexpensive	Results are valid, reliable and reproducible. Easy to standardize. Different speeds and angles could be tested	Assesses muscle function in the whole range of motion. Can be executed using available equipment	No familiarization, easy to use, easy to standardize	Less affected by external factors. Lower day-to-day variability than assessments of MVC
Limitations [42, 70, 150, 151]	Measures only in one angle. Standardization is crucial for validity and reliability	Low availability. Requires expensive equipment. Needs familiarization session	Time consuming and more difficult to standardize than isometric measurements	Measures only handgrip strength	More in the realm of research. Requires expensive equipment

6.3.2 Static Measures: Isometric Muscle Strength Testing

Isometric strength assessment provides information on muscle function at a fixed joint angle and without any change in muscle length. The American Society of Exercise Physiologists recommends to perform at least three contractions interspersed with 1 min of rest, each contraction being held for 4–5 s in order to reach a torque "plateau", with a 1-s transition period at the start of each contraction [68].

Isometric strength can be measured with handheld dynamometers (e.g. Medup™, MicroFET™). These devices are portable, easy to use and relatively inexpensive and can be used at the bedside [48, 69]. They, however, require strict standardization of limb and examiner positions in order to give reliable results [42, 48, 70]. Results also depend on the examiner's skills and strength: isometric strength can be underestimated if the examiner is unable to oppose enough force to keep the limb tested in a fixed position [71].

Isometric torque is another reliable, valid and reproducible measure of static muscle strength [72, 73] that can be obtained from computerized dynamometers (e.g. Biodex™, Cybex™ or Kin-Com™). However, these systems are mostly used for dynamic strength assessment [42] and in research settings since their cost and relative complexity limit their widespread availability in clinical settings.

6.3.3 Dynamic Measures: Isokinetic Strength Testing

Isokinetic strength assessment ensures a fixed angular velocity during a maximal contraction and throughout the whole joint range of motion. The procedure is safe, reliable and valid at numerous angular velocities. 60°/s is the most commonly angular velocity used for quadriceps strength assessment in COPD studies [42], while strength measurement obtained during concentric contractions at 90°/s correlates with functional tests such as the timed up and go test, stair climb power test, and the 30-s sit-to-stand test [74].

6.3.4 Dynamic Measures: Isotonic Strength Testing

Isotonic strength assessment provides information on muscle function when no significant change of load is applied to the tested muscle. It can be executed with hydraulic resistance devices, force transducer platforms adapted to weight machines or one-repetition maximum (1RM) tests [42]. 1RM refers to the maximal weight that one can lift only once through the whole available range of motion and is the most common isotonic measure used with patients with COPD even though it is not purely isotonic [42]. The American College of Sports Medicine recommends a standardized procedure [49], but information on positioning, warm-up, number of trials, velocity of the movement, rest period and familiarization are not always available in COPD studies [42]. A metronome is also useful to set the speed and the amplitude of movement [44], and various training systems can be used for isotonic testing (computerized dynamometer, gymnasium equipment, free weights, pulley systems, elastic bands) [42, 44], which facilitates its assessment in various settings. After positioning the patient and giving the appropriate instructions, a random initial load (ideally close to the suspected maximum) is applied and increased or decreased following the patient's capacity to perform one repetition. Repeated attempts necessary to find the optimal load can however result in muscle fatigue and thus in an underestimation of the true maximal strength. Intra-tester reliability has yet to be investigated in patients with COPD, but 1RM was found to be responsive to pulmonary rehabilitation and to correlate with the 30-s and 1-min sit-to-stand test in this population [75]. It is also a safe and well-tolerated procedure in patients with COPD [76].

6.4 Evaluation of Muscle Endurance

Limb muscle endurance refers to a muscle's ability to sustain or repeat a specific task over time [49]. It reflects the ability to perform tasks requiring a small number of submaximal contractions (e.g. 15–20) such as climbing a set of stairs as well as tasks requiring thousands of submaximal contractions such as bicycling or walking over a long distance. Even though both types of tasks involve the endurance quality of the muscle, it is obvious that the same assessment method cannot be used to evaluate muscle performance in both situations and that no single test can evaluate all aspects of limb muscle endurance [49, 77]. In COPD research, the intensity of the tasks performed for assessing limb muscle endurance is highly variable, resulting in durations from 1 to 20 min [78, 79]. Assessment methods of limb muscle fatigue, which is defined as a reversible reduction in force generated by the muscle during a given task, will also be described since it reflects similar physiological concepts as limb muscle endurance [80, 81]. There is currently a paucity of data to determine the best approaches to assess muscle endurance in patients with COPD. Also, the clinical relevance of muscle endurance measures and their respective normative values have yet to be established.

Limb muscle endurance can be measured with non-volitional and volitional techniques that can be performed with static (isometric) or dynamic strategies (isokinetic, isotonic) and by using either sustained or repeated contractions [77] (Table 6.3). Furthermore, it is important to use standardized conditions, including constant movement speed, fixed posture, familiarization with the device and/or protocol and, before the first evaluation, a warm-up period [49, 51]. Whether or not to provide visual or verbal feedback should be considered.

6.4.1 Non-volitional Measures

Assessments of limb muscle endurance using non-volitional measures in COPD have mainly been performed with repeated isometric contractions using magnetic stimulations of a relaxed muscle. A typical protocol involves a stimulation intensity of 20–30% MVC, at a frequency of 30 Hz, with a duty cycle of 0.4 (2 s on, 3 s off) [82] until a 70–80% reduction in muscle force has been obtained [82–84]. The time required to reach such a reduction in MVC is then used as a measurement of muscle endurance, in which a shorter time to the targeted reduction in force is equivalent to a reduced endurance capacity of the involved muscle [82]. Another approach consists in measuring muscle twitch force, after the completion of a specific task such as walking or cycling [13, 82, 85]. With this methodology, the magnitude of muscle fatigue is quantified by measuring the fall in twitch force occurring during the specific task [86]. One limitation of these non-volitional assessments of limb muscle endurance in patients with COPD is that they cannot be easily applied to muscles other than the quadriceps [77]. Lastly, their reliability in patients with COPD remains to be confirmed.

6.4.2 Static Measures: Isometric Muscle Endurance Testing

Limb muscle endurance can be evaluated using sustained contractions during which the patient is instructed to maintain a tension representing a prespecified intensity of their MVC until exhaustion [78]. In COPD, a single trial is sufficient to obtain a valid assessment which has been performed at intensities corresponding to 50–80% of the individual MVC [62, 78, 87, 88]. Strain gauges [77] and handgrip or hand-held dynamometers have been used to oppose muscle contractions during the procedure [88].

6.4.3 Dynamic Measures: Isokinetic and Isotonic Muscle Endurance Testing

Isokinetic endurance and fatigue assessment protocols are performed at a fixed angular velocity during maximal contraction(s) and throughout the whole joint range of motion. Isokinetic assessment of limb muscle endurance is commonly used to assess quadriceps muscle endurance in patients with COPD [77], but it has also been used for other muscle groups such as the triceps [89] as well as the anterior and posterior deltoid [89, 90]. A wide range of velocities have been used in

COPD studies, from 60°/s up to 300°/s while performing 25–30 maximal contractions [89–93]. Results of isokinetic muscle endurance can be expressed as the total work developed during the procedure, as a fatigue index (e.g. the ratio of work performed during the last ten repetitions to the work performed during the first ten repetitions) [91, 94] or as the decline in muscle work over time [91, 93, 95]. High test-retest reliability has been reported for quadriceps total work measured at 90°/s and 180°/s, while work fatigue index only has been considered reliable at 90°/s [91]. Thus, an angular velocity of 90°/s is recommended for assessment of isokinetic muscle endurance and fatigue in patients with COPD.

Another common strategy to assess limb muscle endurance is to perform tests in which the external loading is constant (i.e. isotonic measurements). In COPD, external loads corresponding to 10% up to 50% of the individual MVC have been used [79, 96–98] during repeated contractions performed until failure. With this method, limb muscle endurance is quantified by reporting the time or number of repetitions performed at failure [77, 98]. The range of motion and speed of movement should be controlled to minimize variation in testing, for example, by using a metronome [44]. An advantage of isotonic muscle testing over isometric and isokinetic techniques is that it could be performed using a variety of equipment such as elastic resistance bands [98], exercise platforms/benches [79, 96, 97] or pulley systems [99]. Isotonic limb muscle endurance assessments have targeted the quadriceps muscle, but other muscle groups including the hamstrings, shoulder, chest, biceps and upper back muscles have also been tested [77, 98, 99]. For all these reasons, we would favour isotonic over isometric and isokinetic techniques to assess muscle endurance.

6.4.4 Alternative Methods to Assess Limb Muscle Endurance

Monitoring surface electromyography (EMG) while performing dynamic or static measurements is an alternative method to quantify muscle fatigue in patients with COPD [78, 79]. However, the feasibility and clinical applicability of EMG measurements of muscle fatigue can be questioned since the equipment requires special knowledge and the procedure is more time consuming than standard methods. It is also uncertain if EMG provides additional information in comparison to the above-described static and dynamic test procedures [100]. Limb muscle endurance could also be assessed with functional tests, performed with or without external loadings, such as sit-to-stand raises and step-up or calf raises [99, 101]. However, the use of functional tests as surrogates for limb muscle strength or endurance warrants some caution. Although these tests may relate to strength or endurance properties of the muscles, the results are procedure specific and do not apply to other conditions.

6.5 Limb Muscles and Exercise Training

Pulmonary rehabilitation is a multidisciplinary, evidence-based and comprehensive approach used to promote better self-management of the disease, minimize symptom burden, optimize functional status and increase participation in activities of daily life [102]. Even though the content of pulmonary rehabilitation may vary depending on factors such as healthcare systems, resources, personnel or settings, individually tailored exercise training is considered the cornerstone of PR [102, 103]. Exercise training within the context of PR is also considered the best available means of improving limb muscle strength and endurance [102]. The "conventional" modalities used to exercise patients with COPD participating in pulmonary rehabilitation programs mainly include aerobic/endurance training and strength/resistive training and a combination of these two training modalities [35, 102, 104]. Continuous or interval aerobic training improves muscle oxidative capacity [7], while specific resistance training has a greater potential to improve muscle mass, strength and function than whole-body aerobic training [6, 105].

6.6 Endurance/Aerobic Training in Pulmonary Rehabilitation

Aerobic training is probably the most common exercise modality in patients with COPD. The main objective of this training modality is to improve aerobic exercise capacity as aerobic activities are part of many everyday tasks and enhance health status and fitness. The general guidelines used to prescribe aerobic training in healthy subjects are also applicable to patients with pulmonary impairments. The frequency, duration and intensity of training are all thought to be important. Even though the optimal intensity is still debatable in COPD, greater physiological and muscle training responses and larger improvements in submaximal exercise tolerance have been obtained when training at high intensity (>60% of maximal work rate) compared to low intensity (below 50% of maximal work rate) [106, 107]. It is generally recommended that aerobic training includes 3 weekly 20–30-min exercise sessions for 8–12 weeks. However, these additional physiologic benefits of a high-intensity training program as compared to low-intensity exercise program do not necessarily translate into additional gains in quality of life [107], and the objective of high-intensity training cannot be achieved in all patients [108]. Therefore, the training intensity should be tailored to the individual's. In the most disabled patients, interval training, where 2–3 min of high-intensity exercise is interspersed with lower-intensity exercise or even rest periods, may allow the patient to reach an adequate training stimulus [109, 110]. Based on the last recommendations of the official American Thoracic Society (ATS)/European Respiratory Society (ERS) statement [102], optimal characteristics of continuous and interval endurance training are summarized in Table 6.4.

The main physiological response to aerobic training consists in structural changes in the cardiovascular and limb muscle systems; this accounts for an improvement in the capacity to transport and utilize oxygen and in exercise capacity [111]. Aerobic exercises, either of interval or constant load modalities, increase muscle cross-sectional area of all fibre types [7, 112–114] and reduce the proportion of type *IIx fibres* in the quadriceps [7, 113, 114]. Metabolic adaptations, such as increased oxidative capacity of the quadriceps muscle and reduction in exercise-induced lactic acid production, are also seen after aerobic training protocols in patients with COPD [7, 35, 113]. Functionally, improved muscle strength and endurance are also consistently observed after aerobic training in patients with COPD [4, 6, 104, 105, 111, 115–119]. All these positive muscle adaptations contribute to the improved exercise tolerance, reduced dyspnoea (i.e. reducing the

Table 6.4 Optimal characteristics of continuous and interval endurance training programs

	Continuous endurance training	Interval endurance training
Frequency	3–4 days/week^{-1}	3–4 days/week^{-1}
Mode	Continuous	Interval modes: • 30 s of exercise, 30 s of rest • 20 s of exercise, 40 s of rest
Intensity	Initially 60–70% of the maximal power rate	Initially 80–100% of the maximal power rate for the first three to four sessions
Duration	Initially 10–15 min for the first three to four sessions	Initially 15–20 min for the first three to four sessions
Progression	• Increase work load by 5–10% as tolerated • Progressively try to reach 80–90% of baseline power rate • Progressively increase exercise duration to 30–40 min	• Increase work load by 5–10% as tolerated • Progressively try to reach 150% of baseline power rate • Progressively increase exercise duration to 45–60 min (including resting time)
Perceived exertion	Try to aim for a perceived exertion on the 10-point Borg scale of 4–6	Try to aim for a perceived exertion on the 10-point Borg scale of 4–6

ventilator requirements for a determined work load) and leg fatigue perception and increase health-related quality of life that is seen after pulmonary rehabilitation [102, 103, 120].

6.7 Resistive Muscle Training

The current ATS/ERS statement on pulmonary rehabilitation recommendations for resistive training is to perform two to four sets of six to twelve repetitions at intensities ranging from 50% to 85% of the one-repetition maximum (1RM), 2–3 days/week [102, 121]. However, considering that limb muscle dysfunction is heterogeneous across patients and that it encompasses not only muscle weakness but also reduced endurance and/or greater muscle fatigability, it is important to tailor the muscle training intervention to the specific needs of the patient. Greater effects on muscle mass and strength are expected with resistance training protocols that use relatively large weights (60–70% of 1RM) and a low number of repetitions (often 8–15 repetitions) [122, 123]. In contrast, limb muscle endurance and resistance to muscle fatigue will be most improved by training strategies using lower weights (45–65% of 1RM) with a high number of repetitions (often 15–25 repetitions). Based on the recommendations of American College of Sports Medicine [124], the characteristics of specific strength training programs are summarized in Table 6.5.

The effects of resistance training on intrinsic muscle changes have been scarcely studied in COPD [125]. In patients with moderately severe COPD and normal whole-body muscle mass, resistance exercise training enhances the expression of muscle IGF-1 and other components of the muscle IGF system and of myogenic regulatory factors [126]. Increases in mid-thigh CSA, diminished inflammation and stimulation of satellite cells (which maintain muscle mass and contribute in muscle fibre regeneration) [127] have all been shown after resistance training regimes in COPD. The pooled results from the three systematic reviews from O'Shea et al. [122], Puhan et al. [128] and Lepsen et al. [129] have shown that rigorous resistance muscle training performed with free weights or exercise equipment is feasible for patients with COPD. High levels of adherence are reported, and few or any adverse events were associated with this intervention. The tolerability of resistance training is also considered to be superior to aerobic training since it results in less exercise-induced dyspnoea, allowing more patients to reach targeted exercise intensities, thus optimizing the training effects. Functionally, resistance exercise alone or in combination with whole-body aerobic exercise helps to improve limb muscle strength and endurance in patients with COPD [4, 6, 105, 122, 128–132], and greater effects on muscle strength are obtained with resistance training in comparison to aerobic training alone or when resistance training is added to an aerobic training protocol [102, 119, 129, 132]

Table 6.5 Optimal characteristics of resistive training programs

	Strength	Strength endurance	Endurance
Loading	80–100% of 1RM	70–85% of 1RM	30–80% of 1RM
Volume	1–3 sets of 1–8 repetitions	3 sets of 8–12 repetitions	1–3 sets of 20–30 repetitions
Rest intervals	2–3 min	1–2 min	1 min
Frequency	4–6 day/week^{-1}	2–4 day/week^{-1} (maintenance 1–2 day week^{-1})	2–4 day/week^{-1}
Progression	2–10% increase	Beginners: 60–70% of 1RM	
Expected benefits			
	Improvement in muscle mass and strength and in bone density	Hypertrophy, improvement in muscle mass and strength and in bone density	Improvement in muscle oxidative capacity and capillarization
		Improvement in muscle endurance and exercise capacity	Improvement in muscle endurance and in exercise capacity

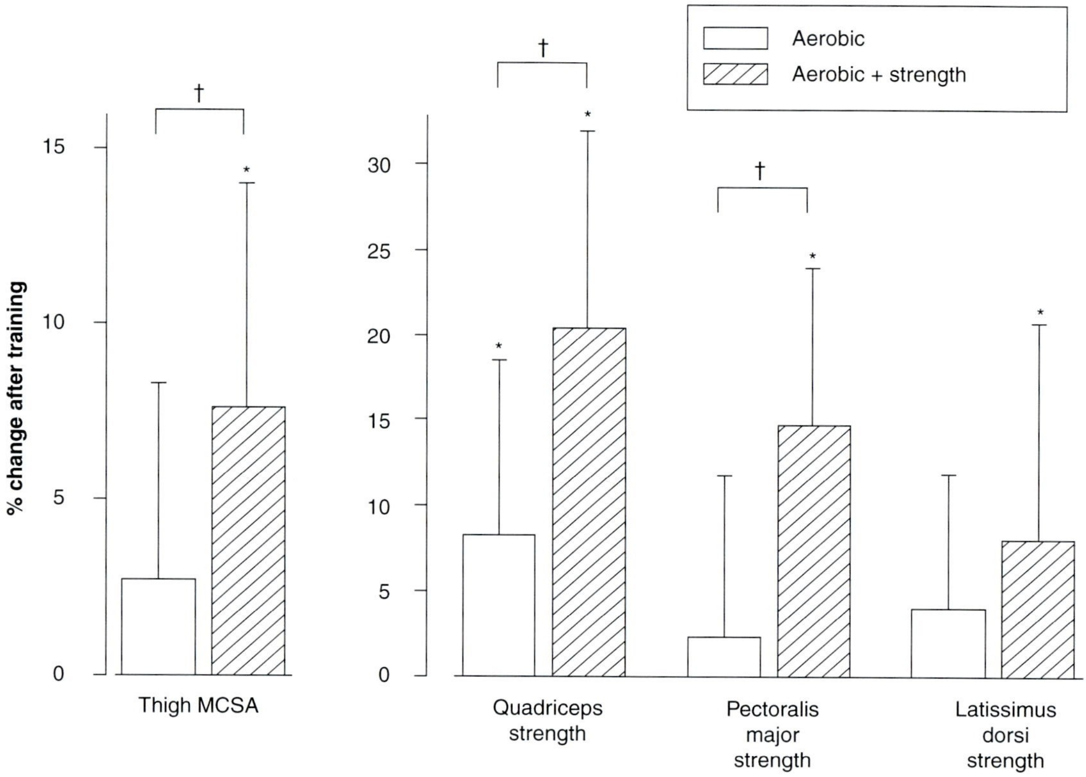

Fig. 6.1 Mean ± SD percent change in bilateral mid-thigh muscle cross-sectional area (MCSA) and in the strength of the quadriceps, pectoralis major and latissimus dorsi muscles before and after training in the aerobic and aerobic + strength groups. The improvement in bilateral mid-thigh MCSA and in the strength of the three muscle groups was statistically significant in the aerobic + strength group. Quadriceps strength also showed a significant increase in the aerobic group. As can be seen, the magnitude of the changes in mid-thigh MCSA and in the strength of the quadriceps and pectoralis major muscles was significantly greater in the aerobic + strength group than in the aerobic group (*$p < 0.05$ for pre- versus post-training within each study group, †$p < 0.05$ for the aerobic group versus the aerobic + strength group) (from Bernard et al. [4] with permission)

(Fig. 6.1). Interestingly, the improvement in muscle function induced by resistance training may translate into better performance of some daily activities [122] and to larger improvement in health-related quality of life than aerobic training [6, 133].

Because limb muscle function is likely to be impaired during exacerbation and hospitalization, several interventions to prevent or counteract muscle impairment during episodes of exacerbation have been successfully considered [86, 103, 125]. Resistance training initiated during the hospitalization may prevent further deterioration in limb muscle function. One study reported increases in quadriceps force and in 6-minute walking distance at discharge when the exercise training intervention is initiated during the hospitalization [125]. This was associated with a more favourable anabolic/catabolic balance in muscle [125]. Moreover, 1 month after discharge, functional status and muscle force remained better in the group that trained during the exacerbation [125]. In spite of short-term effects of resistance training on muscle mass and strength which are well recognized in COPD, the long-term effects of isolated resistance training or sustainability of domestic maintenance training remain to be determined [134].

6.7.1 Neuromuscular Electrical Stimulation Muscle Training

In the last 10 years, neuromuscular electrical stimulation (NMES) has attracted the interests of clinicians as a novel rehabilitative approach. Because of a limited impact on ventilatory requirements and dyspnoea, NMES appears as a promising alternative to general physical reconditioning in patients with advanced COPD. Despite the need to clarify the optimal stimulation parameters (frequency, intensity and duration of stimulation), transcutaneous neuromuscular electrical stimulation (NMES) can be particularly relevant to severely deconditioned or bedbound patients with COPD [135–137]. Increase in mid-thigh muscle and type II fibre cross-sectional area, decrease in fibre type I cross-sectional area, change in fibre-type distribution in favour of type I fibres and decrease in muscle oxidative stress, along with a more favourable anabolic to catabolic balance, have been reported after NMES intervention in patients with COPD [137–139]. From a functional perspective, the most consistent finding of NMES training in COPD is a 20–30% gain in quadriceps strength and endurance as compared with control subjects [137, 140–142]. The magnitude of improvement in walking distance after NMES was recently associated with gains in muscle strength and the ability to tolerate higher stimulation intensity. There also appears to exist a certain NMES intensity threshold below which the likelihood of benefiting from the intervention is reduced [137].

Conclusion

Limb muscle dysfunction is a clinically relevant systemic manifestation of COPD, because it influences important clinical outcomes such as exercise capacity, health-related quality of life and even survival. Assessment of muscle dysfunction and wasting is relevant in this population and can be achieved by several methods. This COPD-associated condition can also be treated successfully with exercise training, the cornerstone of pulmonary rehabilitation. Clinicians are therefore encouraged to assess limb muscle function in patients with COPD.

References

1. Seymour JM, Spruit MA, Hopkinson NS, Natanek SA, Man WD, Jackson A, Gosker HR, Schols AM, Moxham J, Polkey MI, Wouters EF. The prevalence of quadriceps weakness in COPD and the relationship with disease severity. Eur Respir J. 2010;36:81–8.
2. Shrikrishna D, Patel M, Tanner RJ, Seymour JM, Connolly BA, Puthucheary ZA, Walsh SL, Bloch SA, Sidhu PS, Hart N, et al. Quadriceps wasting and physical inactivity in patients with COPD. Eur Respir J. 2012;40:1115–22.
3. Bernard S, Leblanc P, Whittom F, Carrier G, Jobin J, Belleau R, Maltais F. Peripheral muscle weakness in patients with chronic obstructive pulmonary disease. Am J Respir Crit Care Med. 1998;158:629–34.
4. Bernard S, Whittom F, Leblanc P, Jobin J, Belleau R, Bérubé C, Carrier G, Maltais F. Aerobic and strength training in patients with COPD. Am J Respir Crit Care Med. 1999;159:896–901.
5. Sala E, Roca J, Marrades RM, Alonso J, Gonzalez de Suso JM, Moreno A, Barbera JA, Nadal J, de Jover L, Rodriguez-Roisin R, Wagner PD. Effects of endurance training on skeletal muscle bioenergetics in chronic obstructive pulmonary disease. Am J Respir Crit Care Med. 1999;159:1726–34.
6. Ortega F, Toral J, Cejudo P, Villagomez R, Sánchez H, Castillo J, Montemayor T. Comparison of effects of strength and endurance training in patients with chronic obstructive pulmonary disease. Am J Respir Crit Care Med. 2002;166:669–74.
7. Vogiatzis I, Terzis G, Nanas S, Stratakos G, Simoes DC, Georgiadou O, Zakynthinos S, Roussos C. Skeletal muscle adaptations to interval training in patients with advanced COPD. Chest. 2005;128:3838–45.
8. Marquis K, Debigaré R, LeBlanc P, Lacasse Y, Jobin J, Carrier G, Maltais F. Mid-thigh muscle cross-sectional area is a better predictor of mortality than body mass index in patients with COPD. Am J Respir Crit Care Med. 2002;166:809–13.
9. Schols AM, Broekhuizen R, Weling-Scheepers CA, Wouters EF. Body composition and mortality in chronic obstructive pulmonary disease. Am J Clin Nutr. 2005;82:53–9.
10. Swallow EB, Reyes D, Hopkinson NS, Man WD, Porcher R, Cetti EJ, Moore AJ, Moxham J, Polkey MI. Quadriceps strength predicts mortality in patients with moderate to severe chronic obstructive pulmonary disease. Thorax. 2007;62:115–20.
11. Patel MS, Natanek SA, Stratakos G, Pascual S, Martinez-Llorens J, Disano L, Terzis G, Hopkinson NS, Gea J, Vogiatzis I, et al. Vastus lateralis fiber shift is an independent predictor of mortality in chronic obstructive pulmonary disease. Am J Respir Crit Care Med. 2014;190:350–2.
12. Hamilton AL, Killian KJ, Summers E, Jones NL. Muscle strength, symptom intensity and exercise capacity in patients with cardiorespiratory disorders. Am J Respir Crit Care Med. 1995;152:2021–31.

13. Saey D, Debigaré R, LeBlanc P, Mador MJ, Côté C, Jobin J, Maltais F. Contractile leg fatigue after cycle exercise: a factor limiting exercise in patients with COPD. Am J Respir Crit Care Med. 2003;168:425–30.
14. Deschênes D, Pepin V, Saey D, LeBlanc P, Maltais F. Locus of symptom limitation and exercise response to bronchodilation in chronic obstructive pulmonary disease. J Cardiopulm Rehabil Prev. 2008;28:208–14.
15. Engelen MPKJ, Schols AMWJ, Baken WC, Wesseling GJ, Wouters EFM. Nutritional depletion in relation to respiratory and peripheral skeletal muscle function in out-patients with COPD. Eur Respir J. 1994;7:1793–7.
16. Schols AMWJ, Soeters PB, Dingemans MC, Mostert R, Frantzen PJ, Wouters EFM. Prevalence and characteristics of nutritional depletion in patients with stable COPD eligible for pulmonary rehabilitation. Am Rev Respir Dis. 1993;147:1151–6.
17. Eid AA, Ionescu AA, Nixon LS, Lewis-Jenkins V, Mathews SB, Griffiths TL, Shale DJ. The inflammatory response and body composition in chronic obstructive pulmonary disease. Am J Respir Crit Care Med. 2001;164:1414–8.
18. Braun SR, Keim NL, Dixon RM, Clagnaz P, Anderegg A, Shrago ES. The prevalence and determinants of nutritional changes in chronic obstructive pulmonary disease. Chest. 1984;86:558–63.
19. Gray-Donald K, Gibbons L, Shapiro SH, Martin JG. Effect of nutritional status on exercise with chronic obstructive pulmonary disease. Am Rev Respir Dis. 1989;140:1544–8.
20. Schols AMWJ, Slangen J, Volovics L, Wouters EFM. Weight loss is a reversible factor in the prognosis of chronic obstructive pulmonary disease. Am J Respir Crit Care Med. 1998;157:1791–7.
21. Gosselink R, Troosters T, Decramer M. Peripheral muscle weakness contributes to exercise limitation in COPD. Am J Respir Crit Care Med. 1996;153:976–80.
22. Engelen MP, Schols AM, Does JD, Wouters EF. Skeletal muscle weakness is associated with wasting of extremity fat-free mass but not with airflow obstruction in patients with chronic obstructive pulmonary disease. Am J Clin Nutr. 2000;71:733–8.
23. Baarends EM, Schols AM, Mostert R, Wouters EF. Peak exercise response in relation to tissue depletion in patients with chronic obstructive pulmonary disease. Eur Respir J. 1997;10:2807–13.
24. Kobayashi A, Yoneda T, Yoshikawa M, Ikuno M, Takenaka H, Fukuoka A, Narita N, Nezu K. The relation of fat-free mass to maximum exercise performance in patients with chronic obstructive pulmonary disease. Lung. 2000;178:119–27.
25. Schols AMWJ, Mostert R, Soeters PB, Wouters EFM. Body composition and exercise performance in patients with chronic obstructive pulmonary disease. Thorax. 1991;46:695–9.
26. Mostert R, Goris A, Weling-Scheepers C, Wouters EFM, Schols AMW. Tissue depletion and health related quality of life in patients with chronic obstructive pulmonary disease. Respir Med. 2000;94:859–67.
27. Collins PF, Elia M, Stratton RJ. Nutritional support and functional capacity in chronic obstructive pulmonary disease: a systematic review and meta-analysis. Respirology. 2013;18:616–29.
28. van Wetering CR, Hoogendoorn M, Broekhuizen R, Geraerts-Keeris GJ, De Munck DR, Rutten-van Molken MP, Schols AM. Efficacy and costs of nutritional rehabilitation in muscle-wasted patients with chronic obstructive pulmonary disease in a community-based setting: a prespecified subgroup analysis of the INTERCOM trial. J Am Med Dir Assoc. 2010;11:179–87.
29. Steiner MC, Barton RL, Singh SJ, Morgan MD. Bedside methods versus dual energy X-ray absorptiometry for body composition measurement in COPD. Eur Respir J. 2002;19:626–31.
30. Lerario MC, Sachs A, Lazaretti-Castro M, Saraiva LG, Jardim JR. Body composition in patients with chronic obstructive pulmonary disease: which method to use in clinical practice? Br J Nutr. 2006;96:86–92.
31. Siri WE. Body composition from fluid spaces and density: analysis of methods. 1961. Nutrition. 1993;9:480–91; discussion 480, 492.
32. Lukaski HC, Johnson PE, Bolonchuk WW, Lykken GI. Assessment of fat-free mass using bioelectrical impedance measurements of the human body. Am J Clin Nutr. 1985;41:810–7.
33. Schols AMWJ, Wouters EFM, Soeters PB, Westerterp KR. Body composition by bioelectrical-impedance analysis compared with deuterium dilution and skinfold anthropometry in patients with chronic obstructive pulmonary disease. Am J Clin Nutr. 1991;53:421–4.
34. Rutten EP, Spruit MA, Wouters EF. Critical view on diagnosing muscle wasting by single-frequency bio-electrical impedance in COPD. Respir Med. 2010;104:91–8.
35. Maltais F, Decramer M, Casaburi R, Barreiro E, Burelle Y, Debigare R, Dekhuijzen PN, Franssen F, Gayan-Ramirez G, Gea J, et al. An official American Thoracic Society/European Respiratory Society statement: update on limb muscle dysfunction in chronic obstructive pulmonary disease. Am J Respir Crit Care Med. 2014;189:e15–62.
36. Engelen MP, Schols AM, Heidendal GA, Wouters EF. Dual-energy X-ray absorptiometry in the clinical evaluation of body composition and bone mineral density in patients with chronic obstructive pulmonary disease. Am J Clin Nutr. 1998;68:1298–303.
37. Mathur S, Takai KP, Macintyre DL, Reid D. Estimation of thigh muscle mass with magnetic resonance imaging in older adults and people with chronic obstructive pulmonary disease. Phys Ther. 2008;88:219–30.

38. Seymour JM, Ward K, Sidhu PS, Puthucheary Z, Steier J, Jolley CJ, Rafferty G, Polkey MI, Moxham J. Ultrasound measurement of rectus femoris cross-sectional area and the relationship with quadriceps strength in COPD. Thorax. 2009;64:418–23.
39. Maddocks M, Shrikrishna D, Vitoriano S, Natanek SA, Tanner RJ, Hart N, Kemp PR, Moxham J, Polkey MI, Hopkinson NS. Skeletal muscle adiposity is associated with physical activity, exercise capacity and fibre shift in COPD. Eur Respir J. 2014;44:1188–98.
40. Robles PG, Sussman MS, Naraghi A, Brooks D, Goldstein RS, White LM, Mathur S. Intramuscular fat infiltration contributes to impaired muscle function in COPD. Med Sci Sports Exerc. 2015;47:1334–41.
41. Roig M, Eng JJ, MacIntyre DL, Road JD, Reid WD. Deficits in muscle strength, mass, quality, and mobility in people with chronic obstructive pulmonary disease. J Cardiopulm Rehabil Prev. 2011;31:120–4.
42. Robles PG, Mathur S, Janaudis-Fereira T, Dolmage TE, Goldstein RS, Brooks D. Measurement of peripheral muscle strength in individuals with chronic obstructive pulmonary disease: a systematic review. J Cardiopulm Rehabil Prev. 2011;31:11–24.
43. WDc M, Moxham J, Polkey MI. Magnetic stimulation for the measurement of respiratory and skeletal muscle function. Eur Respir J. 2004;24:846–60.
44. Nyberg A, Saey D, Maltais F. Why and how limb muscle mass and function should be measured in patients with COPD. Ann Am Thorac Soc. 2015;12(9):1269–77.
45. Saey D, Troosters T. Measuring skeletal muscle strength and endurance, from bench to bedside. Clin Invest Med. 2008;31:307–11.
46. Meldrum D, Cahalane E, Conroy R, Fitzgerald D, Hardiman O. Maximum voluntary isometric contraction: reference values and clinical application. Amyotroph Lateral Scler. 2007;8:47–55.
47. Andrews AW, Thomas MW, Bohannon RW. Normative values for isometric muscle force measurements obtained with hand-held dynamometers. Phys Ther. 1996;76:248–59.
48. Danneskiold-Samsøe B, Bartels EM, Bülow PM, Lund H, Stockmarr A, Holm CC, Wätjen I, Appleyard M, Bliddal H. Isokinetic and isometric muscle strength in a healthy population with special reference to age and gender. Acta Physiol. 2009;197:1–68.
49. Thompson WR, Gordon NF, Pescatello LS, et al. ACSM's guidelines for exercise testing and prescription. Philadelphia: Wolters Kluwer/Lippincott Williams & Wilkins; 2010.
50. Levinger I, Goodman C, Hare DL, Jerums G, Toia D, Selig S. The reliability of the 1RM strength test for untrained middle-aged individuals. J Sci Med Sport. 2009;12:310–6.
51. Wallerstein LF, Barroso R, Tricoli V, Mello MT, Ugrinowitsch C. The influence of familiarization sessions on the stability of ramp and ballistic isometric torque in older adults. J Aging Phys Act. 2010;18:390–400.
52. Andreacci JL, LeMura LM, Cohen SL, Ea U, Sa C, Von Duvillard SP. The effects of frequency of encouragement on performance during maximal exercise testing. J Sports Sci. 2002;20:345–52.
53. Peacock B, Westers T, Walsh S, Nicholson K. Feedback and maximum voluntary contraction. Ergonomics. 1981;24:223–8.
54. Kellis E. Resistive eccentric exercise: effects of visual feedback on maximum moment of knee extensors and flexors. J Orthop Sports Phys Ther. 1996;23(2):120–4.
55. Hald RD, Bottjen EJ. Effect of visual feedback on maximal and submaximal lsokinetic test measurements of normal quadricem—and hamstrings. J Orthop Sports Phys Ther. 1987;9:86–93.
56. Jung MC, Hallbeck MS. Quantification of the effects of instruction type, verbal encouragement, and visual feedback on static and peak handgrip strength. Int J Ind Ergon. 2004;34:367–74.
57. Amagliani RM, Peterella JK, Jung AP. Type of encouragement influences peak muscle force in college-age women. Int J Exerc Sci. 2015;3(4):165–73.
58. Campenella B, Mattacola CG, Kimura IF. Effect of visual feedback and verbal encouragement on concentric quadriceps and hamstrings peak torque of males and females. Isokinet Exerc Sci. 2000;8:1–6.
59. Man WDC, Soliman MGG, Nikoletou D, Harris ML, Rafferty GF, Mustfa N, Polkey MI, Moxham J. Non-volitional assessment of skeletal muscle strength in patients with chronic obstructive pulmonary disease. Thorax. 2003;58:665–9.
60. Han T-R, Shin H-I, Kim I-S. Magnetic stimulation of the quadriceps femoris muscle: comparison of pain with electrical stimulation. Am J Phys Med Rehabil. 2006;85:593–9.
61. Polkey MI, Kyroussis D, Hamnegard CH, Mills GH, Green M, Moxham J. Quadriceps strength and fatigue assessed by magnetic stimulation of the femoral nerve in man. Muscle Nerve. 1996;19:549–55.
62. CR J, Chen RC. Quadriceps strength assessed by magnetic stimulation of femoral nerve in patients with chronic obstructive pulmonary disease. Chin Med J. 2011;124:2309–15.
63. Wright W. Muscle training in the treatment of infantile paralysis. Boston Med Surgery. 1912;167:567.
64. Hermans G, Clerckx B, Vanhullebusch T, Segers J, Vanpee G, Robbeets C, Casaer MP, Wouters P, Gosselink R, Van Den Berghe G. Interobserver agreement of Medical Research Council sum-score and handgrip strength in the intensive care unit. Muscle Nerve. 2012;45:18–25.
65. Hough CL, Lieu BK, Caldwell ES. Manual muscle strength testing of critically ill patients: feasibility and interobserver agreement. Crit Care. 2011;15:R43.

66. Frese E, Brown M, Norton BJ. Clinical reliability of manual muscle testing. Phys Ther. 1987;67:1072–6.
67. Bohannon RW. Measuring knee extensor muscle strength. Am J Phys Med Rehabil. 2001;80:13–8.
68. Brown L, Weir JP. ASEP procedures recommendation I: accurate assessment of muscular strength and power. J Exerc Physiol Online. 2001;4:1–21.
69. O'Shea SD, Taylor NF, Paratz JD. Measuring muscle strength for people with chronic obstructive pulmonary disease: retest reliability of hand-held dynamometry. Arch Phys Med Rehabil. 2007;88:32–6.
70. Bachasson D, Villiot-Danger E, Verges S, Hayot M, Perez T, Chambellan A, Wuyam B. Maximal isometric voluntary quadriceps strength assessment in COPD. Rev Mal Respir. 2014;31:765–70.
71. Visser J, Mans E, De Visser M, Van Den Berg-Vos RM, Franssen H, JMBV DJ, Van Den Berg LH, JHJ W, De Haan RJ. Comparison of maximal voluntary isometric contraction and hand-held dynamometry in measuring muscle strength of patients with progressive lower motor neuron syndrome. Neuromuscul Disord. 2003;13:744–50.
72. Vieira L, Bottaro M, Celes R, Viegas CA, Silva C. Isokinetic muscle evaluation of quadriceps in patients with chronic obstructive pulmonary disease. Rev Port Pneumol. 2010;16:717–36.
73. Mathur S, Makrides L, Hernandez P. Test-retest reliability of isomeric and isokinetic torque in patients with chronic obstructive pulmonary disease. Physiother Can. 2004;56:94–101.
74. Butcher SJ, Pikaluk BJ, Chura RL, Walkner MJ, Farthing JP, Marciniuk DD. Associations between isokinetic muscle strength, high-level functional performance, and physiological parameters in patients with chronic obstructive pulmonary disease. Int J Chron Obstruct Pulmon Dis. 2012;7:537–42.
75. Zanini A, Aiello M, Cherubino F, Zampogna E, Azzola A, Chetta A, Spanevello A. The one repetition maximum test and the sit-to-stand test in the assessment of a specific pulmonary rehabilitation program on peripheral muscle strength in COPD patients. Int J COPD. 2015;10:2423–30.
76. Kealin ME, Swank AM, Adams KJ, Barnard KL, Berning JM, Green A. Cardiopulmonary responses, muscle soreness, and injury during the one repetition maximum assessment in pulmonary rehabilitation patients. J Cardpulm Rehabil. 1999;19:366–72.
77. Ra E, Kaplovitch E, Beauchamp MK, Dolmage TE, Goldstein RS, Gillies CL, Brooks D, Mathur S. Is quadriceps endurance reduced in COPD? Chest. 2015;147:673.
78. Allaire J, Maltais F, Doyon JF, Noel M, Leblanc P, Carrier G, Simard C, Jobin J. Peripheral muscle endurance and the oxidative profile of the quadriceps in patients with COPD. Thorax. 2004;59:673–8.
79. Coronell C, Orozco-Levi M, Mendez R, Ramirez-Sarmiento A, Galdiz JB, Gea J. Relevance of assessing quadriceps endurance in patients with COPD. Eur Respir J. 2004;24:129–36.
80. Enoka RM, Duchateau J. Muscle fatigue: what, why and how it influences muscle function. J Physiol. 2008;1:11–23.
81. Bigland-Ritchie B, Furbush F, Woods JJ. Fatigue of intermittent submaximal voluntary contractions: central and peripheral factors. J Appl Physiol. 1986;61:421–9.
82. Swallow EB, Gosker HR, Ward KA, Moore AJ, Dayer MJ, Hopkinson NS, Schols AM, Moxham J, Polkey MI. A novel technique for nonvolitional assessment of quadriceps muscle endurance in humans. J Appl Physiol. 2007;103:739–46.
83. Man WD, Natanek SA, Riddoch-Contreras J, Lewis A, Marsh GS, Kemp PR, Polkey MI. Quadriceps myostatin expression in COPD. Eur Respir J. 2010;36:686–8.
84. Natanek SA, Gosker HR, Slot IG, Marsh GS, Hopkinson NS, Moxham J, Kemp PR, Schols AM, Polkey MI. Pathways associated with reduced quadriceps oxidative fibres and endurance in COPD. Eur Respir J. 2013;41:1275–83.
85. Rossman MJ, Venturelli M, McDaniel J, Amann M, Richardson RS. Muscle mass and peripheral fatigue: a potential role for afferent feedback? Acta Physiol (Oxford). 2012;206:242–50.
86. Burtin C, Saey D, Saglam M, Langer D, Gosselink R, Janssens W, Decramer M, Maltais F, Troosters T. Effectiveness of exercise training in patients with COPD: the role of muscle fatigue. Eur Respir J. 2012;40(2):338–44.
87. Zattara-Hartmann MC, Badier M, Guillot C, Tomei C, Jammes Y. Maximal force and endurance to fatigue of respiratory and skeletal muscles in chronic hypoxemic patients: the effects of oxygen breathing. Muscle Nerve. 1995;18:495–502.
88. Shah S, Nahar P, Vaidya S, Salvi S. Upper limb muscle strength & endurance in chronic obstructive pulmonary disease. Indian J Med Res. 2013;138:492–6.
89. Clark CJ, Cochrane LM, Mackay E, Paton B. Skeletal muscle strength and endurance in patients with mild COPD and the effects of weight training. Eur Respir J. 2000;15:92–7.
90. Nyberg A, Lindstrom B, Rickenlund A, Wadell K. Low-load/high-repetition elastic band resistance training in patients with COPD: a randomized, controlled, multicenter trial. Clin Respir J. 2015;9(3):278–88.
91. Ribeiro F, Lepine PA, Garceau-Bolduc C, Coats V, Allard E, Maltais F, Saey D. Test-retest reliability of lower limb isokinetic endurance in COPD: a comparison of angular velocities. Int J Chron Obs Pulmon Dis. 2015;10:1163–72.
92. Malaguti C, Nery LE, Dal Corso S, Napolis L, De Fuccio MB, Castro M, Neder JA. Scaling skeletal muscle function to mass in patients with moderate-to-severe COPD. Eur J Appl Physiol. 2006;98:482–8.
93. Janaudis-Ferreira T, Wadell K, Sundelin G, Lindstrom B. Thigh muscle strength and endurance

in patients with COPD compared with healthy controls. Respir Med. 2006;100:1451–7.
94. Pincivero DM, Lephart SM, Karunakara RA. Reliability and precision of isokinetic strength and muscular endurance for the quadriceps and hamstrings. Int J Sports Med. 1997;18:113–7.
95. Pincivero DM, Gear WS, Sterner RL. Assessment of the reliability of high-intensity quadriceps femoris muscle fatigue. Med Sci Sports Exerc. 2001;33:334–8.
96. Couillard A, Koechlin C, Cristol JP, Varray A, Prefaut C. Evidence of local exercise-induced systemic oxidative stress in chronic obstructive pulmonary disease patients. Eur Respir J. 2002;20:1123–9.
97. Couillard A, Maltais F, Saey D, Debigaré R, Michaud A, Koechlin C, LeBlanc P, Préfaut C. Exercise-induced quadriceps oxidative stress and peripheral muscle dysfunction in patients with COPD. Am J Respir Crit Care Med. 2003;167:1664–9.
98. Nyberg A, Saey D, Martin M, Maltais F. Acute effects of low-load/high-repetition single-limb resistance training in COPD. Med Sci Sports Exerc. 2016;48:2353–61.
99. Clark CJ, Cochrane L, Mackay E. Low intensity peripheral muscle conditioning improves exercise tolerance and breathlessness in COPD. Eur Respir J. 1996;9:2590–6.
100. Nyberg A, Saey D, Martin M, Maltais F. Muscular and functional effects of partitioning exercising muscle mass in patients with chronic obstructive pulmonary disease - a study protocol for a randomized controlled trial. Trials. 2015;16:194.
101. Clark AL, Poole-Wilson PA, Coats AJ. Exercise limitation in chronic heart failure: central role of the periphery. J Am Coll Cardiol. 1996;28:1092–102.
102. Spruit MA, Singh SJ, Garvey C, ZuWallack R, Nici L, Rochester C, Hill K, Holland AE, Lareau SC, Man WD, et al. An official American Thoracic Society/European Respiratory Society statement: key concepts and advances in pulmonary rehabilitation. Am J Respir Crit Care Med. 2013;188:e13–64.
103. McCarthy B, Casey D, Devane D, Murphy K, Murphy E, Lacasse Y. Pulmonary rehabilitation for chronic obstructive pulmonary disease. Cochrane Database Syst Rev. 2015;2:CD003793.
104. Troosters T, Gosselink R, Janssens W, Decramer M. Exercise training and pulmonary rehabilitation: new insights and remaining challenges. Eur Respir Rev. 2010;19:24–9.
105. Spruit MA, Gosselink R, Troosters T, De Paepe K, Decramer M. Resistance versus endurance training in patients with COPD and peripheral muscle weakness. Eur Respir J. 2002;19:1072–8.
106. Casaburi R, Patessio A, Ioli F, Zanaboni S, Donner CF, Wasserman K. Reductions in exercise lactic acidosis and ventilation as a result of exercise training in patients with obstructive lung disease. Am Rev Respir Dis. 1991;143:9–18.
107. Puente-Maestu L, Sanz ML, Sanz P, Cubillo JM, Mayol J, Casaburi R. Comparison of effects of supervised versus self-monitored training programmes in patients with chronic obstructive pulmonary disease. Eur Respir J. 2000;15:517–25.
108. Maltais F, Leblanc P, Jobin J, BÇrubÇ C, Bruneau J, Carrier L, Breton MJ, Falardeau G, Belleau R. Intensity of training and physiologic adaptation in patients with chronic obstructive pulmonary disease. Am J Respir Crit Care Med. 1997;155:555–61.
109. Coppoolse R, Schols AMWJ, Baarends EM, Mostert R, Akkermans MA, Janssen PP, Wouters EFM. Interval versus continuous training in patients with severe COPD: a randomized clinical trial. Eur Respir J. 1999;14:258–63.
110. Vogiatzis I, Nanas S, Roussos C. Interval training as an alternative modality to continuous exercise in patients with COPD. Eur Respir J. 2002;20:12–9.
111. O'Donnell DE, McGuire M, Samis L, Webb KA. General exercise training improves ventilatory and peripheral muscle strength and endurance in chronic airflow limitation. Am J Respir Crit Care Med. 1998;157:1489–97.
112. Whittom F, Jobin J, Simard PM, Leblanc P, Simard C, Bernard S, Belleau R, Maltais F. Histochemical and morphological characteristics of the vastus lateralis muscle in COPD patients. Comparison with normal subjects and effects of exercise training. Med Sci Sports Exerc. 1998;30:1467–74.
113. Vogiatzis I, Stratakos G, Simoes DC, Terzis G, Georgiadou O, Roussos C, Zakynthinos S. Effects of rehabilitative exercise on peripheral muscle TNFalpha, IL-6, IGF-I and MyoD expression in patients with COPD. Thorax. 2007;62:950–6.
114. Vogiatzis I, Terzis G, Stratakos G, Cherouveim E, Athanasopoulos D, Spetsioti S, Nasis I, Manta P, Roussos C, Zakynthinos S. Effect of pulmonary rehabilitation on peripheral muscle fiber remodeling in patients with COPD in GOLD stages II to IV. Chest. 2011;140:744–52.
115. Troosters T, Gosselink R, Decramer M. Short- and long-term effects of outpatient rehabilitation in patients with chronic obstructive pulmonary disease: a randomized trial. Am J Med. 2000;109:207–12.
116. Mador MJ, Kufel TJ, Pineda LA, Steinwald A, Aggarwal A, Upadhyay AM, Khan MA. Effect of pulmonary rehabilitation on quadriceps fatiguability during exercise. Am J Respir Crit Care Med. 2001;163:930–5.
117. Skumlien S, Aure Skogedal E, Skrede Ryg M, Bjortuft O. Endurance or resistance training in primary care after in-patient rehabilitation for COPD? Respir Med. 2008;102:422–9.
118. Man WD, Kemp P, Moxham J, Polkey MI. Exercise and muscle dysfunction in COPD: implications for pulmonary rehabilitation. Clin Sci (Lond). 2009;117:281–91.
119. Vonbank K, Strasser B, Mondrzyk J, Marzluf BA, Richter B, Losch S, Nell H, Petkov V, Haber P. Strength training increases maximum working capacity in patients with COPD--randomized

clinical trial comparing three training modalities. Respir Med. 2012;106:557–63.
120. Spruit MA, Troosters T, Trappenburg JC, Decramer M, Gosselink R. Exercise training during rehabilitation of patients with COPD: a current perspective. Patient Educ Couns. 2004;52:243–8.
121. Nici L, Donner C, Wouters E, Zuwallack R, Ambrosino N, Bourbeau J, Carone M, Celli B, Engelen M, Fahy B, et al. American Thoracic Society/European Respiratory Society statement on pulmonary rehabilitation. Am J Respir Crit Care Med. 2006;173:1390–413.
122. O'Shea SD, Taylor NF, Paratz J. Peripheral muscle strength training in COPD: a systematic review. Chest. 2004;126:903–14.
123. O'Shea SD, Taylor NF, Paratz JD. Progressive resistance exercise improves muscle strength and may improve elements of performance of daily activities for people with COPD: a systematic review. Chest. 2009;136:1269–83.
124. Kraemer WJ, Adams K, Cafarelli E, Dudley GA, Dooly C, Feigenbaum MS, Fleck SJ, Franklin B, Fry AC, Hoffman JR, et al. American College of Sports Medicine position stand. Progression models in resistance training for healthy adults. Med Sci Sports Exerc. 2002;34:364–80.
125. Troosters T, Probst VS, Crul T, Pitta F, Gayan-Ramirez G, Decramer M, Gosselink R. Resistance training prevents deterioration in quadriceps muscle function during acute exacerbations of chronic obstructive pulmonary disease. Am J Respir Crit Care Med. 2010;181:1072–7.
126. Lewis MI, Fournier M, Storer TW, Bhasin S, Porszasz J, Ren SG, Da X, Casaburi R. Skeletal muscle adaptations to testosterone and resistance training in men with COPD. J Appl Physiol. 2007;103:1299–310.
127. Menon MK, Houchen L, Singh SJ, Morgan MD, Bradding P, Steiner MC. Inflammatory and satellite cells in the quadriceps of patients with COPD and response to resistance training. Chest. 2012;142:1134–42.
128. Puhan MA, Schunemann HJ, Frey M, Scharplatz M, Bachmann LM. How should COPD patients exercise during respiratory rehabilitation? Comparison of exercise modalities and intensities to treat skeletal muscle dysfunction. Thorax. 2005;60:367–75.
129. Lepsen UW, Jorgensen KJ, Ringbaek T, Hansen H, Skrubbeltrang C, Lange P. A systematic review of resistance training versus endurance training in COPD. J Cardiopulm Rehabil Prev. 2015;35:163–72.
130. Puente-Maestu L, Sanz ML, Sanz P, Ruiz de Ona JM, Rodriguez-Hermosa JL, Whipp BJ. Effects of two types of training on pulmonary and cardiac responses to moderate exercise in patients with COPD. Eur Respir J. 2000;15:1026–32.
131. Mador MJ, Bozkanat E, Aggarwal A, Shaffer M, Kufel TJ. Endurance and Strength Training in Patients With COPD. Chest. 2004;125:2036–45.
132. Lepsen UWJK, Ringbaek T, Hansen H, Skrubbeltrang C, Lange PA. Combination of resistance and endurance training increases leg muscle strength in COPD: an evidence-based recommendation based on systematic review with meta-analyses. Chron Respir Dis. 2015;12:13.
133. Normandin EA, McCusker C, Connors M, Vale F, Gerardi D, ZuWallack RL. An evaluation of two approaches to exercise conditioning in pulmonary rehabilitation. Chest. 2002;121:1085–91.
134. Houchen L, Steiner MC, Singh SJ. How sustainable is strength training in chronic obstructive pulmonary disease? Physiotherapy. 2009;95:1–7.
135. Vivodtzev I, Lacasse Y, Maltais F. Neuromuscular electrical stimulation of the lower limbs in patients with chronic obstructive pulmonary disease. J Cardiopulm Rehabil Prev. 2008;28:79–91.
136. Sillen MJ, Speksnijder CM, Eterman RM, Janssen PP, Wagers SS, Wouters EF, Uszko-Lencer NH, Spruit MA. Effects of neuromuscular electrical stimulation of muscles of ambulation in patients with chronic heart failure or COPD: a systematic review of the English-language literature. Chest. 2009;136:44–61.
137. Vivodtzev I, Debigare R, Gagnon P, Mainguy V, Saey D, Dube A, Pare ME, Belanger M, Maltais F. Functional and muscular effects of neuromuscular electrical stimulation in patients with severe COPD: a randomized clinical trial. Chest. 2012;141(3):716–25.
138. Dal Corso S, Napolis L, Malaguti C, Gimenes AC, Albuquerque A, Nogueira CR, De Fuccio MB, Pereira RD, Bulle A, McFarlane N, et al. Skeletal muscle structure and function in response to electrical stimulation in moderately impaired COPD patients. Respir Med. 2006;101(6):1236–43.
139. Abdellaoui A, Prefaut C, Gouzi F, Couillard A, Coisy-Quivy M, Hugon G, Molinari N, Lafontaine T, Jonquet O, Laoudj-Chenivesse D, Hayot M. Skeletal muscle effects of electrostimulation after COPD exacerbation: a pilot study. Eur Respir J. 2011;38:781–8.
140. Zanotti E, Felicetti G, Maini M, Fracchia C. Peripheral muscle strength training in bed-bound patients with COPD receiving mechanical ventilation: effect of electrical stimulation. Chest. 2003;124:292–6.
141. Neder JA, Sword D, Ward SA, Mackay E, Cochrane LM, Clark CJ. Home based neuromuscular electrical stimulation as a new rehabilitative strategy for severely disabled patients with chronic obstructive pulmonary disease (COPD). Thorax. 2002;57:333–7.
142. Maddocks M, Nolan CM, Man WD, Polkey MI, Hart N, Gao W, Rafferty GF, Moxham J, Higginson IJ. Neuromuscular electrical stimulation to improve exercise capacity in patients with severe COPD: a randomised double-blind, placebo-controlled trial. Lancet Respir Med. 2016;4:27–36.

143. Vestbo J, Prescott E, Almdal T, Dahl M, Nordestgaard BG, Andersen T, Sorensen TI, Lange P. Body mass, fat-free body mass, and prognosis in patients with chronic obstructive pulmonary disease from a random population sample: findings from the copenhagen city heart study. Am J Respir Crit Care Med. 2006;173:79–83.
144. Coin A, Sergi G, Minicuci N, Giannini S, Barbiero E, Manzato E, Pedrazzoni M, Minisola S, Rossini M, Del Puente A, et al. Fat-free mass and fat mass reference values by dual-energy X-ray absorptiometry (DEXA) in a 20-80 year-old Italian population. Clin Nutr. 2008;27:87–94.
145. Bachasson D, Wuyam B, Pepin JL, Tamisier R, Levy P, Verges S. Quadriceps and respiratory muscle fatigue following high-intensity cycling in COPD patients. PLoS One. 2013;8:e83432.
146. Franssen FM, Broekhuizen R, Janssen PP, Wouters EF, Schols AM. Limb muscle dysfunction in COPD: effects of muscle wasting and exercise training. Med Sci Sports Exerc. 2005;37:2–9.
147. Stark T, Walker B, Phillips JK, Fejer R, Beck R. Hand-held dynamometry correlation with the gold standard isokinetic dynamometry: a systematic review. PM R. 2011;3:472–9.
148. Hartmann A, Knols R, Murer K, De Bruin ED. Reproducibility of an isokinetic strength-testing protocol of the knee and ankle in older adults. Gerontology. 2009;55:259–68.
149. Dourado VZ, Antunes LC, Tanni SE, de Paiva SA, Padovani CR, Godoy I. Relationship of upper-limb and thoracic muscle strength to 6-min walk distance in COPD patients. Chest. 2006;129(3):551–7.
150. Burns SP, Spanier DE. Break-technique handheld dynamometry: relation between angular velocity and strength measurements. Arch Phys Med Rehabil. 2005;86:1420–6.
151. Burns SP, Breuninger A, Kaplan C, Marin H. Handheld dynamometry in persons with tetraplegia: comparison of make- versus break-testing techniques. Am J Phys Med Rehabil. 2005;84:22–9.

7 Assessment of Patient-Reported Outcomes

Anja Frei and Milo Puhan

7.1 Patient-Reported Outcomes: A Long Tradition in Pulmonary Rehabilitation

A patient-reported outcome (PRO) is "any report of the status of a patient's health condition that comes directly from the patient, without interpretation of the patient's response by a clinician or anyone else" [1]. There is a wide range of PROs from single questions on specific symptoms (e.g. shortness of breath) to multi-item questionnaires that capture aspects of health that influence a person's quality of life (i.e. health-related quality of life). PROs have a long tradition in the evaluation of pulmonary rehabilitation, and they have been used for years before they entered research in other clinical areas such as cardiovascular medicine, cancer or diabetes. Petty assessed dyspnoea during activities of daily living and walk tests in his famous study as early as in 1969 [2]. In the very first randomized controlled trial (RCT) by McGavin, patients were asked if their breathlessness, well-being, general activities, cough or sputum has improved over the course of the trial [3]. Up to now, the majority of the 65 RCTs on pulmonary rehabilitation versus usual care in stable COPD patients as well as in the 20 RCTs in patients after an exacerbation used PROs as primary or secondary outcomes [4, 5].

While the first studies used single questions and interviews or daily diaries to address specific symptoms or impairment [2, 3], a major advance towards more standardized and valid assessment of the patients' experience was the development of the Chronic Respiratory Questionnaire (CRQ) in 1987 and the St. George's Respiratory Questionnaire (SGRQ) in 1992 to measure health-related quality of life [6, 7]. These questionnaires were instrumental for the introduction of PROs into clinical research well beyond pulmonary rehabilitation and COPD. Gordon Guyatt, the developer of the CRQ, wrote the seminal paper on health-related quality of life in 1993 where the importance of PROs for patient-centred research and the distinction between generic and disease-specific PRO instruments but also key methodological aspects were highlighted [8]. Thus, much of the introduction of PROs into clinical research was influenced by PROs that were developed and first used in RCTs in the context of pulmonary medicine and pulmonary rehabilitation specifically.

There are a number of purposes to use PROs. The most common use in the context of pulmonary rehabilitation is to assess the difference between the beginning and the end of the rehabilitation program in order to quantify its effects ("evaluative" purpose). For evaluative purpose, PRO instruments need to yield reproducible scores (i.e. good test-retest reliability) and be

A. Frei • M. Puhan (✉)
Epidemiology, Biostatistics und Prevention Institute (EBPI), University of Zurich, Hirschengraben 84, Zurich CH-8001, Switzerland
e-mail: anja.frei@uzh.ch; miloalan.puhan@uzh.ch

© Springer International Publishing AG 2018
E. Clini et al. (eds.), *Textbook of Pulmonary Rehabilitation*,
https://doi.org/10.1007/978-3-319-65888-9_7

able to pick up the change between the beginning and end of pulmonary rehabilitation (i.e. be responsive). PRO instruments vary widely with respect to their responsiveness, and it is of great importance to choose a responsive instrument to avoid false-negative results because the instrument was not able to pick up change. PROs may also be used to predict the probability of success of pulmonary rehabilitation or to predict outcomes of patients with COPD (e.g. exacerbations, mortality) more generally ("predictive" purpose). While the evidence is not strong to support the use of PROs to predict the success of pulmonary rehabilitation and identify individuals who may benefit most, some PROs (e.g. dyspnoea, physical activity or symptoms of anxiety or depression) are predictors of outcomes and have been included in prognostic scores (e.g. BODE, ADO) [9, 10].

Virtually all PRO instruments used in the context of pulmonary rehabilitation and clinical research in general are fully structured questionnaires, i.e. with predefined questions and answer options. Most of them can be completed by patients themselves, while some require an interviewer. Figure 7.1 shows the variety of PROs that can be relevant in patients undergoing pulmonary rehabilitation. They range from specific symptoms in specific situations (e.g. shortness of breath when walking) up to constructs like disease-specific or generic (i.e. not disease-specific) health-related quality of life. Single items (i.e. individual questions and its predefined answer options) can be used to address specific symptoms such as the modified Medical Research Council (MRC) dyspnoea scale. However, many symptoms (e.g. shortness of breath or fatigue) are multifaceted so that a certain number of items are necessary to capture them and express the extent of those symptoms by domain scores. For example, the standardized dyspnoea domain of the CRQ asks patients about shortness of breath in five situations (basic activities of daily living, walking, doing household, participating in social activities and being angry or upset). Thus, five specific questions are asked, which, together, reflect the patient's experience of dyspnoea.

As more symptoms or limitations are addressed, more items are needed that are typically summarized in separate domain scores (e.g. symptoms,

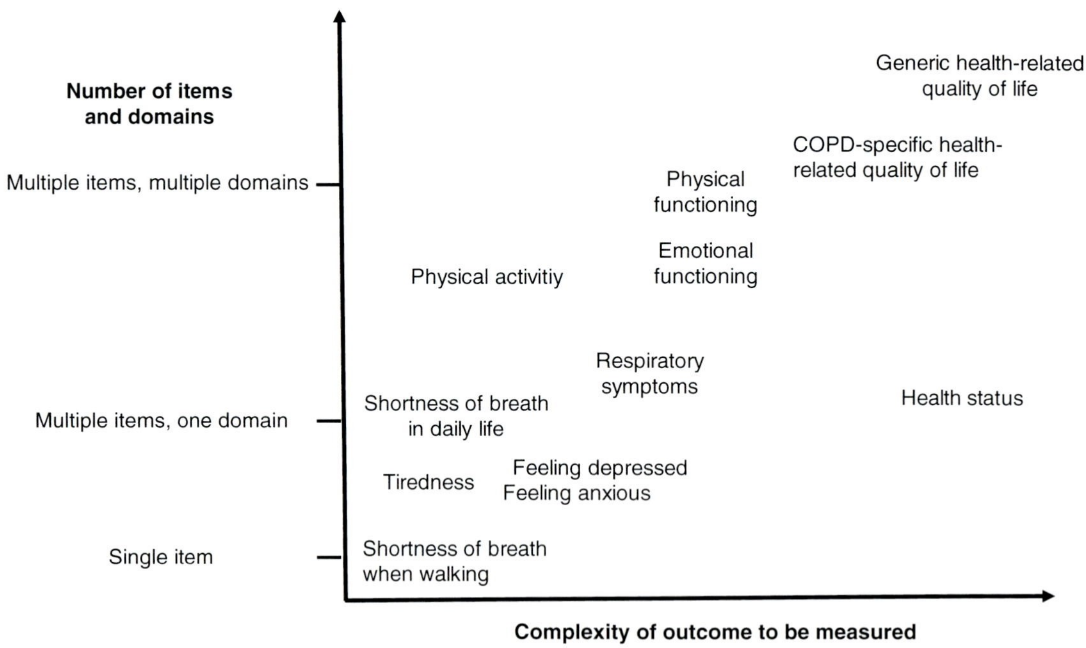

Fig. 7.1 Patient-reported outcomes used in the pulmonary rehabilitation setting according to complexity and number of items and domains. Adapted from: Quality of Life and Pharmacoeconomics in Clinical Trials. Editor: Bert Spilker. 2 Sub Edition. Lippincott Williams & Wilkins; ISBN-13: 978-0781703321

activity and impact domains of the SGRQ) or in a more inclusive score (e.g. physical functioning of the Short Form Health Survey 36 [SF-36] or SGRQ total score). The latter reflects more abstract concepts such as health-related quality of life that are not directly measured but that reflect the patients' perception of the physical, psychological and social burden associated with a specific disease (i.e. disease-specific health-related quality of life) or health (i.e. generic health-related quality of life) more generally. It is important to remember though that most instruments ask about specific symptoms or limitations and not about these more abstract constructs directly, which are difficult to assess in a standardized way across patients.

7.2 PRO Instruments Commonly Used in Respiratory Rehabilitation

A large number of PRO instruments exist, and several databases of commercial or non-commercial providers are available that list them (e.g. https://eprovide.mapi-trust.org/, www.testzentrale.de, http://www.healthmeasures.net/explore-measurement-systems/promis) [11]. Several review articles exist that discuss PRO instruments commonly used in the field of COPD [12–14]. Here, we describe the PRO instruments that are used commonly in respiratory rehabilitation. Further below, we discuss important measurement properties of these instruments including their minimal important difference (MID) and how to select PROs for research and practice.

7.2.1 PRO Instruments to Measure Symptoms of Importance for Patients with COPD

The most commonly used dyspnoea instrument used in trials of respiratory rehabilitation is the dyspnoea domain of the CRQ (24 of the 65 RCTs included in the most recent update of the Cochrane review) [4]. In its original, individualized version, patients were asked to select five situations or activities in which they experience dyspnoea. They then rated the extent of dyspnoea on a Likert-type scale from 1 (extremely severe) to 7 (not severe at all). This individualized version of the CRQ dyspnoea domain is highly responsive to pick up changes of respiratory rehabilitation since it is tailored individually. In 2003, a fully standardized dyspnoea domain became available that is used by most studies since then [15]. The five questions asked patients about the degree of dyspnoea during five situations (basic activities of daily living, walking, doing household, participating in social activities and being angry or upset). The symptom domain of the SGRQ has also been used widely in trials of respiratory rehabilitation and goes beyond dyspnoea. It asks patients about the frequency and severity of cough, sputum, wheezing, shortness of breath and exacerbations.

Other PROs sometimes used to measure dyspnoea as an outcome measure to evaluate the effects of respiratory rehabilitation include the MRC Dyspnoea Scale and the Baseline Dyspnea Index (BDI) and Transition Dyspnea Index (TDI). The original MRC breathlessness scale dates back to the 1950s when it was used in coal miner, postmen and post office employee studies [16]. Patients are asked to pick the statement about breathlessness that applies most to them. The statements range from 1 ("not troubled by breathlessness except on strenuous exercise") to incapacitating dyspnoea (5, "too breathlessness to leave the house, or breathless when undressing"). The modified MRC scale ranges from 0 to 4 but is otherwise the same as the original MRC scale [17]. The MRC is not straightforward to administer. When interviewer administered, interviewers need to make sure patients understand each statement and how the extent of breathlessness and disability varies from 0 to 4. When self-administered, patients sometimes feel uncertain how to pick the statement that applies to them. Four of the five statements are somewhat ambiguous because they list two different situations so that one situation may apply to an individual and the other not. These challenges can lead to measurement error or even systematically different answers when administered differently or used in different populations or contexts.

The BDI is a PRO to quantify dyspnoea in three categories (functional impairment, magnitude of task, magnitude of effort) and uses a scale from 0 to 4 resulting in a score from 0 to 12 [18, 19]. Its purpose is to discriminate between patients with more or less dyspnoea. The TDI quantifies changes in dyspnoea from a baseline state in the same three categories. It uses a scale from −3 (major deterioration) to 3 (major improvement) with 0 representing no change and results in a score ranging from −9 to 9. Originally developed as a physician interview with the patient, self-administered, computer-based and paper and pencil versions have been introduced later. A common dyspnoea score used in respiratory rehabilitation is the Borg scale. However, it should be noted that the purpose of using the Borg scale is mostly for guiding the intensity of exercise training. Patients are asked, during or after exercise and an exercise test, to express their level of breathlessness on a scale from 0 to 10 (there are multiple versions with different numerical values).

Another respiratory symptom score used in COPD research but unfrequently in the context of respiratory rehabilitation is the EXAcerbations of Chronic Pulmonary Disease Tool (EXACT-PRO). The EXACT-PRO is a 14-item daily diary PRO measure that evaluates the frequency, severity and duration of symptoms of COPD exacerbations [20]. Thus, a possible use of the EXACT-PRO in respiratory rehabilitation could be as part of post-exacerbation trials in order to get a detailed assessment of how the symptoms change with post-exacerbation rehabilitation or as a monitoring tool to capture exacerbations as important outcomes. The breathlessness, cough and sputum scale also measures the severity of respiratory symptoms (breathlessness, cough and sputum) and can be used as a daily diary [21]. But as with the EXACT-PRO and other PROs, it has rarely been used in patients undergoing respiratory rehabilitation.

Finally, aspects of mental health are of great importance for COPD patients and respiratory rehabilitation programs. A substantial proportion of COPD patients suffers from symptoms of depression and anxiety. Of course, major depression and anxiety disorders occur in COPD patients irrespective of COPD, but the majority of patients have symptoms of depression and anxiety as a consequence of being chronically ill for many years as it is the case for patients with other chronic diseases. Respiratory rehabilitation has been shown to reduce symptoms of depression and anxiety to a clinically meaningful extent. The most commonly used PRO instrument is the Hospital Anxiety and Depression Scale (HADS) [22]. Its 14 items (7 for items of depression and anxiety each) ask patients on a scale from 0 to 3 about symptoms of depression and anxiety, and the domain score ranges from 0 to 21. The questionnaire is self-administered and straightforward for patients to complete. There are many other PROs to measure mental health, but the HADS has been used most commonly in respiratory rehabilitation.

7.2.2 PRO Instruments to Measure Health-Related Quality of Life

The CRQ or SGRQ has been used in two thirds of all RCTs comparing respiratory rehabilitation and usual care in stable COPD patients and in patients after an exacerbation. Both PRO instruments are disease specific as they address symptoms and limitations that are typical for patients with COPD or chronic respiratory disease. The CRQ has 20 items and four domains. The dyspnoea and fatigue domains address common symptoms of COPD patients, while the emotional function domain captures mental health, mainly symptoms of depression. Finally, the mastery domain asks patients how they cope with COPD. The developers of the CRQ always suggested to report the four CRQ domains separately and advised against a total score because it may mask important information from the domain scores. Nevertheless, a total score has been used by many investigators but been calculated differently (either as sum of the 20 items or as average of the four domain scores). Nowadays, the self-administered standardized version of the CRQ is mostly used, which facilitates comparisons across studies [15].

The SGRQ has originally 50 items and measures health-related quality of life in patients with chronic airflow limitation [7]. The refined 40-item version has been developed for COPD patients and is nowadays mostly used. The SGRQ has three domains (symptoms, activity and impact) and a total score, each of which are calculated from the specific items that are weighted differently. The symptom domain captures the frequency and severity of respiratory symptoms including cough, sputum, wheezing, shortness of breath and exacerbations. The activity domain asks patients about limitations in activities of daily living, and the impact domain assesses how patients experience the respiratory disease in terms of the impact of symptoms and activity limitations on their daily life. In comparison to the CRQ that focuses mostly on symptoms and coping as major and disease-specific determinants of health-related quality of life, the SGRQ also considers contextual factors from the patients' everyday life.

Other COPD-specific PROs exist, but they have been used less frequently in the context of respiratory rehabilitation. The Clinical COPD Questionnaire (CCQ) has ten items the patients can complete themselves and gives domain scores symptoms, functional state and mental state [23]. It has been developed for the primary care setting, but it does have measurement properties that would make it a suitable tool for the evaluation of respiratory rehabilitation. Similarly, the COPD Assessment Test (CAT) is a simple PRO instrument that quantifies symptoms of COPD patients and that is responsive to pick up the effects of respiratory rehabilitation [24].

Finally, there are non-COPD-specific PROs to measure health-related quality of life. The Short Form Health Survey, probably the most widely used PRO instrument in the medical field, has been used in respiratory rehabilitation [25]. Both the 36- and the 12-item versions have been used to derive different domain scores that do, however, not address specific problems of COPD patients. The Short Form Health Survey has been developed as a discriminative measure, and it is able to show differences in health-related quality of life of patients with mild, moderate or severe disease, but it has limited value for the evaluation of respiratory rehabilitation because of limited responsiveness. This is generally true for generic health-related quality of life instruments that are substantially less responsive than the disease-specific CRQ or SGRQ [26]. Of note, a simple PRO instrument, the feeling thermometer (FT), is an exception because it is more responsive to treatment changes than other generic instruments. The FT is a modified visual analogue scale with numerical values that range from 0 (worst imaginable health state) to 100 (best imaginable health state). Patients are asked to draw a line between 0 and 100 on the FT that reflects their health status on the past 7 days. The FT is part of the EuroQol-5D [27], a commonly used instrument with five items to derive utilities for cost analyses, and has been used repeatedly in the context of respiratory rehabilitation [26, 28].

7.3 Key Measurement Properties of PRO Instruments for Pulmonary Rehabilitation

It is essential that PRO instruments validly assess the outcome they intend to assess, that they assess the intended outcomes consistently and that their specific purpose (i.e. evaluative, discriminative or predictive) is clear. In the context of pulmonary rehabilitation, the evaluative properties are arguably most important, and instruments need to be able to detect changes over time caused by the rehabilitation. Moreover, clinicians and researchers are interested in whether a specific change score of a PRO instrument derived from assessments before and after rehabilitation actually reflects a difference that is relevant for the patient. These requirements are expressed by the measurement properties of PRO instruments, the reliability, validity, responsiveness and minimal important difference. However, measurement properties are not only relevant for the validation process but provide the basis for the entire development process of new PROs.

7.3.1 Development of PROs

The development of PRO instruments is an iterative process for which different strategies and methods can be used. Nevertheless, at the beginning of the process, developers should clearly define the concept the PRO should assess, the population it is targeted to, the purpose it should fulfil (e.g. being able to detect changes over time or to discriminate between persons) and whether the PRO instrument should meet specific requirements regarding its format (e.g. self-administered or interviewer administered, maximum time required for completion, etc.). The intended purpose of the instruments determines the required validation methods. For example, the validity for instruments with a discriminative purpose should be assessed cross-sectionally, whereas the validity for an instrument with an evaluative aim should be tested in a longitudinal design.

In the last years, both the US Food and Drug Administration (FDA) and European Medicines Agency (EMA) have developed guidance documents or recommendations on the appropriate development, validation and use of PRO instruments [1, 29, 30]. This illustrates the growing acknowledgement of PRO measurements in the evaluation of therapies by the regulatory bodies, i.e. the importance of whether or not the patient actually perceives an improvement of his or her state. The FDA guidance document describes how the FDA reviews and evaluates the adequacy of PRO instruments that are intended to be used as endpoints in labelling claims. Besides the measurement properties of the instrument, a main aspect that the FDA evaluates is whether evidence is given for patient input during item generation and testing to ensure content validity. Also the International Society for Pharmacoeconomics and Outcomes Research (ISPOR) published recommendations on establishing content validity of newly designed PRO instruments [31, 32]. Content validity refers to the extent to which the concepts of interest are comprehensively represented by the items of the PRO. It can only be established during the development process of a new instrument.

Another main aspect that the FDA evaluates is whether the instrument is based on a conceptual framework. The conceptual framework explicitly defines the concepts measured by the instrument and describes, using a diagram, the relationships between single items (e.g. dyspnoea during walking on level ground), sub-domains (e.g. dyspnoea), domains (e.g. symptoms) and concepts (e.g. health-related quality of life) measured as well as the score(s) obtained from the PRO instrument. An inadequate or lacking conceptual framework questions the grouping of items into domains and the analysis and the interpretation of PRO scores, and it may be unclear what is actually measured [33]. The conceptual framework should be drafted by the developers based on literature reviews and expert opinion at the beginning and will usually be adapted and confirmed over the course of instrument development based on patient input [29].

Many PROs which are used in pulmonary rehabilitation were developed prior to the publication of the FDA guidelines and are unlikely to completely fulfil all requirements. More recently, PROs have been developed in larger initiatives and in collaboration between COPD specialists, instrument development experts and the regulatory bodies, such as the daily diary EXACT-PRO. Another example is the Innovative Medicines Initiative's (IMI) PROactive project undertaken by a consortium of academic organizations and pharmaceutical companies with formal input from the FDA and EMA.

The background of the PROactive project was the growing evidence on the negative effect of physical inactivity in COPD patients, particularly regarding progression of disease, incidence of exacerbations and mortality [34]. The need for a tool to capture patient-relevant dimensions of physical activity emerged that fulfils the methodological requirements for PRO instruments to be used in academic or industry clinical trials. The aim of PROactive was to develop and validate two PRO instruments to capture experience of physical activity in patients with COPD, one for the daily assessment of physical activity and one for use during clinical study visits. These instruments, the D-PPAC and C-PPAC (daily and clinical visit versions of the PROactive physical activity in COPD instruments), are also presented in Chap. 8, "Assessment of Physical Activity". In short, they capture the experience of physical activity on the two domains "amount of physical activity" and "difficulty with physical activity" [35, 36]. The instruments are hybrid tools combining a short PRO questionnaire and two activity monitor variables. The D-PPAC refers to daily physical activity (recall today) and includes nine items; the C-PPAC refers to physical activity during the last 7 days and includes 14 items. Each item is scored from 0 to 4, and the raw scores are scaled to two domain scores ranging from 0 to 100. Although physical activity PROs might have limited purposes for use during pulmonary rehabilitation, they can be crucial to look beyond pulmonary rehabilitation into daily life of patients.

In the following, we exemplify the development process of new PROs by the description of the development of the PROactive instruments, since within the PROactive project, a systematic approach has been used and recommendations by the regulatory bodies were followed. Figure 7.2 shows the entire development and validation process of new PROs.

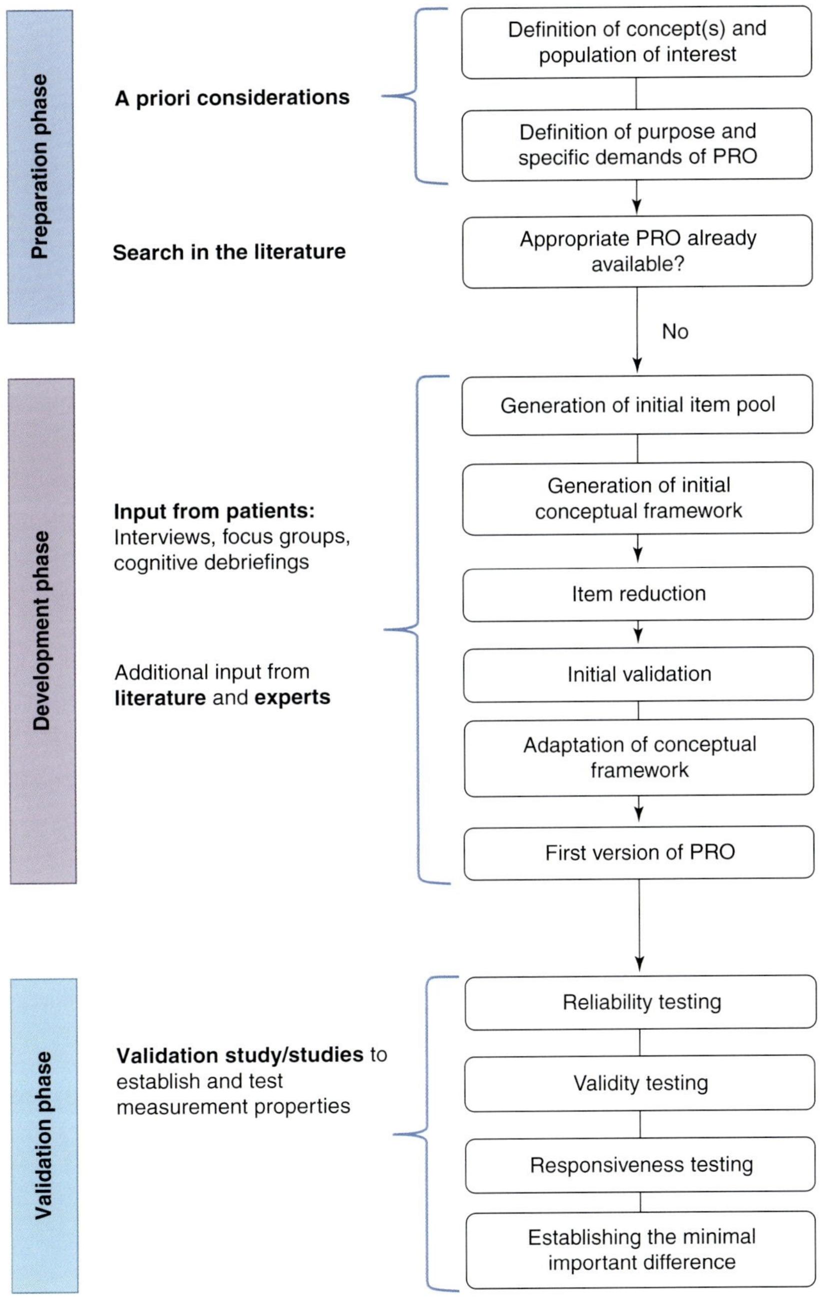

Fig. 7.2 Overview of development and validation process of new PRO instruments

7.3.1.1 Development and Initial Validation Steps: Illustrated by the PROactive Instruments

Before undertaking the time-consuming and cost-intensive process of developing a new PRO, it is recommended to conduct a thorough or even *systematic literature search* to learn whether a suitable PRO is already available that assesses the concept of interest and fulfils the methodological requirements for the purpose it is intended to be used.

Within the PROactive project, several systematic reviews of the literature were conducted regarding the relevant topics of the project, namely, the existence, characteristics and methodological quality of PRO instruments and activity monitors to assess physical activity. The systematic reviews showed that although many PRO instruments exist to assess physical activity in chronically ill or elderly persons covering a broad range of physical activity content, there was no consensus on content and format of the PROs [37]. For the majority of the PROs, the development process lacked important aspects such as patient input for item identification and reduction that would have ensured content validity [38]. None of the instruments was developed based on a conceptual framework of physical activity [39], and the quality of the initial validation varied widely between instruments. Particularly responsiveness to change was assessed only for a minority and the minimal important difference for just a fraction of the instruments. Thus, the systematic reviews showed that no PRO instrument was developed according to the state-of-the-art methodology and that none was specifically designed to detect small but important treatment changes in COPD patients. Therefore, the reviews justified the development of a new PRO. The results of the systematic reviews also supported the draft of an initial PROactive conceptual framework and informed and added to the initial item pool.

Items can be generated by different sources such as literature reviews, experts (clinicians, researchers), family members or close persons, but most importantly *item generation* should include input from the target patient population in order to ensure content validity. Input from patients is also crucial to inform the *conceptual framework* of the new PRO. Qualitative methods such as interviews, focus groups and cognitive debriefings can be used to detect relevant concepts and to generate item wordings, to evaluate the completeness of item coverage and to assess clarity and readability. Item generation ideally includes the input of a wide range of patients with the condition of interest to represent a wide variety of the patients' characteristics so that content validity is ensured.

Within the PROactive project, all these qualitative methods have been applied in studies with COPD patients from four European countries. One-to-one interviews provided information on how patients experience physical activity. The results were used to develop an initial conceptual framework and a discussion guide for the focus groups. Focus groups were conducted to evaluate whether any additional themes related to physical activity were missing and to discuss the preferred format of the questionnaire. Based on the transcripts of the interviews and focus groups, a draft item list was generated and integrated in an e-PRO device to undergo cognitive debriefings with patients. In cognitive debriefings, the patients' understanding of the draft items and instructions is assessed by targeting mental processes (i.e. comprehension, retrieval, judgement and response) the patients use when completing the PRO instrument. This information is used to revise the items and instructions. Three themes emerged from the qualitative studies: the impact of COPD on amount of physical activity, symptoms experienced during physical activity and adaptations made to facilitate physical activity. These themes emerged similarly irrespective of country, demographic or disease characteristics. Iterative rounds of appraisal and refinement of candidate items resulted in 30 items with a daily recall period (draft daily version) and 34 items with a 7-day recall period (draft clinical version) which represented the pivotal basis for the subsequent empirically based item reduction and validation [35]. In order to capture the complete patient experience with physical activity, activity monitors have also been considered to contribute to the development of the instruments. As a result of the literature review [40] and additionally conducted laboratory validation studies [41, 42], two activity monitors showed to accurately assess physical activity in the target population of COPD patients and were selected to be used in the subsequent study.

The next step of the development process is *item reduction*. The initially generated items are applied to the target patient population in order to assess quantitatively how the individual items are answered by the patients: using quantitative methods such as Rasch analysis and classical item-response theory, it is assessed how the answers to the items cover the continuum of the possible responses, how the items are able to distinguish between different patients or how items correlate between each other and the total score. Subsequently, factor analyses can be used to test whether the actual measures reflect the hypothesized dimensions of the new PRO. Results from these quantitative methods together with qualitative input from patients and experts contribute to the item reduction process.

In the PROactive project, an initial validation study was performed in order to reduce the item pool, to confirm the conceptual framework and to initially validate the PROactive tools. The 6-week, randomized, two-way crossover, multicentre study assessed in 236 COPD patients from five European centres the daily and clinical versions of the draft PROactive instruments and the two selected activity monitors [36]. The items of the draft daily and clinical versions were reduced from 30 to 7 and from 35 to 12 items based on several statistical criteria, and both versions were supplemented with two variables from the activity monitors, resulting in the final version of the instruments, the D-PPAC and C-PPAC.

Subsequently, the D-PPAC and C-PPAC have been further validated in six longitudinal studies, performed by Academia and EFPIA partners, including over 1000 COPD patients. In summary, the conceptual framework has been confirmed, and both PPAC instruments have demonstrated construct validity. The available data showed indication of responsiveness and allowed identification of the minimal important difference (MID).

7.3.2 Key Measurement Properties to Be Tested in Validation Studies

In the following, we will describe the key measurement properties reliability, validity, responsiveness and MID, illustrated by the two most frequently used health-related quality of life PROs in COPD, the CRQ and SGRQ. Both instruments have extensively been used in COPD trials and in the pulmonary rehabilitation setting but were developed years before the FDA guidance document was published. However, both instruments have been recommended by the EMA as a suitable health-related quality of life instrument that can be used in COPD drug development programs and clinical trials, and the SGRQ has been mentioned as a suitable endpoint in the COPD draft guidance by the FDA [12]. Both instruments have been validated in several studies. A recent systematic review on psychometric properties of quality of life measurements in COPD detected 23 papers assessing psychometric properties of the CRQ and 26 papers assessing psychometric properties of the SGRQ, and the authors rated the overall evidence based on the criteria number of studies, the methodological quality of the studies and the consistency of the results [43].

7.3.2.1 Reliability

Reliability refers to the overall consistency of a measure, i.e. the extent to which an instrument produces consistent results for stable individuals on different occasions or by different observers. Measures of reliability include internal consistency, test-retest reliability and, for interviewer-administered PROs, inter-rater reliability.

Internal consistency describes the extent to which all the items of a PRO scale or PRO subscales reflect the same underlying concept. It is most commonly assessed by Cronbach's alpha which represents the average correlation among the items of the scale and/or subscales, respectively. Good internal consistency measures have been proposed to have Cronbach's alpha values of 0.70 to 0.90 or 0.95. Too low values indicate a lack of correlation between the items which questions the summarizing of the items into a scale; a very high value indicates redundancy of information across items. Cronbach's alpha also depends on the number of items in the scale; with an increasing number of items, the value increases [44].

Test-retest reliability relates to the degree to which repeated measurements in stable persons provide similar answers. The time interval between the repeated assessments should be long enough to prevent recall and short enough to ensure that no real change has occurred. Test-retest reliability is usually assessed by intra-class correlation coefficient (ICC) expressed as a ratio between 0 and 1 ($\geq$0.7 recommended [44]) and by Bland-Altman plots. Correlation coefficients (e.g. Pearson or Spearman rank) are not enough to assess test-retest reliability since they can miss systematic differences between the first and subsequent measurements.

Both the CRQ and SGRQ demonstrated good to high internal consistency and test-retest reliability [12]. Weldam et al. rated for the CRQ strong evidence for internal consistency and moderate evidence for test-retest reliability and for the SGRQ moderate evidence for internal consistency and strong evidence for test-retest reliability [43].

7.3.2.2 Validity

Validity describes the extent to which the instrument measures the construct it is intended to measure. As already described, content validity refers to the extent to which the concepts of interest are comprehensively represented by the items of the PRO. It can only be established during the development process of a new instrument.

The CRQ was developed including review of current literature, input from clinical respiratory specialist and patient interviews by using classical test theory. The original 50-item version of the SGRQ was developed with patient input, and the 40-item version was derived from the original version after detailed analysis of data from large studies in COPD. Using Rasch modelling, weaker items were removed and the measurement properties of the instrument improved. For both instruments, there was strong evidence summarized for content validity [12, 43].

Construct validity is a measure of the extent to which scores on the new instrument relate to other measures or characteristics of patients conform to a priori stated hypotheses concerning the strength of the relationship. The specific hypotheses usually are stated either about the expected strength of the correlations between the measures (e.g. $r > 0.6$, high; $r = 0.4$–0.6, moderate; $r < 0.4$, weak) or about the expected differences in scores between "known groups" (i.e. known-group validity).

Measures that were used to assess the construct validity of the CRQ and SGRQ were on the one hand PRO instruments assessing dyspnoea such as the BDI/TDI or modified MRC dyspnoea scale, general health-related quality of life such as the SF-36 or mental constructs such as the HADS. On the other hand, lung function measures such as FEV1 and exercise capacity measures such as six-minute walk test were used. Since the two instruments assess similar constructs, both have been used to assess construct validity of each other. Summarized, both instruments usually show good construct validity since observed correlations with validation instruments met expected correlations. Weldam et al. rated strong evidence for the CRQ and moderate evidence for the SGRQ for construct validity and hypothesis testing.

7.3.2.3 Responsiveness

Responsiveness describes the extent to which an instrument can detect changes over time. In order to detect true treatment effects, it is crucial that PROs, which are used to evaluate the effects of pulmonary rehabilitation, are responsive. Poor responsiveness could either reflect that the treatment was truly ineffective or that the treatment was actually effective but the tool insensitive to detect changes (false-negative result). Responsiveness is best assessed in a situation where an effect is strongly expected to occur. Pulmonary rehabilitation offers a good setting since many randomized trials have shown its effects [4]. If a PRO indeed shows a relevant before-after difference (e.g. effect size $\geq$ 0.5) in such situations, it is considered responsive.

One study directly compared the responsiveness of the CRQ with the responsiveness of the SGRQ after pulmonary rehabilitation in a sample of lung disease patients, primarily COPD, and showed that both instruments were responsive to the rehabilitation. However, the CRQ subscales were more responsive than the SGRQ subscales, and total score and the highest effect sizes were observed for the CRQ dyspnoea domain [26].

7.3.2.4 Minimal Important Difference

The minimal important difference (MID) refers to the smallest change in the score of a PRO measure that is perceived by patients as beneficial or harmful. There is no clear consensus for the best practice approach for determining the MID of a PRO, but a frequently used approach to establish an MID is combining anchor-based methods with distribution-based methods and to triangulate on a single value or small range of values for the MID. Anchor-based approaches use an external indicator (e.g. clinical or another established PRO) with a demonstrated MID in the target patient populations as the anchor, distribution-based methods include statistical criteria such as effect sizes or the standard error of measurement. Confidence in a specific MID usually evolves over time and is confirmed by additional evidence, and MID may vary by population and context [45].

For both instruments, the CRQ and the SGRQ MIDs have been well-established, for the CRQ domains an improvement of 0.5 points and for the SGRQ domains and total scores an improvement of 4 points [12]. Results from the recent systematic review on pulmonary rehabilitation for COPD [4] showed that a statistically significant improvement for the CRQ domains and the SGRQ domains and total score were shown in patients after rehabilitation compared to those allocated to control groups. The meta-analyses indicated that these changes exceeded the MID of 0.5 or 4 points, respectively.

7.4 Selection of PROs for Pulmonary Rehabilitation

This section describes how to select an appropriate PRO instrument for the pulmonary rehabilitation setting. There exists no single correct answer. We suggest a selection approach that is based on several predefined criteria and will illustrate the approach using the example of a hypothetical RCT. Let's assume that the RCT aims to compare the effect of a home-based, supervised pulmonary rehabilitation program versus an outpatient-based supervised pulmonary rehabilitation program in COPD patients after suffering from an exacerbation. The investigators have chosen psychological well-being or mental health as the primary outcome and need to select the instrument. For the assessment of the psychological well-being or mental health, the following potential PRO instruments may be used: the emotional function domain of the CRQ, the symptoms domain of the SGRQ, the FT, the SF-36 or the HADS. There are, of course, a number of other instruments, but we restrict our example for selecting a PRO to these tools for simplicity since they have been described above.

The suggested selection criteria are summarized in Table 7.1 together with our ratings applied to the example, with +++ meaning that the respective criterion is fully met, ++ moderately, + partly

Table 7.1 Criteria for selecting a PRO instrument applied to the RCT example for the outcome psychological well-being/mental health

Criteria	CRQ	SGRQ	SF-36	FT	HADS
Measures what it is intended to measure	++	–	++	+	+++
Matches measures of existing trials	+++	+++	+	+	++
Can be measured reliably	+++	+++	+++	++	+++
Has shown validity	+++	+++	+++	++	+++
Is responsive to change	+++	+++	+	++	++
Has an established MID	+++	+++	+	++	++
Is efficient to measure	++	+	+	+++	++

Abbreviations: *CRQ* Chronic Respiratory Questionnaire, *SGRQ* St. George's Respiratory Questionnaire, *SF-36* Short Form Health Survey, *FT* feeling thermometer, *HADS* Hospital Anxiety and Depression Scale
Ratings from +++ (criterion fully met) to – (not met)

met and – not met. We would like to highlight, however, that the relevance of some criteria is also depending on the kind of study in which the PRO is used. In contrast to the current example where a PRO is used to evaluate an intervention, a study that aims to distinguish between patients with different degree of psychological well-being would have cross-sectional or known-group validity as a criterion rather than responsiveness or an established MID.

A key criterion is whether the PRO *measures what it is intended to measure*; for our example, this means whether the PRO assesses psychological well-being or mental health in COPD patients. The HADS specifically addresses symptoms of depression and anxiety and provides two distinct domain scores. Although it was not specifically developed for COPD patients, it is widely used in the COPD research field. The CRQ and SGRQ both are disease-specific health-related quality of life instruments specifically developed for COPD patients. The SGRQ however has no specific psychological well-being or mental health domain, although some of its items address emotional disturbances. The CRQ in contrast provides an individual emotional function domain that captures mental health, mainly symptoms of depression, with seven items. The FT and SF-36 are both generic instruments. The FT reflects the general health status on the past 7 days and is not specific to emotional well-being. In contrast, the SF-36 consists of a mental health and role emotional subscale as well as a mental component summary score.

The second selection criterion we suggest refers to the question whether the PRO *matches measures of existing trials*, which means for our example whether and how frequently the specific instrument has been applied in RCTs including COPD patients undergoing pulmonary rehabilitation setting. This criterion is important to ensure that the results of the RCT can be compared to the existing body of evidence. Both the CRQ and SGRQ were frequently used as outcome instruments in pulmonary rehabilitation trials on stable COPD patients and patients after exacerbations [4, 5]. The HADS is the most commonly used PRO instrument to assess symptoms of anxiety and depression in studies including COPD patients but was less frequently used as an outcome measure in RCTs than the CRQ or SGRQ. This also applies to the generic SF-36 and FT which were even more rarely used in these trials.

The criteria whether the PRO *can be measured reliably* and whether *validity has been shown* can be rated to be fully met for the CRQ and SGRQ, as already outlined in Sect. 7.3.2. Both instruments demonstrated good to high internal consistency and test-retest reliability in COPD patients and good construct validity and conform to a priori stated hypotheses concerning the strength of the relationship. Only few studies evaluated the reliability and validity of the FT in COPD patients but showed good test-retest reliability and validity. For the SF-36 and the HADS, good internal consistency and construct validity have been shown in different patient populations, but only very few studies specifically included COPD populations.

The next criterion is whether the PRO *is responsive to detect changes* after pulmonary rehabilitation. Usually disease-specific instruments are more responsive to change than generic instruments. The disease-specific CRQ and SGRQ showed good responsiveness to rehabilitation in pulmonary rehabilitation trials including COPD patients. In contrast, the few studies that examined responsiveness for the SF-36 after rehabilitation in COPD patients demonstrated either only low to moderate changes in the SF-36 subscales and component summary scores or no improvement [46]. This pattern was also shown in a study which directly compared the responsiveness of the CRQ, SGRQ, FT and SF-36 in COPD patients after respiratory rehabilitation, where higher responsiveness was found for the disease-specific CRQ and SGRQ compared to the generic FT and SF-36. In particular, the CRQ emotional function domain was significantly more responsive than the SF-36 mental composite score [26]. Only few studies assessed the responsiveness of the FT and the HADS in COPD patients after rehabilitation. However, good responsiveness was shown for both instruments; for the HADS domains, the responsiveness was even comparable to the SGRQ total score [47].

Analogous to responsiveness, the *MID* has been well-*established* in COPD patients for the CRQ and the SGRQ using anchor- and distribution-based approaches. The MID has also been established for the FT and the HADS in COPD patients but in fewer studies. To our knowledge, even if the MID has been established for the SF-36 subscales and component summary scores for some patient populations, none has been established so far specifically for COPD patients.

The final criterion on how to choose a PRO is whether it is *efficient to measure* which refers to the time it takes for administration, to the mode of administration and to the calculation of scores. All five PROs are fully structured questionnaires with clear instructions for administration. The FT, which consists of one single rating using a modified visual analogue scale with numerical values, takes very little time for the patient to fill in and does not have to be scored. The HADS with 14 items, the CRQ with 20 items, the SF-36 with 36 and the SGRQ with 40 items take increasingly more time to fill in. The depression and anxiety domain scores of the HADS and the CRQ domain scores can be easily computed, for the HADS by summing up the item values and for the CRQ domain scores by averaging the items of the specific domains. The scoring for the SF-36 and the SGRQ is slightly more complex. For the SF-36, the item values are recoded according to a scoring key so that each item is scored on a 0 to 100 range, and then the items in the same scale are averaged together. Also the SGRQ domain and total scores are transformed into a 0 to 100 scale after weights have been assigned to the single item answers. However, for the SGRQ, an Excel-based scoring calculator is provided by the authors facilitating the scoring.

Based on these criteria, either the emotional function domain of the CRQ or the HADS appears to be an appropriate choice for the RCT. The HADS offers a more comprehensive assessment of mental health aspects and offers two distinct domains, anxiety and depression, whereas the CRQ emotional domain is a simpler assessment of mental health representing merely depression symptoms. However, the CRQ offers also the assessment of other aspects of health-related quality of life, was specifically developed for COPD patients and more widely validated in this population compared to the HADS. Again, the criteria and judgements need to be adapted to the study question at issue and are subjective, but such an approach helps to find an appropriate tool based on the outcome to be measured, existing evidence and practical considerations.

7.5 Key Points/Conclusion

- PROs, from specific symptoms to health-related quality life, have been important outcome measures in pulmonary rehabilitation for a long time and paved the way for their use in clinical research in general.
- A thorough development process provides the necessary basis for the validity and other measurement properties of PROs.
- In the context of pulmonary rehabilitation and its evaluation, evaluative PRO instruments are usually the first choice that are responsive to change and have an established MID. Disease-specific PROs like the CRQ or SGRQ are more responsive and thus more suitable than generic PROs.
- The selection of a PRO instrument is greatly facilitated if a systematic approach with predefined criteria about the content, measurement properties and practical aspects is followed.

References

1. US Department of Health and Human Services; Food and Drug Administration. Guidance for industry: patient-reported outcome measures: use in medical product development to support labeling claims. 2009. http://www.fda.gov/downloads/Drugs/Guidances/UCM193282.pdf. Accessed 24 Oct 2016.
2. Petty TL, et al. A comprehensive care program for chronic airway obstruction. Methods and preliminary evaluation of symptomatic and functional improvement. Ann Intern Med. 1969;70(6):1109–20.
3. McGavin CR, et al. Physical rehabilitation for the chronic bronchitic: results of a controlled trial of exercises in the home. Thorax. 1977;32(3):307–11.
4. McCarthy B, et al. Pulmonary rehabilitation for chronic obstructive pulmonary disease. Cochrane Database Syst Rev. 2015;2:CD003793.

5. Puhan MA, et al. Pulmonary rehabilitation following exacerbations of chronic obstructive pulmonary disease. Cochrane Database Syst Rev. 2016;1:CD005305.
6. Guyatt GH, et al. A measure of quality of life for clinical trials in chronic lung disease. Thorax. 1987;42(10):773–8.
7. Jones PW, et al. A self-complete measure of health status for chronic airflow limitation. The St. George's Respiratory Questionnaire. Am Rev Respir Dis. 1992;145(6):1321–7.
8. Guyatt GH, Feeny DH, Patrick DL. Measuring health-related quality of life. Ann Intern Med. 1993;118(8):622–9.
9. Celli BR, et al. The body-mass index, airflow obstruction, dyspnea, and exercise capacity index in chronic obstructive pulmonary disease. N Engl J Med. 2004;350(10):1005–12.
10. Puhan MA, et al. Expansion of the prognostic assessment of patients with chronic obstructive pulmonary disease: the updated BODE index and the ADO index. Lancet. 2009;374(9691):704–11.
11. Emery M-P, Perrier L-L, Acquadro C. Patient-reported outcome and quality of life instruments database (PROQOLID): frequently asked questions. Health Qual Life Outcomes. 2005;3:12.
12. Cazzola M, et al. A review of the most common patient-reported outcomes in COPD—revisiting current knowledge and estimating future challenges. Int J Chron Obstruct Pulmon Dis. 2015;10:725–38.
13. Ekström M, Sundh J, Larsson K. Patient reported outcome measures in chronic obstructive pulmonary disease: which to use? Expert Rev Respir Med. 2016;10(3):351–62.
14. Jones P, et al. Beyond FEV_1 in COPD: a review of patient-reported outcomes and their measurement. Int J Chron Obstruct Pulmon Dis. 2012;7:697–709.
15. Schünemann HJ, et al. A comparison of the original chronic respiratory questionnaire with a standardized version. Chest. 2003;124(4):1421–9.
16. Fletcher CM, et al. The significance of respiratory symptoms and the diagnosis of chronic bronchitis in a working population. Br Med J. 1959;2(5147):257–66.
17. Mahler DA, Wells CK. Evaluation of clinical methods for rating dyspnea. Chest. 1988;93(3):580–6.
18. Eakin EG, et al. Reliability and validity of dyspnea measures in patients with obstructive lung disease. Int J Behav Med. 1995;2(2):118–34.
19. Mahler DA, et al. The measurement of dyspnea. Contents, interobserver agreement, and physiologic correlates of two new clinical indexes. Chest. 1984;85(6):751–8.
20. Leidy NK, et al. Development of the EXAcerbations of Chronic Obstructive Pulmonary Disease Tool (EXACT): a patient-reported outcome (PRO) measure. Value Health. 2010;13(8):965–75.
21. Leidy NK, et al. The breathlessness, cough, and sputum scale: the development of empirically based guidelines for interpretation. Chest. 2003;124(6):2182–91.
22. Zigmond AS, Snaith RP. The hospital anxiety and depression scale. Acta Psychiatr Scand. 1983;67(6):361–70.
23. van der Molen T, et al. Development, validity and responsiveness of the Clinical COPD questionnaire. Health Qual Life Outcomes. 2003;1:13.
24. Jones PW, et al. Development and first validation of the COPD assessment test. Eur Respir J. 2009;34(3):648–54.
25. Tarlov AR, et al. The medical outcomes study. An application of methods for monitoring the results of medical care. JAMA. 1989;262(7):925–30.
26. Puhan MA, et al. Relative responsiveness of the Chronic Respiratory Questionnaire, St. Georges Respiratory Questionnaire and four other health-related quality of life instruments for patients with chronic lung disease. Respir Med. 2007;101(2):308–16.
27. The EuroQol Group. EuroQol-a new facility for the measurement of health-related quality of life. Health Policy. 1990;16(3):199–208. http://www.ncbi.nlm.nih.gov/pubmed/10109801.
28. Puhan MA, et al. Measurement of agreement on health-related quality of life changes in response to respiratory rehabilitation by patients and physicians—a prospective study. Respir Med. 2004;98(12):1195–202.
29. Bottomley A, Jones D, Claassens L. Patient-reported outcomes: assessment and current perspectives of the guidelines of the Food and Drug Administration and the reflection paper of the European Medicines Agency. Eur J Cancer. 2009;45(3):347–53.
30. European Medicines Agency. Committee for medicinal products for human use (CHMP). Reflection paper on the regulatory guidance for the use of health-related quality of life (HRQL) measures in the evaluation of medicinal products. 2005. http://www.ema.europa.eu/docs/en_GB/document_library/Scientific_guideline/2014/06/WC500168852.pdf. Accessed 24 Oct 2016.
31. Patrick DL, et al. Content validity—establishing and reporting the evidence in newly developed patient-reported outcomes (PRO) instruments for medical product evaluation: ISPOR PRO Good Research Practices Task Force report: part 1—eliciting concepts for a new PRO instrument. Value Health. 2011a;14(8):967–77.
32. Patrick DL, et al. Content validity—establishing and reporting the evidence in newly developed patient-reported outcomes (PRO) instruments for medical product evaluation: ISPOR PRO Good Research Practices Task Force Report: part 2—assessing respondent understanding. Value Health. 2011b;14(8):978–88.
33. Rothman ML, et al. Patient-reported outcomes: conceptual issues. Value Health. 2007;10:S66–75.
34. Garcia-Aymerich J, et al. Regular physical activity reduces hospital admission and mortality in chronic obstructive pulmonary disease: a population based cohort study. Thorax. 2006;61(9):772–8.

35. Dobbels F, et al. The PROactive innovative conceptual framework on physical activity. Eur Respir J. 2014;44(5):1223–33.
36. Gimeno-Santos E, et al. The PROactive instruments to measure physical activity in patients with chronic obstructive pulmonary disease. Eur Respir J. 2015;46(4):988–1000.
37. Williams K, et al. Patient-reported physical activity questionnaires: a systematic review of content and format. Health Qual Life Outcomes. 2012;10:28.
38. Frei A, et al. A comprehensive systematic review of the development process of 104 patient-reported outcomes (PROs) for physical activity in chronically ill and elderly people. Health Qual Life Outcomes. 2011;9:116.
39. Gimeno-Santos E, et al. Validity of instruments to measure physical activity may be questionable due to a lack of conceptual frameworks: a systematic review. Health Qual Life Outcomes. 2011;9:86.
40. Van Remoortel H, Giavedoni S, et al. Validity of activity monitors in health and chronic disease: a systematic review. Int J Behav Nutr Phys Act. 2012a;9:84.
41. Rabinovich RA, et al. Validity of physical activity monitors during daily life in patients with COPD. Eur Respir J. 2013;42(5):1205–15.
42. Van Remoortel H, Raste Y, et al. Validity of six activity monitors in chronic obstructive pulmonary disease: a comparison with indirect calorimetry. PLoS One. 2012b;7(6):e39198.
43. Weldam SWM, et al. Evaluation of Quality of Life instruments for use in COPD care and research: a systematic review. Int J Nurs Stud. 2013;50(5):688–707.
44. Terwee CB, et al. Quality criteria were proposed for measurement properties of health status questionnaires. J Clin Epidemiol. 2007;60(1):34–42.
45. Revicki D, et al. Recommended methods for determining responsiveness and minimally important differences for patient-reported outcomes. J Clin Epidemiol. 2008;61(2):102–9.
46. Limsuwat C, et al. Pulmonary rehabilitation improves only some domains of health-related quality of life measured by the Short Form-36 questionnaire. Ann Thorac Med. 2014;9(3):144–8.
47. Smid DE, et al. Responsiveness and MCID estimates for CAT, CCQ, and HADS in patients with COPD undergoing pulmonary rehabilitation: a prospective analysis. J Am Med Dir Assoc. 2017;18(1):53–8.

8 Assessment of Physical Activity

Heleen Demeyer and Henrik Watz

The present chapter will describe methods to measure physical activity in patients with COPD. We will mainly focus on the measurement of physical activity using the conventional (physiological) definition in which physical activity is defined as "Any bodily movement produced by skeletal muscles that result in energy expenditure" [1]. We will provide an overview of subjective (questionnaires, part A) and objective (activity monitoring, part B) ways of measuring physical activity in patients, together with their advantages and disadvantages both for research and clinical practice. In the last part (C), the measurement of physical activity beyond the purely physiological definition will be expanded. Table 8.1 summarizes advantages and disadvantages of the proposed instruments to quantify physical activity together with recommendations provided by the authors.

H. Demeyer
Department of Rehabilitation Sciences, KU Leuven, Leuven B-3000, Belgium

Centre for Research in Environmental Epidemiology (CREAL), IS Global, Barcelona, Spain
e-mail: Heleen.demeyer@faber.kuleuven.be

H. Watz (✉)
Pulmonary Research Institute at Lungen Clinic Grosshandorf, Airway Research Center North, German Center for Lung Research, Grosshansdorf, Germany
e-mail: H.Watz@pulmoresearch.de

© Springer International Publishing AG 2018
E. Clini et al. (eds.), *Textbook of Pulmonary Rehabilitation*, https://doi.org/10.1007/978-3-319-65888-9_8

8.1 Questionnaires to Measure the Amount of Physical Activity

By using questionnaires, the measurement of physical activity can be performed in an inexpensive and easy way. These advantages make the use of questionnaires interesting for epidemiological studies and large clinical trials [2]. Questionnaires can be collected remotely (e.g., sent via the Internet), making this a time-efficient way of information collection. This self-report or subjective data collection can be used to obtain insight in the physical activity behavior of patients, both in research and in the clinical practice.

Many questionnaires, frequently available in different versions, have already been used as a measure of daily activity. A thorough systematic review concluded that, currently, 104 different questionnaires are available to measure dimensions of physical activity or related constructs in elderly and chronically ill people [3]. These patient-reported outcome tools could include different aspects of physical activity such as amount, type, duration, and intensity, and they can also capture other aspects of the lifestyle of patients and physical activity-related limitations that may not be captured by an objective activity monitoring [4].

The physical activity recommendations provided by the World Health Organization (WHO) state that healthy adults should engage in at least 150 min of moderate-intensity aerobic physical activity throughout the week, in bouts of at least

Table 8.1 Overview of advantages and disadvantages of instruments to measure physical activity in chronic respiratory disease together with recommendations provided by the authors

Instrument	Pros	Cons	Recommendations
Questionnaires	– Low cost – Easy to administer (can be done remotely)	– Risk for biased results – Poor responsiveness	Questionnaires can be used to classify patients in large epidemiological trials and to screen for severe inactivity. These instruments are not recommended to measure PA in an individual patient, especially not when aiming for measuring changes over time
Doubly labeled water	– Accurate measurement of total energy expenditure	– Expensive – Complex measurement setup – Total daily energy expenditure needs to be corrected for resting energy expenditure	Use for specific research purposes
Pedometers	– Cheap – Ready-to-use devices with a simple metric	– No assessment of other activities or intensity of walking – No assessment of wearing time	Good motivational tools
Accelerometers	– More comprehensive assessment of physical activity including duration and intensity of physical activity	– Purchase costs – Validity in patients with chronic respiratory diseases might not be given in all devices available	Accelerometers are generally recommended for an objective and more comprehensive assessment of physical activity
Wearables	– Availability, consumer friendly – Integration in tele-coaching because of remote data collection and transmission	– No validation in COPD	Potentially helpful in clinical practice due to the widespread use of smartphones; further data in patients with chronic respiratory disease are needed

10-min duration [5]. When interested in classifying patients based on these recommendations, one would probably choose questionnaires including at least measures of duration and frequency of physical activity, not specified to a certain setting (e.g., only work or leisure time activity). However, in other settings, people could possibly be more interested in physical activity-related constructs (e.g., the patients' ability to perform activities of daily living).

When **choosing a questionnaire**, it is important to assure that:

– The questionnaire fits the aim of the measurement in the population of interest ("qualitative attributes of the questionnaires") [4, 6].
– The questionnaire has strong measurement properties in terms of reliability, validity, and responsiveness [3, 7].

When measuring physical activity in patients with chronic respiratory disease such as COPD, it is recommended to choose a questionnaire including measures of light-intense activity. This measure is essential in this inactive population because most of the patients' activities are performed in light intensity [8, 9]. Not having this information in the questionnaire can preclude the classification of patients. For more detailed information, we invite the reader to go to the systematic review by Williams et al. providing an extensive overview of the content of the available physical activity questionnaires for elderly and chronic diseased people [4] and the review by Frei et al. summarizing their measurement properties [3]. For the present chapter, we will focus on self-reported questionnaires aiming to quantify physical activity.

Importantly, the use of physical activity questionnaires comes with **several limitations**, which can lead to biases in the results. These biases limit the use of the questionnaires for individual measurements in clinical practice. In healthy adults, it has been estimated that physical activity questionnaires fail to explain more than 45% of the variance in the measures of physical activity [10]. The most important limitations are the accuracy of the measurement, the effect of social desirability, and the lack of responsiveness.

8.1.1 Accuracy of the Measurement

Information obtained by questionnaires relies on the patients' **recall ability**. The period of recall of questionnaires ranges from as short as 1 h to as long as a lifetime [2]. The accuracy of the measurement depends on the recall period. Questionnaires with a shorter recall period tend to show better results in validation trials as compared to longer periods [11]. Asking for the last week shows better results as when asking for "a usual" PA behavior [12]. In addition, the salience of the activity that has to be recalled is influencing the reliability of the recall [10]. In adults, when comparing to an objective measurement of physical activity, correlations differed slightly with higher correlations for vigorous activity as compared to light activity [12]. Importantly, older adults are more likely to engage in light- to moderate-intense physical activity, which is thus the most difficult type of activity to be assessed by questionnaires. Finally, the magnitude of the recall bias depends on subject characteristics such as education, age, and gender. As a result of completion of a 1-day logbook of activities, 69% of patients with COPD overestimated their walking time, when compared to an objective physical activity measurement [13]. Interestingly, when patients with COPD had to recall their physical activity behavior immediately after a standardized 1-h protocol, they significantly underestimated the time spent sitting [13]. This could potentially be explained by the lower cognitive function in patients with COPD [14] as well as by social desirability (see further).

Some **validation studies** of physical activity questionnaires have been performed in patients with COPD. More information of these questionnaires can be found in Table 8.2. Garfield et al. [15] compared four physical activity questionnaires (Stanford 7-day physical activity recall questionnaire, Baecke questionnaire, physical activity scale for the elderly (PASE), and Zutphen questionnaire) to objectively measured physical activity. These authors concluded that the Stanford 7-day physical activity recall questionnaire, the only questionnaire significantly related to the objective PA measurement, was not accurate enough to make individual recommendations on physical activity. However, the questionnaire was able to identify patients at extremes of the physical activity spectrum.

Donaire-Gonzalez et al. [16] analyzed the relation between the Yale Physical Activity Survey and 7 days of objective PA measurement using the SenseWear Armband. In line with the previous paper, the authors concluded that the questionnaire was a valid tool to classify but not to quantify physical activity in patients with COPD. The questionnaire was able to identify patients with sedentarism (defined as <30-min activity per day), especially when using the summary index of the questionnaire, which showed the best validity properties.

Depew et al. [17] aimed to identify tools to screen for severely inactive patients with COPD. The authors concluded a) a modest relation between the score as measured with the PASE questionnaire and objectively measured physical activity and b) that the PASE questionnaire could be used as a valid tool to screen for severe inactivity in this patient population. The authors investigated as well the test-retest reliability 5 days apart and concluded a good reliability for the PASE and a fair reliability for the Stanford Brief Activity Scale (SBAS). Using SBAS showed a worse predicting ability for severe inactivity as compared to the PASE.

Of note, health status questionnaires, frequently containing a domain related to physical activity, are only loosely related to an objective measurement of physical activity in patients with COPD and not able to show a correct presentation of the physical activity level at an individual patient level [18].

Table 8.2 Physical activity questionnaires included in the present chapter

Questionnaire	Characteristics
Modified Baecke physical activity questionnaire for older adults	The questionnaire assesses leisure, household, and sport activities. The section about household activity (e.g., cleaning, preparing meals) consists of ten questions. In addition patients can report any leisure or sport activities. An intensity code is used to convert the duration and frequency into the overall questionnaire score. The modified Baecke questionnaire asks about "habitual" physical activity and should be interviewer administered
Physical activity scale for the elderly (PASE)	The PASE is a brief questionnaire including 12 items. The questionnaire combines information on leisure, household, and occupational activity. The PASE score is calculated by multiplying the amount of time spent in each activity (hours a day) by the respective weights (more weight is given to activities performed by elderly as compared to sport activity). The higher the score (range 0–360), the higher the physical activity. The PASE has a 1-week recall period and can be self- or interviewer administered
Zutphen physical activity questionnaire (ZPAC)	The ZPAC asks about the frequency and duration of walking and bicycling during the previous week, the average amount of time spent weekly on hobbies and gardening in both summer and winter, and the average amount of time spent monthly on jobs and sports. The hours a day of activity are multiplied with an intensity code. The focus of the questionnaire lies on assessing energy expenditure and the amount of minutes in light, moderate, and intense activity. The questionnaire provides a summary kcal score in units of kcal/kg of body mass/day depending on the frequency, intensity, and duration of the activities. The recall period varies across questions; the questionnaire is self-administered
Stanford 7-day physical activity recall questionnaire	The questionnaire is based on a 15–20-min interview with patients. During the interview, patients report the approximate number of hours they slept and spent in moderate, hard, and very hard activity during the previous week. Total daily energy expenditure is calculated as the average hours per day in each activity category multiplied by an assigned MET value and body weight in kilograms. The Stanford questionnaire uses a recall of 7 days and is interviewer led
YALE physical activity survey (YPAS)	The YPAS consists of 32 items, including different domains of activities (work, yard work, caretaking, exercise, recreational activities, vigorous activity, leisure walking, moving, standing, sitting, flight, seasonal adjustment). The YPAS reflects the volume, frequency, and intensity of physical activity. From the questionnaire, several summarizing parameters can be retrieved (e.g., time in activity per day, energy expenditure, intensity). The summary index is based on seven questions asking for frequency and intensity of activities in general and ranges between 0 and 137 (higher score, higher activity). The questionnaire uses a recall period of 4 weeks and is interviewer administered
Stanford brief activity scale (SBAS)	The SBAS is a two-item physical activity questionnaire (focusing on leisure and occupational activity). The patient chooses between various descriptions of physical activities that best represents his/her activity. The score is categorical and ranges from "inactive" to "very hard-intensity activity." The questionnaire asks about the past year

8.1.2 Social Desirability

Social desirability is "the tendency of individuals to provide socially desirable information" [19]. This personality trait may affect the self-reporting of physical activity and lead toward an overreporting of activity [19]. Social desirability leading to a bias has also been shown in, for example, the self-report of dietary information, resulting in a significant underreporting of calorie intake [20].

8.1.3 Responsiveness

Responsiveness (or sensitivity) is an important measurement property of an instrument. Responsiveness has been defined as "the ability of an instrument to detect changes over time that are known to occur" [6]. Especially when the aim of the measurement is to measure changes over time, the validation of the change over time is a crucial measurement property, besides reliability and validity. In systematic reviews on measurement properties of physical activity questionnaires in healthy adults and elderly, responsiveness was judged as poor [7, 12]. Of note, responsiveness was only reported in the minority of studies [3, 7, 12]. In patients with COPD, there is at date no specific information about the responsiveness of physical activity questionnaires.

In summary, the use of self-report to measure physical activity in patients with chronic respiratory disease should be performed with caution. Questionnaires can be used to classify patients because the data show the ability to identify patients at extremes of the physical activity spectrum. This makes the questionnaires valid to be used in epidemiological studies using the questionnaire data as the physical activity exposure. In line with this, physical activity questionnaires can be used as a screening tool for severe inactivity. This chapter has summarized questionnaires validated for this purpose. However, the questionnaires are not recommended to make an assessment of the individual patient's physical activity level because of the risk for a biased assessment. Especially when one is interested in measuring changes over time, the lack of responsiveness is a base of not recommending this.

8.2 Objective Physical Activity Measurement

8.2.1 Doubly Labeled Water

The doubly labeled water technique is generally thought to be the most accurate method to measure total energy expenditure [21]. For the assessment of total energy expenditure, deuterium (^{2}H) and ^{18}O are ingested. Once ingested, ^{2}H is eliminated as water, and ^{18}O is eliminated as water and carbon dioxide [22]. The excess disappearance rate of ^{18}O relative to ^{2}H is a measure of the carbon dioxide production rate, which is a direct measure of total energy expenditure [21]. Normally, the measurement is performed for a period of 2 weeks [21].

The doubly labeled water technique has several disadvantages. First, total energy expenditure as measured by doubly labeled water technique needs to be corrected for resting energy expenditure in order to quantify the activity-related energy expenditure. Resting energy expenditure (or basal metabolic rate) in turn needs to be measured by, e.g., indirect calorimetry at rest [21]. Second, doubly labeled water does not quantify the duration, frequency, and intensity of physical activity performed [2]. Finally, it is a very expensive method with a rather complex setup.

8.2.2 Activity Monitors

8.2.2.1 Step Counters

Pedometers are small, relatively inexpensive devices usually worn at the waist that record the number of steps walked per day [23, 24]. Walking is something that most people can do, and steps per day is a simple metric for assessing physical activity [25]. Pedometers are most accurate at step counting but less accurate in distance or energy expenditure estimates [22]. Importantly, when using pedometers, one should be aware that pedometers might underestimate steps during walking at slow speeds, which has been shown in as well healthy elderly as patients with COPD [26–29].

Pedometers are increasingly used as motivational tools to improve physical activity levels [22]. An important predictor of an increase of physical activity in general population is having a step goal of 10,000 steps per day [23], which is not only associated with significant increases in physical activity but also significant decreases in body mass index and blood pressure [23]. For patients with COPD, more individual step goals need to be defined. A 12-week pedometer-based exercise counseling strategy effectively enhanced daily physical activity, physical fitness, and health-related quality of life in COPD outpatients who did not participate in a rehabilitation program [30]. In line with this, a 4-month pedometer Internet-mediated walking program increased physical activity and quality of life in COPD patients [31]. Demeyer et al. recently showed the effectiveness of a 12-week semiautomated activity coaching program on the physical activity levels in patients with COPD [32]. This intervention consisted of a step counter and a project-tailored application installed on a smartphone [32]. Patients received an automatic calculated goal, based on their own achievements, and could contact their coaches if they wanted so [32]. In these intervention studies, daily step count (measured by the step counter) was used as an incentive to patients, to provide an individual goal setting. The latter can be performed during face-to-face contacts [30] or using a remote tele-coaching approach [31, 32].

8.2.2.2 Accelerometers

Accelerometers are portable electronic devices that are worn on the body to detect acceleration and thereby reflect bodily movement [22]. They quantify activity counts and may provide an estimate of time spent above or below a prespecified activity level, number of steps, and energy expenditure [2, 22]. The use of accelerometers has received increasing interest since they add objective data which cannot be obtained from questionnaires or pedometers [22]. Accelerometers have emerged as an important means of assessing the duration and intensity of physical activity and have served to define primary outcome measures in several studies in COPD [24] as well as in other chronic respiratory diseases [33–35].

Several types (uni-, bi-, or triaxial accelerometers) generating different output measures are available [2, 22, 24]. Integrated multisensor systems combine accelerometry with other sensors that capture body responses to exercise (e.g., heart rate or skin temperature) in an attempt to optimize physical activity assessments and to obtain reasonably valid estimates of energy expenditure [24]. The validity of accelerometers for assessment of physical activity in patients with COPD has been the subject of many investigations in recent years [22]. Three devices, the DynaPort MoveMonitor (McRoberts BV, the Hague, the Netherlands), the Actigraph GT3X (Actigraph, Pensacola, FL, USA), and the SenseWear Armband (BodyMedia, Inc., Pittsburgh, PA, USA) (all employing triaxial accelerometers), were valid and responsive for use in COPD [22, 36, 37].

8.2.2.3 Smartphone Applications and Wearable Devices

Smartphone applications and wearable devices with a more consumer-friendly appeal are increasingly being used by the general population [38] and might also have a more prominent role in the future in patient with COPD. Because of their capability of Bluetooth or USB transmission, data tele-coaching interventions, as highlighted above, become possible. The majority of the currently available smartphone applications and wearable devices have been shown to provide relatively accurate estimates of step counts, when compared with a direct observation of the step counts [38]. However, thorough validation studies of these devices are lacking in respiratory disease. With advancing technology, it is likely that also different types of activities, intensity of activities, and related energy expenditure will become valid readouts of these devices.

8.2.3 Measurement Characteristics and Post-processing of Data

In addition to the choice of monitor, decisions in measurement properties and post-processing of data and challenges in the interpretation are important to consider when using an objective measurement of physical activity. The use of activity monitoring provides researchers and clinicians with a wealth of data on different variables, with a high variability in the signal. The way of handling these data is important to obtain an interpretable, reliable, and valid physical activity measurement. Of note, the less sophisticated and less expensive devices often do not include information on wearing time, which precludes any quality control of the measurement based on this. We will discuss (1) the definition of a valid day, (2) the recommended number of days of measurement, and (3) the challenges in the interpretation of physical activity data.

8.2.3.1 Valid Days of Measurement

When measuring physical activity, two sampling frames are typically used; either a 24-h assessment, including both sleep and waking times, or a measurement of the waking hours [39]. This choice will be mainly driven by the aim of the assessment. For example, if one is interested in the assessment of sedentary behavior, defined as "any waking behavior characterized by an energy expenditure of <1.5 MET in a sitting or reclining posture" [40], asking patients to wear the monitor during waking hours will be sufficient and more appropriate.

Compliance with wearing the device is a prerequisite of obtaining a reliable assessment. In population-based research, it is generally accepted to use the cutoff of 10 h/day as the minimum wearing time to define a valid day [39]. This cutoff is also used in COPD research [22]. One study showed that defining the minimum of wearing time as at least 8 h between 7 AM and 8 PM resulted in similar results [41]. Practically seen, when retrieving data from an activity monitor, deleting days with an insufficient (too low) wearing time should be the first step of data handling. Of note, many step counters do not include wearing time in the output. Therefore, clinicians should take into account that this important quality control cannot be performed when using these devices.

8.2.3.2 Number of Days of Measurement

Because of the high day-by-day variability in free-living physical activity, the number of days physical activity is measured is an important factor influencing the reliability of the assessment. In population-based research, activity monitors are typically worn for a 7-day period [39]. In patients with COPD, the needed number of days of assessment has been estimated between 2 and 7 days based on cross-sectional data [8, 41–45]. Two papers excluded weekend days in this estimation and concluded both a reliable assessment with having at least 2 weekdays of measurement [8, 41], whereas others defined assessment period with weekend days [42, 43]. Patients with COPD are remarkably less active on Sundays as compared to other days in the week [43]. Therefore, it is recommended to include weekends when one is interested in the characterization of the physical activity level of a patient. Watz et al. concluded that 2–3 days of measurement will result in a reliable measurement in patients in GOLD stage IV, whereas 5 days were needed to obtain a reliable assessment in patients in GOLD stage I [43]. When the aim is to detect changes, 4 days of measurement excluding the weekends were recommended in moderate to severe patients with COPD following pulmonary rehabilitation [41]. Exclusion of weekend days did not affect the magnitude of the effect but decreased the variability of the measurement. Therefore, weekend days can be deleted for this purpose. Screening for valid measurements and deleting invalid assessment are important second steps in the processing of data.

A multicenter observational study investigated the compliance of patients wearing an activity monitor in a measurement of 8 consecutive days using a 24-h sampling [46]. The authors concluded an excellent compliance of wearing the activity monitor in this patient population. In more than 94% of patients, a valid physical activity measurement (defined as 5 measurement days with a valid at least 22 h wearing time) was obtained.

It is important to provide clear instructions to patients at the start of the physical activity measurement. It is recommended to instruct patients to wear the monitor all the time, besides when taking a bath or a shower when using the 24-h sampling or during all waking hours besides these personal care activities when aiming for a measurement during waking hours. Patient should be motivated to wear the devices, even when taking a rest during the day or when experiencing health problems.

8.2.3.3 Challenges in the Interpretation of Physical Activity Data

The Influence of the Season of the Measurement

The physical activity level is highly depending on external influences such as the season in which the measurement has been done (lowest physical activity in winter) [47]. Sewell et al. showed that the effect of pulmonary rehabilitation on physical activity was influenced by the season in which

COPD patients started the rehabilitation program. More specifically, patients who started in winter time and finished the rehabilitation in a milder season showed the largest intervention effect [47]. In line with this, Alahmari et al. showed that in COPD patients, in cold days, step count was reduced by 43.3 steps/day per lower °C and that the activity was lower on rainy than dry days and on overcast compared to sunny days [48]. Therefore, adjusting for season when investigating intervention effects can be important, especially when looking to within-patient effects of an intervention. One study showed that by including the duration of daylight as a covariate in the analyses investigating the effect of pulmonary rehabilitation on physical activity, a more robust outcome was obtained, which leads to a lower sample size requirement [41].

The Choice of the Physical Activity Variable

When overviewing physical activity literature, it becomes clear that multiple physical activity variables exist and that these are used across trials. Frequently used physical activity variables are the number of daily steps, energy expenditure, time in different postures (e.g., walking, sitting, lying), and time above a certain intensity threshold (e.g., moderate-intense activity). The lack of uniformity across trials makes it difficult to compare results. This has, for example, been shown by a review summarizing the effect of pulmonary rehabilitation in patients with COPD [49]. In addition to the variety in possible variables that can be obtained by activity monitors, the lack in uniformity in the definition of different variables across devices complicates the comparability [50].

Several software programs, delivered with the activity monitor, give the option of defining the threshold of each intensity of interest (e.g., SenseWear Pro Armband (BodyMedia, Pittsburgh, PA, USA), Actigraph GT3X (Actigraph LLC Pensacola, FL, USA)). In this case, it is important to specify the detailed settings when reporting the results. One study highlighted the large differences in classification of patients when using different cutoffs to define "moderate intensity," all based on different guidelines [51]. Of note, the use of step count is probably less depending on proprietary algorithms and therefore potentially a more comparable outcome across devices.

Finally the choice of the variables used as an outcome can influence the found results. One study concluded that the daily number of steps and time in light intensity were more sensitive outcomes as compared to time in moderate-intense activity and daily mean MET level when investigating the effect of rehabilitation on physical activity [41].

The Interpretation of the Physical Activity Data

When the aim of the activity measure is to classify patients, the found results can be compared with the step count classification as proposed by Tudor-Locke et al. [52], the recommendations provided by the World Health Organization based on the physical activity level (PAL, ratio between whole-night sleep energy expenditure and the total daily energy expenditure) [43], or recommendations based on the time in at least moderate-intense activity [5]. In 2013, sex- and age-specific normative step data were published [53]. However, it should be noted that these normative values were based on data collected by the Actigraph GT3X accelerometer and post-processed in a specific way to step counter measurements, known to possibly be an underestimation.

When investigating changes in physical activity, the minimal important difference (MID) is the standard approach of the interpretation of clinically relevant changes of an intervention. Recently the first MID for objectively measured physical activity in patients with COPD has been estimated as being between 600 and 1100 steps per day, as a result of a rehabilitation program [54].

8.3 Physical Activity from a Patient Perspective

Up till now, the present chapter has focused on the measurement of physical activity using the widely known definition of physical activity as

"Any bodily movement produced by skeletal muscles that result in energy expenditure" [1]. However, it should be acknowledged that this physiological definition misses out the patients' experience with physical activity.

In a recent review, it has been shown that none of 15 questionnaires with the aim of measuring dimensions of physical activity or related constructs in patients with COPD was based on a conceptual framework defining the concept (i.e., physical activity) from a patient's perspective [55]. In 2014 Dobbels et al. published a paper defining physical activity from a patient's perspective [56]. Based on interviews with patients in combination with expert input, the authors concluded that the conceptual framework of physical activity comprises the amount of physical activity, the symptoms experienced during physical activity, and the adaptations made to facilitate physical activity [56].

Based on this definition, the same group of researcher developed a patient-reported outcome tool capturing the physical activity from a patient's perspective in patients with COPD [57]. The instruments (one with a daily recall and the other with a weekly recall) combine classical items ("questions") with data derived from an activity monitor. The instruments consist of two domains (i.e., amount of physical activity and difficulty during physical activity) that are scored separately and were found to be reliable and valid [57].

References

1. Caspersen CJ, Powell KE, Christenson GM. Physical activity, exercise, and physical fitness: definitions and distinctions for health-related research. Public Health Rep. 1985;100(2):126–31.
2. Pitta F, Troosters T, Probst VS, Spruit MA, Decramer M, Gosselink R. Quantifying physical activity in daily life with questionnaires and motion sensors in COPD. Eur Respir J. 2006;27(5):1040–55.
3. Frei A, Williams K, Vetsch A, Dobbels F, Jacobs L, Rudell K, et al. A comprehensive systematic review of the development process of 104 patient-reported outcomes (PROs) for physical activity in chronically ill and elderly people. Health Qual Life Outcomes. 2011;9:116.
4. Williams K, Frei A, Vetsch A, Dobbels F, Puhan MA, Rudell K. Patient-reported physical activity questionnaires: a systematic review of content and format. Health Qual Life Outcomes. 2012;10:28.
5. Haskell WL, Lee IM, Pate RR, Powell KE, Blair SN, Franklin BA, et al. Physical activity and public health: updated recommendation for adults from the American College of Sports Medicine and the American Heart Association. Circulation. 2007;116(9):1081–93.
6. Terwee CB, Mokkink LB, van Poppel MN, Chinapaw MJ, van Mechelen W, de Vet HC. Qualitative attributes and measurement properties of physical activity questionnaires: a checklist. Sports Med. 2010;40(7):525–37.
7. Forsen L, Loland NW, Vuillemin A, Chinapaw MJ, van Poppel MN, Mokkink LB, et al. Self-administered physical activity questionnaires for the elderly: a systematic review of measurement properties. Sports Med. 2010;40(7):601–23.
8. Pitta F, Troosters T, Spruit MA, Probst VS, Decramer M, Gosselink R. Characteristics of physical activities in daily life in chronic obstructive pulmonary disease. Am J Respir Crit Care Med. 2005;171(9):972–7.
9. Troosters T, Sciurba F, Battaglia S, Langer D, Valluri SR, Martino L, et al. Physical inactivity in patients with COPD, a controlled multi-center pilot-study. Respir Med. 2010;104(7):1005–11.
10. Durante R, Ainsworth BE. The recall of physical activity: using a cognitive model of the question-answering process. Med Sci Sports Exerc. 1996;28(10):1282–91.
11. Bonnefoy M, Normand S, Pachiaudi C, Lacour JR, Laville M, Kostka T. Simultaneous validation of ten physical activity questionnaires in older men: a doubly labeled water study. J Am Geriatr Soc. 2001;49(1):28–35.
12. van Poppel MN, Chinapaw MJ, Mokkink LB, van Mechelen W, Terwee CB. Physical activity questionnaires for adults: a systematic review of measurement properties. Sports Med. 2010;40(7):565–600.
13. Pitta F, Troosters T, Spruit MA, Decramer M, Gosselink R. Activity monitoring for assessment of physical activities in daily life in patients with chronic obstructive pulmonary disease. Arch Phys Med Rehabil. 2005;86(10):1979–85.
14. Inc A, Marra C, Giordano A, Calcagni ML, Cappa A, Basso S, et al. Cognitive impairment in chronic obstructive pulmonary disease--a neuropsychological and spect study. J Neurol. 2003;250(3):325–32.
15. Garfield BE, Canavan JL, Smith CJ, Ingram KA, Fowler RP, Clark AL, et al. Stanford seven-day physical activity recall questionnaire in COPD. Eur Respir J. 2012;40(2):356–62.
16. Donaire-Gonzalez D, Gimeno-Santos E, Serra I, Roca J, Balcells E, Rodriguez E, et al. Validation of the Yale Physical Activity Survey in chronic obstructive pulmonary disease patients. Arch Bronconeumol. 2011;47(11):552–60.
17. DePew ZS, Garofoli AC, Novotny PJ, Benzo RP. Screening for severe physical inactivity in chronic obstructive pulmonary disease: the value of simple measures and the validation of two physical activity questionnaires. Chron Respir Dis. 2013;10(1):19–27.

18. Demeyer H, Duenas-Espin I, De JC, Louvaris Z, Hornikx M, Gimeno-Santos E, et al. Can health status questionnaires be used as a measure of physical activity in COPD patients? Eur Respir J. 2016;47(5):1565–8.
19. Adams SA, Matthews CE, Ebbeling CB, Moore CG, Cunningham JE, Fulton J, et al. The effect of social desirability and social approval on self-reports of physical activity. Am J Epidemiol. 2005;161(4):389–98.
20. Hebert JR, Clemow L, Pbert L, Ockene IS, Ockene JK. Social desirability bias in dietary self-report may compromise the validity of dietary intake measures. Int J Epidemiol. 1995;24(2):389–98.
21. Manini TM, Everhart JE, Patel KV, Schoeller DA, Colbert LH, Visser M, et al. Daily activity energy expenditure and mortality among older adults. JAMA. 2006;296(2):171–9.
22. Watz H, Pitta F, Rochester CL, Garcia-Aymerich J, ZuWallack R, Troosters T, et al. An official European Respiratory Society statement on physical activity in COPD. Eur Respir J. 2014;44(6):1521–37.
23. Bravata DM, Smith-Spangler C, Sundaram V, Gienger AL, Lin N, Lewis R, et al. Using pedometers to increase physical activity and improve health: a systematic review. JAMA. 2007;298(19):2296–304.
24. Watz H. Physical activity. In: Kolb M, Vogelmeier CF, editors. Outcomes in clinical trials, European Respiratory Monographs. Lausanne: European Respiratory Society; 2013. p. 117–26.
25. Moy ML, Danilack VA, Weston NA, Garshick E. Daily step counts in a US cohort with COPD. Respir Med. 2012;106(7):962–9.
26. Furlanetto KC, Bisca GW, Oldemberg N, Sant'anna TJ, Morakami FK, Camillo CA, et al. Step counting and energy expenditure estimation in patients with chronic obstructive pulmonary disease and healthy elderly: accuracy of 2 motion sensors. Arch Phys Med Rehabil. 2010;91(2):261–7.
27. Karabulut M, Crouter SE, Bassett DR Jr. Comparison of two waist-mounted and two ankle-mounted electronic pedometers. Eur J Appl Physiol. 2005;95(4):335–43.
28. Melanson EL, Knoll JR, Bell ML, Donahoo WT, Hill JO, Nysse LJ, et al. Commercially available pedometers: considerations for accurate step counting. Prev Med. 2004;39(2):361–8.
29. Moy ML, Janney AW, Nguyen HQ, Matthess KR, Cohen M, Garshick E, et al. Use of pedometer and Internet-mediated walking program in patients with chronic obstructive pulmonary disease. J Rehabil Res Dev. 2010;47(5):485–96.
30. Mendoza L, Horta P, Espinoza J, Aguilera M, Balmaceda N, Castro A, et al. Pedometers to enhance physical activity in COPD: a randomised controlled trial. Eur Respir J. 2015;45(2):347–54.
31. Moy ML, Collins RJ, Martinez CH, Kadri R, Roman P, Holleman RG, et al. An internet-mediated pedometer-based program improves health-related quality-of-life domains and daily step counts in COPD: a randomized controlled trial. Chest. 2015;148(1):128–37.
32. Demeyer H, Louvaris Z, Frei A, Rabinovich RA, de Jong C, Gimeno-Santos E, et al. Physical activity is increased by a 12-week semiautomated telecoaching programme in patients with COPD: a multicentre randomised controlled trial. Thorax. 2017;72(5):415–23.
33. Bahmer T, Kirsten AM, Waschki B, Rabe KF, Magnussen H, Kirsten D, et al. Clinical correlates of reduced physical activity in idiopathic pulmonary fibrosis. Respiration. 2016;91(6):497–502.
34. Bahmer T, Watz H, Waschki B, Gramm M, Magnussen H, Rabe KF, et al. Reduced physical activity in lymphangioleiomyomatosis compared with COPD and healthy controls: disease-specific impact and clinical correlates. Thorax. 2016;71(7):662–3.
35. Bahmer T, Waschki B, Schatz F, Herzmann C, Zabel P, Kirsten AM, et al. Physical activity, airway resistance and small airway dysfunction in severe asthma. Eur Respir J. 2017;49(1):1601827.
36. Rabinovich RA, Louvaris Z, Raste Y, Langer D, Van RH, Giavedoni S, et al. Validity of physical activity monitors during daily life in patients with COPD. Eur Respir J. 2013;42(5):1205–15.
37. Van Remoortel H, Raste Y, Louvaris Z, Giavedoni S, Burtin C, Langer D, et al. Validity of six activity monitors in chronic obstructive pulmonary disease: a comparison with indirect calorimetry. PLoS One. 2012;7(6):e39198.
38. Case MA, Burwick HA, Volpp KG, Patel MS. Accuracy of smartphone applications and wearable devices for tracking physical activity data. JAMA. 2015;313(6):625–6.
39. Matthews CE, Hagstromer M, Pober DM, Bowles HR. Best practices for using physical activity monitors in population-based research. Med Sci Sports Exerc. 2012;44(1 Suppl 1):S68–76.
40. Gibbs BB, Hergenroeder AL, Katzmarzyk PT, Lee IM, Jakicic JM. Definition, measurement, and health risks associated with sedentary behavior. Med Sci Sports Exerc. 2015;47(6):1295–300.
41. Demeyer H, Burtin C, Van Remoortel H, Hornikx M, Langer D, Decramer M, et al. Standardizing the analysis of physical activity in patients with COPD following a pulmonary rehabilitation program. Chest. 2014;146(2):318–27.
42. Steele BG, Holt L, Belza B, Ferris S, Lakshminaryan S, Buchner DM. Quantitating physical activity in COPD using a triaxial accelerometer. Chest. 2000;117(5):1359–67.
43. Watz H, Waschki B, Meyer T, Magnussen H. Physical activity in patients with COPD. Eur Respir J. 2009;33(2):262–72.
44. Hecht A, Ma S, Porszasz J, Casaburi R. Methodology for using long-term accelerometry monitoring to describe daily activity patterns in COPD. COPD. 2009;6(2):121–9.
45. Sugino A, Minakata Y, Kanda M, Akamatsu K, Koarai A, Hirano T, et al. Validation of a compact motion sensor for the measurement of physical activity in patients with chronic obstructive pulmonary disease. Respiration. 2012;83(4):300–7.

46. Waschki B, Spruit MA, Watz H, Albert PS, Shrikrishna D, Groenen M, et al. Physical activity monitoring in COPD: compliance and associations with clinical characteristics in a multicenter study. Respir Med. 2012;106(4):522–30.
47. Sewell L, Singh SJ, Williams JE, Morgan MD. Seasonal variations affect physical activity and pulmonary rehabilitation outcomes. J Cardiopulm Rehabil Prev. 2010;30(5):329–33.
48. Alahmari AD, Mackay AJ, Patel AR, Kowlessar BS, Singh R, Brill SE, et al. Influence of weather and atmospheric pollution on physical activity in patients with COPD. Respir Res. 2015;16:71.
49. Mantoani LC, Rubio N, McKinstry B, MacNee W, Rabinovich RA. Interventions to modify physical activity in patients with COPD: a systematic review. Eur Respir J. 2016;48(1):69–81.
50. Butte NF, Ekelund U, Westerterp KR. Assessing physical activity using wearable monitors: measures of physical activity. Med Sci Sports Exerc. 2012;44(1 Suppl 1):S5–12.
51. Van Remoortel H, Camillo CA, Langer D, Hornikx M, Demeyer H, Burtin C, et al. Moderate intense physical activity depends on selected Metabolic Equivalent of Task (MET) cut-off and type of data analysis. PLoS One. 2013;8(12):e84365.
52. Tudor-Locke C, Craig CL, Thyfault JP, Spence JC. A step-defined sedentary lifestyle index: <5000 steps/day. Appl Physiol Nutr Metab. 2013;38(2):100–14.
53. Tudor-Locke C, Schuna JM Jr, Barreira TV, Mire EF, Broyles ST, Katzmarzyk PT, et al. Normative steps/day values for older adults: NHANES 2005-2006. J Gerontol A Biol Sci Med Sci. 2013;68(11):1426–32.
54. Demeyer H, Burtin C, Hornikx M, Camillo CA, Van RH, Langer D, et al. The minimal important difference in physical activity in patients with COPD. PLoS One. 2016;11(4):e0154587.
55. Gimeno-Santos E, Frei A, Dobbels F, Rudell K, Puhan MA, Garcia-Aymerich J. Validity of instruments to measure physical activity may be questionable due to a lack of conceptual frameworks: a systematic review. Health Qual Life Outcomes. 2011;9:86.
56. Dobbels F, de Jong C, Drost E, Elberse J, Feridou C, Jacobs L, et al. The PROactive innovative conceptual framework on physical activity. Eur Respir J. 2014;44(5):1223–33.
57. Gimeno-Santos E, Raste Y, Demeyer H, Louvaris Z, de Jong C, Rabinovich RA, et al. The PROactive instruments to measure physical activity in patients with chronic obstructive pulmonary disease. Eur Respir J. 2015;46(4):988–1000.

Global Assessment

9

Sally Singh

9.1 Global Assessment

The initial assessment of the patient is critical to the overall success of pulmonary rehabilitation, it is important to invest time with the patient and if possible the carer/partner to secure a comprehensive evaluation of the patient, their social circumstances and their willingness and barriers to engagement. Furthermore the exercise and education components of the programme, delivered by the multidisciplinary team require specific detail information on exercise limitation and symptom burden to prescribe an exercise training programme to maximise the opportunities for a successful outcome for both the individual and the service delivering the programme.

The comprehensive assessment of the individual prior to a course of rehabilitation is critical to the success of the programme at an organisational and individual level. It is incumbent upon the multidisciplinary team to ensure that the participant has been fully assessed for suitability (including patient safety, physical and emotional well-being, symptom burden) for the programme. The measures collected at the time of the assessment may have different meanings for the participant, the healthcare professional and the provider (payer) of the service (Fig. 9.1).

This chapter will review aspects of the assessment not necessarily covered in the proceeding chapters that have specifically examined physical function with respect to muscle strength, exercise capacity, physical activity and emotional well-being.

The overarching aim of the assessment is for the healthcare provider in collaboration with the participant to:

1. Confirm that the participant understands the process and principles of rehabilitation and the level of engagement required from the individual in collaboration with the healthcare professionals.
2. Understand the impact of the disease upon the individual (symptoms, physical, psychological, social).

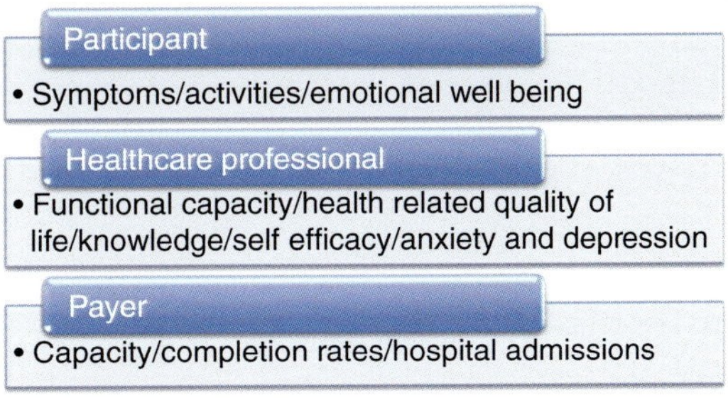

Fig. 9.1 Aspects of the measurements assessed during the process of rehabilitation for the participant, the healthcare professional and the payer

S. Singh
Centre for Exercise and Rehabilitation Science,
University Hospitals of Leicester NHS Trust,
Glenfield Hospital, Groby Road,
Leicester LE3 9QP, UK
e-mail: Sally.singh@uhl-tr.nhs.uk

© Springer International Publishing AG 2018
E. Clini et al. (eds.), *Textbook of Pulmonary Rehabilitation*,
https://doi.org/10.1007/978-3-319-65888-9_9

3. Understand the level of disability the patient is experiencing.
4. Understand the level of pre-existing disease knowledge and how this may influence engagement in the programme.
5. Identify the goals/aspirations of the patient and how these might be achieved within a rehabilitation programme.
6. Identify other important disease processes that may impact upon the success of the rehabilitation programme.
7. Ensure patient safety to participate in the programme.

The purpose of the assessment for the multidisciplinary team includes all of the above points but in addition should facilitate a greater understanding of:

1. The patients' physical capacity and their exercise tolerance, their response to the exercise test(s) and limitations to exercise
2. The patients' psychological well-being
3. The challenges patients face completing daily tasks
4. The level of motivation to participate in the programme
5. Potential barriers to engagement
6. Factors that need to be considered to prescribe an appropriate exercise programme with reference to baseline exercise capacity and important comorbidities

Furthermore the healthcare professional will regard the initial assessment as an opportunity to collect outcome measures that are appropriate and feasible to collect pre- and post rehabilitation allowing the value of the intervention for the individual and for the service to be evaluated over a predefined period. This data collection should be embedded in a process of benchmarking and quality assurance. If the centre is research active, the complexity of the initial assessment may be reflected in a more sophisticated suite of outcome measures that rely on expensive equipment and trained staff.

The payer for the service may have different data requirements of the assessment process and may anticipate a broad ranging service report that not only includes measures of clinical effectiveness but also data in terms of the overall process of rehabilitation. The multidisciplinary team will be responsible for collecting 'process' data around the time of the assessment that could include:

1. Waiting times for the initial assessment
2. Number of patients who do not attend an initial assessment despite being referred by their physician
3. Waiting times to progress onto the programme (as a measure of programme capacity)
4. Numbers of patients assessed every year
5. Number of patients that are deemed appropriate for rehabilitation as a percentage of those referred for an assessment
6. Number of patients that complete a final assessment (a measure of dropouts is often required)
7. Data describing the clinical effectiveness of the programme using a selection of the parameters described above

The discharge assessment completed at the final stages of the rehabilitation programme may also be multidisciplinary. All measures taken initially may not be repeated at this stage but importantly a core set of measures should be identified, ideally at a national level to allow a degree of benchmarking. The final assessment is also important for the individual it presents an opportunity to formally record the outcome and share these with the patients. Improved performance of an exercise test may be particularly motivating for the individual with an objective measure of capacity. This will facilitate a discussion by the multidisciplinary team to consider options post rehabilitation and agree a maintenance strategy.

The multidisciplinary team have an obligation to formally evaluate the results of the programme to confirm the quality of the programme and identify areas for improvement. The results of the programme can be expressed using a variety of approaches. It is common to report mean changes of the outcomes, and ensure that the programme is reaching predefined minimum clinically important differences that have been reported.

An alternative approach is to define the percentage of the population that achieve the threshold values. Spruit et al. have described the importance of a multicomponent assessment [1]. Complex mathematical modelling revealed an intricate matrix of responses. There was a non-uniform response to a set of outcomes. Interestingly there was a differential response to the two exercise tests that had been deployed; consequently if only one of the tests had been used, the response rate would have been lower. Furthermore the data identified patients that uniquely responded positively to the activity of daily living scale but no other measures.

The response rate of different outcome measures can be challenging to compare, for example, quality of life measures have different domains and different scoring systems. Using the effect size allows a standardised comparison of measures (the mean difference between two groups, and then divide the result by the pooled standard deviation). Kon et al. [2] identified that for their rehabilitation programme, the St Georges respiratory questionnaire had an effect size of −0.33, whilst the COPD assessment test (CAT) had an effect size of −0.25 and the chronic respiratory disease questionnaire had an effect size of 0.62. This is true for the assessment of exercise capacity too; different tests respond differently, a number of studies have deployed the 6-minute walking test, alongside the incremental and endurance shuttle walking tests [3–5]. Different exercise tests and the likely reasons for these diverging values will be fully described in a different chapter. Briefly a constant work rate test, be it cycling or walking (treadmill or the endurance shuttle walking test), is consistently more sensitive to change compared to an incremental (bike, treadmill or shuttle walking test) or self-paced test (6-minute walking test) [6].

The assessment of the participant prior to embarking on a course of pulmonary rehabilitation is critical to the success of the programme, not only for the individual but also to allow the centre to report results more widely to the insurers or commissioners of the service to ensure a high-quality service is being provided for the individuals referred. It is important that various aspects of patients' well-being are assessed to formulate a treatment plan. There is no clear international guidance as to who should conduct the initial assessment or perhaps more controversially no predefined competencies that certify an individual adequately trained to conduct the assessment. Arguably more than one member of the multidisciplinary team may contribute to the initial assessment. Indeed there is a real variation in how the programme is delivered not only in terms of structure, but content, delivery and referral pathways [7–9]. Furthermore there are no reported national training programmes to deliver training for professional staff engaged in the delivery of pulmonary rehabilitation. The reasons for this are complex and reflect the modest profile that pulmonary rehabilitation has in many countries amongst those who fund rehabilitation services within the healthcare system.

The composition of the multidisciplinary team alters not only between centres, but there is significant international variation (Fig. 9.2). The contribution of the multidisciplinary team was reported in an international survey of pulmonary rehabilitation programmes. The survey recorded a number of healthcare professionals involved; these included respiratory physician, physiotherapist, occupational therapist, social worker, psychologist, dietician, exercise physiologist, internist, cardiologist, general practitioner, pharmacist, nurse and respiratory therapist with their representation across Europe and North America varying; the most commonly reported were doctors, physiotherapists, occupational therapists, social workers, psychologists, pharmacists and cardiologists; and less well represented in the teams were general practitioners (which is probably a reflection on the location of the programme) and interns. The median number of team members in the centres participating in the survey was six in Europe and four in North America. Overall the contributions appear encouraging but obviously in any centre there is limited access, if any at all, to a number of members of the multidisciplinary team that have historically been valued in statements describing the delivery of pulmonary rehabilitation [7].

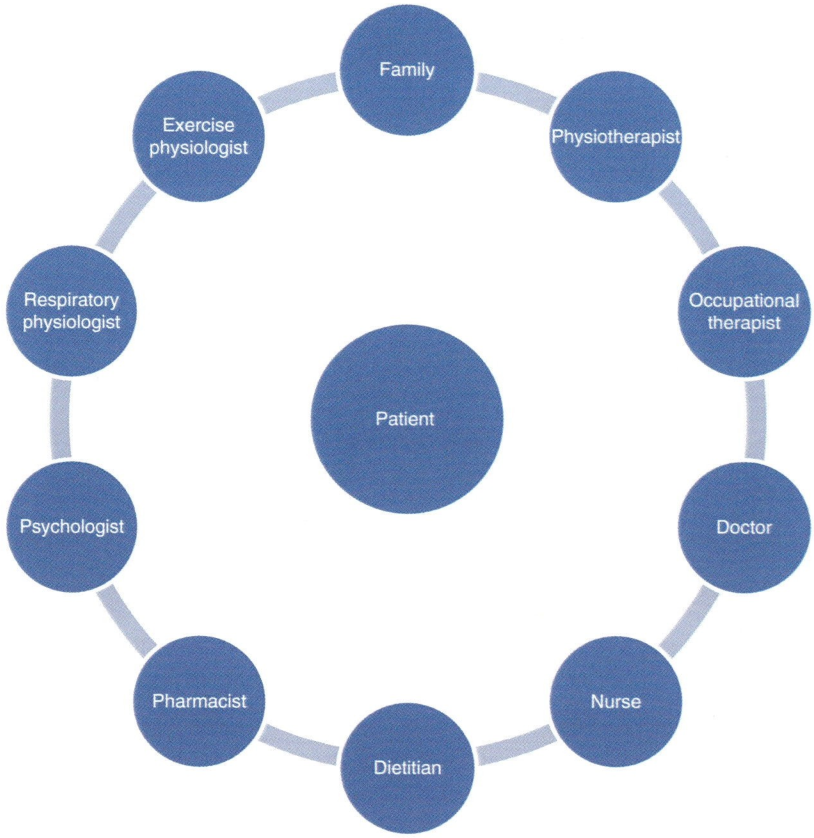

Fig. 9.2 The multidisciplinary team

Various aspects of an assessment will be reviewed in this chapter, and it is often decided at a local level who is best placed to conduct the assessment either in full or as part of a multidisciplinary assessment. Given the focus of that particular component of the assessment it is usually obvious who would have the expertise to fulfil that role.

The fundamental requirement of the referral is one of safety to participate in the programme. There is usually a medically qualified professional (respiratory physician/general practitioner) who oversees the programme, but this is not ubiquitous. The contribution of the medical team may be negligible for the formal assessment, but the safe referral and optimisation of medical therapy is critical to the success of the programme. Medical support is an important resource during the time of the assessment for advice, and expert opinion should there be unexpected complications during the exercise tests. In many centres where a laboratory-based cardiopulmonary exercise test is conducted, a doctor may need to be present.

The core component of the assessment will be conducted by a member of the pulmonary rehabilitation team, but access to a wider team is of course important to address the specific issues, for example, a dietitian may not be a core member of the team but is an essential member of the team to ensure optimal management of weight and nutrition and access to a psychologist for well-being, motivation and behaviour change techniques.

The initial aspects of the assessment comprise the confirmation of patient demographic and anthropometric measures if not recently reported in the medical notes. This includes height, weight, age, gender, ethnicity (language spoken), comorbidities and confirmation of the respiratory diagnosis. To do this it is important that someone in the team is able to conduct quality assured spirometry to confirm the diagnosis (if not available in the medical notes), failing this the individual will need to be assessed by the **respiratory physiology** team. In addition to these characteristics, it is important to confirm their social circumstances, housing and social support networks. Data from the British Thoracic Society National Pulmonary Rehabilitation Audit identified that access to rehabilitation seemed to be proportionally lower in those from a lower socioeconomic group, but the outcome to rehabilitation is equitable across all socioeconomic groups [10].

The sections below identify perhaps the most commonly involved staff in the multidisciplinary assessment, not discussed in terms of importance rather the flow of the assessment.

The **pharmacist** brings expertise in medicines management, device use and drug interactions. At the time of the initial assessment, it is important to assess inhaler technique (a skill that all members of the multidisciplinary team should have) and correct where necessary but where there is doubt about the therapeutic regime, the patient should be referred either back to the medical team or the pharmacist involved with the programme. At this stage the pharmacist will assess the patient and be involved in device and dose change of medicines (potentially both respiratory and nonrespiratory), compliance reviews and further treatment as required (e.g. mucolytic trials).

9.2 Specific Assessment

The **physiotherapists** frequently perform the assessment of exercise capacity using a field-based exercise test, physical activity and muscle function (both respiratory and peripheral) (described in a different chapter). The tests are commonly field-based exercise tests either the 6-minute walking test (6MWT) or the incremental shuttle walking test (ISWT). A complementary test to the incremental shuttle walking test is the endurance shuttle walking test (ESWT). The 6MWT and the ISWT are employed to measure exercise capacity, to understand the limitation to exercise, identify any desaturation that may need remedial actions and support the prescription of an exercise programme. The ISWT and the 6MWT are not interchangeable and the 6MWT is conducted along a 30-m course and is self-paced, whilst the ISWT is externally paced and requires 10 m of corridor and has an incremental protocol, with the speed of walking every minute to provoke a symptom limited performance. The ESWT is conducted along the same course as the ISWT, but rather than having an incremental protocol, the test is again externally paced but the speed of walking is constant. The test defines the constant work rate performance and is helpful to confirm the speed of the exercise prescription. For the exercise tests, it is important to conduct them in line with the ERS guidance [11]. Pre- and post-baseline measures should include heart rate, oxygen saturation, breathlessness score and blood pressure. Post-exercise measures should include all those collected previously and the reason why patients terminated the test. Comorbidities should be taken into account prior to the exercise test.

However if a physiotherapist is unavailable, other members of the team who have been trained and assessed as competent by the service lead can perform these tests. Exercise physiologists may also participate in the programme, but it is important that the assessor has clinical experience to manage the complex COPD patient that may have a number of comorbidities. Each centre should have a competency framework to assess the necessary skills and knowledge to conduct these tests.

Measurements of strength should be collected; peripheral muscle strength is reflected most commonly with quadriceps strength of the dominant leg. The measurements can be relatively simple to secure (e.g. using a handheld dynamometer) through to a more complex measure that can be taken with an isokinetic dynamometer. Handgrip strength has also been reported, but is less likely to change as a consequence of the intervention.

There is increasing importance in the assessment of balance and frailty. Patients may have disturbed balance and therefore at greater risk of falls; it is therefore important to ask the patient whether there is a history of falls. Balance can be assessed using a number of available scales, including the Berg Balance Scale [12] or the activities-specific balance confidence scale [13], and the fear of falling can also be assessed [14]. The physical assessment of balance can be made with the short physical performance battery [15] that has a component of balance within it. A more sophisticated assessment of gait disturbances can be made with an accelerometer that can detect abnormalities of weight transfer and lateral movements contributing to unsteadiness.

The role of the **nurse** within the rehabilitation programme can be fairly extensive; in many units the COPD nurse specialist may conduct or participate in the initial assessment, components of which have been outlined in a number of chapters.

At the initial assessment, particularly if it is at the post-exacerbation phase, advice about exacerbation detection and action planning may need to be reinforced. Furthermore the need to check medicines and inhaler technique is an important component of the assessment.

The nurse (and the rest of the team) should be prepared to discuss and address issues of sexual health with the candidate for rehabilitation and their partner. It is important to make no assumptions about an individual's willingness to discuss their sexual feelings or sexuality [16]. Vincent and Singh [17] restated that sexual expression is an important part of individuals' identity, and that nurses should consider whether or not poor sexual health has a direct effect on their patients' quality of life. If the topic is approached objectively, it should not be awkward for either the healthcare professional or the patient. It may be particularly helpful for these discussions if the patients' partner is involved in the discussion. Nurses may be well placed to consider and support patients to discuss advance care planning processes and their desire to make informed decisions about their future healthcare, in collaboration with carers and loved ones. Prognosis is rarely discussed in the outpatient consultation and it may be something that arises during the course of the assessment. Alternatively the subject may arise during the programme itself.

Whoever is responsible for conducting the initial assessment, that individual must be competent for the tasks being undertaken and have worked with the multidisciplinary team to identify when further structured support may be required. Many aspects will be discussed in accompanying chapters of this text. For example, a **dietitian** may be involved to supporting individuals who are over- or underweight. This is usually defined by their BMI, but in more sophisticated centres there may be the option of measuring fat-free mass. It is important to question the patient about any weight loss; this has been defined as a drop of 5% in the last 6 months [18].

The assessment of the educational needs of the patient is a shared responsibility of the multidisciplinary team. Specific educational needs may be assessed within the context of the rehabilitation programme itself. It is important to remember that the educational component of rehabilitation occupies usually 50% of the contact time for patients within a rehabilitation programme and therefore should be reflected in the initial assessment of the participant. This should be part of the core assessment. Knowledge is the most accessible to assess with a number of endorsed scores. There is a small choice of questionnaires that have been reported to assess COPD specific knowledge, the Bristol Knowledge Questionnaire [19] and the Lung Information Needs Questionnaire [20] both have been deployed in pulmonary rehabilitation programmes and have shown gains post intervention. At this stage it is important to consider the participants reading age, and asking when they left school may give some indication of educational qualifications but obviously not a complete picture. The capacity of the individual to participate with an educational-based intervention requires an assessment of cognitive skills; this again can be completed by a number of team members. Suitable scores may include the Montreal Cognitive Assessment (MoCA) [21], Mini-Mental State Exam (MMSE) [22] and [23]. Of increasing importance is the emerging concept of health literacy, which can be evaluated but is not commonly applied to the field of pulmonary rehabilitation. Health literacy is defined as an individual's ability to read, understand and act on healthcare information and affects their ability to access and use healthcare, to interact with care providers and health professionals and to make sound decisions for their own health [24]. As a service there is increasing potential to assess the individuals' desired mode of delivery for the educational component of rehabilitation, for example, would the participants prefer group sessions, written information, DVD's they could use at home with family of a digital solution to knowledge enhancement. As yet this is untested but with a broadening scope of rehabilitation it is entirely feasible that the face-to-face educational sessions will be supplemented or enhanced with other modes of learning [25].

In addition to their level of knowledge, we should also endeavour to clarify the patients' perceptions of benefit of the programme and their own health beliefs that may set artificial boundaries for engagement that may need negotiating. Barriers and enablers to participation in pulmonary rehabilitation have been described in the literature [26, 27]; participation in physical activity may provoke a particular set of beliefs and barriers that limit active participation particularly beyond the confines of the supervised programme [28] and should be openly discussed, either as part of the initial assessment or embedded within the educational component during the early stages of the programme. These barriers or misconceptions can fall into a number of categories that are broadly intervention related, individual participant related, disease related, health system related and influenced by the socioeconomic factors present. The aim would be to address many of these barriers at the outset to improve adherence with the programme, but this is clearly a 'work in progress' for many centres aiming to maximise the potential gains for the individual.

Overall engagement in activities that support positive behaviour change requires a degree of self-efficacy. This concept is thought to be a strong predictor of health behaviours [29] and can be measured in COPD in relation specifically to pulmonary rehabilitation [30].

An important aspect of the educational sessions is to help patients self-manage their disease. Competency to self-manage is rarely assessed. The assumption is broadly that knowledge transfer leads to skill acquisition and behaviour change. There are questionnaires available that assess other long-term conditions competency to self-manage, heart failure self-management tools, e.g. Self-Care of Heart Failure Index (SCHFI; [31]), the Self-Management of Heart Failure Instrument [32] and the European Heart Failure Self-Care Behaviour Scale (EHFScBS; [33]), but these are not widely reported in the respiratory literature. Motivation to change behaviour is pivotal to the immediate and ongoing success of the rehabilitation programme. Successful modification can contribute to the acquisition of behaviours that deliver successful health outcomes; the most obvious examples are smoking cessation and engagement in the exercise programme. Motivation whilst widely discussed is rarely measured, although reports are emerging in the literature [34, 35], and this may become an important outcome measure for multidisciplinary team in the future.

It is important to consider the composition of the population participating in rehabilitation. For example, it has been well documented that although successful [36], recruitment to post-acute exacerbation rehabilitation is poor [37], and the team data may be limited in this group compared to the eligible population. It is a challenge to all multidisciplinary rehabilitation teams to support patients post hospitalisation to take up the opportunity of rehabilitation in the early stages of recovery. For the routine rehabilitation for patients with stable disease may have mixed pathology (COPD, interstitial pulmonary fibrosis). In this case the selection of outcome measures may require careful consideration to be appropriate for the participant, for example, the COPD Bristol Knowledge Questionnaire [19] is inappropriate for individuals with interstitial lung disease.

Improvement initiatives centred around pulmonary rehabilitation often employ the data collected by the multidisciplinary team at the time of the initial and discharge assessment and is an important function of the team, but itself is a complex activity. There is a vast literature on quality improvement [38] that is worthy of consideration. Broadly the dimensions of healthcare that are considered under this umbrella are for the service to be safe, effective, patient centred, timely, efficient and equitable [39]. Without observing the data collected from these assessments, it is impossible to understand the potential problem, and this may extend to understanding the processes and systems. Armed with this data from the multidisciplinary assessment, the rehabilitation team can interrogate the flow of patients through the programme and the clinical effectiveness and areas for improvement.

References

1. Spruit MA, Augustin IM, Vanfleteren LE, Janssen DJ, Gaffron S, Pennings H, et al. Differential response to pulmonary rehabilitation in COPD: multidimensional profiling. Eur Respir J. 2015;46(6):1625–35.
2. Kon SS, Dilaver D, Mittal M, Nolan CM, Clark AL, Canavan JL, et al. The Clinical COPD Questionnaire: response to pulmonary rehabilitation and minimal clinically important difference. Thorax. 2014;69(9):793–8.
3. Revill SM, Morgan MD, Singh SJ, Williams J, Hardman AE. The endurance shuttle walk: a new field test for the assessment of endurance capacity in chronic obstructive pulmonary disease. Thorax. 1999;54(3):213–22.
4. Eaton T, Young P, Nicol K, Kolbe J. The endurance shuttle walking test: a responsive measure in pulmonary rehabilitation for COPD patients. Chron Respir Dis. 2006;3(1):3–9.
5. Dodd JW, Hogg L, Nolan J, Jefford H, Grant A, Lord VM, et al. The COPD assessment test (CAT): response to pulmonary rehabilitation. A multicentre, prospective study. Thorax. 2011;66(5):425–9.
6. Singh SJ, Puhan MA, Andrianopoulos V, Hernandes NA, Mitchell KE, Hill CJ, et al. An official systematic review of the European Respiratory Society/American Thoracic Society: measurement properties of field walking tests in chronic respiratory disease. Eur Respir J. 2014;44(6):1447–78.
7. Spruit MA, Pitta F, Garvey C, ZuWallack RL, Roberts CM, Collins EG, et al. Differences in content and organisational aspects of pulmonary rehabilitation programmes. Eur Respir J. 2014;43(5):1326–37.
8. Garvey C, Fullwood MD, Rigler J. Pulmonary rehabilitation exercise prescription in chronic obstructive lung disease: US survey and review of guidelines and clinical practices. J Cardiopulm Rehabil Prev. 2013;33(5):314–22.
9. Desveaux L, Janaudis-Ferreira T, Goldstein R, Brooks D. An international comparison of pulmonary rehabilitation: a systematic review. COPD. 2015; 12(2):144–53.
10. Steiner MC, Lowe D, Beckford K, Blakey J, Bolton CE, Elkin S, et al. Socioeconomic deprivation and the outcome of pulmonary rehabilitation in England and Wales. Thorax. 2017;72(6):530–7.
11. Holland AE, Spruit MA, Troosters T, Puhan MA, Pepin V, Saey D, et al. An official European Respiratory Society/American Thoracic Society technical standard: field walking tests in chronic respiratory disease. Eur Respir J. 2014;44(6):1428–46.
12. Berg KO, Wood-Dauphinee SL, Ivan Williams J, Maki B. Measuring balance in the elderly: validation of an instrument. Can J Public Health. 1992;83:S11.
13. Myers AM, Fletcher PC, Myers AH, Sherk W. Discriminative and evaluative properties of the activities-specific balance confidence (ABC) scale. J Gerontol A Biol Sci Med Sci. 1998;53(4):M294.
14. Horak FB, Wrisley DM, Frank J. The balance evaluation systems test (BESTest) to differentiate balance deficits. Phys Ther. 2009;89(5):484–98.
15. Patel MS, Clark AL, Ingram KA, Fowler RP, Donaldson AV, Kon SS, et al. S74 Effect of pulmonary rehabilitation on the Short Physical Performance Battery (SPPB) in COPD. Thorax. 2010;65(Suppl 4):A35.
16. Wells P. No sex please, I'm dying. A common myth explored. Eur J Palliat Care. 2002;9(3):119–22.
17. Vincent EE, Singh SJ. Review article: addressing the sexual health of patients with COPD: the needs of the patient and implications for health care professionals. Chron Respir Dis. 2007;4(2):111–5.
18. Schols AM, Ferreira IM, Franssen FM, Gosker HR, Janssens W, Muscaritoli M, et al. Nutritional assessment and therapy in COPD: a European Respiratory Society statement. Eur Respir J. 2014;44(6):1504–20.
19. White R, Walker P, Roberts S, Kalisky S, White P. Bristol COPD Knowledge Questionnaire (BCKQ): testing what we teach patients about COPD. Chron Respir Dis. 2006;3(3):123–31.
20. Jones RC, Wang X, Harding S, Bott J, Hyland M. Educational impact of pulmonary rehabilitation: lung Information Needs Questionnaire. Respir Med. 2008;102(10):1439–45.
21. Nasreddine ZS, Phillips NA, Bedirian V, Charbonneau S, Whitehead V, Collin I, et al. The montreal cognitive assessment, MoCA: a brief screening tool for mild cognitive impairment. J Am Geriatr Soc. 2005;53(4):695–9.
22. Folstein M, Folstein S, McHugh P. Mini-mental state: a practical method for grading the cognitive state of patients for the clinician. J Psychiatr Res. 1975;12(3):189–98.
23. Royall DR, Cordes JA, Polk M. CLOX: an executive clock drawing task. J Neurol Neurosurg Psychiatry. 1998;64(5):588–94.
24. Shum J, Poureslami I, Doyle-Waters MM, FitzGerald JM. The application of health literacy measurement tools (collective or individual domains) in assessing chronic disease management: a systematic review protocol. Syst Rev. 2016;5(1):97.

25. Ward S, Sewell L, Singh S. P144 Evaluation of multidisciplinary pulmonary rehabilitation education delivered by either DVD or spoken talk. Thorax. 2011;66(Suppl 4):A126.
26. Sohanpal R, Steed L, Mars T, Taylor SJ. Understanding patient participation behaviour in studies of COPD support programmes such as pulmonary rehabilitation and self-management: a qualitative synthesis with application of theory. NPJ Prim Care Respir Med. 2015;25:15054.
27. Thorpe O, Johnston K, Kumar S. Barriers and enablers to physical activity participation in patients with COPD: a systematic review. J Cardiopulm Rehabil Prev. 2012;32(6):359–69.
28. Kosteli MC, Heneghan NR, Roskell C, Williams SE, Adab P, Dickens AP, et al. Barriers and enablers of physical activity engagement for patients with COPD in primary care. Int J COPD. 2017;12:1019–31.
29. Bandura A. Self-efficacy: toward a unifying theory of behavioral change. Psychol Rev. 1977;84:191–215.
30. Vincent E, Sewell L, Wagg K, Deacon S, Williams J, Singh S. Measuring a change in self-efficacy following pulmonary rehabilitation: an evaluation of the PRAISE tool. Chest. 2011;140(6):1534–9.
31. Riegel B, Lee C, Dickson VV, Carlson B. An update on the self-care of heart failure index. J Cardiovasc Nurs. 2009;24(6):485–97.
32. Riegel B, Carlson B, Glaser D. Development and testing of a clinical tool measuring self-management of heart failure. Heart Lung. 2000;29(1):4–15.
33. Jaarsma T, Stromberg A, Martensson J, cup K. Development and testing of the European heart failure self-care behaviour scale. Eur J Heart Fail. 2003;5(3):363–70.
34. Mesquita R, Nakken N, Janssen DJA, van den Bogaart EHA, Delbressine JML, Essers JMN, et al. Activity levels and exercise motivation in COPD patients and their resident loved ones. Chest. 2017;151(5):1028–38.
35. Roberts NJ, Kidd L, Dougall N, Patel IS, McNarry S, Nixon C. Measuring patient activation: the utility of the Patient Activation Measure within a UK context-Results from four exemplar studies and potential future applications. Patient Educ Couns. 2016;99(10):1739–46.
36. Puhan M, Scharplatz M, Troosters T, Walters EH, Steurer J. Pulmonary rehabilitation following exacerbations of chronic obstructive pulmonary disease. Cochrane Database Syst Rev. 2009;1:CD005305.
37. Jones SE, Green SA, Clark AL, Dickson MJ, Nolan AM, Moloney C, et al. Pulmonary rehabilitation following hospitalisation for acute exacerbation of COPD: referrals, uptake and adherence. Thorax. 2014;69(2):181–2.
38. The Health Foundation. Quality improvement made simple: what everyone should know about health care quality improvement. The Health Foundation; 2013 August.
39. Institute of Medicine. Crossing the quality chasm: a new health system for the 21st century. Washington, DC: National Academy Press; 1990.

Part IV

Program Components

Exercise Training in Pulmonary Rehabilitation

10

Chris Burtin and Richard ZuWallack

10.1 Exercise and Pulmonary Rehabilitation: Concepts

10.1.1 Exercise and Activity

Higher levels of exercise capacity and physical activity are each independently related to health in individuals in general and COPD patients in particular [1]. Exercise and physical activity, however, while sharing some features, are separate concepts: exercise is considered a subset of physical activity. Physical activity refers to any bodily movement produced by skeletal muscles that results in energy expenditure. In contrast, exercise is planned, structured, typically repetitive, and done with a particular goal in mind [2]. Increases in both exercise capacity and physical activity are important goals of pulmonary rehabilitation, although the methods (and success) of achieving these goals are different.

C. Burtin
Faculty of Medicine and Life Sciences, Rehabilitation Research Centre, Biomedical Research Institute, Hasselt University, Diepenbeek, Belgium
e-mail: chris.burtin@uhasselt.be

R. ZuWallack (✉)
Saint Francis Hospital and Medical Center, University of Connecticut, Farmington, USA
e-mail: rzuwalla@stfranciscare.org

10.1.2 Pulmonary Rehabilitation

Pulmonary rehabilitation is defined as "… a comprehensive intervention based on a thorough patient assessment followed by patient-tailored therapies that include, but are not limited to, exercise training, education, and behavior change, designed to improve the physical and psychological condition of people with chronic respiratory disease and to promote the long-term adherence to health-enhancing behaviors" [3]. Exercise and education aimed at behavior change are the two pillars of comprehensive pulmonary rehabilitation. Exercise training is necessary, but not sufficient, to achieve the fullest benefit from the pulmonary rehabilitation intervention. The two components, exercise training and education, are complementary: (1) patients' perceptions of improvements in exercise capacity during exercise training may lead to a better "buy-in" to the educational efforts aimed at collaborative self-management, while (2) increased self-efficacy resulting from education may lead to better long-term adherence to the exercise training prescription.

Exercise training for COPD patients—as for individuals in general—does not refer to a single modality; rather, it includes varied methods such as endurance exercise training, interval exercise training, walking exercise, Nordic walking (designed as an off-season training for athletes, requiring walking with specially designed poles [4]), resistance training, aquatic exercise, classroom calisthenics, and Tai Chi [5]. Adding to this complexity, training

© Springer International Publishing AG 2018
E. Clini et al. (eds.), *Textbook of Pulmonary Rehabilitation*, https://doi.org/10.1007/978-3-319-65888-9_10

intensities can be high or low [6, 7], the intervention is focused on specific patient deficits, and its duration varies widely among patients, again dependent on their specific requirements. Truly, one size does not fit all. It is the responsibility of the pulmonary rehabilitation professionals to tailor the intervention to the individual patient.

10.1.3 The Problem of Translating Increases in Exercise Capacity Realized in the Pulmonary Rehabilitation Area to Meaningful and Sustained Increases in the Home and Community Settings

Increased exercise capacity resulting from exercise training, while permissive of increased physical activity, is not directly translated into this latter, important goal [8]. Most likely changes in self-efficacy resulting from educational efforts are important for eventual increases in physical activity in the home and community setting. This increase in physical activity probably has a different (flatter) trajectory than the change in exercise capacity realized in the pulmonary laboratory, leading one editorial writer to quip that "...one needs 3 months to train the muscle, but 6 months to train the brain" [9]. As with exercise training, this underscores the need for incorporation of education aimed at promoting self-efficacy in optimizing physical outcomes. Promoting sustained increases in exercise capacity and meaningful physical activity remain major challenges to pulmonary rehabilitation.

10.1.4 Mechanisms of Exercise Capacity Limitation in COPD

Exercise capacity is often substantially reduced in individuals with chronic respiratory disease. Exercise limitation in this setting usually is due to exertional dyspnea and fatigue from the disease, its systemic effects, and common comorbid conditions. Often underappreciated by clinicians is the contribution of these comorbid conditions—such as cardiovascular disease, anxiety or depression, exercise-limiting dyspnea, or fatigue in chronic respiratory disease. For example, anxiety, which is epidemic in the COPD population, aggravates the dyspnea sensation resulting from the physiologic disturbances of the respiratory disease. The symptom burden and the resultant decrease in exercise capacity contribute substantially to reductions in functional status and quality of life in this disease.

Table 10.1 Physiologic and psychologic causes of dyspnea in patients with chronic lung disease

• Increased resistive work of breathing from airflow limitation
• Increased elastic work of breathing and "pseudo-restriction" from static and dynamic hyperinflation
• Physical and cardiovascular deconditioning from sedentarism
• Gas exchange abnormalities: hypoxemia and increased physiologic dead space
• Cardiovascular limitations: cardiac or peripheral vascular comorbidity, leading to early lactate production with exercise
• Skeletal muscle abnormalities: decreased mass, fiber-type alterations (reduction in Type I, increase in Type IIx), capillarization defect, decreased oxidative enzymes, also leading to early lactate production with exercise [68]
• Coexisting obesity, increasing workload requirements for a specific task
• Anxiety associated with dyspnea-producing activity

Table 10.1 lists some of these physiologic and psychologic disturbances that may cause or aggravate dyspnea in individuals with chronic lung disease. The typical patient has several derangements which lead to dyspnea, and a number of them respond to the comprehensive pulmonary rehabilitation intervention. Furthermore, some of these mechanisms clearly overlap, such as physical deconditioning, cardiovascular limitation, and decreased muscle mass and oxidative enzymes.

10.1.5 The Vicious Circle of Dyspnea, Inactivity, Deconditioning, and Increased Dyspnea in COPD

Thus, exertional dyspnea in COPD is caused by multiple factors, including increased resistive work of breathing from airflow limitation, increased elastic work of breathing from static and dynamic hyperinflation, increased dead space ventilation, gas exchange abnormalities with exercise-induced hypoxemia, cardiovascular limitations, anxiety associated with dyspnea-producing activities, functional respiratory muscle weakness resulting from a mechanical disadvantage and increased loading from hyperinflation, and abnormalities of the ambulatory muscles, including depletion of muscle mass and reductions in oxidative enzymes. The latter may result from nutritional disturbances, physical deconditioning, systemic inflammation, oxidative stress, corticosteroid use, and low anabolic steroid levels [3]. The ambulatory muscle dysfunction results in increased production of lactic acid during exercise; buffering of this acid further increases the ventilatory demands on the compromised system [7].

The unpleasant symptoms of dyspnea and fatigue lead to conscious or unconscious decreases in exercise and physical activity by the patient. Prolonged physical inactivity, in turn, leads to further increases in dyspnea and fatigue, increasing physical deconditioning. Thus, a vicious circle of dyspnea/fatigue leads to inactivity, leading to deconditioning, leading to increased dyspnea/fatigue ensues. Comprehensive pulmonary rehabilitation can interrupt this vicious circle.

10.1.6 A Brief History of Exercise Training in COPD

Exercise training remains, by far, the best intervention to enhance skeletal muscle function in COPD [10–12]. Enhancement of exercise capacity realized from exercise training occurs predictably without corresponding direct improvement in lung physiology [13, 14]. This apparent paradox undoubtedly led to a delay in the acceptance of pulmonary rehabilitation by the general medical community. Prior to the 1990s, clinicians—who failed to think outside the box—believed COPD patients were ventilatory (i.e., pump) limited and because of this could not attain the levels of exercise intensity needed for a physiologic training effect.

The rationale behind the effectiveness of exercise training in pulmonary rehabilitation began to change in 1991, when Casaburi and colleagues [7] showed, in a very small trial comparing high- and low-intensity exercise training interventions in patients with COPD, that (1) individuals often were physiologically deconditioned, leading to lactate production (which has to be buffered by the increased ventilation) from even low levels of physical exercise; (2) exercise training led to demonstrable physiologic training effects; and (3) the physiologic effect of exercise training was dose-dependent: higher intensity led to greater benefit than lower intensity.

Shortly after the above study, work by Maltais and colleagues demonstrated that oxidative enzymes were reduced in the skeletal muscles of the lower extremities of COPD patients [15]. Furthermore, these enzymes could be increased by exercise training [12]. This established some of the metabolic underpinnings to the exercise limitation and the benefits from skeletal muscle training.

Subsequently, exercise training was demonstrated to *indirectly* reduce dynamic hyperinflation in patients with COPD: a physiologic training effect reduces lactate production from the exercising (ambulatory) muscles at iso-time or iso-work levels; this in turn reduces ventilatory demand, allowing for a lower respiratory rate, more time for emptying of the lung at the end of each exhalation, and less dynamic hyperinflation [16]. Expanding on this concept, these investigators demonstrated that oxygen supplementation increases exercise capacity in COPD, probably through, in part, less dynamic hyperinflation [17], and that supplemental oxygen can increase exercise capacity even in non-hypoxemic patients [18].

These studies underscore the complex nature of exercise capacity limitation in COPD and the varied mechanisms through which exercise training may work.

10.1.7 Increasing Exercise Capacity from Different Perspectives

Pharmacologic therapy, such as administration of inhaled bronchodilators, tends to increase exercise capacity in patients with COPD, probably through reducing the resistive work of breathing (bronchodilation) and/or the elastic work of breathing (reducing dynamic hyperinflation). However, the effect of pharmacologic interventions on exercise capacity in these patients, although significant, is often of a relatively low magnitude. Exercise training, as a major component of pulmonary rehabilitation, on the other hand, often produces relatively greater increases in exercise capacity than drug therapy. Much of this improvement results from direct effects on ambulatory muscles from the formal exercise training intervention. However, other aspects of comprehensive pulmonary rehabilitation, such as promotion of adherence to regular exercise and regular physical activity, pacing and energy-conserving techniques, and desensitization to dyspnea, probably also contribute to this salutatory effect [19–23].

Additionally, pharmacologic therapy and exercise training should be considered complementary: exercise training will further increase exercise capacity in patients whose lung function is optimized with bronchodilators, and optimal bronchodilation will allow for greater intensity and duration of exercise training in pulmonary rehabilitation, thereby augmenting its effectiveness. This relationship was demonstrated in a randomized, controlled study by Casaburi and colleagues [24], who showed that the group of COPD patients given long-acting bronchodilator therapy had greater increases in exercise capacity from pulmonary rehabilitation exercise training than the control group, which took only as-needed short-acting beta-agonist therapy.

Besides bronchodilators, other therapies may enhance the effectiveness of exercise training in COPD. Supplemental oxygen is virtually universally prescribed for patients with significant and sustained hypoxemia, based on studies demonstrating its effect on prolonging survival [25]. Although results are somewhat mixed, supplemental oxygen may increase the beneficial effects of high-intensity exercise training in COPD patients with and (remarkably) even without significant hypoxemia associated with exercise [26]. The proposed mechanism underlying its potential effectiveness as an exercise training enhancer in COPD is that oxygen supplementation reduces dyspnea, resulting in a decreased respiratory rate and prolonged expiratory time during exercise, allowing for more complete emptying of the lung in hyperinflated COPD patients [18, 27]. Other potential nonpharmacologic exercise enhancers include the use of rollators (rolling walkers), which may enhance the mechanical advantage of the accessory muscles of ventilation with fixation of the arm or reduce the metabolic cost of ambulation, [28] unloading the respiratory muscles using noninvasive ventilation or a helium-oxygen mixture [28].

Hormonal supplements such as anabolic steroids or growth hormone have been used as supplements to exercise training in COPD patients. In general, the administration of testosterone or its analogs has shown increases in muscle mass, but not necessarily muscle strength [29–31]. One small, short-term trial in COPD patients compared four treatments: testosterone alone, strength training alone, both, and neither. Both single intervention treatments resulted in increased muscle mass and strength, and their combination showed additive effects in these areas. Other outcomes, such as exercise endurance capacity or health status, were not tested. Two small studies of growth hormone treatment in COPD have demonstrated increase in lean (muscle) mass increases, but no functional improvement [32, 33]. Certainly, in view of the limited effectiveness and potential side effects, further and longer-term studies would be necessary before these therapies would be indicated.

Partitioning of the exercising muscle mass during exercise training is another potential method for enhancing its effectiveness in COPD patients. Near whole-body exercise training imposes a substantial increased ventilatory load in patients who may already be severely "pump limited," thereby limiting the intensity or duration of the training. By partitioning the muscle mass of the exercise muscles to a smaller exercising mass, such as with one-leg cycle training (versus two-leg simultaneous exercise), peak power and peak oxygen consumption can be increased [34, 35]. This technique can be readily incorporated into a pulmonary rehabilitation program [36].

Noninvasive positive pressure ventilation (NPPV) has also been successfully used as an adjunct to exercise training in the pulmonary rehabilitation of patients with COPD. In this setting, NPPV can be used either (1) during exercise training, to help unload the respiratory muscles which are often at a mechanical disadvantage because of hyperinflation and thereby promote increased exercise intensity, or (2) at night, presumably to help rest the respiratory muscles. In general, the use of NPPV in these two applications appears to be successful [37], especially in those patients with severe disease. Practically, since NPPV requires special expertise and is labor-intensive, its use as an exercise performance enhancer should probably be reserved for those COPD patients with severe airflow obstruction, hyperinflation, and functional limitation.

10.2 Exercise Training Principles

10.2.1 Aerobic Training

Aerobic training is generally considered the core component of exercise training in patients with COPD [3]. It is most frequently performed on a cycle ergometer and/or a stationary treadmill, but stair climbing, stepping, free walking, Nordic walking, and swimming are possible and effective alternatives or complements. Upper limb aerobic training can be a valuable addition to lower limb training in light of optimizing the performance of activities of daily living [38]. In general, recommendations of the American College of Sports Medicine in terms of training parameters (frequency, intensity, time, and mode) have been successfully applied in patients with different disease severities [39]. Programs including three to five weekly aerobic training sessions of 20–60 min at moderate-to-high intensity (>60% of maximal work capacity) yield optimal training results in terms of exercise tolerance and health-related quality of life [3]. Session duration and intensity are built up gradually throughout the training program.

Endurance-based exercise (exercise bouts > 10 min) has historically been the aerobic training method of choice in patients with COPD. Higher training intensities are typically associated with larger physiological improvements, as more overload is provided at the peripheral muscle level [7, 40]. However, a proportion of patients are not able to reach sufficiently high intensity during endurance efforts, mostly due to symptoms of dyspnea, leg fatigue, or anxiety. In these patients, high-intensity interval training can be an interesting alternative strategy. This modality typically consists of short bouts of cycling exercise (30 s to 2 min) at high relative intensity (80–100% of maximum workload), alternated with short periods of active rest at very low intensities [41]. This approach provides a strong stimulus to the peripheral muscle, with somewhat lower cardiorespiratory responses and limited lactate accumulation, allowing a prolonged exercise session with possibly decreased symptom scores [41, 42].

Evidence indicates that high-intensity interval training results in similar improvements of peak oxygen consumption, 6-min walking distance, and health-related to quality of life compared to traditional endurance training, given that the performed work (workload x exercise time) is identical [43, 44]. In line with this, local peripheral muscle adaptations (e.g., increased cross-sectional area of type I and type IIa muscle fibers, increased capillary-to-fiber ratio, increased oxidative enzyme activity) are similar after both interventions [45]. High-intensity interval training appears to be feasible even in patients with severe disease but requires excellent patient motivation and close supervision.

An alternative approach to provide an aerobic stimulus to the leg muscles with limited ventilatory load is one-legged cycling. By partitioning working muscle mass, a similar metabolic stimulus can be provided in the leg muscles with a lower minute ventilation and lower dyspnea scores [34]. Pilot studies indicate that this training method enhances peak oxygen consumption and decreases submaximal heart rate and ventilation to a larger extent compared to two-legged endurance cycling, indicating an enhanced cardiovascular and/or muscular training effect [35]. Importantly, this training modality does not extend the duration of the training session, as it appears sufficient to train each leg for half of the bi-legged cycling time. Practically, however, this modality requires modification of a typical cycle ergometer, since the generally used freewheeling mechanism needs to be blocked (to avoid excessive "pulling" activity from the hamstring) and bars need to be attached to rest the non-exercising leg. Nevertheless, one-legged cycling might optimize training response in a similar time frame as endurance training and therefore is an appealing strategy in patients that have difficulties to achieve high intensity during endurance exercise or patients that have troubles to induce peripheral muscle fatigue during exercise.

Eccentric exercise training is another alternative training modality for patients with COPD. Body movements typically include both concentric and eccentric contractions. When focusing on eccentric effort, higher muscle forces can be generated and the lengthening contractions are associated with a higher risk of muscle micro-damage [46]. Pilot projects in COPD have shown that eccentric cycling can elicit similar effect in terms of physical fitness than concentric cycling but with lower symptom scores [47]. Similarly, eccentric walking enhanced the development of quadriceps contractile fatigue in patients with COPD, with lower cardiovascular load and lower dyspnea scores [48]. Importantly, these trials indicated that delayed onset muscle soreness was not reported by patients and creatine kinase levels stayed within normal levels. The downside of these modalities is the fairly large cost of adapted equipment. Identification of specific patients that might respond well to this intervention (e.g., patients that cannot induce muscle fatigue with standard training) seems to be warranted.

In whole-body exercise modalities that are performed at higher intensities (e.g., high-intensity interval training), training duration is generally decreased and subdivided in a number of exercise bouts. Even though in general a choice of intensity and duration (i.e., shorter bouts at high to maximal intensity or longer bouts at moderate to high intensity) is consistently made for the whole training program (both in research settings as clinical programs), it may be beneficial to vary these parameters over time. A randomized controlled trial investigating the effectiveness of nonlinear exercise training in patients with advanced COPD reported enhanced results in terms of whole-body endurance capacity and health-related quality of life compared to traditional combined endurance-based aerobic training and resistance training [49]. The nonlinear program varied between sessions (not within sessions!) in terms of intensity and duration of cycle training and attempted to attain different adaptations of the neuromuscular system (both aerobic and anaerobic components). The clinical implementation of this "athlete" training approach is however challenging and needs further attention.

10.2.1.1 How to Start Your First Aerobic Training Session

Initially, training intensity during the first few sessions should be somewhat lower than the targeted optimal intensity, to customize patients to the training routine. This might especially be necessary in patients who are naïve to exercise training and patients who will perform treadmill walking exercise for the first time. During the first sessions, extensive attention should be paid to the safe use of the exercise training apparatus (including strategies to climb on and off a cycle ergometer, walking position and optimal use of upper limb support, and safety procedures during treadmill walking) and to breathing strategies during exercise.

Optimally, training intensity during cycling ergometry is based on cardiopulmonary exercise test (CPET) results. Aerobic training at 60% of maximal workload during CPET is often and successfully used as target intensity for aerobic training [50]. Treadmill walking speed can be based on field walking test performance. For example, a target walking speed of 70% of incremental shuttle walk speed or 80–85% of the average speed during the 6-min walk test speed can be used. While exercise tests allow an adequate estimation of optimal intensity, symptom scores (i.e., modified Borg scores) must be used to optimally titrate training intensity to the individual patients. A modified Borg score for dyspnea and/or fatigue ranging from 4 to 6 generally corresponds to moderate to high intensity exercise during whole-body exercise training [51]. Importantly, it is not recommended to use heart rate or heart rate reserve as marker for training intensity in patients with ventilatory exercise limitation.

During exercise, transcutaneous oxygen saturation and heart rate are measured regularly to ensure safety. In patients who desaturate below predetermined cutoff values (oftentimes oxygen saturation < 90%), supplemental oxygen should be used to exercise safely and increase training intensity. In patients who keep on desaturating despite adequate oxygen support, it is appropriate to divide the exercise session into multiple short bouts, allowing transcutaneous oxygen saturation to recover and stay in a safe range.

At every two to three sessions, an attempt should be made to increase the performed work during training by increasing workload (e.g., by increasing resistance on a cycle, increasing speed, or introduction of an inclination on a treadmill) or duration. Increasing both workload and duration in one session is not recommended.

10.2.2 Resistance Training

Resistance, or strength, training implies training of local muscle groups by repetitive lifting of relatively high loads. Compared to aerobic training, resistance training elicits lower cardiorespiratory responses (e.g., oxygen consumption and ventilation) and less dyspnea, which is particularly desirable in patients with more advanced COPD [52]. According to the American College of Sports Medicine, 1–3 sets of 8–12 repetitions should be performed on 2–3 days/week to obtain optimal benefits in terms of muscle strength [39]. Intensity should be sufficient to induce muscle fatigue; protocols with an intensity equaling 60–70% of one-repetition maximum (1-RM) are frequently used [50]. Adequate high-intensity resistance training primarily results in increased muscle strength and muscle mass but also has the potential to improve (sub)maximal exercise tolerance [53].

It has preference to perform resistance training on state-of-the-art equipment. This facilitates resistance training at an optimal intensity and allows for adequately monitoring the performed work. If such equipment is not available, training with free weight and therabands (elastic bands) could be considered as alternatives. Recently, whole-body vibration has been introduced as a promising modality to enhance the effects of resistance exercises in terms of functional status [54].

In line with aerobic training principles, intensity and duration are also inversely related in resistance training. High-intensity training with a low number of repetitions (as suggested by the ACSM, see above) targets muscle strength and power, while low-to-moderate intensity training with a high number of repetitions targets muscle endurance characteristics. The latter is less frequently used in the context of pulmonary rehabilitation, but combination of high- and low-intensity resistance training might be an interesting approach to optimize the local muscle stimulus.

10.2.2.1 How to Start Your First Resistance Training Session

The intensity of equipment-based resistance training is typically based on a direct measurement or estimation of the 1-RM on the same device. Even though target intensity is 60–70% of 1-RM (when aiming to increase muscle strength), it is advisable to start off at a somewhat lower intensity, to customize patients with the equipment, performed movement, and breathing strategy. Workload can then be rather quickly increased throughout the first training sessions. Training intensity in free weight or theraband-based training is typically set based on clinical expertise and symptom scores. Regardless of the modality, it is important to perform warming-up exercises in muscle that will be involved in high-intensity resistance training to avoid musculoskeletal injuries. In light of that, it is practical to perform aerobic exercise ahead of resistance exercises focusing on the same muscle groups.

Regular increase of the performed work (e.g., every week) is of crucial importance to keep on inducing overload to the skeletal muscles. Mostly, an increase of work is obtained by increasing workload (i.e., weight). The decision to increase the workload can be based on the modified Borg score on muscle fatigue (score 4–6) and the quality of the performed repetitions [51]. Patients should be able to perform a controlled movement over full range of motion, without overt compensation or trembling. Breathing pattern should be adequately linked with the exercise (i.e., expiration during the concentric phase and inspiration during the eccentric phase) to avoid dysfunctional breathing or Valsalva maneuvers.

10.2.3 Combined Aerobic and Resistance Training

Evidence suggests that aerobic training positive influences skeletal muscle strength, while resistance training improves aerobic exercise tolerance to some extent. Nevertheless, optimal effects in both muscle strength and aerobic exercise tolerance are only achieved by combining resistance and aerobic training, respectively, in line with the specificity of training principle [55]. Most pulmonary rehabilitation programs include one or more aerobic training modalities and resistance training of the large lower limb muscles (leg press, leg extension, leg flexion). Upper limb endurance and resistance training is a useful addition in patients that report difficulties to performed upper limb-based activities of daily living [38].

10.2.4 Low-Intensity Training

As stated above, exercise training in COPD follows general principles of exercise training in general, including greater gains in muscle function from greater intensity and duration of effort. However, patients may not be able to maintain higher intensities for prolonged durations, and long-term adherence with rigorous training schedules may be problematic. As a result, lower-intensity training, such as classroom calisthenics, may, on occasion, be considered. In one comparative study addressing these two approaches, although high-intensity training in pulmonary rehabilitation led to predictably greater improvements in exercise performance than low-intensity training, both approaches resulted in similar improvements in questionnaire-rated dyspnea, functional performance, and health status [6]. However, in general, higher-intensity exercise, as tolerated, is more commonly employed in pulmonary rehabilitation.

10.3 Systematic Reviews on Exercise Training in COPD

The most recent joint statement on pulmonary rehabilitation of the American Thoracic Society and European Respiratory Society provides an extensive overview of the published literature on comprehensive pulmonary rehabilitation [3]. Recent meta-analyses summarize the effects of aerobic and/or resistance training in patients with COPD [56, 57], while a review by Gloeckl et al. provides an interesting overview of practical recommendations for exercise training in these patients [50]. A systematic review of Camillo et al. summarizes the additional effect of several add-on interventions on top of aerobic exercise training (REF expected soon). In general, these reviews provide a strong level of scientific support for the effectiveness of exercise training across multiple outcome areas.

10.4 Selection of Appropriate Exercise Interventions for Individual Patients

10.4.1 Frail Patients

Frail patients might not be able to perform traditional aerobic and resistance training. Neuromuscular electrical stimulation of the upper leg muscles is a feasible intervention that increases muscle strength and functional status [58] and might be a start-up intervention in severely impaired patients, to allow the performance of more dynamic exercises in a next stage. Patients with balance issues can benefit from specific balance and transfer training [59].

10.4.2 Patients with Severe Exertional Breathlessness (e.g., With Advanced Disease or During Exacerbations)

Breathlessness symptoms might prevent patients from performing aerobic exercise. It is important to rule out oxygen desaturation as a cause of breathlessness, and supplemental oxygen should be provided in patients with decreased transcutaneous oxygen saturation (generally if < 90%). Also, as stated earlier, providing supplemental oxygen even for those COPD patients without exercise hypoxemia might allow for higher training intensity, probably through reducing the sensation of dyspnea, resulting in a lower respiratory rate and less dynamic hyperinflation. Resistance training and neuromuscular electrical stimulation are alternative strategies that positively influence muscle structure, while symptoms of breathlessness and fatigue are within the accepted limits [60, 61]. In patients experiencing a temporary increase in symptoms (e.g., during an exacerbation), the early initiation of high-intensity exercise training during recovery (as part of a pulmonary rehabilitation program) generates clinically relevant results in terms of exercise tolerance, quality of life, and use of health-care resources [62].

10.4.3 Patients with Comorbidities

Most patients with COPD attending pulmonary rehabilitation have one or more significant comorbid conditions [63]. This association is especially pronounced for several conditions, including cardiovascular disease, diabetes, lung cancer, anxiety, and depression [64]. In general, comorbid conditions are not, by definition, a sufficient reason to exclude patients from participating in exercise training. Only those comorbid conditions that would place the patient at undue risk from exercising or those conditions that would prevent meaningful exercise training would be considered as contraindications. Furthermore, and importantly, training results are generally not influenced by the presence of comorbidities [65]. Of course, every comorbidity should be taken into account when prescribing exercise, monitoring safety, and offering education, self-management strategies, and multidisciplinary care.

10.4.4 Exercise Training Based on ADL Impairments

As stated earlier, despite the positive results of exercise-based pulmonary rehabilitation on exercise performance, training effects do not always translate into a more satisfying performance of activities of daily living (ADL). During the course of the training program, it is important to identify ADLs that are impaired in the individual patient and important to that patient. Functional training should then, if possible, focus on those limited and important activities (e.g., stair climbing, sweeping, overhead arm movements, etc.).

10.5 Future Directions for Exercise Training in Pulmonary Rehabilitation

The science, rationale, and methodology underpinning exercise training in pulmonary rehabilitation have advanced dramatically over the past three decades. This remarkable progress is in contrast with that of the second pillar of pulmonary rehabilitation and education, where considerably more research is necessary to determine the optimal intervention for the specific patient. Nevertheless, further research in exercise training in pulmonary rehabilitation is certainly warranted, especially to fine-tune this already-proven therapy. Some areas that would seem particularly fruitful in this area include:

1. Determining the optimal mode, intensity, and duration of exercise training for the non-COPD respiratory patient
2. Evaluating exercise training in the peri-hospital period for the COPD exacerbation

3. Further studies on the potential usefulness, safety, role, and indications of non-center-based exercise training (such as home-based exercise) in pulmonary rehabilitation [66]
4. Further evaluating potential adjuncts to exercise training, evaluating methods to enhance the long-term adherence to the post-rehabilitation exercise prescription, including telemedicine [67]
5. Determining ways to better translate the gains made in exercise capacity into meaningful and sustained increases in physical activity in the home and community settings

References

1. Garcia-Rio F, Rojo B, Casitas R, Lores V, Madero R, Romero D, Galera R, Villasante C. Prognostic value of the objective measurement of daily physical activity in copd patients. Chest. 2012;142(2):338–46.
2. Caspersen CJ, Powell KE, Christenson GM. Physical activity, exercise, and physical fitness: definitions and distinctions for health-related research. Public Health Rep. 1985;100:126–31.
3. Spruit MA, Singh SJ, Garvey C, Zuwallack R, Nici L, Rochester C, Hill K, Holland AE, Lareau SC, Man WD, Pitta F, Sewell L, Raskin J, Bourbeau J, Crouch R, Franssen FM, Casaburi R, Vercoulen JH, Vogiatzis I, Gosselink R, Clini EM, Effing TW, Maltais F, van der Palen J, Troosters T, Janssen DJ, Collins E, Garcia-Aymerich J, Brooks D, Fahy BF, Puhan MA, Hoogendoorn M, Garrod R, Schols AM, Carlin B, Benzo R, Meek P, Morgan M, Rutten-van Molken MP, Ries AL, Make B, Goldstein RS, Dowson CA, Brozek JL, Donner CF, Wouters EF. An official american thoracic society/european respiratory society statement: key concepts and advances in pulmonary rehabilitation. Am J Respir Crit Care Med. 2013;188:e13–64.
4. Breyer MK, Breyer-Kohansal R, Funk GC, Dornhofer N, Spruit MA, Wouters EF, Burghuber OC, Hartl S. Nordic walking improves daily physical activities in copd: A randomised controlled trial. Respir Res. 2010;11:112.
5. Andrianopoulos V, Klijn P, Franssen FM, Spruit MA. Exercise training in pulmonary rehabilitation. Clin Chest Med. 2014;35:313–22.
6. Normandin EA, McCusker C, Connors M, Vale F, Gerardi D, ZuWallack RL. An evaluation of two approaches to exercise conditioning in pulmonary rehabilitation. Chest. 2002;121:1085–91.
7. Casaburi R, Patessio A, Ioli F, Zanaboni S, Donner CF, Wasserman K. Reductions in exercise lactic acidosis and ventilation as a result of exercise training in patients with obstructive lung disease. Am Rev Respir Dis. 1991;143:9–18.
8. Mador MJ, Patel AN, Nadler J. Effects of pulmonary rehabilitation on activity levels in patients with chronic obstructive pulmonary disease. J Cardiopulm Rehabil Prev. 2011;31:52–9.
9. Polkey MI, Rabe KF. Chicken or egg: Physical activity in copd revisited. Eur Respir J. 2009;33:227–9.
10. Sala E, Roca J, Marrades RM, Alonso J, Gonzalez De Suso JM, Moreno A, Barbera JA, Nadal J, de Jover L, Rodriguez-Roisin R, Wagner PD. Effects of endurance training on skeletal muscle bioenergetics in chronic obstructive pulmonary disease. Am J Respir Crit Care Med. 1999;159:1726–34.
11. Bernard S, Whittom F, Leblanc P, Jobin J, Belleau R, Berube C, Carrier G, Maltais F. Aerobic and strength training in patients with chronic obstructive pulmonary disease. Am J Respir Crit Care Med. 1999;159:896–901.
12. Maltais F, LeBlanc P, Simard C, Jobin J, Berube C, Bruneau J, Carrier L, Belleau R. Skeletal muscle adaptation to endurance training in patients with chronic obstructive pulmonary disease. Am J Respir Crit Care Med. 1996;154:442–7.
13. Franssen FM, Broekhuizen R, Janssen PP, Wouters EF, Schols AM. Effects of whole-body exercise training on body composition and functional capacity in normal-weight patients with copd. Chest. 2004;125:2021–8.
14. Spruit MA, Gosselink R, Troosters T, De Paepe K, Decramer M. Resistance versus endurance training in patients with copd and peripheral muscle weakness. Eur Respir J. 2002;19:1072–8.
15. Maltais F, Simard AA, Simard C, Jobin J, Desgagnes P, LeBlanc P. Oxidative capacity of the skeletal muscle and lactic acid kinetics during exercise in normal subjects and in patients with copd. Am J Respir Crit Care Med. 1996;153:288–93.
16. O'Donnell DE. Hyperinflation, dyspnea, and exercise intolerance in chronic obstructive pulmonary disease. Proc Am Thorac Soc. 2006;3:180–4.
17. Somfay A, Porszasz J, Lee SM, Casaburi R. Effect of hyperoxia on gas exchange and lactate kinetics following exercise onset in nonhypoxemic copd patients. Chest. 2002;121:393–400.
18. Emtner M, Porszasz J, Burns M, Somfay A, Casaburi R. Benefits of supplemental oxygen in exercise training in nonhypoxemic chronic obstructive pulmonary disease patients. Am J Respir Crit Care Med. 2003;168:1034–42.
19. Aliverti A, Macklem PT. The major limitation to exercise performance in copd is inadequate energy supply to the respiratory and locomotor muscles. J Appl Physiol. 2008;105:749–51; discussion 755–747
20. Debigare R, Maltais F. The major limitation to exercise performance in copd is lower limb muscle dysfunction. J Appl Physiol. 2008;105:751–3. discussion 755-757
21. O'Donnell DE, Webb KA. The major limitation to exercise performance in copd is dynamic hyperin-

flation. J Appl Physiol. 2008;105:753–5; discussion 755-757
22. Garcia-Aymerich J, Hernandez C, Alonso A, Casas A, Rodriguez-Roisin R, Anto JM, Roca J. Effects of an integrated care intervention on risk factors of copd readmission. Respir Med. 2007;101:1462–9.
23. Nici L, ZuWallack R. They can't bury you while you're still moving: A review of the european respiratory society statement on physical activity in chronic obstructive pulmonary disease. Pol Arch Med Wewn. 2015;125:771–8.
24. Nici L, ZuWallack R. Chronic obstructive pulmonary disease-evolving concepts in treatment: advances in pulmonary rehabilitation. Semin Respir Crit Care Med. 2015;36:567–74.
25. Continuous or nocturnal oxygen therapy in hypoxemic chronic obstructive lung disease: a clinical trial. Nocturnal oxygen therapy trial group. Ann Intern Med 1980;93:391–398.
26. Ries AL, Bauldoff GS, Carlin BW, Casaburi R, Emery CF, Mahler DA, Make B, Rochester CL, Zuwallack R, Herrerias C. Pulmonary rehabilitation: Joint accp/aacvpr evidence-based clinical practice guidelines. Chest. 2007;131:4S–42S.
27. Somfay A, Porszasz J, Lee SM, Casaburi R. Dose-response effect of oxygen on hyperinflation and exercise endurance in nonhypoxaemic copd patients. Eur Respir J. 2001;18:77–84.
28. Hill KHA. Strategies to enhance the benefits of exercise training in the respiratory patient. Clin Chest Med. 2013;35:323–36.
29. Ferreira IM, Verreschi IT, Nery LE, Goldstein RS, Zamel N, Brooks D, Jardim JR. The influence of 6 months of oral anabolic steroids on body mass and respiratory muscles in undernourished copd patients. Chest. 1998;114:19–28.
30. Schols AM, Soeters PB, Mostert R, Pluymers RJ, Wouters EF. Physiologic effects of nutritional support and anabolic steroids in patients with chronic obstructive pulmonary disease. A placebo-controlled randomized trial. Am J Respir Crit Care Med. 1995;152:1268–74.
31. Yeh SS, DeGuzman B, Kramer T. Reversal of COPD-associated weight loss using the anabolic agent oxandrolone. Chest. 2002;122:421–8.
32. Burdet L, de Muralt B, Schutz Y, Pichard C, Fitting JW. Administration of growth hormone to underweight patients with chronic obstructive pulmonary disease. A prospective, randomized, controlled study. Am J Respir Crit Care Med. 1997;156:1800–6.
33. Pape GS, Friedman M, Underwood LE, Clemmons DR. The effect of growth hormone on weight gain and pulmonary function in patients with chronic obstructive lung disease. Chest. 1991;99:1495–500.
34. Dolmage TE, Goldstein RS. Response to one-legged cycling in patients with copd. Chest. 2006;129:325–32.
35. Dolmage TE, Goldstein RS. Effects of one-legged exercise training of patients with copd. Chest. 2008;133:370–6.
36. Evans RA, Dolmage TE, Mangovski-Alzamora S, Romano J, O'Brien L, Brooks D, Goldstein RS. One-legged cycle training for chronic obstructive pulmonary disease. A pragmatic study of implementation to pulmonary rehabilitation. Ann Am Thorac Soc. 2015;12:1490–7.
37. Corner E, Garrod R. Does the addition of non-invasive ventilation during pulmonary rehabilitation in patients with chronic obstructive pulmonary disease augment patient outcome in exercise tolerance? A literature review. Physiother Res Int. 2010;15:5–15.
38. Janaudis-Ferreira T, Hill K, Goldstein R, Wadell K, Brooks D. Arm exercise training in patients with chronic obstructive pulmonary disease: a systematic review. J Cardiopulm Rehabil Prev. 2009;29:277–83.
39. Garber CE, Blissmer B, Deschenes MR, Franklin BA, Lamonte MJ, Lee IM, Nieman DC, Swain DP. American college of sports medicine position stand. Quantity and quality of exercise for developing and maintaining cardiorespiratory, musculoskeletal, and neuromotor fitness in apparently healthy adults: guidance for prescribing exercise. Med Sci Sports Exerc. 2011;43:1334–59.
40. Probst VS, Kovelis D, Hernandes NA, Camillo CA, Cavalheri V, Pitta F. Effects of 2 exercise training programs on physical activity in daily life in patients with copd. Respir Care. 2011;56:1799–807.
41. Vogiatzis I, Nanas S, Roussos C. Interval training as an alternative modality to continuous exercise in patients with copd. Eur Respir J. 2002;20:12–9.
42. Sabapathy S, Kingsley RA, Schneider DA, Adams L, Morris NR. Continuous and intermittent exercise responses in individuals with chronic obstructive pulmonary disease. Thorax. 2004;59:1026–31.
43. Varga J, Porszasz J, Boda K, Casaburi R, Somfay A. Supervised high intensity continuous and interval training vs. Self-paced training in copd. Respir Med. 2007;101:2297–304.
44. Kortianou EA, Nasis IG, Spetsioti ST, Daskalakis AM, Vogiatzis I. Effectiveness of interval exercise training in patients with copd. Cardiopulm Phys Ther J. 2010;21:12–9.
45. Vogiatzis I, Terzis G, Nanas S, Stratakos G, Simoes DC, Georgiadou O, Zakynthinos S, Roussos C. Skeletal muscle adaptations to interval training in patients with advanced copd. Chest. 2005;128:3838–45.
46. Tidball JG. Mechanisms of muscle injury, repair, and regeneration. Compr Physiol. 2011;1:2029–62.
47. Rocha Vieira DS, Baril J, Richard R, Perrault H, Bourbeau J, Taivassalo T. Eccentric cycle exercise in severe copd: feasibility of application. COPD. 2011;8:270–4.
48. Camillo CA, Burtin C, Hornikx M, Demeyer H, De Bent K, van Remoortel H, Osadnik CR, Janssens W, Troosters T. Physiological responses during downhill walking: a new exercise modality for subjects with chronic obstructive pulmonary disease? Chron Respir Dis. 2015;12:155–64.

49. Klijn P, van Keimpema A, Legemaat M, Gosselink R, van Stel H. Nonlinear exercise training in advanced chronic obstructive pulmonary disease is superior to traditional exercise training. A randomized trial. Am J Respir Crit Care Med. 2013;188:193–200.
50. Gloeckl R, Marinov B, Pitta F. Practical recommendations for exercise training in patients with copd. Eur Respir Rev. 2013;22:178–86.
51. Borg GA. Psychophysical bases of perceived exertion. Med Sci Sports Exerc. 1982;14:377–81.
52. Probst VS, Troosters T, Pitta F, Decramer M, Gosselink R. Cardiopulmonary stress during exercise training in patients with copd. Eur Respir J. 2006;27:1110–8.
53. O'Shea SD, Taylor NF, Paratz J. Peripheral muscle strength training in copd: a systematic review. Chest. 2004;126:903–14.
54. Gloeckl R, Heinzelmann I, Kenn K. Whole body vibration training in patients with copd: a systematic review. Chron Respir Dis. 2015;12:212–21.
55. Ortega F, Toral J, Cejudo P, Villagomez R, Sanchez H, Castillo J, Montemayor T. Comparison of effects of strength and endurance training in patients with chronic obstructive pulmonary disease. Am J Respir Crit Care Med. 2002;166:669–74.
56. McCarthy B, Casey D, Devane D, Murphy K, Murphy E, Lacasse Y. Pulmonary rehabilitation for chronic obstructive pulmonary disease. Cochrane Database Syst Rev. 2015;2:CD003793.
57. Iepsen UW, Jorgensen KJ, Ringbaek T, Hansen H, Skrubbeltrang C, Lange P. A combination of resistance and endurance training increases leg muscle strength in copd: an evidence-based recommendation based on systematic review with meta-analyses. Chron Respir Dis. 2015;12:132–45.
58. Sillen MJ, Speksnijder CM, Eterman RM, Janssen PP, Wagers SS, Wouters EF, Uszko-Lencer NH, Spruit MA. Effects of neuromuscular electrical stimulation of muscles of ambulation in patients with chronic heart failure or copd: a systematic review of the english-language literature. Chest. 2009;136:44–61.
59. Beauchamp MK, O'Hoski S, Goldstein RS, Brooks D. Effect of pulmonary rehabilitation on balance in persons with chronic obstructive pulmonary disease. Arch Phys Med Rehabil. 2010;91:1460–5.
60. Troosters T, Probst VS, Crul T, Pitta F, Gayan-Ramirez G, Decramer M, Gosselink R. Resistance training prevents deterioration in quadriceps muscle function during acute exacerbations of chronic obstructive pulmonary disease. Am J Respir Crit Care Med. 2010;181:1072–7.
61. Neder JA, Sword D, Ward SA, Mackay E, Cochrane LM, Clark CJ. Home based neuromuscular electrical stimulation as a new rehabilitative strategy for severely disabled patients with chronic obstructive pulmonary disease (copd). Thorax. 2002;57:333–7.
62. Puhan MA, Gimeno-Santos E, Scharplatz M, Troosters T, Walters EH, Steurer J. Pulmonary rehabilitation following exacerbations of chronic obstructive pulmonary disease. Cochrane Database Syst Rev. 2011;1:CD005305.
63. Vanfleteren LE, Spruit MA, Groenen M, Gaffron S, van Empel VP, Bruijnzeel PL, Rutten EP, Op't Roodt J, Wouters EF, Franssen FM. Clusters of comorbidities based on validated objective measurements and systemic inflammation in patients with chronic obstructive pulmonary disease. Am J Respir Crit Care Med. 2013;187:728–35.
64. Divo M, Cote C, de Torres JP, Casanova C, Marin JM, Pinto-Plata V, Zulueta J, Cabrera C, Zagaceta J, Hunninghake G, Celli B, Group BC. Comorbidities and risk of mortality in patients with chronic obstructive pulmonary disease. Am J Respir Crit Care Med. 2012;186:155–61.
65. Mesquita R, Vanfleteren LE, Franssen FM, Sarv J, Taib Z, Groenen MT, Gaffron S, Bruijnzeel PL, Pitta F, Wouters EF, Spruit MA. Objectively identified comorbidities in copd: Impact on pulmonary rehabilitation outcomes. Eur Respir J. 2015;46:545–8.
66. Maltais F, Bourbeau J, Lacasse Y, Shapiro S, Perrault H, Penrod JR, Baltzan M, Rouleau M, Julien M, Paradis B, Audet R, Hernandez P, Levy RD, Camp P, Lecours R, Picard D, Bernard S. A canadian, multicentre, randomized clinical trial of home-based pulmonary rehabilitation in chronic obstructive pulmonary disease: rationale and methods. Can Respir J. 2005;12:193–8.
67. Troosters T, Gosselink R, Janssens W, Decramer M. Exercise training and pulmonary rehabilitation: new insights and remaining challenges. Eur Respir Rev. 2010;19:24–9.
68. Caron MATM, Debigare R, Maltais F. Skeletal muscle dysfunction. In: Nici L, Richard ZW, editors. Chronic obstructive pulmonary disease: co-morbidities and systemic consequences. New York: Humana Press; 2012. p. 137–60.

11 Nutrition in Pulmonary Rehabilitation

Annemie Schols

11.1 Introduction

Nutrition has been the topic of extensive scientific research in chronic obstructive pulmonary disease (COPD). This chapter examines the impact that dietary habits, nutritional status and nutritional interventions may have in COPD. This chapter is largely based and partly overlapping with the ERS statement 'Nutritional assessment and therapy in COPD' [1] but updated in the context of pulmonary rehabilitation.

11.1.1 Scope

COPD is an important global health problem. Next to pulmonary impairment, systemic disease manifestations and acute exacerbations influence disease burden and mortality risk. Extending the classical descriptions of the 'pink puffer' and 'blue bloater', recent unbiased statistical approaches [2, 3] support the concept that body weight and body composition discriminate for pulmonary phenotypes and are predictors of outcome independent of lung function impairment. Incorporation of body composition in nutritional assessment has been a major step forwards in understanding systemic COPD pathophysiology and nutritional potential. While initially being considered as an indicator of inevitable and terminal progression of the disease process, there is now convincing evidence that unintended weight loss is not an adaptive mechanism to decrease metabolic rate in advanced COPD but an independent determinant of survival, arguing for weight maintenance in patient care. An important role of muscle loss and a decreased muscle oxidative metabolism in impaired physical performance has been demonstrated providing new leads for nutritional supplementation as adjunct to exercise training, not only confined to advanced disease but also in earlier disease stages. In addition, a pivotal role of osteoporosis, visceral adiposity and poor dietary quality in COPD risk and progression has emerged which positions dietary awareness and intervention as integral part of disease management, from prevention to chronic respiratory failure.

A. Schols
Department of Respiratory Medicine, NUTRIM School of Nutrition and Translational Research in Metabolism, Maastricht University Medical Centre, Maastricht, The Netherlands
e-mail: a.schols@maastrichtuniversity.nl

11.1.2 Nutritional Assessment

To develop and evaluate effective prevention and intervention strategies, stratification of the patient population into specific metabolic phenotypes is

© Springer International Publishing AG 2018
E. Clini et al. (eds.), *Textbook of Pulmonary Rehabilitation*, https://doi.org/10.1007/978-3-319-65888-9_11

required. While it is accepted that body weight and body composition variables represent a continuous spectrum, clear definitions and reference values for phenotypes that predict outcome and response to treatment have been developed over the past decade as shown in Table 11.1. These different conditions reflect a complex interaction between the effects of (epi)genetics, lifestyle and disease triggers on muscle, bone and adipose tissue. In view of the coexistence of different metabolic phenotypes during the disease trajectory, the ERS taskforce on 'nutrition and respiratory disease' has established a nutritional risk profile, based on prospective assessment of body weight (change) and body composition [1]. This nutritional risk stratification diaphragm will be useful in clinical trial design and in individually tailoring nutritional management. In this risk profile, an adapted WHO classification for BMI is used based on the lowest standardized rate of death from recent population studies [4, 5]. As a rule of thumb, involuntary weight loss >5% during the last 6 months is considered clinically significant taking natural variations into account. Recent weight loss can be assessed by patient recollection, although standardized weight measurements at regular intervals by caregivers and self-monitoring are often incorporated and more informative. Weight changes and BMI classification do not take body compositional shifts, including fat mass (FM) and distribution, lean mass (LM) and distribution and bone mineral density (BMD) into account. To distinguish between low and normal fat-free mass (FFM = LM + BMD), body composition needs to be assessed. Appropriate measurements of body composition and surrogate markers in research and clinical practice are presented in Table 11.2. In normal to underweight COPD patients, age- and gender-adjusted FFMI (=FFM (kg)/height^2(m)) <10th percentile is defined as abnormally low based on well-established adverse effects of low FFMI on physical performance and survival. In the age range of most Caucasian COPD patients at risk, this corresponds to a FFMI <17 kg/m^2 for males and <15 kg/m^2 for females as clinically useful proxy in normal to underweight patients with COPD [6]. Sarcopenia is characterized by low skeletal muscle index (SMI) defined as a lean appendicular mass (assessed by DEXA)/height^2 equal or below the mean minus 2 SD of that of healthy persons between 20 and 30 years of age of the same ethnic group [7]. Sarcopenia imposes additional risk for skeletal muscle weakness in an increasing proportion of older and overweight patients including COPD [8, 9]. An important difference between the risk stratification diagram and conventional nutritional risk scores, e.g. the malnutrition universal screening tool (MUST) [10] or mini nutritional assessment (MNA) [11], is that the latter are primarily focused on malnutrition and do not take abnormal body composition into account.

Table 11.1 Metabolic phenotypes, definition and clinical risks

Metabolic phenotype	Definition	Clinical risk
Obesity	BMI 30–35 kg/m^2	Increased cardiovascular risk
Morbid obesity	BMI > 35 kg/m^2	Increased cardiovascular risk Impaired physical performance
Sarcopenic obesity	BMI 30–35 kg/m^2 and SMI < 2SD below mean SMI of young (m) and (f) reference groups[111]	Increased cardiovascular risk Impaired physical performance
Sarcopenia	SMI < 2SD below mean SMI of young (m) and (f) reference groups	Increased mortality risk Impaired physical performance
Cachexia	Unintentional weight loss >5% in6 months and FFMI < 17 kg/m^2 (m)<15 kg/m^2 (f)	Increased mortality risk Impaired physical performance
Precachexia	Unintentional weight loss >5%in 6 months	Increased mortality risk

BMI body mass index: weight/height^2, *SMI* appendicular skeletal muscle index: appendicular lean mass/height^2, *FFMI* fat-free mass index: fat-free mass/height^2, *m* male, *f* female

Table 11.2 Appropriate measurements of body composition and surrogate markers in research and clinical practice

Variable	Research	Clinical practice
Fat-free mass/fat mass	Deuterium dilution (^2H_2O)	DEXA, single-frequency BIA
Intracellular mass	^2H_2O combined with bromide dilution	Anthropometry (sum of four skinfolds)
		Multifrequency BIA
Muscle mass	Computed tomography (CT)	DEXA
	Magnetic resonance imaging (MRI)	Ultrasonography
	Biomarkers (i.e. D_3 creatine dilution)	Biomarkers (i.e. creatine height index)
		Anthropometry (mid-arm muscle circumference)
Abdominal fat	CT	DEXA
Abdominal visceral fat	MRI	Anthropometry (i.e. sagittal diameter and/or waist/hip circumference)
	Biomarkers (i.e. PAI-1)	Ultrasonography
Bone mass and density	DEXA	DEXA
		HRCT
Muscle strength and related physical performance	Isokinetic quadriceps strength	One-repetition maximum
	(Repetitive) magnetic stimulation	Handgrip strength
	Timed up and go test	Timed up and go test
	Stair climb power test	Stair climb power test
	Cycle ergometry	

BIA bioelectrical impedance, *DEXA* dual-energy X-ray absorptiometry, *HRCT* high-resolution CT scan

11.2 Metabolic Phenotypes and Nutritional Risk Profile in COPD

Recent large population studies have revealed that the age-standardized rate of death from any cause was lowest among participants with a BMI of 22.5–24.9 kg/m^2 and of 20–25 kg/m^2 in analyses restricted to those who never smoked [4, 5]. In patients with moderate to severe airflow obstruction, a BMI <25 kg/m^2 was consistently associated with increased mortality risk relative to overweight and even obese patients [12–14]. This prognostic advantage of increased BMI also referred to as 'obesity paradox' in COPD could be related to the direct effect of adipose tissue on lung mechanics (e.g. relative reduction in static volumes in obese COPD patients [15]). However, it might also be an epiphenomenon for other yet unknown disease characteristics that confer both a reduced mortality risk and preserved FM and/or FFM. Furthermore, it is not yet clear whether it is excessive fat or preserved FFM that contributes to the survival advantage in COPD, since low FFM index (<10th percentile) independent of BMI and FM is a strong predictor of mortality [16]. The prevalence of underweight in COPD increases with disease severity [16] and is also clearly associated with the presence of emphysema [17]. In normal to overweight patients, a low FFMI implies a proportionally high FMI. Furthermore, FM may be redistributed from the subcutaneous to visceral adipose tissue which has been associated with increased cardiovascular risk in mild-to-moderate COPD [18]. COPD patients with underweight or low FFM are more prone to loss of BMD than overweight patients [19]. DEXA is most appropriate for combined screening of both osteoporosis, FFM and FM. Although distinction between abdominal visceral and subcutaneous fat mass requires more advanced imaging technologies (e.g. computed tomography (CT) and magnetic resonance imaging (MRI)), a clinically useful estimate can be derived by DEXA.

11.3 Pathophysiology of Abnormal Body Composition and Targets for Nutritional Intervention

Understanding the pathophysiology and cross talk of muscle loss and adiposity in COPD is essential for the development of targeted nutritional interventions to address specific metabolic phenotypes.

11.3.1 Fat Loss

Loss of body weight and fat mass occurs when energy expenditure exceeds energy availability. Eating *per se* is an activity that can adversely affect haemoglobin saturation and increase dyspnoea in patients with severe COPD [20]. Ageing is also a contributing factor to reduced dietary intake in COPD due to symptoms (e.g. loss of taste, poor dentition, dysphagia, poor chewing and swallowing ability, poor appetite or food aversion) and social problems (e.g. living or eating alone or poverty) and the inability to self-feed [21]. Anorexia is however not the primary trigger of a disturbed energy balance in clinically stable disease, since generally a normal appetite to even increased dietary intake is reported in underweight patients [22, 23]. Moreover, while the normal response to semi-starvation is a reduced metabolic rate and depressed whole-body protein turnover, weight losing of COPD patients may display elevated resting energy expenditure (REE) and increased whole-body protein turnover [24]. Furthermore, in addition to an increased cost of ventilation due to abnormal pulmonary mechanics, a higher ATP cost of muscular contraction [25] may contribute to decreased mechanical efficiency of lower limb exercise [26] and elevated daily energy requirements in some COPD patients [27]. In support of this, weight gain after lung volume reduction surgery was associated with improved lung function and reduced work of breathing [28]. Collectively, this indicates a hypermetabolic state that may contribute to weight loss if energy requirements are not fully met and provides a convincing rationale for caloric supplementation to maintain or increase fat mass. Early concerns about adverse effects of carbohydrate (CHO) supplementation in COPD due to increased CO_2 production, resulting from CHO oxidation loading ventilation, have not been substantiated in more recent studies but were only observed after hyperalimentation [29]; this is in practice unlikely to happen with oral nutrition, especially in patients with poor appetite, and can easily be avoided by smaller meal portions well spread over the day.

11.3.2 Muscle Loss

Muscle mass is determined by the net balance of muscle protein synthesis and protein breakdown. There is evidence for increased muscle protein degradation rate in cachectic COPD patients characterized by low BMI and low FFMI [30]. Analyses of the effector pathways of protein degradation showed consistent elevation of components of the ubiquitin 26S-proteasome system and enhanced autophagy [31]. Conversely, distal protein synthesis signalling cues (IGF-I and phospho-Akt expression levels) are mainly unaltered or adaptively increased [30]. More research is required to exclude any impairment in protein synthesis signalling (i.e. its responsiveness to catabolic triggers), but assuming this is not the case [32], stimulating protein synthesis more proximally using nutritional intervention to counterbalance elevated proteolysis may contribute to muscle mass maintenance in the presence of increased protein turnover in cachectic patients. Stimulation of protein synthesis depends on the availability of AA in the blood stream. COPD patients with low FFM have low plasma levels of branched-chain amino acids (BCAA) compared with age-matched controls [33]. It is well known that BCAA, in particular leucine, are able to stimulate muscle protein synthesis. Further research is required to investigate if the anabolic potential of high-quality protein is less in chronic respiratory failure or in the cachectic susceptible emphysematous phenotype, since the latter also exhibited a blunted whole-body protein turnover after acute exercise [34].

11.3.3 Loss of Bone Mineral Density

Osteoporosis is a skeletal disease characterized by low bone mass and micro-architectural deterioration with a net increase in bone fragility and hence susceptibility to fracture [35]. Hip fractures are directly related to falls causing hospitalization and excess mortality. Vertebral fractures occur more often silently and are thought to result from routine activities such as bending or lifting. In patients with COPD, vertebral and rib cage fractures may lead to increased kyphosis, reduced rib cage mobility and further reduction of pulmonary function. COPD and osteoporosis often coincide. Prevalence data are varying from 5 to 60% depending on the diagnostic methods, the population setting and the severity of the disease [36]. One reason for this association is the presence of common risk factors such as ageing, smoking, underweight, sarcopenia and physical or functional limitation. Additionally, systemic inflammation, the use of systemic corticosteroids and the high prevalence of vitamin D deficiency, which are frequently observed in more severe stages of COPD, unequivocally contribute to a further loss of bone and muscle mass [37, 38]. Observational studies also suggest that emphysema represents a particular phenotype that is associated with musculoskeletal impairment, but the underlying mechanisms still remain unclear [39–41]. Bone tissue is continuously renewed throughout life. After reaching a peak bone mass at the age of 25–30 years, bone formation balances back to resorption with an annual loss of 0.5–1%. Vitamin D plays a key role in the regulation of calcium and bone homeostasis, but other factors including several pro-inflammatory cytokines also act on this pathway. Significant associations between low 25-OHD levels and bone mineral density (BMD) have been shown in different populations, including COPD patients [42]. Low 25-OHD levels are also associated with muscle weakness and increased risk of falls, so that sufficient intake of vitamin D and calcium, in addition to life style modifications (increased physical activity, spending more time outside, smoking cessation and limited alcohol use), still composes the basis of all prevention and treatment strategies of osteoporosis [43].

11.3.4 Adiposity

In patients with advanced disease, respiratory failure is the most common cause of death, with sarcopenia and cachexia as important risk factors. In contrast, in patients with mild-to-moderate disease, the primary cause of death is ischaemic cardiovascular disease, for which adiposity is an important lifestyle-induced risk factor [44]. There is increasing evidence that adipose tissue in COPD patients with relative or absolute fat abundance is a significant contributor to the systemic inflammatory load [45]. Abdominal visceral fat is more strongly associated with cardiovascular risk than subcutaneous fat, which could be related to a higher inflammatory capacity. In mild-to-moderate nonobese COPD patients, a fat redistribution was shown towards more abdominal visceral fat compared to controls despite comparable total fat mass [18]. It is yet unclear to what extent this redistribution reflects unhealthy lifestyle or is disease induced and whether the two act synergistically [46]. Obese COPD patients have increased dyspnoea at rest and poorer health status compared to normal-weight patients, while static lung hyperinflation is reduced, irrespective of the severity of disease [15]. The combined effects of obesity and COPD on exercise tolerance seem to depend on the type of exercise (weight bearing versus non weight bearing) that is performed. While peak cycling capacity is preserved in obese COPD patients compared to nonobese and dyspnoea, ratings are consistently lower during cycling in obese patients, the distance covered during a 6-min walk test (6MWD) is reduced, and the degree of fatigue is increased in obese patients [47]. No studies have systematically investigated the effects of weight loss interventions on adiposity, functionality and systemic inflammatory profile in patients with COPD. Although weight maintenance after a short-term period of weight loss is reported as major challenge in other risk populations, even modest reductions in weight can reduce the cardiovascular disease risk through improvements in body fat distribution [48]. A combination of dietary intervention and aerobic exercise may achieve this goal best as aerobic exercise training improves insulin sensitivity, induces mitochondrial biogenesis in skeletal muscle and induces loss of visceral fat mass [46]. Feasibility and efficacy of this approach however may be limited in advanced COPD by ventilatory restraints on exercise intensity. Alternatively or as adjunct, intervention with bioactive nutrients (e.g. polyphenols, polyunsaturated fatty acids and nitrate) has been proposed to boost muscle mitochondrial metabolism and limit ectopic fat accumulation [49], but this requires adequate clinical trials in COPD in the future.

11.3.5 Acute Exacerbations

Weight loss and wasting of muscle and bone tissue may be induced or accelerated during severe acute exacerbations requiring hospitalization, due to convergence of different catabolic stimuli including malnutrition [50], physical inactivity [51], hypoxia, inflammation [52] and systemic glucocorticoids [53]. Moreover, this may be a time when energy intake may be compromised by practical difficulties in providing adequate nutrition due to breathlessness or other treatments such as noninvasive ventilation. Furthermore, impaired responsiveness to signalling cues of muscle regeneration and protein synthesis [32] may delay recovery and increase the risk for readmission [54]. In the acute phase of respiratory exacerbations, loss of appetite and reduced dietary intake are often experienced in concert with elevated systemic levels of the appetite-regulating hormone leptin and pro-inflammatory cytokines [50, 52]. Next to nutritional risk screening and early intervention in primary care, hospitalizations could be considered as an additional opportunity for detailed nutritional assessment and implementation of longer-term nutritional management as it represents a period of heightened 'nutritional risk' which may require intensive nutritional therapy [55]. The impact of such intensive regimes on clinical outcomes and underlying mechanisms is yet to be clearly established.

11.4 Dietary Management and Nutritional Supplementation

Due to the ubiquitous nature of nutrition and the multiple metabolic effects induced by each food, nutrient or micronutrient, randomized clinical trials in this area are facing specific obstacles. By nature, some obstacles are difficult to resolve, such as having a placebo or proper blinding of food. Due to the multiple metabolic impacts of nutrients, choosing a primary outcome and the determination of sample size are particularly difficult. Nutritional research on single foods is also complex because it exploits a multitude of bioactive compounds acting on an extensive network of interacting processes.

11.4.1 Treatment of Weight Loss in COPD

A patient in a negative energy balance and losing weight will need to increase energy intake, as additional reduction of energy expenditure is highly undesirable in COPD. A suitable energy- and protein-enriched diet can be achieved by several small portions spread throughout the whole day [56]. The energy- and protein-enriched diet often has a higher fat content (45% of total energy) than in recommendations for healthy individuals. Due to the high proportion of fat, consideration needs to be given to the quality of fat, especially in choice of fat used for cooking, to minimize the proportion of saturated fat. It is generally recommended in current guidelines that protein should provide 20% of the total energy intake. Fortification products can be used to increase energy and protein content in different meals [57]. A dietician can tailor the energy- and protein-enriched diet considering each subject's eating habits, lifestyle, symptoms, likes and dislikes. At low energy intakes, it can be hard to fulfil the needs for vitamins, minerals and trace elements. Oral nutritional supplements (as powders, puddings or liquids) can be used to supplement the diet when nutrient requirements cannot be satisfied through normal food and drink.

While the rationale for nutritional support to maintain or increase energy availability and muscle protein synthesis in weight losing and underweight COPD patients is compelling, randomized clinical trials investigating the clinical efficacy are generally small, and initial meta-analyses revealed small estimates of effect only. The updated Cochrane review [58] and two other meta-analyses [59, 60] consistently showed that nutritional supplementation promotes weight gain among patients with COPD, especially if undernourished. Furthermore, significant positive findings were reported for total energy intake, handgrip and quadriceps strength. Five out of 17 trials included in the updated meta-analysis [58], specifically the trials that had FFM as an outcome, had nutritional supplementation combined with exercise. It is likely that the benefits of supplementation will be maximized if combined with exercise, although based on the current literature, the effects of nutrition and exercise cannot clearly be distinguished, which is a subject for future research.

11.4.2 Nutrition as Ergogenic Aid

The importance of nutrition to enhance performance and training has long been recognized in the fields of sports and athletics. There is evidence for the benefits of ensuring adequate carbohydrate and protein intake (depending on the athletic discipline) in optimizing performance and evidence that some specific nutrients (e.g. creatine, nitrate) may enhance physical performance. Enhancing physical performance is a key therapeutic goal in COPD, and therefore there are theoretical reasons for hypothesizing that nutritional intervention might improve performance in this population or enhance the outcome of exercise training, an intervention that is of proven clinical and physiological benefit in COPD. Aerobic exercise training is of established efficacy in COPD, but it remains uncertain whether the magnitude of benefit is comparable to similar aged healthy subjects. Moreover, lower limb muscles in COPD are characterized by a decreased proportion of type I muscle fibres associated with decreased levels of muscle oxidative metabolic markers and nutrient-sensing regulators of cellular energy state (e.g. PGC1, PPAR, AMPK and sirtuins) [61]. These observations support the rationale for augmenting exercise training with nutritional therapies, and there are a limited number of trials investigating the impact of nutritional therapies on exercise performance or training in COPD. These involved a variety of interventions including carbohydrate and fat-rich supplements [62], essential amino acids [63], whey protein (rich in BCAA) [64], creatine [65–67] and PUFA (natural ligands of PPARs) [68] nitrate [69–73]. The literature is characterized by considerable heterogeneity in the nature and duration of the intervention, the populations enrolled and the exercise outcomes that were studied. Many studies were underpowered and most were single-centre investigations. Early macronutrient studies involving fat-rich supplements did not suggest a performance advantage in the intervention groups, but subsequent studies using a carbohydrate-rich supplement and PUFAs suggested the outcome or exercise training might be enhanced in selected patients [62, 68]. Small pilot investigations have suggested potential benefit of whey protein and carnitine but had insufficient statistical power for wider conclusions to be drawn. Three trials have tested the effect of creatine supplementation during exercise training in COPD with no consistent positive effect as confirmed by a subsequent systematic review and meta-analysis [74]. Five trials investigated the acute effect of nitrate supplementation on several outcome measures including blood pressure and exercise performance with no consistent effects to suggest being a promising adjunct to pulmonary rehabilitation [69–73]. In a group of overall non-wasted COPD patients, protein and carbohydrate supplementation post-resistance exercise did not augment functional or molecular exercise responses [75]. The NUTRAIN trial showed that high-intensity exercise training is successful in improving lower limb muscle strength and cycle exercise performance in COPD patients with moderate airflow obstruction but low muscle mass and sufficient dietary protein intake. Additional specific nutritional supplementation enriched with vitamin D, n-3 fatty acids and leucine had beneficial effects on body weight, plasma nutrient status and (non-trained) inspiratory muscle strength and positively influenced physical activity [76]. The observed dissociation between effects of exercise training and nutritional intervention on physical performance and physical activity warrants further investigation.

11.5 Dietary Quality and Nutrient Deficiencies

Vitamin D deficiency and insufficient intake of vitamins with antioxidant capacity (vitamins A, C and E) have been reported in COPD. Vitamin D has an important role in bone and calcium homeostasis, but effects may occur beyond bone health as anti-inflammatory, anti-infectious and antitumoural actions, as well as neuromuscular improvements, have been attributed to vitamin D [77]. Vitamin D status is assessed by the measurement of 25-OHD serum levels, a precursor of the active hormone. In a general population, vitamin D status is an independent predictor of all-cause mortality, upper airway respiratory infections and pulmonary function. For COPD, conflicting evidence exists on whether 25-OHD levels correlate with lung function decline, infectious exacerbations and muscular function [78–81]. Vitamin D status is determined by the synthesis capacity of the skin, hours of sun (UV) exposure, genetic variation in key enzymes of the involved pathway and supplemental intake by food. In COPD, vitamin D deficiency frequently occurs because of smoke-induced skin ageing, reduced outdoor activity and low-quality dietary intake. Based on international accepted cut-offs, vitamin D deficiency (25-OHD levels <20 ng/mL) is highly prevalent in COPD and increases with disease severity. The hypothesis that such deficiency may also causally contribute to pathogenesis of COPD is much debated, but recent prospective epidemiologic evidence associates vitamin D deficiency to an increased incidence of COPD and a more rapid decline of pulmonary function in subjects with COPD [82]. The higher prevalence in more advanced COPD and in nutritionally depleted states suggests that screening for vitamin D deficiency may be of value in these populations. It may restrict lifelong supplementation to vitamin D-deficient patients in whom beneficial effects on the bone and fall prevention, especially if combined with calcium intake, are proven. Daily intakes in addition to a minimal amount of UV exposure vary with age, but a dose of 800 IU with 1 g of calcium is largely sufficient. The potential of high-dose supplementation to obtain other than calcaemic effects, including lung function decline and COPD exacerbations, needs further exploration [83].

Insufficient intake of fresh fruits and vegetables may result in deficiency of vitamins with antioxidant capacity. Conversely, long-term supplementation with vitamin E has been shown to reduce the risk of COPD [84], but no evidence exists on the positive effects of additional vitamin intake on clinical outcome in a COPD population. As smoking and lung inflammation in COPD are known to cause significant oxidative stress, a reduction of the antioxidative capacity may have negative effects on the course of COPD. Large population-based epidemiological studies have shown that a prudent diet is associated with better pulmonary function, less lung function decline and reduced risk of COPD [85–87]. More specifically, greater intake of dietary fibre has been consistently associated with reduced COPD risk, better lung function and reduced respiratory symptoms [88]. Three studies have reported associations between frequent or high consumption of cured meats and increased risk of developing COPD [85, 89, 90]. A recent study has extended this association to include the evolution of the disease, revealing that high-cured meat consumption is linked to a higher risk of readmission to hospital with COPD [91]. Finally, albeit rarely assessed in clinical practice, iron deficiency often occurs in COPD which may be caused by several factors including systemic inflammation, malabsorption of iron from the gut, renal failure (as a consequence of concomitant chronic kidney disease or diabetes mellitus) and medications such as ACE inhibitors and corticosteroids [92]. Overall, the evidence indicates that a well-balanced diet with sufficient intake of fresh fruits and vegetables is beneficial to COPD patients, not only for its potential benefits on the lung but also for its proven benefits on metabolic and cardiovascular risk.

11.6 Nutrition as Part of Integrated Disease Management

Nutritional intervention has so far been studied either as single treatment or as adjunct to exercise training in depleted COPD patients, often in the context of pulmonary rehabilitation. The efficacy of nutritional supplementation could be enhanced by additional interventions including smoking cessation, correction of hypoxemia and/or hypercapnia with long-term oxygen therapy and/or noninvasive ventilation, reduction of static and dynamic hyperinflation by long-acting bronchodilators or lung volume reduction or androgens either to correct hypogonadism or to boost muscle anabolism. Two studies have shown the potential of a multimodal rehabilitation programme consisting nutritional supplementation, androgens and exercise training in improving clinical outcome and even survival in malnourished patients with advanced COPD [93, 94]. Long-term multimodal intervention studies are lacking to demonstrate if these modalities are indeed able to significantly change the natural history of weight loss and muscle wasting and reduce morbidity and mortality. Attempts to prevent or correct weight loss during acute exacerbations are scarce, and in fact, only one placebo-controlled randomized clinical trial so far proved feasibility and efficacy of nutritional supplementation in hospitalized COPD patients in maintaining energy balance and increasing protein intake [50]. The added value of enteral nutritional support for COPD patients, who do not respond to oral nutritional supplementation, has not been systematically investigated.

Recommendations by the ERS Task Force

1. Nutritional status is an important determinant of outcome of COPD.
2. Nutritional risk can be assessed by longitudinal measurement of body weight and body composition.
3. The prevalence of vitamin D nutrient deficiency is high in COPD and could be incorporated in nutritional risk screening.
4. The nutritional risk profiles associated with different metabolic phenotypes of COPD patients could be useful in patient counselling.
5. Nutritional intervention is likely to be effective in undernourished patients (based on current meta-analyses) and is probably most effective if combined with an exercise programme.
6. Providing evidence of the cost-effectiveness of nutritional intervention is required to support reimbursement of, and thus increase access to, nutritional intervention.
7. Overall, the evidence indicates that a well-balanced diet with sufficient intake of fresh fruits and vegetables is beneficial to COPD patients, not only for its potential benefits on the lung but also for its proven benefits on metabolic and cardiovascular risk.

Acknowledgements ERS task force 'nutrition and respiratory disease': Ivonne Ferreira, Frits Franssen, Harry Gosker, Wim Janssens, Mauricio Muscaritoli, Christophe Pison C, Mauren Rutten-van Mölken, Frode Slinde F, Mick Steiner, Ruzena Tkacova R and Sally Singh.

References

1. Schols AM, Ferreira IM, Franssen FM, Gosker HR, Janssens W, Muscaritoli M, Pison C, Rutten-van Mölken M, Slinde F, Steiner MC, Tkacova R, Singh SJ. Nutritional assessment and therapy in COPD. A European Respiratory Society Statement. Eur Respir J. 2014;44(6):1504–20.
2. Vanfleteren LE, Spruit MA, Groenen M, Gaffron S, van Empel VP, Bruijnzeel PL, Rutten EP, Op 't Roodt J, Wouters EF, Franssen FM. Clusters of comorbidities based on validated objective measurements and systemic inflammation in patients with chronic obstructive pulmonary disease. Am J Respir Crit Care Med. 2013;187(7):728–35.
3. Burgel PR, Paillasseur JL, Peene B, Dusser D, Roche N, Coolen J, Troosters T, Decramer M, Janssens W. Two distinct chronic obstructive pulmonary disease (COPD) phenotypes are associated with high risk of mortality. PLoS One. 2012;7(12):e51048.

4. Berrington de Gonzalez A, Hartge P, Cerhan JR, Flint AJ, Hannan L, MacInnis RJ, Moore SC, Tobias GS, Anton-Culver H, Freeman LB, Beeson WL, Clipp SL, English DR, Folsom AR, Freedman DM, Giles G, Hakansson N, Henderson KD, Hoffman-Bolton J, Hoppin JA, Koenig KL, Lee IM, Linet MS, Park Y, Pocobelli G, Schatzkin A, Sesso HD, Weiderpass E, Willcox BJ, Wolk A, Zeleniuch-Jacquotte A, Willett WC, Thun MJ. Body-mass index and mortality among 1.46 million white adults. N Engl J Med. 2010;363(23):2211–9.
5. Whitlock G, Lewington S, Sherliker P, Clarke R, Emberson J, Halsey J, Qizilbash N, Collins R, Peto R. Body-mass index and cause-specific mortality in 900 000 adults: collaborative analyses of 57 prospective studies. Lancet. 2009;373(9669):1083–96.
6. Vestbo J, Prescott E, Almdal T, Dahl M, Nordestgaard BG, Andersen T, Sorensen TI, Lange P. Body mass, fat-free body mass, and prognosis in patients with chronic obstructive pulmonary disease from a random population sample: findings from the Copenhagen City Heart Study. Am J Respir Crit Care Med. 2006;173(1):79–83.
7. Morley JE, Abbatecola AM, Argiles JM, Baracos V, Bauer J, Bhasin S, Cederholm T, Coats AJ, Cummings SR, Evans WJ, Fearon K, Ferrucci L, Fielding RA, Guralnik JM, Harris TB, Inui A, Kalantar-Zadeh K, Kirwan BA, Mantovani G, Muscaritoli M, Newman AB, Rossi-Fanelli F, Rosano GM, Roubenoff R, Schambelan M, Sokol GH, Storer TW, Vellas B, von Haehling S, Yeh SS, Anker SD. Sarcopenia with limited mobility: an international consensus. J Am Med Dir Assoc. 2011;12(6):403–9.
8. Bool v d, Rutten EP, Franssen FM, Wouters EF, Schols AM. Antagonistic effects of sarcopenia and abdominal obesity on physical performance in COPD. Eur Respir J. 2015;46(2):336–45.
9. Joppa P, Tkacova R, Franssen FM, et al. Sarcopenic Obesity, functional outcomes and systemic inflammation in patients with chronic obstructive pulmonary disease. J Am Med Dir Assoc. 2016;17(8): 712–8.
10. Stratton RJ, Hackston A, Longmore D, Dixon R, Price S, Stroud M, King C, Elia M. Malnutrition in hospital outpatients and inpatients: prevalence, concurrent validity and ease of use of the 'malnutrition universal screening tool' ('MUST') for adults. Br J Nutr. 2004;92(5):799–808.
11. Vellas B, Villars H, Abellan G, Soto ME, Rolland Y, Guigoz Y, Morley JE, Chumlea W, Salva A, Rubenstein LZ, Garry P. Overview of the MNA—Its history and challenges. J Nutr Health Aging. 2006;10(6):456–63; discussion 463–455
12. Landbo C, Prescott E, Lange P, Vestbo J, Almdal TP. Prognostic value of nutritional status in chronic obstructive pulmonary disease. Am J Respir Crit Care Med. 1999;160(6):1856–61.
13. Schols AM, Slangen J, Volovics L, Wouters EF. Weight loss is a reversible factor in the prognosis of chronic obstructive pulmonary disease. Am J Respir Crit Care Med. 1998;157(6 Pt 1):1791–7.
14. Lainscak M, von Haehling S, Doehner W, Sarc I, Jeric T, Ziherl K, Kosnik M, Anker SD, Suskovic S. Body mass index and prognosis in patients hospitalized with acute exacerbation of chronic obstructive pulmonary disease. J Cachex Sarcopenia Muscle. 2011;2(2):81–6.
15. Ora J, Laveneziana P, Wadell K, Preston M, Webb KA, O'Donnell DE. Effect of obesity on respiratory mechanics during rest and exercise in COPD. J Appl Physiol 2011: 111(1): 10–19.
16. Schols AM, Broekhuizen R, Weling-Scheepers CA, Wouters EF. Body composition and mortality in chronic obstructive pulmonary disease. Am J Clin Nutr. 2005;82(1):53–9.
17. Engelen MP, Schols AM, Lamers RJ, Wouters EF. Different patterns of chronic tissue wasting among patients with chronic obstructive pulmonary disease. Clin Nutr. 1999;18(5):275–80.
18. van den Borst B, Gosker HR, Koster A, Yu B, Kritchevsky SB, Liu Y, Meibohm B, Rice TB, Shlipak M, Yende S, Harris TB, Schols AM. The influence of abdominal visceral fat on inflammatory pathways and mortality risk in obstructive lung disease. Am J Clin Nutr. 2012;96(3):516–26.
19. Bolton CE, Ionescu AA, Shiels KM, Pettit RJ, Edwards PH, Stone MD, Nixon LS, Evans WD, Griffiths TL, Shale DJ. Associated loss of fat-free mass and bone mineral density in chronic obstructive pulmonary disease. Am J Respir Crit Care Med. 2004;170(12):1286–93.
20. Schols A, Mostert R, Cobben N, Soeters P, Wouters E. Transcutaneous oxygen saturation and carbon dioxide tension during meals in patients with chronic obstructive pulmonary disease. Chest. 1991;100(5):1287–92.
21. Gronberg AM, Slinde F, Engstrom CP, Hulthen L, Larsson S. Dietary problems in patients with severe chronic obstructive pulmonary disease. J Hum Nutr Diet. 2005;18(6):445–52.
22. Goris AH, Vermeeren MA, Wouters EF, Schols AM, Westerterp KR. Energy balance in depleted ambulatory patients with chronic obstructive pulmonary disease: the effect of physical activity and oral nutritional supplementation. Br J Nutr. 2003;89(5):725–31.
23. Schols AM, Soeters PB, Mostert R, Saris WH, Wouters EF. Energy balance in chronic obstructive pulmonary disease. Am Rev Respir Dis. 1991;143(6):1248–52.
24. Kao CC, Hsu JW, Bandi V, Hanania NA, Kheradmand F, Jahoor F. Resting energy expenditure and protein turnover are increased in patients with severe chronic obstructive pulmonary disease. Metabolism. 2011;60(10):1449–55.
25. Layec G, Haseler LJ, Hoff J, Richardson RS. Evidence that a higher ATP cost of muscular contraction contributes to the lower mechanical efficiency associated with COPD: preliminary findings. Am J Phys Regul Integr Comp Phys. 2011;300(5):R1142–7.
26. Baarends EM, Schols AM, Akkermans MA, Wouters EF. Decreased mechanical efficiency in clinically stable patients with COPD. Thorax. 1997;52(11):981–6.

27. Baarends EM, Schols AM, Pannemans DL, Westerterp KR, Wouters EF. Total free living energy expenditure in patients with severe chronic obstructive pulmonary disease. Am J Respir Crit Care Med. 1997;155(2):549–54.
28. Kim V, Kretschman DM, Sternberg AL, DeCamp MM Jr, Criner GJ. Weight gain after lung reduction surgery is related to improved lung function and ventilatory efficiency. Am J Respir Crit Care Med. 2012;186(11):1109–16.
29. Efthimiou J, Mounsey PJ, Benson DN, Madgwick R, Coles SJ, Benson MK. Effect of carbohydrate rich versus fat rich loads on gas exchange and walking performance in patients with chronic obstructive lung disease. Thorax. 1992;47(6):451–6.
30. Kneppers AEM, Langen RC, Gosker HR, et al. Increased myogenic and protein turnover signaling in skeletal muscle in chronic obstructive pulmonary disease patients with sarcopenia. J Am Med Dir Assoc. 2017;18(7):637.e1–637.e11.
31. Rutten EP, Franssen FM, Engelen MP, Wouters EF, Deutz NE, Schols AM. Greater whole-body myofibrillar protein breakdown in cachectic patients with chronic obstructive pulmonary disease. Am J Clin Nutr. 2006;83(4):829–34.
32. Jonker R, Deutz NE, Erbland ML, Anderson PJ, Engelen MP. Hydrolyzed casein and whey protein meals comparably stimulate net whole-body protein synthesis in COPD patients with nutritional depletion without an additional effect of leucine co-ingestion. Clin Nutr. 2014;33(2):211–20.
33. Engelen MP, Wouters EF, Deutz NE, Menheere PP, Schols AM. Factors contributing to alterations in skeletal muscle and plasma amino acid profiles in patients with chronic obstructive pulmonary disease. Am J Clin Nutr. 2000;72(6):1480–7.
34. Engelen MP, Deutz NE, Mostert R, Wouters EF, Schols AM. Response of whole-body protein and urea turnover to exercise differs between patients with chronic obstructive pulmonary disease with and without emphysema. Am J Clin Nutr. 2003;77(4):868–74.
35. Sambrook P, Cooper C. Osteoporosis. Lancet. 2006;367(9527):2010–8.
36. Lehouck A, Boonen S, Decramer M, Janssens W. COPD, bone metabolism, and osteoporosis. Chest. 2011;139(3):648–57.
37. Graat-Verboom L, Wouters EF, Smeenk FW, van den Borne BE, Lunde R, Spruit MA. Current status of research on osteoporosis in COPD: a systematic review. Eur Respir J. 2009;34(1):209–18.
38. Graat-Verboom L, Smeenk FW, van den Borne BE, Spruit MA, Donkers-van Rossum AB, Aarts RP, Wouters EF. Risk factors for osteoporosis in Caucasian patients with moderate chronic obstructive pulmonary disease: a case control study. Bone. 2012;50(6):1234–9.
39. Bon J, Fuhrman CR, Weissfeld JL, Duncan SR, Branch RA, Chang CC, Zhang Y, Leader JK, Gur D, Greenspan SL, Sciurba FC. Radiographic emphysema predicts low bone mineral density in a tobacco-exposed cohort. Am J Respir Crit Care Med. 2011;183(7):885–90.
40. Makita H, Nasuhara Y, Nagai K, Ito Y, Hasegawa M, Betsuyaku T, Onodera Y, Hizawa N, Nishimura M. Characterisation of phenotypes based on severity of emphysema in chronic obstructive pulmonary disease. Thorax. 2007;62(11):932–7.
41. Ohara T, Hirai T, Muro S, Haruna A, Terada K, Kinose D, Marumo S, Ogawa E, Hoshino Y, Niimi A, Chin K, Mishima M. Relationship between pulmonary emphysema and osteoporosis assessed by CT in patients with COPD. Chest. 2008;134(6):1244–9.
42. Franco CB, Paz-Filho G, Gomes PE, Nascimento VB, Kulak CA, Boguszewski CL, Borba VZ. Chronic obstructive pulmonary disease is associated with osteoporosis and low levels of vitamin D. Osteoporos Int. 2009;20(11):1881–7.
43. Rachner TD, Khosla S, Hofbauer LC. Osteoporosis: now and the future. Lancet. 2011;377(9773):1276–87.
44. McGarvey LP, John M, Anderson JA, Zvarich M, Wise RA. Ascertainment of cause-specific mortality in COPD: operations of the TORCH Clinical Endpoint Committee. Thorax. 2007;62(5):411–5.
45. van den Borst B, Gosker HR, Wesseling G, de Jager W, Hellwig VA, Snepvangers FJ, Schols AM. Low-grade adipose tissue inflammation in patients with mild-to-moderate chronic obstructive pulmonary disease. Am J Clin Nutr. 2011;94(6):1504–12.
46. van den Borst B, Gosker HR, Schols AM. Central fat and peripheral muscle: partners in crime in chronic obstructive pulmonary disease. Am J Respir Crit Care Med. 2013;187(1):8–13.
47. Bautista J, Ehsan M, Normandin E, Zuwallack R, Lahiri B. Physiologic responses during the six minute walk test in obese and non-obese COPD patients. Respir Med. 2011;105(8):1189–94.
48. Chaston TB, Dixon JB. Factors associated with percent change in visceral versus subcutaneous abdominal fat during weight loss: findings from a systematic review. Int J Obes. 2008;32(4):619–28.
49. Schols AM. Translating nutritional potential of metabolic remodelling to disease-modifying nutritional management. Curr Opin Clin Nutr Metab Care. 2013;16(6):617–8.
50. Vermeeren MA, Schols AM, Wouters EF. Effects of an acute exacerbation on nutritional and metabolic profile of patients with COPD. Eur Respir J. 1997;10(10):2264–9.
51. Ehsan M, Khan R, Wakefield D, Qureshi A, Murray L, Zuwallack R, Leidy NK. A longitudinal study evaluating the effect of exacerbations on physical activity in patients with chronic obstructive pulmonary disease. Ann Am Thorac Soc. 2013;10(6):559–64.
52. Creutzberg EC, Wouters EF, Vanderhoven-Augustin IM, Dentener MA, Schols AM. Disturbances in leptin metabolism are related to energy imbalance during acute exacerbations of chronic obstructive pulmonary disease. Am J Respir Crit Care Med. 2000;162(4 Pt 1):1239–45.
53. Saudny-Unterberger H, Martin JG, Gray-Donald K. Impact of nutritional support on functional status during an acute exacerbation of chronic obstructive pulmonary disease. Am J Respir Crit Care Med. 1997;156(3 Pt 1):794–9.

54. Pouw EM, Ten Velde GP, Croonen BH, Kester AD, Schols AM, Wouters EF. Early non-elective readmission for chronic obstructive pulmonary disease is associated with weight loss. Clin Nutr. 2000;19(2):95–9.
55. Lainscak M, Gosker HR, Schols AM. Chronic obstructive pulmonary disease patient journey: hospitalizations as window of opportunity for extra-pulmonary intervention. Curr Opin Clin Nutr Metab Care. 2013;16(3):278–83.
56. Broekhuizen R, Creutzberg EC, Weling-Scheepers CA, Wouters EF, Schols AM. Optimizing oral nutritional drink supplementation in patients with chronic obstructive pulmonary disease. Br J Nutr. 2005;93(6):965–71.
57. Weekes CE, Emery PW, Elia M. Dietary counselling and food fortification in stable COPD: a randomised trial. Thorax. 2009;64(4):326–31.
58. Ferreira IM, Brooks D, White J, Goldstein R. Nutritional supplementation for stable chronic obstructive pulmonary disease. Cochrane Database Syst Rev. 2012;12:CD000998.
59. Collins PF, Stratton RJ, Elia M. Nutritional support in chronic obstructive pulmonary disease: a systematic review and meta-analysis. Am J Clin Nutr. 2012;95(6):1385–95.
60. Collins PF, Elia M, Stratton RJ. Nutritional support and functional capacity in chronic obstructive pulmonary disease: a systematic review and meta-analysis. Respirology. 2013;18(4):616–29.
61. Schols AM. Nutrition as a metabolic modulator in COPD. Chest. 2013;144(4):1340–5.
62. Steiner MC, Barton RL, Singh SJ, Morgan MD. Nutritional enhancement of exercise performance in chronic obstructive pulmonary disease: a randomised controlled trial. Thorax. 2003;58(9):745–51.
63. Baldi S, Aquilani R, Pinna GD, Poggi P, De Martini A, Bruschi C. Fat-free mass change after nutritional rehabilitation in weight losing COPD: role of insulin, C-reactive protein and tissue hypoxia. Int J Chron Obstruct Pulmon Dis. 2010;5:29–39.
64. Sugawara K, Takahashi H, Kashiwagura T, Yamada K, Yanagida S, Homma M, Dairiki K, Sasaki H, Kawagoshi A, Satake M, Shioya T. Effect of anti-inflammatory supplementation with whey peptide and exercise therapy in patients with COPD. Respir Med. 2012;106(11):1526–34.
65. Deacon SJ, Vincent EE, Greenhaff PL, Fox J, Steiner MC, Singh SJ, Morgan MD. Randomized controlled trial of dietary creatine as an adjunct therapy to physical training in chronic obstructive pulmonary disease. Am J Respir Crit Care Med. 2008;178(3):233–9.
66. Fuld JP, Kilduff LP, Neder JA, Pitsiladis Y, Lean ME, Ward SA, Cotton MM. Creatine supplementation during pulmonary rehabilitation in chronic obstructive pulmonary disease. Thorax. 2005;60(7):531–7.
67. Faager G, Soderlund K, Skold CM, Rundgren S, Tollback A, Jakobsson P. Creatine supplementation and physical training in patients with COPD: a double blind, placebo-controlled study. Int J Chron Obstruct Pulmon Dis. 2006;1(4):445–53.
68. Broekhuizen R, Wouters EF, Creutzberg EC, Weling-Scheepers CA, Schols AM. Polyunsaturated fatty acids improve exercise capacity in chronic obstructive pulmonary disease. Thorax. 2005;60(5):376–82.
69. Berry MJ, Justus NW, Hauser JI, Case AH, Helms CC, Basu S, Rogers Z, Lewis MT, Miller GD. Dietary nitrate supplementation improves exercise performance and decreases blood pressure in COPD patients. Nitric Oxide. 2015;48:22–30.
70. Curtis KJ, O'Brien KA, Tanner RJ, Polkey JI, Minnion M, Feelisch M, Polkey MI, Edwards LM, Hopkinson NS. Acute dietary nitrate supplementation and exercise performance in COPD: a double-blind, placebo-controlled, randomised controlled pilot study. PLoS One. 2015;10(12):e0144504.
71. Kerley CP, Cahill K, Bolger K, McGowan A, Burke C, Faul J, Cormican L. Dietary nitrate supplementation in COPD: an acute, double-blind, randomized, placebo-controlled, crossover trial. Nitric Oxide. 2015;44:105–11.
72. Leong P, Basham JE, Yong T, Chazan A, Finlay P, Barnes S, Bardin PG, Campbell DA. double blind randomized placebo control crossover trial on the effect of dietary nitrate supplementation on exercise tolerance in stable moderate chronic obstructive pulmonary disease. BMC Pulm Med. 2015;15:52.
73. Shepherd AI, Wilkerson DP, Dobson L, Kelly J, Winyard PG, Jones AM, Benjamin N, Shore AC, Gilchrist M. The effect of dietary nitrate supplementation on the oxygen cost of cycling, walking performance and resting blood pressure in individuals with chronic obstructive pulmonary disease: a double blind placebo controlled, randomised control trial. Nitric Oxide. 2015;48:31–7.
74. Al-Ghimlas F, Todd DC. Creatine supplementation for patients with COPD receiving pulmonary rehabilitation: a systematic review and meta-analysis. Respirology. 2010;15(5):785–95.
75. Constantin D, Menon MK, Houchen-Wolloff L, Morgan MD, Singh SJ, Greenhaff P, Steiner MC. Skeletal muscle molecular responses to resistance training and dietary supplementation in COPD. Thorax. 2013;68(7):625–33.
76. Van de Bool C, Rutten E, van Helvoort A, Franssen FM, Wouters EFM, Schols AMWJ. A randomized clinical trial investigating the efficacy of targeted nutrition as adjunct to exercise training in COPD. J Cachex Sarcopenia Muscle. 2017; doi:10.1002/jcsm.12219.
77. Janssens W, Lehouck A, Carremans C, Bouillon R, Mathieu C, Decramer M. Vitamin D beyond bones in chronic obstructive pulmonary disease: time to act. Am J Respir Crit Care Med. 2009;179(8):630–6.
78. Black PN, Scragg R. Relationship between serum 25-hydroxyvitamin d and pulmonary function in the third national health and nutrition examination survey. Chest. 2005;128(6):3792–8.
79. Ginde AA, Mansbach JM, Camargo CA Jr. Association between serum 25-hydroxyvitamin D level and upper respiratory tract infection in the Third National Health and Nutrition Examination Survey. Arch Intern Med. 2009;169(4):384–90.

80. Kunisaki KM, Niewoehner DE, Singh RJ, Connett JE. Vitamin D status and longitudinal lung function decline in the Lung Health Study. Eur Respir J. 2011;37(2):238–43.
81. Lange NE, Sparrow D, Vokonas P, Litonjua AA. Vitamin D deficiency, smoking, and lung function in the Normative Aging Study. Am J Respir Crit Care Med. 2012;186(7):616–21.
82. Afzal S, Lange P, Bojesen SE, Freiberg JJ, Nordestgaard BG. Plasma 25-hydroxyvitamin D, lung function and risk of chronic obstructive pulmonary disease. Thorax. 2013; doi:10.1136/thoraxjnl-2013-203682.
83. Lehouck A, Mathieu C, Carremans C, Baeke F, Verhaegen J, Van Eldere J, Decallonne B, Bouillon R, Decramer M, Janssens W. High doses of vitamin D to reduce exacerbations in chronic obstructive pulmonary disease: a randomized trial. Ann Intern Med. 2012;156(2):105–14.
84. Agler AH, Kurth T, Gaziano JM, Buring JE, Cassano PA. Randomised vitamin E supplementation and risk of chronic lung disease in the Women's Health Study. Thorax. 2011;66(4):320–5.
85. Varraso R, Jiang R, Barr RG, Willett WC, Camargo CA Jr. Prospective study of cured meats consumption and risk of chronic obstructive pulmonary disease in men. Am J Epidemiol. 2007;166(12):1438–45.
86. Varraso R, Fung TT, Barr RG, Hu FB, Willett W, Camargo CA Jr. Prospective study of dietary patterns and chronic obstructive pulmonary disease among US women. Am J Clin Nutr. 2007;86(2):488–95.
87. Varraso R, Willett WC, Camargo CA Jr. Prospective study of dietary fiber and risk of chronic obstructive pulmonary disease among US women and men. Am J Epidemiol. 2010;171(7):776–84.
88. Fonseca Wald EL, van den Borst B, Gosker HR, Schols AM. Dietary fibre and fatty acids in chronic obstructive pulmonary disease risk and progression: a systematic review. Respirology. 2014;19(2):176–84.
89. Jiang R, Camargo CA Jr, Varraso R, Paik DC, Willett WC, Barr RG. Consumption of cured meats and prospective risk of chronic obstructive pulmonary disease in women. Am J Clin Nutr. 2008;87(4):1002–8.
90. Chow CK. Consumption of cured meats and risk of chronic obstructive pulmonary disease. Am J Clin Nutr. 2008;88(6):1703; author reply 1704
91. de Batlle J, Mendez M, Romieu I, Balcells E, Benet M, Donaire-Gonzalez D, Ferrer JJ, Orozco-Levi M, Anto JM, Garcia-Aymerich J. Cured meat consumption increases risk of readmission in COPD patients. Eur Respir J. 2012;40(3):555–60.
92. Silverberg DS, Mor R, Weu MT, Schwartz D, Schwartz IF, Chernin G. Anemia and iron deficiency in COPD patients: prevalence and the effects of correction of the anemia with erythropoiesis stimulating agents and intravenous iron. BMC Pulm Med. 2014;14(1):24.
93. Schols AM, Soeters PB, Mostert R, Pluymers RJ, Wouters EF. Physiologic effects of nutritional support and anabolic steroids in patients with chronic obstructive pulmonary disease. A placebo-controlled randomized trial. Am J Respir Crit Care Med. 1995;152(4 Pt 1):1268–74.
94. Pison CM, Cano NJ, Cherion C, Caron F, Court-Fortune I, Antonini MT, Gonzalez-Bermejo J, Meziane L, Molano LC, Janssens JP, Costes F, Wuyam B, Similowski T, Melloni B, Hayot M, Augustin J, Tardif C, Lejeune H, Roth H, Pichard C. Multimodal nutritional rehabilitation improves clinical outcomes of malnourished patients with chronic respiratory failure: a randomised controlled trial. Thorax. 2011;66(11):953–60.

Occupational Therapy and Pulmonary Rehabilitation

12

Louise Sewell

12.1 Introduction

Occupational therapists (OTs) are concerned with helping people to gain or regain independence in functional activities. These activities are referred to as 'occupations', but to an OT, the term occupation means much more than activities only related to productivity or work. OTs consider occupation to mean any meaningful and purposeful activity that allows someone to live as independently as possible and gives them a sense of identity [1]. This is a large remit and often leads to misunderstanding with regard to the role of an OT. People who attend pulmonary rehabilitation programmes often do so with a desire not only to regain exercise capacity but crucially to improve their ability to carry out their activities of daily living (ADLs) (or their occupations) that are restricted because of the impact of their respiratory disease. Most commonly this is due to breathlessness or fatigue. It is therefore a crucial element of any PR programme to ensure that any improvements made in exercise performance are translated into improvements in the person's ability to carry out activities of daily living.

L. Sewell, Ph.D.
School of Health, Coventry University, Coventry, UK
e-mail: ab1214@coventry.ac.uk

© Springer International Publishing AG 2018
E. Clini et al. (eds.), *Textbook of Pulmonary Rehabilitation*,
https://doi.org/10.1007/978-3-319-65888-9_12

This chapter will explore how the OT is central to achieving this aim in pulmonary rehabilitation (PR). It will describe the main barriers to activities of daily living faced by people with chronic respiratory disease and will examine assessments and outcome measures used to assess these. This chapter will then go on to investigate some of the main areas for interventions delivered by an OT in PR, namely, energy conservation, environmental modification and anxiety management.

12.2 Understanding Occupation

Occupation refers to all activities of daily living (ADLs) that we need, are expected or would like to complete. OTs recognise that it is these activities that define who we are and what we would like to be and describe this concept as 'occupational identity' [2]. The American Occupational Therapy Association [3] has described the following categories of ADLS:

- Basic ADLs: These are self-care activities that we need to complete in function. These include tasks such as eating, bathing and showering, personal hygiene and grooming, toileting, functional mobility (tasks such as walking, transferring out of a bed and a chair) and sexual activity.
- Instrumental ADLs: These are activities that support the way in which we are able to func-

tion at home and our wider environment and include activities such as housework, caring for others (e.g. children), driving and moving around the community, managing finances, shopping, health management, meal preparation and religious activities.

- Activities related to paid and voluntary employment.
- Educational activities.
- Leisure activities.
- Social participation activities.
- Play.
- Rest and sleep.

The concept of occupational performance describes the outcome of the complex interaction between the person, the occupation and the environment [4]. OTs recognise that it is futile to only consider the impact of the respiratory disease upon the person's ability to successfully complete the chosen occupation or ADL but it is also essential to consider the influence of personal and environmental factors. For instance, two people who attend PR may have an identical respiratory diagnosis and similar lung function. In addition, they may both identify the same functional goal (or occupation) of being able to walk to the shops. Differences in their environment (such as social environment or who they live with) and personal factors (such as levels of motivation and self-efficacy) will determine each person's ability to reach the goal of walking to the shop.

The World Health Organisation has proposed the International Classification of Functioning, Disability and Health (ICF) to describe these complexities. [5] The ICF acknowledges the interaction between the impact the respiratory disease has upon the ability to complete activities and also recognises the restrictions that may be placed upon someone's ability to complete activities and also how the person is able to participate in life situations. Underpinning these three elements are environmental and personal factors that influence the interplay between the respiratory condition and the three elements of body functions and structure, activity and participation (Fig. 12.1).

12.3 Barriers to Activities of Daily Living

The reasons why activities of daily living become difficult for people who attend PR will inevitably vary because of differences in environmental and personal contexts. It is beyond the scope of this chapter to document and discuss all of these but some common barriers have been identified in the literature.

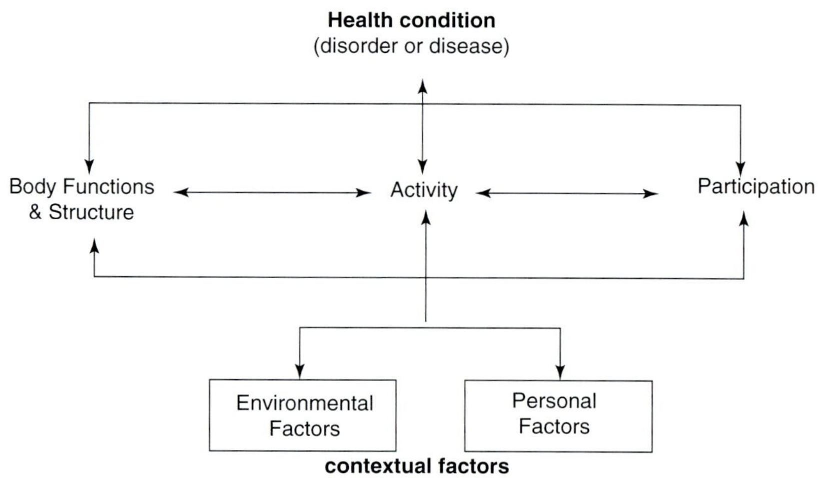

Fig. 12.1 The international classification of functioning, disabilities and health (WHO 2001) [5]

12.3.1 Breathlessness

Breathlessness is clearly cited as the most significant barrier to completion of activities of daily for people who have chronic respiratory disease [6]. Most people who first seek medical advice regarding their increasing breathlessness will commonly describe how their daily lives are affected. For example, "I can't walk up the stairs now without having to stop and catch my breath" or "I used to be able to do all my own gardening but now I have to ask for help because I get so breathless". The importance of these occupations is therefore captured from the very beginning of a person's involvement in PR.

A gradual reduction in daily activities can often be the result of avoiding breathlessness on exertion. This can happen over a period of some years and results in what has become known as the disability or deconditioning spiral [7]. This is a process in which ADLs are slowly reduced in an attempt to reduce or manage the distressing problem of breathlessness on exertion. It has been shown that breathlessness has a negative impact upon activities such as walking, household tasks and social participation activities [8] (Fig. 12.2).

12.3.2 Anxiety

It is known that anxiety levels are higher in people who attend PR compared to an age-matched population [9]. In addition, anxiety is likely to impact negatively upon engagement

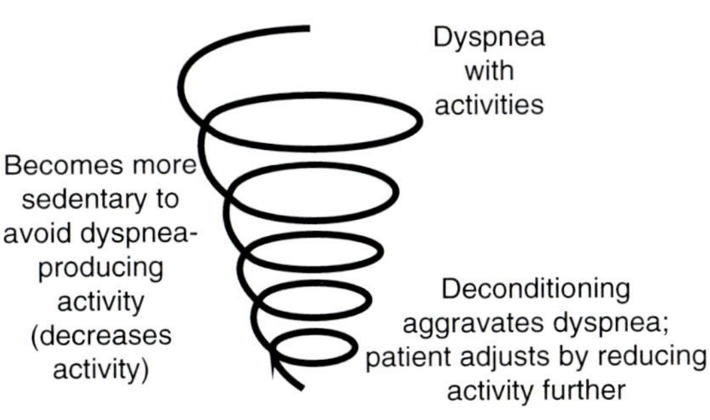

Fig. 12.2 The disability spiral (reproduced from Reardon, Lareau and ZuWallack 2006 [7])

in ADLs. It can be the fear of breathlessness (rather than experienced breathlessness) during ADLs that can become a barrier to occupational performance. This fear may be rooted in the memory of an occasion when a certain activity produced more pronounced and frightening levels of breathlessness than previously experienced. This phenomenon is difficult to confirm in large scale studies but a relationship between levels of anxiety in people who have COPD and ADL scores have been documented [10]. In a large cross-sectional study, Doyle and colleagues have recently shown that patients who had lower functional status and higher levels of anxiety were more likely to have higher levels of breathlessness [11]. However, a more in depth understanding has been provided by studies that have employed qualitative methodology. There is evidence from these studies that anxiety regarding the fear of breathlessness has directly led to a gradual disengagement in activities [12].

12.3.3 Fatigue

Fatigue is also a common barrier to ADLs for people attending a PR, but the mechanisms and predictors are poorly understood. Theander and colleagues [13] have shown that fatigue was reported as the worst or one of the worst symptoms in 51% of a sample of patients with COPD compared to only 27% of healthy controls. This has been confirmed by Lewko et al. [14] who also demonstrated in a cross-sectional study that fatigue levels are significantly higher in people with COPD when compared with an aged matched population. There is also evidence to suggest that the time of the day may be an important factor in managing fatigue. Kapella et al. [15] examined subjective fatigue in patients with COPD using self-reported measures. They concluded that fatigue in COPD is closely related to breathlessness during activity and is experienced more in the afternoon that morning. They also documented that fatigue had a negative effect upon functional performance.

12.4 Common Assessments Used by Occupational Therapists

Assessments used by the OT should always be integrated into the wider assessment process of a PR programme. Approaches to assessing occupational performance can be seen on a continuum that ranges from quantifiable, objectively monitored activity to self-reported performance in individually selected ADLs (Fig. 12.3). There is often a 'time' versus 'depth of data' trade-off when collecting this information. For instance, a device such as an accelerometer does not require much time from the OT other than to issue the device and download the data, whereas sitting down during a PR assessment and speaking with someone about their current difficulties with ADLs and how they would rate these demands time.

Directly monitored daily activity by pedometers or accelerometers has attracted much interest in recent years. Advances in technology mean that accelerometer hardware is readily available in smartphones and fitness trackers, and access to these devices is increasing in the PR population. This approach is potentially of interest to the OT as it can provide a plot of daily activity via directly measured by step count or derived values such as energy expenditure [16]. Such measures would be extremely useful to help identify if there are peaks and troughs of daily activity (see Fig. 12.4) to help to establish if energy conservation advice is required. However this approach does not provide any information with regard to individual task completion.

Standardised functional status measures do provide some indication of which daily tasks are able to be completed. These are completed by patients attending PR and consist of a list of common ADLs, and participants are asked to rate how well they are currently able to complete these tasks. A number of ADLs scales have been validated for use in PR. These include:

- Pulmonary function status and dyspnoea questionnaire—modified [17]
- Manchester respiratory activities of daily living scale [18]
- London Chest Activities of Daily Living scale [19]
- Nottingham extended activities of daily living scale [20]
- Pulmonary function status scale [21]

The list of activities rated in these scales is predetermined and normally cover a range of both basic and instrumental ADLs. Items have usually been selected for inclusion following a robust qualitative process.

Individualised measures of ADL performance allow the participant to identify those ADLs that are most relevant and important. The Canadian

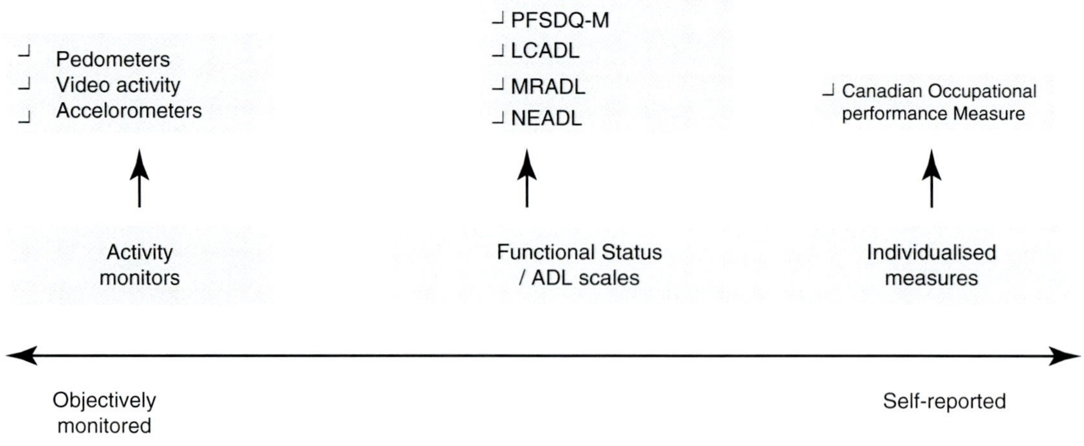

Fig. 12.3 Approaches to ADL assessment

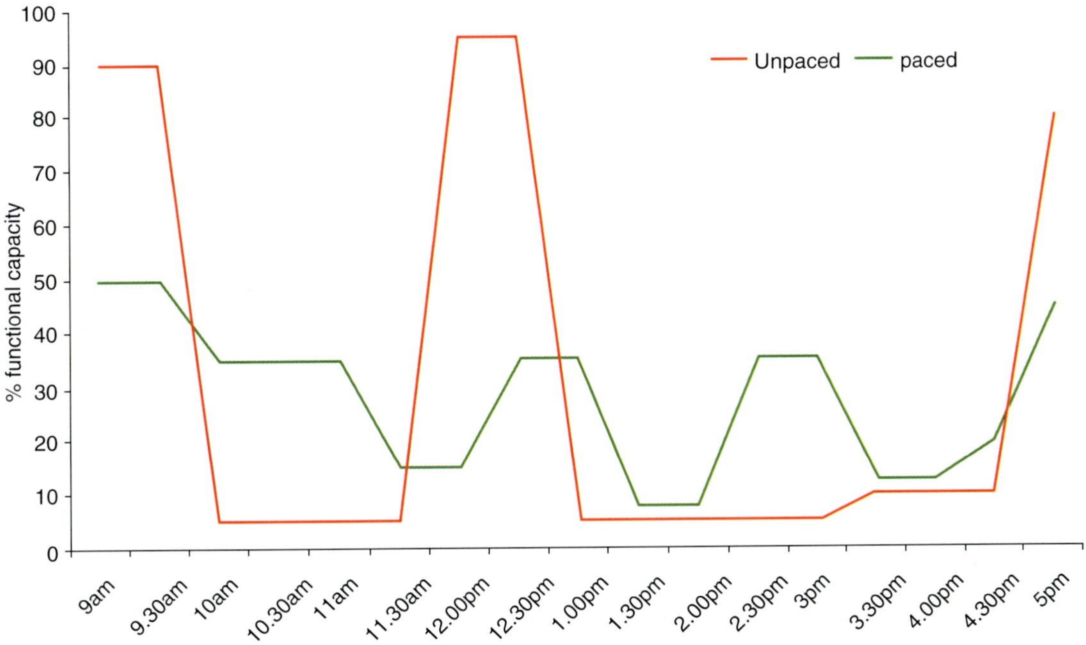

Fig. 12.4 Unpaced vs. paced daily activity

Occupational Performance Measure (COPM) [22] is an individualised measure that has been shown to be both reliable [23] and sensitive to change following PR [24]. Participants identify the five most important self-care, productivity or leisure activities and then rate how well they feel they perform these tasks and how satisfied they are if how well they complete them. Dyspnoea scores are obtained via similar individualised process in the Chronic Respiratory Disease Questionnaire [25].

12.5 Occupational Therapy Interventions

12.5.1 Energy Conservation

Energy conservation advice is recommended in international PR guidelines [26, 27], and it is a commonplace for OTs to deliver these sessions. The rationale for this intervention is to reduce the metabolic demands of daily tasks by changing the way these are completed, for instance, to complete activities in a seated, rather than a standing position, etc. This type of advice has been shown to reduce both the energy cost and level of breathlessness experienced in common ADLs [28].

The premise for energy conservation could be seen as contradictory to the overall aim of PR. Often energy conservation education sessions take place after an exercise session in a PR programme. During that session, they have been encouraged to increase their physical activity, and this is followed by an OT encouraging them to conserve energy and seemingly do less activity. At first sight, this seems to be a confusing message to deliver and can be difficult to reconcile this with the primary aim of PR programmes which is to increase performance capacity. In order to understand this, the important energy costs that are faced by a person attending a PR programme must be understood.

12.5.2 Energy Costs

12.5.2.1 Daily Activities

Each daily occupation has an energy cost. There is evidence to suggest that, in relative terms, daily activities are more costly in terms of oxygen uptake when compared with people who did not have COPD [29]. Both basic and instrumental ADLs all have a measurable metabolic cost, and people attending PR programmes report that they have to think carefully about which activities they will complete if energy levels are low. It should therefore be recognised that engaging in a PR programme will be a significant 'energy cost' for many patients.

12.5.2.2 Anxiety

People attending PR may experience situations that increase their levels of anxiety. These situations are often linked to the fear of breathlessness. For instance, people with attending PR can become anxious at the thought of a shopping trip because they may be worried about whether they will be able to walk far enough to reach the shops or be faced with a flight of stairs that they may struggle to climb. These anxieties can be based upon a fear of becoming breathless and memories of similar past situations can fuel these fears. This anxiety response is described as the 'fight or flight response' to deplete the body's energy stores.

12.5.2.3 Exercise

Embarking upon an exercise programme will become a significant energy cost to PR participants. Some people embark on PR with long-standing reduced levels of energy for the reasons outlined above. It is therefore unsurprising that when faced with the addition of an exercise programme, they find it difficult to commence, maintain or continue to exercise.

12.5.2.4 Strategies to Assist in Energy Conservation

An energy budget: A really useful way to help patients to understand how their energy is affected by their respiratory disease is to explain the idea of an energy budget. This is the idea that we all have a limited amount of energy to last the day. OTs often explain this in terms of monetary value to encourage PR participants to dive each daily task a metaphorical monetary cost, i.e. "Let's say that we all have £50 worth of energy to last the day. How will you spend this?"

The overall aims of energy conservation can be summarised by the three 'P's: **P**lan, **P**rioritise and **P**ace.

Plan: As is the case with a financial budget, living within the constraints of an energy budget takes careful planning. OTs encourage patients who attend PR to consider how they schedule their days and week. For instance, do they tend to schedule energy-intensive weekly tasks such as completing their weekly shopping on a Monday and then vacuuming the whole house on a Tuesday on consecutive days? This exercise should also be completed with a daily focus to establish if activities that carry a high 'energy cost' are completed in a fairly narrow time frame leaving the individual exhausted for the rest of the day.

Notably, attending a PR programme may mean that tasks that were previously within someone's capacity suddenly feel unachievable. Unfortunately some people may withdraw from PR in an effort to maintain their independence in activities of daily living. It is therefore incumbent on the OT on the PR team to help the person to plan their overall daily activity in order to manage all of these tasks and gain maximum benefit from PR.

Prioritise: PR participants may be forced to make decisions about where their 'energy spending' priorities may lie. People with severe disease may be compelled to prioritise basic ADLs over instrumental ADLs or leisure tasks [30], and this may impact negatively on overall quality of life. OTs is well placed to help PR patients to identify those activities that they enjoy and assist in helping the patient to set achievable goals. It is also the role of the OT to help the patient to understand that if the PR exercise programme becomes a priority in terms of the patient's energy spent, then this could be viewed as an 'investment' as they become fitter and therefore increase their overall energy budget in time.

The process of **goal setting** is a critical intervention to translate gains in physical exercise capacity into patient identified improvements in occupational performance. Changes to daily routine, habits and roles are difficult to achieve and often require a regular reflection and discussion. Sustained contact with the OT and the rest of the PR team may help to achieve this but these changes are likely to take some time develop (Box 12.1).

Pace: Pacing daily activity is a crucial focus of energy conservation advice. Building in rest periods during ADLs and allowing the person to complete them at a steadier pace can also be helpful and avoid energy depleting sustained peaks of activity (see Fig. 12.4).

Changing the way in which daily activities are completed demands a change of overall approach. This is difficult as the way in which we approach such as personal care tasks, and housework is often influenced by daily routines and habits that have been the same for many years. These tasks are therefore completed with little conscious thought. Minimising breathlessness during completion of these tasks can be the outcome from effective pacing.

One approach to achieving this is by offering advice regarding equipment provision. For people with respiratory disease, the aim of providing assistive technology and equipment is solely based around helping the person to pace a specific task. For instance, most people with respiratory disease are able to stand in the shower unaided, but the provision of a shower seat enables that task to be completed more slowly and makes it easier to pause and pace the task of showering.

Box 12.1: Case Study 1 (John)

John is a 73-year-old retired teacher who has COPD and has just commenced a pulmonary rehabilitation programme. He lives alone in house and struggles to complete all his household and gardening tasks. John's daughter lives nearby and has offered to help with the gardening, but John has declined these offers as although he doesn't particularly enjoy gardening; he still wishes to remain as independent as possible. John has enjoyed his pulmonary rehabilitation programme so far, but he has found it difficult to manage his home exercise programme. He also finds Thursdays very tiring as he usually meets his friends in the morning to play bowls and then attends his pulmonary rehabilitation session in the afternoon. He finds that he needs to rest all day on Friday just to recover and is considering whether it is worth attending pulmonary rehabilitation if it leaves him feeling this tired.

After spending some time talking to the occupational therapist, John thinks about his weekly routine. He realises that if he doesn't complete the exercise programme, then he is unlikely to see any improvement in his breathlessness. He decides to ask his friends if they would be able to meet on a Wednesday morning whilst he attends pulmonary rehabilitation programme. He also chats to her daughter and takes up her offer of mowing his lawn for the next few weeks.

John meets up with the occupational therapist towards the end the pulmonary rehabilitation programme. He was able tell him that without having to spend his energy on gardening he has been able to complete his home exercise programme and now feels considerably fitter and can walk further without becoming breathless. His friends have noticed an improvement in John's level of breathlessness, and they were happy to keep their bowls session to Wednesday mornings.

12.5.3 Environmental Modification and Equipment to Assist in Activities of Daily Living

Some people who attend PR programmes may benefit from assistive equipment or technology that will reduce the overall 'energy cost' of any individual task or activity. This may include equipment that can help a person to remain in a seated position whilst performing tasks that are usually completed in standing or equipment that are designed to help the individual to avoid bending.

Examples of assistive equipment that people attending PR find useful:

- Perching stool: an adjustable height stool with a sloping seat that enables activities that are normally completed in standing to be completed in a sitting position. It is commonly used in either the kitchen (to use when preparing meals, washing dishes, etc.) or in the bathroom (when washing at the bathroom sink).

- Shower board (for use in a shower that is positioned over a bath) or shower seat in a shower cubicle. This helps to pace the task of showering as the person is able to sit and rest for short periods.
- A wheeled rollator: this can often be used as a temporary measure to help people achieve longer continuous walking distances during their PR programme. The rollator reduces the overall work of walking by supporting the upper body. It is also useful for people who require ambulatory oxygen as the oxygen cylinder can be carried in basket that is fixed to the rollator.
- Long-handled reacher: this avoids bending, e.g. when picking up mail, clothes from the floor or washing from washing machine.
- Dressing equipment such as a long-handled shoe horn, elastic shoe laces and sock aids. These reduce the need to bend when dressing.
- Long-handled gardening tools

12.5.3.1 Environmental Modifications

People with more severe disease attending a PR programme often have questions regarding possible home modifications that may be of help to them. OTs are often employed by social care

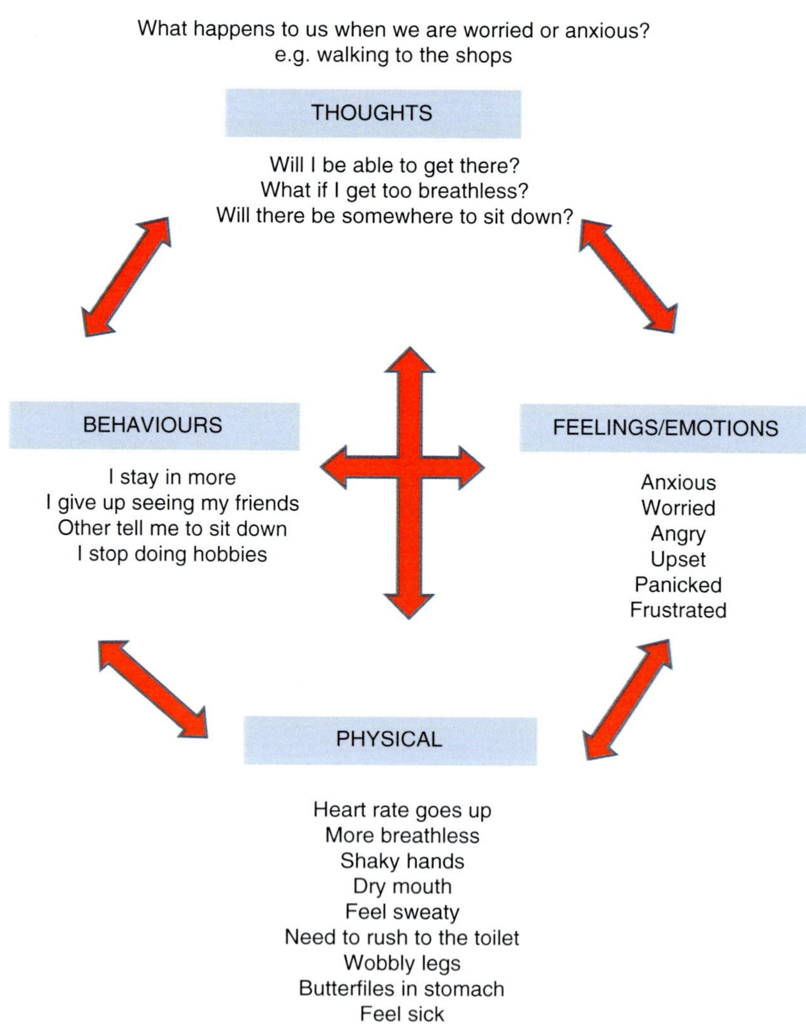

Fig. 12.5 The anxiety response

agencies to assess and offer advice regarding the suitability of major adaptations. Home adaptations or modifications that could be suitable for PR patients include the provision of:

- Stair lifts
- Through floor lifts
- Ground floor bathrooms, toilets or wet rooms
- Modifications to widen doorways if wheelchair access is required
- Installation of ramps and/or rails to enable improved property access

Decisions regarding this advice should be carefully considered with the patient at the very centre of these discussions. Factors such as the level of social support, future housing needs and disease severity are clearly important and each case will be different. People should be encouraged to consider the advantages of housing modifications against the future loss of physical activity. For instance, the provision of a stair lift may considerably reduce levels of breathlessness but may also result in loss of lower limb strength with the reduced need to climb stairs.

These issues should be actively discussed in a PR programme, especially for people who have more severe disease or a poorer prognosis. Major adaptations can take time to organise and fund. Therefore, regular assessment by the OT of how ADLs are being managed will monitor the need for this type of intervention. The process required to fund a major home adaptation differs from country to country but can take time to organise. A referral to an OT who specialises in housing adaptions should be completed at the earliest opportunity in order to address this.

12.5.4 Anxiety Management and Relaxation Training

It has previously been discussed in this chapter that anxiety can increase symptoms of breathlessness and is a significant barrier to maintaining independence in ADLs for some people who attend PR. It is crucial to recognise and address issues related to anxiety in order to ensure meaningful improvement in functional status. This could start during the assessment for entry onto a PR programme with an early assessment of psychological status.

Education sessions in PR that discuss symptoms of anxiety and breathlessness are recommended in PR guidelines [26] and offer opportunities to explore anxiety management strategies. These are often completed in group interventions, but this support could also be delivered on an individual basis. Key to this process is an understanding of the 'fight or flight' response and the physiological, cognitive and behavioural effects of this. This intervention is rooted in the cognitive behavioural approach to managing anxiety. This discussion is most usefully based around explaining the model outlined in Fig. 12.5, and these sessions are more generally successful when the interaction of the group is used to populate this model. PR group members are asked to share their experiences and feelings about a time when they felt anxious. These sessions should be facilitated by therapists who are skilled in group work.

Relaxation training is also recommended as an educational intervention in PR [26]. A recent systematic review concluded that relaxation therapy may have a moderate effect upon psychological well-being but accepted that the studies included in the review had a high heterogeneity. Qualitative evidence seems to support the inclusion of relaxation training as part of occupational therapy intervention for people with COPD [12].

There are differing relaxation techniques, and there is not yet any evidence to suggest which is preferable for people attending PR programmes. These include Progressive Muscle Relaxation (PMR) and guided imagery. PMR encourages increased awareness of muscle tension by firstly tensing certain muscle groups, holding the position of tension so that this can be remembered and then purposefully relaxing the muscle groups that the contrast in feeling can be recognised. This is usually completed by working down from the head to the feet until all muscles groups have been relaxed.

Guided imagery involves the visualisation of a pleasant and relaxing situation. This has similarities to the recent development of 'mindfulness' as people are encouraged to fully immerse themselves in this mental image. These sessions are usually directed by either an audio recording or the therapist describing a situation that the whole group will usually regard as relaxing such as walking along a beach on a warm summer's day or relaxing in front of a fire in a cosy armchair.

There are number of points to note when facilitating relaxation groups. Time should be taken at the beginning of the session to carefully explain the process and ensure that all distractions are minimised (e.g. mobile phones switched to silent, etc.). In addition it should be recognised that often people may initially feel uncomfortable about closing their eyes in an unfamiliar group situation, and reassurance should be given that this isn't compulsory. The end of the session is to ensure that all participants have had their blood pressure return to normal levels before they continue with any exercise or exertion. This can normally be achieved by taking some time after the relaxation training to offer some advice about relaxation that can be practised at home. The OT should explain that relaxation techniques take practice and only by completing relaxation training on daily basis at home can these techniques help them to manage breathlessness in daily situations.

Conclusion

This chapter has explored the contribution that an OT can bring to a multidisciplinary PR team. People who attend pulmonary rehabilitation programmes face many barriers to occupational performance, and this requires careful individual assessment. Interventions are often delivered as part of the PR group but one-to-one intervention advice also be considered in order to maximise benefit. OTs are integral to ensuring that any improvements made in functional capacity are translated into tangible benefits in the ability to maintain or regain independence in ADLs.

References

1. College of Occupational Therapists. What is Occupational Therapy? 2011.; https://www.cot.co.uk/ot-helps-you/what-occupational-therapy. Accessed 24 Sept 2016.
2. Duncan EAS. Introduction. In: Duncan EAS, editor. Foundations for Practice in Occupational Therapy. 5th ed. Edinburgh: Churchill Livingstone/Elsevier; 2012. p. 3.
3. American Occupational Therapy Association. Occupational therapy practice framework: domain & process 3rd edition. Am J Occup Ther. 2014;68: S1–S48.
4. Christiansen C, Baum C, Bass J. The person-environment-occupational performance (PEOP) model. In: Duncan EAS, editor. Foundations for practice in occupational therapy. 5th ed. Edinburgh: Churchill Livingstone/Elsevier; 2012. p. 93.
5. World Health Organisation. International classification of functioning, disabilities and health: ICF. 2001.
6. Bourbeau J. Activities of life: the COPD patient. COPD. 2009;6(3):192.
7. Reardon JZ, Lareau SC, ZuWallack R. Functional status and quality of life in chronic obstructive pulmonary disease. Am J Med. 2006;119(10 Suppl 1):32–7.
8. Williams V, Bruton A, Ellis-Hill C, McPherson K. The effect of pulmonary rehabilitation on perceptions of breathlessness and activity in COPD patients: a qualitative study. Prim Care Respir J. 2010;19(1):45–51.
9. Eisner MD, Blanc PD, Yelin EH, Katz PP, Sanchez G, Iribarren C, et al. Influence of anxiety on health outcomes in COPD. Thorax. 2010;65(3):229–34.
10. Karakurt P, Unsal A. Fatigue, anxiety and depression levels, activities of daily living of patients with chronic obstructive pulmonary disease. Int J Nurs Pract. 2013;19(2):221–31.
11. Doyle T, Palmer S, Johnson J, Babyak MA, Smith P, Mabe S, et al. Association of anxiety and depression with pulmonary-specific symptoms in chronic obstructive pulmonary disease. Int J Psychiatry Med. 2013;45(2):189–202.
12. Chan SC. Chronic obstructive pulmonary disease and engagement in occupation. Am J Occup Ther. 2004;58(4):408–15.
13. Theander K, Jakobsson P, Torstensson O, Unosson M. Severity of fatigue is related to functional limitation and health in patients with chronic obstructive pulmonary disease. Int J Nurs Pract. 2008;14(6):455–62.
14. Lewko A, Bidgood PL, Garrod R. Evaluation of psychological and physiological predictors of fatigue in patients with COPD. BMC Pulm Med. 2009;9:47.
15. Kapella MC, Larson JL, Patel MK, Covey MK, Berry JK. Subjective fatigue, influencing variables, and consequences in chronic obstructive pulmonary disease. Nurs Res. 2006;55(1):10–7.
16. Sewell L, Herbert S, Singh S. Daily activity patterns and energy conservation advice in patients with COPD. Eur Respir J. 2010;36(Suppl. 54):612.

17. Lareau SC, Meek PM, Roos PJ. Development and testing of the modified version of the pulmonary functional status and dyspnea questionnaire (PFSDQ-M). Heart Lung. 1998;27(3):159–68.
18. Yohannes AM, Roomi J, Winn S, Connolly MJ. The Manchester respiratory activities of daily living questionnaire: development, reliability, validity, and responsiveness to pulmonary rehabilitation. J Am Geriatr Soc. 2000;48(11):1496–500.
19. Garrod R, Bestall JC, Paul EA, Wedzicha JA, Jones PW. Development and validation of a standardized measure of activity of daily living in patients with severe COPD: the London Chest Activity of Daily Living scale (LCADL). Respir Med. 2000;94(6):589–96.
20. Lincoln NB, Gladman JR. The extended activities of daily living scale: a further validation. Disabil Rehabil. 1992;14(1):41–3.
21. Chen YJ, Narsavage GL, Culp SL, Weaver TE. The development and psychometric analysis of the short-form Pulmonary Functional Status Scale (PFSS-11). Res Nurs Health. 2010;33(6):477–85.
22. Law M, Baptiste S, Carswell A, et al. The Canadian occupational performance measure. CAOT. 2005.
23. Sewell L, Singh SJ. The Canadian occupational performance measure: is it a reliable measure in clients with chronic obstructive pulmonary disease? Br J Occup Ther. 2001;64(6):305.
24. Sewell L, Singh SJ, Williams JE, Collier R, Morgan MD. Can individualized rehabilitation improve functional independence in elderly patients with COPD? Chest. 2005;128(3):1194.
25. Williams JE, Singh SJ, Sewell L, Morgan MD. Health status measurement: sensitivity of the self-reported Chronic Respiratory Questionnaire (CRQ-SR) in pulmonary rehabilitation. Thorax. 2003;58(6):515–8.
26. Bolton CE, Bevan-Smith E, Blakey JD, Crowe P, Elkin SL, Garrod R, et al. British thoracic society guideline on pulmonary rehabilitation in adults. Thorax. 2013;68(2):ii1.
27. Spruit MA, Singh SJ, Garvey C, ZuWallack R, Nici L, Rochester C, et al. An official American Thoracic Society/European Respiratory Society statement: key concepts and advances in pulmonary rehabilitation. Am J Respir Crit Care Med. 2013;188(8):e13–64.
28. Velloso M, Jardim JR. Study of energy expenditure during activities of daily living using and not using body position recommended by energy conservation techniques in patients with COPD. Chest. 2006;130(1):126–32.
29. Vaes AW, Wouters EF, Franssen FM, Uszko-Lencer NH, Stakenborg KH, Westra M, et al. Task-related oxygen uptake during domestic activities of daily life in patients with COPD and healthy elderly subjects. Chest. 2011;140(4):970–9.
30. ZuWallack R. How are you doing? What are you doing? Differing perspectives in the assessment of individuals with COPD. COPD. 2007;4(3):293–7.

13 Psychological Considerations in Pulmonary Rehabilitation

Samantha Louise Harrison and Noelle Robertson

13.1 The Psychological Dimensions of Chronic Obstructive Pulmonary Disease (COPD)

Given the impact of COPD on patients' ability to fully engage in everyday tasks, it is not surprising that quality of life experienced by patients is often compromised and associated with psychological co-morbidities, notably, symptoms of anxiety and depression [1].

It is well documented that individuals with COPD report elevated levels of anxiety and depression when compared to their healthy elderly counterparts [2, 3]. A critical review of the literature estimates the prevalence of anxiety as 36% and 40% for depression [4]. These figures are further elevated following an acute exacerbation of COPD (AECOPD) with 53% and 43% of patients displaying at least a probable presence of anxious and depressed symptoms, respectively [5].

S.L. Harrison, Ph.D., M.C.S.P. (✉)
School of Health and Social Care Institute, Teesside University, Tees Valley, Middlesbrough TS1 3BX, UK
e-mail: S.L.Harrison@tees.ac.uk

N. Robertson, Ph.D., D.Clin.Psy.
School of Psychology, University of Leicester, Leicester, UK
e-mail: nr6@leicester.ac.uk

For those experiencing an AECOPD, particularly one that necessitates hospitalisation, fears of death and helplessness may be traumatising, and AECOPD have been linked to post-traumatic stress symptoms (PTSS), related to post-traumatic stress disorder (PTSD) [6]. Such PTSS have been noted in over 33% of patients following an AECOPD with prevalence increasing in those who experience two or more exacerbations in a 12-month period [6]. In a pulmonary rehabilitation (PR), cohort PTSD is present in 8% of patients and is associated with worse health status [7].

However, the psychological impact of COPD may extend beyond the more frequently assessed for and researched presentations of anxiety, depression and panic. As the role of personal behaviour and lifestyle choices has been emphasised in disease aetiology and progression, social judgements and stigma may also contribute to distress. Reflection on personal culpability for COPD and attributions of self-blame regarding smoking may evoke guilt, shame and regret [8]. A view of COPD as a self-inflicted disease, strengthened by the media representation of smoking behaviour, may elicit little sympathy from strangers, friends, family or even healthcare professionals (HCPs). Indeed, a substantial proportion of physicians believe patients with COPD are to blame for their disease [9]. If condemnatory or discouraging views are communicated to patients, they may undermine adherence, prompt

© Springer International Publishing AG 2018
E. Clini et al. (eds.), *Textbook of Pulmonary Rehabilitation*,
https://doi.org/10.1007/978-3-319-65888-9_13

avoidance of consultation and challenge patients' perceived legitimacy for dedicated care.

Individuals with COPD appear acutely aware of stigma [10]. Self-conscious emotions such as guilt, shame and embarrassment are frequently expressed [11] and have been linked to poor disease management including reduced help-seeking, reduced adherence to oxygen therapy and refusal of PR [12–14]. Such negative emotional responses appear to be associated not only with self-blame for the condition but also from visible differences, particularly socially undesirable symptoms (coughing, sputum production and severe breathlessness) and dependency on devices (rollators and oxygen therapy) [15, 16]. Patients may attempt to hide their disease, socially isolating themselves, with adverse consequences for mood and wellbeing.

13.2 Psychological Factors Through the Stages of PR

13.2.1 Initial Engagement with PR

PR is well recognised to be of benefit, yet a large proportion of people choose not to participate. Between 8% and 50% of patients referred to PR never attend [17], and following an AECOPD 45% refuse a referral to PR, and, of those who do accept, a further 45% do not attend the initial assessment for PR [5].

Evidence derived from a systematic review suggests that patients' belief in lack of benefit from PR is largely responsible for poor uptake [17]. Even following an AECOPD, which might be expected to emphasise the importance of actively engaging in treatment, PR is considered indifferently as irrelevant [5]. Lack of perceived benefit might arise from feelings of reduced self-worth associated with ageing, and an insidious onset of disease may imply little to make a difference; "it will get worse, because your lungs are getting more older and worn out, along with everything else" [14]. Indeed, during an AECOPD feelings of fear associated with symptoms of breathlessness accompany beliefs that the disease is too advanced to allow participation in exercise; "I wasn't just short of breath, I was gasping" [18].

Increasingly, PR services have started to encompass the use of patient testimonies. These accounts of positive peer experiences maybe useful to challenge beliefs about lack of benefit and encourage participation in PR as they have with exercise [19]. A recent retrospective analysis of 711 patients also highlights the importance of social support on patients' willingness to attend PR [20]. Family members, friends and carers are integral to supporting initial engagement with PR. Such interpersonal systems should be understood when offering a referral, and whenever possible family members and peers ought to be involved in conversations concerning acceptance of PR.

Patient characteristics are not the only factor adversely affecting PR uptake; HCPs who initiate referral are also key [21]. HCPs can adopt a positive approach to PR and be mindful that, particularly during an AECOPD, patients seem sensitive to insufficient time offered in key consultation, "they want the beds for other people", and apparently dismissive behaviour [14]. HCPs capacity to fully empathise with patients is attributable to their repeated exposure to symptomatic patients and pressures from the healthcare service to treat high numbers [22], yet by openly exhibiting empathy and compassion during consultations, HCPs can ensure they promote feelings of safety and trust.

Sensitivity can also be shown by HCPs carefully considering timing and context of offering a referral to PR. Promoting an intervention which emphasises exercise and induces shortness of breath, at a time when patients fear breathlessness, may suggest that they fail to understand the seriousness of symptoms which patients feel are life-threatening. Instead a referral to PR maybe best offered at a time when acute breathlessness has been resolved.

13.2.2 Adherence to PR

Once a referral to PR is accepted, the next challenge faced by patients and PR providers is to manage adherence to the programme. Adherence to PR is very poor with approximately 20–60% of those eligible failing to complete programmes [23–27].

Non-completion rates have been ascribed to symptoms of anxiety and depression. A systematic review noted that in conjunction with smoking status, only the presence of depressed symptoms could predict non-adherence to PR [17], although a more recent study including 111 patients with COPD concluded that this was true only for women [28]. However, two large retrospective analyses identified that neither anxious nor depressed symptoms as measured using the hospital anxiety and depression scale (HADS) were able to successfully predict those able to complete PR [20, 27].

A better correlate of PR adherence may be patients' appraisals of their disease as articulated by the common sense model [29] which forms the base of the Illness Perceptions Questionnaire-Revised (IPQ-R) [30]. This questionnaire comprises eight domains: *identity* assessing the number of symptoms associated with the disease, *consequences* relating to disease severity, *timeline acute/chronic* indicating the disease duration, *timeline cyclical* relating to whether the disease is stable or fluctuating, *personal control* measuring the amount of control a person feels he or she has over his or her disease, *treatment control* relating to the efficacy of treatment, *illness coherence* referring to understanding of the disease and *emotional representations* assessing impact on emotional wellbeing.

Beliefs about controllability of treatment for patients with stable COPD can differentiate those adhering to a PR programme and those displaying only low adherence [23]. These results complement findings derived from qualitative studies, which found that a lack of perceived benefit (akin to treatment control) could successfully predict poor adherence to PR [17]. More recent data revealed patients enrolled in PR ascribed their continued attendance to experiencing noticeable changes in mobility and gaining greater understanding of the disease process [18]. By offering sustained encouragement for patients to monitor their own progress and by fully discussing and supporting any observed improvements, HCPs may have a positive influence on patients' willingness to complete PR.

The experience of an AECOPD appears to further diminish the likelihood of completing PR, with only 9% of all patients admitted to hospital completing PR within a 6-month follow-up period [5, 31]. Understanding of the reasons behind non-completion in patients' post-AECOPD is scant; however, psychological profiling using the IPQ-R has been useful to highlight variation in illness appraisals within this population [5]. Of 128 patients who had been admitted to hospital with an AECOPD, three groups were identified. Patients in Group 1 (n = 52) were labelled 'in control', and despite having higher perceived personal control and lesser emotional representations, they did not view their disease to have serious consequences [5]. This has been identified as a key factor in predicting attendance at cardiac rehabilitation (CR) [32]. Patients in Group 2 (n = 36) were characterised as 'disengaged' and associated more symptoms with their disease but reported fewer consequences, had less understanding of their condition and had lower personal control. Importantly, those patients who perceived their condition as controllable were more likely to attend CR [32]. Finally, patients in Group 3 (n = 40) were considered to be 'distressed' reporting elevated emotional representations from the perception of the disease as highly symptomatic with severe consequences. Such findings argue for a greater profiling of the psychological status of those embarking on PR and offering more nuanced and tailored forms of the programmes to meet their specific needs [5].

13.3 Psychological Assessment Within PR

13.3.1 Psychometric Measures

13.3.1.1 The Hospital and Anxiety Depression Scale

In both clinical practice and research, the HADS is one of the most commonly applied tools to assess psychological wellbeing in individuals with COPD [4]. Fourteen statements are scored on a four point Likert scale ranging from zero to three and are divided into two subscales: (anxiety (α = 0.68) and depression (α = 0.91)) each of which are scored between zero and 21 [33]. Scores of zero to seven are considered to be in the normal range, a score of eight to ten is suggestive of anxiety or depression and scores higher than 11 indicate a presence of psychological 'caseness'. The minimal clinically important difference (MCID) for a change in each subscale has been established in patients with COPD and quoted as −1.5 [34].

Despite its popularity the appropriateness of the HADS for patients with respiratory disease has been questioned. Items may confound physical with psychological status. For example, one item asks patients to indicate how often 'they feel slowed down'. The majority of patients with COPD often feel slowed down as a result of their disease leading clinicians to question its utility and precision to indicate psychological distressed state in this population.

13.3.1.2 Anxiety Inventory for Respiratory Disease

Willgoss et al. have developed a disease-specific, non-somatic anxiety scale to mitigate overlap of somatic symptoms of anxiety with physical symptoms of COPD and side-effects of medications (i.e. breathlessness, fatigue and heart palpitations) [35]. The Anxiety Inventory for Respiratory Disease (AIR) comprises ten items with scores ranging from 0 to 30 (α = 0.92). A higher score indicates greater severity of anxious symptoms with the MCID quoted as 5.55 [36].

13.3.1.3 Brief IPQ

The HADS and the AIR can screen for psychological morbidity but offer little information to guide focus of any intervention. The IPQ-R, as described previously, provides a comprehensive investigation of patients' illness appraisals with over 80 items. Where time constraints exist, a shorter version of the questionnaire is available comprising nine items assessed on a continuous scale. The brief IPQ was found to be valid and reliable when compared to the IPQ-R [37]. The brief IPQ has been administered to patients over 80 years, with a wide range of illnesses including COPD. Scores correlate with anxiety, depression and quality of life, and it is sensitive to change after intervention [38].

13.3.1.4 Self-Conscious Emotions

As awareness of the potential role of stigma, shame and guilt in living with COPD is growing, a number of questionnaires can be used to assess self-conscious emotions in patients with COPD [11]. These include the Brief Fear of Negative Evaluation Scale [39], the Shame and Guilt Scale [40] and the Self-Compassion Scale Short-Form [41]. However, since these assessment tools were validated in psychiatric populations, there is scope to develop more niche tools appropriate for those with long-term conditions. Ten disease-specific items have been developed for individuals with COPD, enquiring about issues pertaining to self-blame, embarrassment associated with disease visibility, concerns about the views of others and grief, although these items are yet to be validated. That said, assessment of self-conscious emotions through self-reported measures is limited given such emotions are rarely experienced on the conscious level [42]. Instead such emotions are more likely to arise through conversing with patients [11].

13.3.2 Clinical Interview

The clinical interview of patients is a cornerstone of assessment taking place prior to and following PR. It is 'a conversation with a purpose' and may uncover any concerns related to the disease and/or attending PR through a dialogue with the patient.

Given that patients with COPD may be anxious, distressed or self-conscious, there are a number of important factors that ought to be taken into consideration when conducting a clinical interview. Placing a patient at ease is paramount, and a quiet and nonthreatening space is essential to facilitating frank dialogue. Conducting the interview in a busy physiotherapy gym would not be appropriate and may appear dismissive. Sitting behind a desk or computer creates an unwelcome physical barrier and power differential, and some patients may feel less able to convey their concerns or ask questions. Starting an interview by reassuring patients that their conversation is completely confidential helps to build trust and encourages an open and honest exchange. Using open-ended questions also allows patients to tell their own story with time to think and respond, and can give clinicians time to attend to non-verbal cues such as posture and the tone of voice, giving a complete view of communication.

Given the previously discussed barriers to engaging with and adhering to PR (lacking the belief that PR will be of benefit [17] and reduced social support [20]), both should be explicitly addressed when offering a referral to PR.

13.4 Psychological Impact of COPD on Carers and Supportive Intervention

For many individuals with COPD, family members provide the primary source of support [43] helping to manage symptoms, assisting with mobility and performing personal care [44]. However, giving such support can impose significant burden [45, 46]. Grant and colleagues' review explored the impact of caring for those with COPD revealing adverse physical and emotional consequences: notably difficulty of staying alert throughout the night and anxiety about symptom knowledge and trajectory of the disease [45]. These findings resonate with a later synthesis documenting the physical (e.g. fatigue), social (e.g. the necessity of planning everyday activities) and financial burdens (e.g. need for expensive medications and loss of patients income) experienced [46].

Given the profound emotional, physical and social consequences of caring for individuals with COPD, it is unsurprising that carers, like patients, report psychological distress. Anxiety and depression have been detected in 63% and 34% of family members of patients with COPD, respectively [47]. Physical distress and psychological morbidity in carers are likely to affect the quality of care that family members are able to offer, both in routine care (i.e. everyday tasks such as washing and dressing) and at the time of an AECOPD. During an AECOPD, when symptoms of breathlessness are prominent, patients have described both intense fear of family members, "Oh God hes's panic stricken he is, he's useless, absolutely useless" [48] and complacency "According to him I can breathe and its normal" [48].

Despite carers' role in facilitating a patients' attendance at PR and their reported distress, to date only one study has tested the effectiveness of a family intervention, integrated into a PR programme. Zakrisson and colleagues invited family members to attend one session of a 6-week PR programme and conducted interviews to explore their views towards the intervention [49]. Carers reported numerous benefits notably relief from the burden of caring by translating strategies learned in PR to home activities and strategies to help their own wellbeing gleaned from others in a similar situation. However, family members did report increased vigilance towards patients' response to observed breathlessness and reduced strength, and their feelings of anxiety were also heightened through confirmation of the disease progression [49]. More research is required to explore interventions to support carers for those with COPD, particularly since the provision of education alone is not sufficient and can even promote feelings of anxiety and personal vulnerability.

13.5 The Impact of PR on Psychological Symptoms

An explicit function of PR is to provide psychosocial support and address distress [50]. To date, the multifactorial nature of a PR programme makes it difficult to explore which components of the programme may be most effective in reducing symptoms of anxiety and depression and improving quality of life. It is possible to theorise that in addition to the benefits of exercise on reducing physical impairment (behavioural activation), the educational component increasing coping skills as well as the role of social support may also be important.

Meta-analysis has revealed that PR is effective at reducing symptoms of anxiety and depression in COPD. However, the mean symptoms scores of distress at the intervention's outset were only mild [51]. With the conclusion of benefit limited to those with less marked symptoms [51]. A more recent study exploring the effectiveness of PR across varying levels of anxiety and depression revealed that the greatest reductions in HADS scores were evident in patients displaying the most severe symptoms of anxiety and depression. By contrast those reporting few symptoms of anxiety and depression showed no significant change in HADS score after PR. This may suggest that the impact of PR has been underestimated, and those who may derive the most benefit are those patients disclosing most distress [27].

Whilst this study showed that PR appears to diminish reported anxiety and depression in those with the most severe psychological symptoms, a percentage of patients still had a possible presence of psychological symptoms following PR. Furthermore 47% and 40% of patients who had a 'presence' of anxious and depressed symptoms, respectively, before PR still had a 'presence' of symptoms despite the programmes completion. These patients may need further interventions to reduce symptoms of anxiety and depression to within the normal range.

A small minority of patients may report increased distress, possibly through increased focus on challenge to breathing and hypervigilance. Arguably an education programme, discussing disease trajectory, can increase awareness of the disease process and its terminal nature, often visible in other group members with more advanced disease. Indeed identifying with patients whose symptoms are more disabling (downward assimilation) has been recognised in a PR population and found to enhance social comparisons and anxious mood [52].

The impact of PR on how patients perceive their disease appears equally complex and yet is important as negative illness perceptions (i.e. a cyclical timeline, higher emotional representations and greater consequences) prior to treatment have been shown to predict reduced exercise capacity and poorer self-reported wellbeing post-PR [53]. Overall PR has little effect on patients' perceptions of their disease assessed using the IPQ-R which is unsurprising given PR, delivered in its current form, does not explicitly address how patients appraise their disease. However, following a programme, patients viewed their disease as more episodic rather than unrelenting which likely stems from an increased awareness of AECOPD gleaned from personal experience, from witnessing others, from increased attention to bodily symptoms promoted through relaxation or from the education provided during PR [54]. Increases in personal control were also noted and are likely linked to an increase in self-efficacy, which is known to improve following PR [55].

13.6 Psychological Interventions for Individuals with COPD

To enhance the capacity of PR to treat psychological morbidity, national guidelines have incorporated support for the development of psychological interventions to improve patients' wellbeing [50].

13.6.1 Cognitive Behavioural Therapy (CBT) and COPD

CBT has been recommended for inclusion in the care of patients with COPD, driven by the evidence base in the management of chronic conditions and its therapeutic dominance in current healthcare delivery. The premise of CBT is that changing unhelpful thinking leads to behaviour change. Patients are encouraged to identify and challenge their beliefs and replace errors in thinking (i.e. magnifying negatives, minimising positives and catastrophising) with more adaptive and effective thoughts, mitigating emotional distress. CBT helps patients to challenge their way of thinking to promote adaptive, coping skills, emotions, cognitions and behaviours through a number of techniques including education, relaxation, cognitive therapy, behavioural therapy, behavioural activation, exposure therapy and sleep management skills [56].

Effectiveness of CBT, delivered to those living with COPD, has been synthesised in a review from four studies exploring the impact on anxiety and depression [57]. Meta-analysis revealed equivocal findings with only small improvements in anxiety and depression noted associated with active intervention [57]. Despite these premature results, a number of lessons can be gleaned from the studies included in the review. Firstly, although psychological symptoms were significantly reduced following treatment in the group receiving CBT versus COPD education, these differences were not evident at follow-up perhaps indicating the importance of long-term face-to-face delivery [58]. Secondly, that results revealed CBT to be effective in reducing clinically significant symptoms in patients with COPD with reductions maintained after eight months, suggesting CBT may be more effective in patients with psychological symptoms reaching clinical caseness [56]. Finally, only one study exploring the effect of CBT on panic pathology in individuals with COPD delivered the intervention on an individual basis. Significant differences were noted in the frequency of panic disorder and panic attacks in favour of the intervention compared to the usual care group [59]. Those who received CBT were asymptomatic post-intervention and remained so for 18 months highlighting both treatment effect and the preventative impact of CBT and emphasising the importance of one-to-one delivery [59].

It would seem that the impact of CBT compared to an active intervention (i.e. COPD education) is still unclear [60]. Most individuals are at least 40 years of age when they develop symptoms of COPD although it occurs most often in older adults. Many of the limitations of CBT pertain to its application in older adult populations. A key component of CBT is problem solving, yet the ability to problem solve appears diminished with age [61, 62]. Furthermore, following an AECOPD patients express intense levels of arousal associated with symptoms of breathlessness heightening fears of dying. Such fears may not be unrealistic and attempts to modify these beliefs may serve to further heighten anxious affect. Routine adoption of CBT for elderly patients with COPD may need to focus on supporting patients to accept these challenges to health rather than attempting to alter such cognitions [63]. However, acceptance is not a component always emphasised by a CBT approach, rather it is more aligned with the technique of mindfulness.

13.6.2 Mindfulness and COPD

Mindfulness is an approach to life and therapeutic vehicle that has been gaining popularity in recent years and appears well suited to the needs of older adults. With ageing it becomes necessary to reappraise our expectations in the face of age-related losses, which are magnified in the presence of a debilitating chronic condition. Patients with COPD suffer from a gradual loss of function as a result of their condition—these losses may activate a grieving process [64]. Yet wellbeing can be enhanced by the ability to disengage from unattainable goals (i.e. returning to work in heavy construction) and re-engaging in alternative goals that are realistic (i.e. gardening and playing with grandchildren). Disengagement is not seen as hopeless, 'giving up' or a reflection of personal inadequacy, but instead it involves actively seeking out alternative opportunities to maximise control, protecting patients' sense of 'self' and emotional wellbeing.

Mindfulness's relevance to COPD has been considered through a systematic review of four randomised controlled trials exploring mindfulness delivered to patients with respiratory conditions [65]. Meta-analysis revealed no benefit of the intervention compared to a control group on disease-specific HRQOL, mindful awareness or stress levels. Indeed adherence to mindfulness appears challenging for those with COPD; only around 60% were able to complete the recommended number of sessions perhaps explaining the observed lack of effect [66, 67]. However, improvements in emotional function were observed in those who completed six or more sessions [66]. Since traditional mindfulness involves the redirection of attention towards one's own breath, this may be problematic for patients with symptoms of dyspnoea. Drawing attention to breathing may magnify hypervigilance to breathless symptoms and lead to heightened emotional arousal and agitation. The evidence thus far on potential benefits of mindfulness-based approaches is scant, and a growing evidence base will help establish whether this is a fruitful therapeutic tool.

13.6.3 Motivational Interviewing

Motivational interviewing is described as a focused and goal-oriented, client-centred counselling style for eliciting behaviour change by helping clients to explore and resolve ambivalence [68]. Importantly motivation to change behaviour must come from the client, and any attempt from the HCP to confront resistance is likely to be met with further resistance. Instead patients should be encouraged to express ambivalence, i.e. 'I know going to PR might help me to walk further but I don't want to feel breathless when exercising'. The HCPs' role is to clarify this ambivalence and work in partnership with the patient to resolve it by being attentive and responsive in a respectful manner that encompasses compassion [68].

Interventions that incorporate components of MI seem able to enhance positive behaviour change in patients with COPD. MI can be successfully merged with self-management, a key component of PR, and pilot testing has shown it to be feasible and valued by patients with COPD [69]. The principles of MI have also been incorporated into a PR programme as part of lifestyle physical activity counselling with feedback from a pedometer [70]. The group receiving lifestyle counselling increased the number of steps performed per day compared to a control group who actually had a reduced number of steps [70].

When combined with mindfulness, MI might be an effective intervention to encourage attendance at PR. In a recent randomised controlled trial consisting of 215 patients hospitalized with an AECOPD, attendance to PR was increased in those assigned to MI-based health coaching compared to those who received only usual care. In part, increased attendance to PR may be responsible for the significant differences in favour of the intervention group observed on the risk of re-hospitalisation at one, three and six months follow-up and on HRQOL at 6 and 12 months follow-up [71].

13.7 Where Do We Go Next?

There is substantial evidence that psychological distress commonly accompanies COPD and those attending PR, and international guidelines include psychological support in the parameters of PR [50]. However, delivered in its current form, PR is not sufficient to treat those with severe psychological symptoms. This has led to arguments for more nuanced understanding of those who are the most psychologically vulnerable and more tailoring of interventions and applications of more focused psychological interventions, notably CBT, mindfulness and MI, in individuals with COPD. Unfortunately the complexities of the disease, issues with adherence and uncertainty around the manner in which to deliver psychological support mean a proven psychological intervention for individuals with COPD is still requiring development. When considering psychological therapy for people with COPD, the following points require consideration.

13.7.1 Adapting PR to Meet the Needs of Those with Psychological Symptoms

PR provides a comprehensive model of care delivered by members of a multidisciplinary team; however, it may need to evolve to effectively meet the individual needs of patients, particularly those with psychological co-morbidity.

13.7.1.1 Individual Versus Group Therapy

Traditionally PR programmes are delivered in a group format with all patients receiving treatment in the same manner and with little focus on the additional needs of those with heightened psychological symptoms. Group therapies are often cost driven, yet despite a blanket approach and assumed homogeneity, this is not always the most effective means of promoting positive health outcomes. A recent review of the literature exploring psychologically based interventions for patients with COPD revealed that all interventions, with the exception of one, had been delivered within a group setting [57]. One intervention delivered individually noted positive effects of CBT on panic psychopathology [59], whereas other group interventions' impact was more circumscribed, in alleviating symptoms of anxiety and depression [57]. The specific needs of the individual need more detailed assessment and formulation to maximise the effectiveness of psychological strategies for patients with COPD. This is a concept now endorsed by the international guidelines for PR [50], and programmes are becoming more individually focused. Psychological therapy maybe best delivered alongside PR in a stepped-care fashion which would enable the delivery of treatment within a group setting, increasing cost-effectiveness and feasibility but still attending to the individual needs of the patient. Incorporating psychological support into PR is also likely to reduce any possible stigma and encourage patients to adhere to such support.

13.7.1.2 Hospital Versus Home Delivery

A large proportion of patients do not attend PR, missing important factors of care. Psychological symptoms likely contribute to patients' unwillingness to engage with PR presenting an argument for offering psychological support prior to a referral to PR for those experiencing marked distress. Furthermore, optimising patients in terms of their psychological wellbeing prior to enrolment in PR maybe important in ensuring clinically significant gains are obtained [72].

Psychological interventions could form part of a prehabilitation programme. Many patients are reluctant to attend the hospital for care, especially following an AECOPD, due to issues with transport and fear of picking up another infection [5]. Psychological therapies that require few resources could be applied within the home environment, perhaps improving adherence [59].

13.7.1.3 Patients with High Levels of Distress Versus All Individuals Eligible for PR

There appears to be reluctance among patients to engage in psychological interventions, demonstrated via poor adherence rates in previous studies, and this could be attributed to the fact that most researchers have targeted all patients, irrespective of psychological status. Contrary to assumed behaviour, those who are most distressed do not appear most motivated to engage in interventions to address their symptoms. Indeed Chan et al. noted that attendance was highest in those with low levels of anxiety perhaps because these patients were better practically and emotionally able to attend [66].

The diversity and complexity of psychological symptoms experienced by patients presents another challenge for targeted therapy. As discussed previously psychological presentations in COPD may extend beyond anxiety and depression and encompass emotions such as guilt, shame, self-blame and embarrassment. These emotions may not be detected using traditional methods of assessment, i.e. the HADS. Instead by taking the time to talk and listen to patients, HCPs may find themselves better placed to make judgements regarding patients' psychological needs [73].

References

1. Cully JA, Graham DP, Stanley MA, Ferguson CJ, Sharafkhaneh A, Souchek J, et al. Quality of life in patients with chronic obstructive pulmonary disease and comorbid anxiety or depression. Psychosomatics. 2006;47(4):312–9.
2. Karajgi B, Rifkin A, Doddi S, Kolli R. The prevalence of anxiety disorders in patients with chronic obstructive pulmonary disease. Am J Psychiatry. 1990;147(2):200–1.
3. van Ede L, Yzermans CJ, Brouwer HJ. Prevalence of depression in patients with chronic obstructive pulmonary disease: a systematic review. Thorax. 1999;54(8):688–92.
4. Yohannes AM, Willgoss TG, Baldwin RC, Connolly MJ. Depression and anxiety in chronic heart failure and chronic obstructive pulmonary disease: prevalence, relevance, clinical implications and management principles. Int J Geriatr Psychiatry. 2010;25(12):1209–21.

5. Harrison SL, Robertson N, Graham CD, Williams J, Steiner MC, Morgan MDL, et al. Can we identify patients with different illness schema following an acute exacerbation of COPD: a cluster analysis. Respir Med. 2014;108(2):319–28.
6. Teixeira PJ, Porto L, Kristensen CH, Santos AH, Menna-Barreto SS, Do Prado-Lima PA. Post-traumatic stress symptoms and exacerbations in COPD patients. COPD. 2015;12(1):90–5.
7. Jones RC, Harding SA, Chung MC, Campbell J. The prevalence of posttraumatic stress disorder in patients undergoing pulmonary rehabilitation and changes in PTSD symptoms following rehabilitation. J Cardiopulm Rehabil Prev. 2009;29(1):49–56.
8. Halding AG, Heggdal K, Wahl A. Experiences of self-blame and stigmatisation for self-infliction among individuals living with COPD. Scand J Caring Sci. 2011;25(1):100–7.
9. Winstanley L, Daunt M, Macfarlane J. Doctors' attitude towards current smokers with chronic obstructive pulmonary disease and its impact on delivering smoking cessation advice. J Smok Cessat. 2008;3(02):133–5.
10. Berger BE, Kapella MC, Larson JL. The experience of stigma in chronic obstructive pulmonary disease. West J Nurs Res. 2011;33(7):916–32.
11. Harrison SL, Robertson N, Goldstein RS, Brooks D. Exploring self-conscious emotions in individuals with chronic obstructive pulmonary disease: a mixed-methods study. Chron Respir Dis. 2016;14(1):22–32.
12. Earnest MA. Explaining adherence to supplemental oxygen therapy: the patient's perspective. J Gen Intern Med. 2002;17(10):749–55.
13. Arne M, Emtner M, Janson S, Wilde-Larsson B. COPD patients perspectives at the time of diagnosis: a qualitative study. Prim Care Respir J. 2007;16(4):215–21.
14. Harrison SL, Robertson N, Apps L, C Steiner M, Morgan MD, Singh SJ. "We are not worthy"—understanding why patients decline pulmonary rehabilitation following an acute exacerbation of COPD. Disabil Rehabil. 2015;37(9):750–6.
15. Arnold E, Bruton A, Donovan-Hall M, Fenwick A, Dibb B, Walker E. Ambulatory oxygen: why do COPD patients not use their portable systems as prescribed? A qualitative study. BMC Pulm Med. 2011;11(1):1–7.
16. Hill K, Goldstein R, Gartner EJ, Brooks D. Daily utility and satisfaction with rollators among persons with chronic obstructive pulmonary disease. Arch Phys Med Rehabil. 2008;89(6):1108–13.
17. Keating A, Lee A, Holland AE. What prevents people with chronic obstructive pulmonary disease from attending pulmonary rehabilitation? A systematic review. Chron Respir Dis. 2011;8(2):89–99.
18. Guo SE, Bruce A. Improving understanding of and adherence to pulmonary rehabilitation in patients with COPD: a qualitative inquiry of patient and health professional perspectives. PLoS One. 2014;9(10):e110835.
19. Cameron-Tucker HL, Wood-Baker R, Owen C, Joseph L, Walters EH. Chronic disease self-management and exercise in COPD as pulmonary rehabilitation: a randomized controlled trial. Int J Chron Obstruct Pulmon Dis. 2014;9:513–23.
20. Hayton C, Clark A, Olive S, Browne P, Galey P, Knights E, et al. Barriers to pulmonary rehabilitation: characteristics that predict patient attendance and adherence. Respir Med. 2013;107(3):401–7.
21. Arnold E, Bruton A, Ellis-Hill C. Adherence to pulmonary rehabilitation: a qualitative study. Respir Med. 2006;100(10):1716–23.
22. Belcher VN, Fried TR, Agostini JV, Tinetti ME. Views of older adults on patient participation in medication-related decision making. J Gen Intern Med. 2006;21(4):298–303.
23. Fischer MJ, Scharloo M, Abbink JJ, van't Hul AJ, van Ranst D, Rudolphus A, et al. Drop-out and attendance in pulmonary rehabilitation: the role of clinical and psychosocial variables. Respir Med. 2009;103(10):1564–71.
24. Garrod R, Marshall J, Barley E, Jones PW. Predictors of success and failure in pulmonary rehabilitation. Eur Respir J. 2006;27(4):788–94.
25. Hogg L, Garrod R, Thornton H, McDonnell L, Bellas H, White P. Effectiveness, attendance, and completion of an integrated, system-wide pulmonary rehabilitation service for COPD: prospective observational study. COPD. 2012;9(5):546–54.
26. Selzler AM, Simmonds L, Rodgers WM, Wong EY, Stickland MK. Pulmonary rehabilitation in chronic obstructive pulmonary disease: predictors of program completion and success. COPD. 2012;9(5):538–45.
27. Harrison SL, Greening NJ, Williams JE, Morgan MD, Steiner MC, Singh SJ. Have we underestimated the efficacy of pulmonary rehabilitation in improving mood? Respir Med. 2012;106(6):838–44.
28. Busch AM, Scott-Sheldon LA, Pierce J, Chattillion EA, Cunningham K, Buckley ML, et al. Depressed mood predicts pulmonary rehabilitation completion among women, but not men. Respir Med. 2014;108(7):1007–13.
29. Leventhal H, Diefenbach M, Leventhal EA. Illness cognition: Using common sense to understand treatment adherence and affect cognition interactions. Cogn Ther Res. 1992;16(2):143–63.
30. Moss-Morris R, Weinman J, Petrie K, Horne R, Cameron L, Buick D. The revised illness perception questionnaire (IPQ-R). Psychol Health. 2002;17(1):1–16.
31. Jones SE, Green SA, Clark AL, Dickson MJ, Nolan A-M, Moloney C, et al. Pulmonary rehabilitation following hospitalisation for acute exacerbation of COPD: referrals, uptake and adherence. Thorax. 2014;69(2):181–2.
32. French DP, Cooper A, Weinman J. Illness perceptions predict attendance at cardiac rehabilitation following acute myocardial infarction: a systematic review with meta-analysis. J Psychosom Res. 2006;61(6):757–67.

33. Zigmond AS, Snaith RP. The hospital anxiety and depression scale. Acta Psychiatr Scand. 1983;67(6): 361–70.
34. Puhan MA, Frey M, Büchi S, Schünemann HJ. The minimal important difference of the hospital anxiety and depression scale in patients with chronic obstructive pulmonary disease. Health Qual Life Outcomes. 2008;6(1):1–6.
35. Willgoss TG, Goldbart J, Fatoye F, Yohannes AM. The development and validation of the anxiety inventory for respiratory disease. Chest. 2013;144(5):1587–96.
36. Yohannes AM, Dryden S, Hanania NA. The responsiveness of the anxiety inventory for respiratory disease scale following pulmonary rehabilitation. Chest. 2016;150(1):188–95.
37. Broadbent E, Petrie KJ, Main J, Weinman J. The brief illness perception questionnaire. J Psychosom Res. 2006;60(6):631–7.
38. Broadbent E, Wilkes C, Koschwanez H, Weinman J, Norton S, Petrie KJ. A systematic review and meta-analysis of the brief illness perception questionnaire. Psychol Health. 2015;30(11):1361–85.
39. Leary MR. A brief version of the fear of negative evaluation scale. Personal Soc Psychol Bull. 1983;9(3):371–5.
40. Marschall D, Sanftner J, Tangney JP. The state shame and guilt scale. Fairfax: George Mason University; 1994.
41. Neff KD. The development and validation of a scale to measure self-compassion. Self Identity. 2003;2(3):223–50.
42. Strang S, Farrell M, Larsson L-O, Sjöstrand C, Gunnarsson A, Ekberg-Jansson A, et al. Experience of guilt and strategies for coping with guilt in patients with severe COPD: a qualitative interview study. J Palliat Care. 2014;30(2):108–15.
43. Seamark DA, Blake SD, Seamark CJ, Halpin DM. Living with severe chronic obstructive pulmonary disease (COPD): perceptions of patients and their carers. An interpretative phenomenological analysis. Palliat Med. 2004;18(7):619–25.
44. Gardiner C, Gott M, Payne S, Small N, Barnes S, Halpin D, et al. Exploring the care needs of patients with advanced COPD: an overview of the literature. Respir Med. 2010;104(2):159–65.
45. Grant M, Cavanagh A, Yorke J. The impact of caring for those with chronic obstructive pulmonary disease (COPD) on carers' psychological well-being: a narrative review. Int J Nurs Stud. 2012;49(11): 1459–71.
46. Cruz J, Marques A, Figueiredo D. Impacts of COPD on family carers and supportive interventions: a narrative review. Health Soc Care Community. 2017;25(1):11–25.
47. Jacome C, Figueiredo D, Gabriel R, Cruz J, Marques A. Predicting anxiety and depression among family carers of people with chronic obstructive pulmonary disease. Int Psychogeriatr. 2014;26(7):1191–9.
48. Halpin D, Hyland M, Blake S, Seamark C, Pinnuck M, Ward D, et al. Understanding fear and anxiety in patients at the time of an exacerbation of chronic obstructive pulmonary disease: a qualitative study. JRSM Open. 2015;6(12):2054270415614543.
49. Zakrisson AB, Theander K, Anderzen-Carlsson A. The experience of a multidisciplinary programme of pulmonary rehabilitation in primary health care from the next of kin's perspective: a qualitative study. Prim Care Respir J. 2013;22(4):459–65.
50. Spruit MA, Singh SJ, Garvey C, ZuWallack R, Nici L, Rochester C, et al. An official American thoracic society/European respiratory society statement: key concepts and advances in pulmonary rehabilitation. Am J Respir Crit Care Med. 2013;188(8):e13–64.
51. Coventry PA, Hind D. Comprehensive pulmonary rehabilitation for anxiety and depression in adults with chronic obstructive pulmonary disease: systematic review and meta-analysis. J Psychosom Res. 2007;63(5):551–65.
52. Petersen S, Taube K, Lehmann K, Van den Bergh O, von Leupoldt A. Social comparison and anxious mood in pulmonary rehabilitation: the role of cognitive focus. Br J Health Psychol. 2012;17(3):463–76.
53. Zoeckler N, Kenn K, Kuehl K, Stenzel N, Rief W. Illness perceptions predict exercise capacity and psychological well-being after pulmonary rehabilitation in COPD patients. J Psychosom Res. 2014;76(2):146–51.
54. Fischer M, Scharloo M, Abbink J, van't Hul A, van Ranst D, Rudolphus A, et al. The dynamics of illness perceptions: testing assumptions of Leventhal's common-sense model in a pulmonary rehabilitation setting. Br J Health Psychol. 2010;15(Pt 4):887–903.
55. Vincent E, Sewell L, Wagg K, Deacon S, Williams J, Singh S. Measuring a change in self-efficacy following pulmonary rehabilitation: an evaluation of the PRAISE tool. Chest. 2011;140(6):1534–9.
56. Hynninen MJ, Bjerke N, Pallesen S, Bakke PS, Nordhus IH. A randomized controlled trial of cognitive behavioral therapy for anxiety and depression in COPD. Respir Med. 2010;104(7):986–94.
57. Smith SMS, Sonego S, Ketcheson L, Larson JL. A review of the effectiveness of psychological interventions used for anxiety and depression in chronic obstructive pulmonary disease. BMJ Open Respir Res. 2014;1(1):e000042.
58. Kunik ME, Braun U, Stanley MA, Wristers K, Molinari V, Stoebner D, et al. One session cognitive behavioural therapy for elderly patients with chronic obstructive pulmonary disease. Psychol Med. 2001;31(4):717–23.
59. Livermore N, Sharpe L, McKenzie D. Prevention of panic attacks and panic disorder in COPD. Eur Respir J. 2010;35(3):557–63.
60. Kunik ME, Veazey C, Cully JA, Souchek J, Graham DP, Hopko D, et al. COPD education and cognitive behavioral therapy group treatment for clinically significant symptoms of depression and anxiety in COPD patients: a randomized controlled trial. Psychol Med. 2008;38(3):385–96.

61. Diehl M, Willis SL, Schaie KW. Everyday problem solving in older adults: observational assessment and cognitive correlates. Psychol Aging. 1995;10(3):478–91.
62. Burton CL, Strauss E, Hultsch DF, Hunter MA. Cognitive functioning and everyday problem solving in older adults. Clin Neuropsychol. 2006;20(3):432–52.
63. Laidlaw K, Thompson LW, Gallagher-Thompson D. Comprehensive conceptualization of cognitive behaviour therapy for late life depression. Behav Cogn Psychother. 2004;32(4):389–99.
64. Boer LM, Daudey L, Peters JB, Molema J, Prins JB, Vercoulen JH. Assessing the stages of the grieving process in chronic obstructive pulmonary disease (COPD): validation of the Acceptance of Disease and Impairments Questionnaire (ADIQ). Int J Behav Med. 2014;21(3):561–70.
65. Harrison SL, Lee A, Janaudis-Ferreira T, Goldstein RS, Brooks D. Mindfulness in people with a respiratory diagnosis: a systematic review. Patient Educ Couns. 2016;99(3):348–55.
66. Chan RR, Giardino N, Larson JL. A pilot study: mindfulness meditation intervention in COPD. Int J Chron Obstruct Pulmon Dis. 2015;10:445–54.
67. Mularski RA, Munjas BA, Lorenz KA, Sun S, Robertson SJ, Schmelzer W, et al. Randomized controlled trial of mindfulness-based therapy for dyspnea in chronic obstructive lung disease. J Altern Complement Med. 2009;15(10):1083–90.
68. Rollnick S, Miller WR. What is motivational interviewing? Behav Cogn Psychother. 2009;23(4):325–34.
69. Benzo RP. Mindfulness and motivational interviewing: two candidate methods for promoting self-management. Chron Respir Dis. 2013;10(3):175–82.
70. de Blok BM, de Greef MH, ten Hacken NH, Sprenger SR, Postema K, Wempe JB. The effects of a lifestyle physical activity counseling program with feedback of a pedometer during pulmonary rehabilitation in patients with COPD: a pilot study. Patient Educ Couns. 2006;61(1):48–55.
71. Benzo R, Vickers K, Novotny PJ, Tucker S, Hoult J, Neuenfeldt P, et al. Health coaching and COPD Re-hospitalization: a randomized study. Am J Respir Crit Care Med. 2016;194(6):672–80.
72. Carreiro A, Santos J, Rodrigues F. Impact of comorbidities in pulmonary rehabilitation outcomes in patients with chronic obstructive pulmonary disease. Rev Port Pneumol. 2013;19(3):106–13.
73. Torheim H, Kvangarsnes M. How do patients with exacerbated chronic obstructive pulmonary disease experience care in the intensive care unit? Scand J Caring Sci. 2014;28(4):741–8.

14 The Respiratory Nurse in Pulmonary Rehabilitation

Vanessa M. McDonald, Mary Roberts, and Kerry Inder

14.1 Introduction

Pulmonary rehabilitation is an effective evidencebased intervention for people with Chronic Obstructive Pulmonary Disease (COPD), as well as other chronic lung conditions including asthma, bronchiectasis, interstitial lung disease, and pulmonary hypertension [1]. The definition of pulmonary rehabilitation has been dealt with in previous chapters, in brief the most recent and complete definition is that pulmonary rehabilitation is "*a comprehensive intervention based on a thorough patient assessment followed by patient tailored therapies that include, but are not limited to, exercise training, education, and behavior change, designed to improve the physical and psychological condition of people with chronic respiratory disease and to promote the long-term adherence to health-enhancing behaviors*" [1]. This revised definition highlights the multidimensional nature of effective pulmonary rehabilitation, which importantly not only includes exercise training but places a high value on behavioral change to address the multicomponent consequences of chronic lung disease. Is it well recognized that in order to achieve these goals of pulmonary rehabilitation, interdisciplinary teams of motivated, committed, and experienced health care professionals are required. While the optimal make up of the team has not been defined there are key disciplines involved in the delivery of programs, these include, but are not limited to, physiotherapists, medical practitioners, respiratory therapists, exercise physiologists, psychologists, nutritionists, occupational therapists, social workers, and **respiratory nurses**. As it is acknowledged that not one group of health care professionals possess all of the skills and

V.M. McDonald
School of Nursing and Midwifery,
The University of Newcastle,
New Lambton, NSW, Australia

Centre of Excellence for Severe Asthma,
The University of Newcastle,
New Lambton, NSW, Australia

Priority Research Centre for Healthy Lungs,
The University of Newcastle,
New Lambton, NSW, Australia
e-mail: vanessa.mcdonald@newcastle.edu.au; Vanessa.McDonald@hnehealth.nsw.gov.au

M. Roberts
Department of Respiratory and Sleep Medicine,
Westmead Hospital, Westmead, NSW, Australia

Ludwig Engel Centre of Respiratory Research,
Westmead, NSW, Australia

Westmead Institute for Medical Research,
Westmead, NSW, Australia

K. Inder
School of Nursing and Midwifery,
The University of Newcastle,
New Lambton, NSW, Australia

Centre of Excellence for Severe Asthma,
The University of Newcastle,
New Lambton, NSW, Australia

© Springer International Publishing AG 2018
E. Clini et al. (eds.), *Textbook of Pulmonary Rehabilitation*,
https://doi.org/10.1007/978-3-319-65888-9_14

knowledge required for optimal delivery of pulmonary rehabilitation, collaboration between these disciplines is vital. Respiratory nurses play a central role in pulmonary rehabilitation in terms of assessment, symptom management and monitoring and disease management.

The role of the nurse varies depending on the setting, structure, and operationalization of the specific program. In some rural and remote regions where staffing is minimal they may be the sole providers of pulmonary rehabilitation, but generally, in most parts of the world, the nurse works within the team previously described.

At the core of nursing is the therapeutic nurse—patient relationship, this has been defined as "*a helping relationship that's based on mutual trust and respect, the nurturing of faith and hope, being sensitive to self and others, and assisting with the gratification of the patient's physical, emotional, and spiritual needs through nursing knowledge and skill*" [2]. This key principle of nursing practice ideally places members of the profession to deliver a high standard of care that is centered around the goals of pulmonary rehabilitation. Respiratory nurses in particular have a unique set of skills and expert knowledge that enables delivery of person centered care to patients with chronic lung disease; they have an important role in the provision of patient education and self-management, symptom management and primary and secondary prevention strategies to improve health and prevent deterioration. It should be noted that some of the roles and responsibilities described within this chapter are not necessarily exclusive to the respiratory nurse's role, however their knowledge, training, and skill set facilitates a high standard of care. The role of the respiratory nurse in pulmonary rehabilitation may involve case management, assessment (at baseline, throughout the program and for outcomes), delivery of interventions and referral to other services and disciplines as appropriate. These specific roles will be explored in this chapter.

14.2 Chronic Disease Management and Case Management

Chronic disease management has developed as an approach to the care of chronic conditions, and can be applied in a range of patient populations in both specialist and generalist services. Disease management can broadly be defined as a comprehensive strategy for improving overall health status and reducing health care costs [3]. This is a key role of respiratory nurses.

Disease management is recommended as part of the pulmonary rehabilitation model. It takes a holistic approach, treating patients as individuals throughout the clinical course of a disease rather than viewing their care as a series of discrete episodes [4]. Patient education and self-management, implementation of practice guidelines, appropriate consultation, and supplies of medications and services are intregal to the disease management approach [4].

Case management is a component of many disease management programs, it is defined as "*a collaborative process of assessment, planning, facilitation, care coordination, evaluation, and advocacy for options and services to meet an individual's and family's comprehensive health needs through communication and available resources to promote quality cost-effective outcomes*" [5]. In many cases, the role of the case manager is the nurse's responsibility, since through their specialist skills and collaborative methods they can ensure the goals of case management including optimization of health, access to care and appropriate and effective use of resources are met. Critical to this role however is appropriate training and acquisition of skills relating to communication, collaboration, and coordination of multidisciplinary teams, a high level of disease specific knowledge and expertise and the ability to foster behavior change in individuals. According to Bourbeau and colleagues COPD case management nurses should have at least specific training in behavioral change techniques, self-management education, and good communication [6]. An essential part of the triad of disease management, case management, and pulmonary rehabilitation is assessment and there are many areas where the skills of respiratory nurses can enhance the pulmonary rehabilitation program leading to better patient outcome.

14.3 Assessment and Individualized Management

A multidimensional and multidisciplinary assessment of a person with chronic respiratory disease prior to commencement of pulmonary rehabilitation is recommended [1], and enables the delivery of care that is tailored to the characteristics of the individual. From this assessment a personalized care plan can be developed and implemented throughout the course of the pulmonary rehabilitation program.

The role of the nurse in the baseline and ongoing assessment may include, but is not limited to, an evaluation of: disease knowledge; inhaler device proficiency and medication management including an assessment of adherence; exacerbation frequency; skills for management of such exacerbations and whether a written action plan has been prescribed; risk factors such as physical inactivity, nutrition, smoking and substance use; symptom and comorbidity management and psychological state (Fig. 14.1).

The respiratory nurse's role in pulmonary rehabilitation outcome assessment is similar to that of their initial assessment role. Following completion of the pulmonary rehabilitation program, in collaboration with the pulmonary rehabilitation team, the nurse can reassess the patient and ensure that their self-management plan remains current and appropriate, making alterations as required. The respiratory nurse can also reassess the patient's disease knowledge; inhaler device proficiency; and medication management. If deficiencies are identified, they can be addressed or refer the patient on for long-term support and follow-up.

A small Australian study that evaluated the effect of multidimensional assessment and individualized management, facilitated by an expert nurse case manager within a pulmonary rehabilitation program, found that this approach led to highly significant outcomes compared with usual care pulmonary rehabilitation [7]. A mean (95% CI) of 10.5 (9.7 to 11.2) clinical management problems were identified during a multidimensional assessment, participants had an

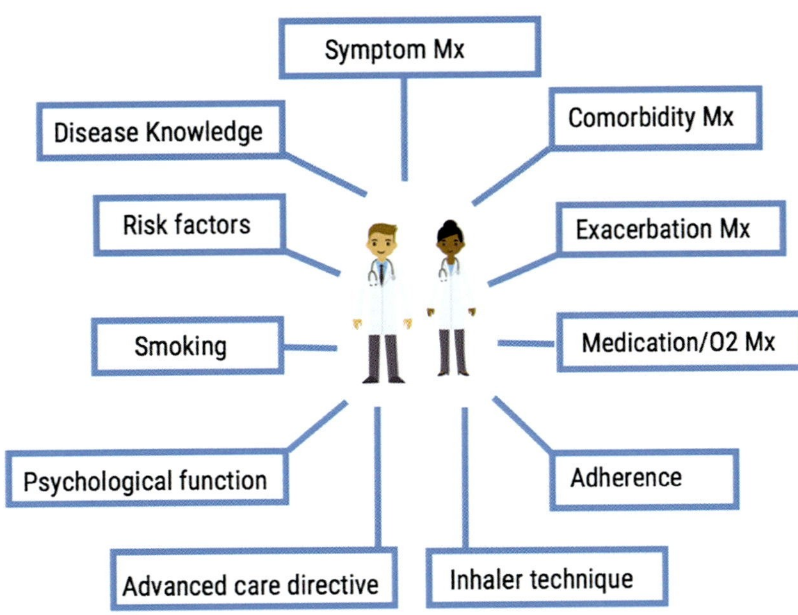

Fig. 14.1 Respiratory nurses role in assessment and management. Key: *Mx* management, O_2 oxygen

individualized care plan developed and targeted interventions delivered in partnership with the patient over the course of their pulmonary rehabilitation. Health status improved in the intervention group, the mean (95% CI) difference in St George's Respiratory Questionnaire was 14 (20.7 to 8.5) versus 3.5 units (−3.8 to 10.8) for the control group; $p = 0.0003$ [7]. Within this study, participants were involved in the development of the care plan; they were provided with a list of clinical problems identified during the multidimensional assessment and asked by the nurse to rate the importance of each of these problems; their physician was asked to do the same [8]. The nurse then engaged the participants in a discussion providing information about their given clinical problems, presented the priorities of the physician, gave advice on the management of the problems and then came to an agreement about the development the care plan with the patient and the multidisciplinary team, and coordinated the delivery of the plan [7, 8]. Interestingly there was a significant level of discordance between the physician and the participants in terms of the importance of clinical management problems, with participants ranking the importance of self-management skills including inhaler device technique lower than that of the physicians, suggesting that patients have an erroneous understanding of the importance of prescribed therapies [7, 8]. This highlights the integral role of the nurse in the assessment and management of these important therapeutic interventions.

14.3.1 Disease Knowledge

In addition to understanding the pathophysiology, causes, common presentations and disease trajectory of chronic respiratory diseases and the subsequent diversity and complexity of these diseases, respiratory nurses should have an understanding of the epidemiology and burden of chronic respiratory disease at a local, national, and global level. Specifically this includes knowledge about the incidence and prevalence of chronic respiratory conditions; rates of mortality and morbidity, including disability associated with chronic respiratory diseases; common risk factors; diagnosis, prognosis, treatment, and disease management strategies; as well as primary and secondary prevention measures. Long-term consequences and complications of these diseases and their management are important to understand as well as being aware of the cost to individuals and their families and the community, both in personal and financial terms. This knowledge will allow effective communication with patients to improve their own knowledge of their disease.

This knowledge is also dynamic; it will change and develop over time as a result of ongoing research and changes and advances in technology that impact on the diagnosis or management of chronic respiratory diseases. Evidence-based practice is therefore the cornerstone of providing quality, safe care to people with chronic respiratory disease and their families.

14.3.2 Disease Management Skills

14.3.2.1 Medication Management and Inhaler Device Proficiency

Pharmacotherapy is one of the fundamental strategies used in the management of respiratory disease and can lead to improved outcomes such as symptoms, exercise capacity, and overall health status [9, 10]. Further, appropriate pharmacotherapy can also reduce the frequency and severity of acute exacerbations [11]. In the case of chronic respiratory disease, individuals will more often than not be diagnosed with other medical conditions or comorbidities. In an observational study of 213 COPD patients, nearly all patients (97.7%) had one or more comorbidity and over 50% of patients had at least four [12]. Similarly in a US survey of 1003 COPD patients, almost 50% reported 6–10 comorbid diagnoses [13, 14]. This being the case patients attending pulmonary rehabilitation are likely to be prescribed multiple treatments for both the respiratory condition and their comorbidities and as such have complex medication regimens [15]. This situation can lead to poor adherence [16] and can also increase the risk of drug–drug interactions and adverse treatment side effects [17]. Nurses in the pulmonary rehabilitation program can ensure patients have a thorough understanding of what the prescribed treatments are, the rationale for their use, and ways to minimize potential side effects. These strategies may lead to better outcomes for patients.

Inhaled Medication

Delivery of medication via the inhaled route is the cornerstone of pharmacological treatment for chronic respiratory diseases such as COPD and asthma, as it offers an ideal balance between efficacy and safety [9]. Unfortunately inadequate inhalation technique and inhaler device polypharmacy are common [18] and this can lead to reduced treatment efficacy [19]. In a group of COPD patients recruited from a tertiary care center, 48.5% were deemed to have inadequate inhaler technique and 50% had inhaler device polypharmacy, defined as the use of three or more different inhaler devices [18]. Other studies have reported rates of poor inhaler techniques as high as 90% [20, 21]. This issue is becoming increasingly problematic as the progressive number of new devices become available. Proficiency in inhaler device competency and minimization of the number of inhaler devices used is required in order for patients to receive the maximum benefit from their inhaled medication therapy [22]. Observation of medication delivery and patient education regarding pharmacotherapy is standard practice for respiratory nurses and as such is an ideal role for the respiratory nurse working in pulmonary rehabilitation programs. Nurses generally work in clinics with physicians and can collaborate to ensure that the devices prescribed meet the patient's needs in terms of their ability, dexterity, vision, and inspiratory flow [9]. The role of the nurse in doing this is to ensure the patient receives adequate education including a practical demonstration of the correct technique with written and or video instruction to refer back to. Once the technique is demonstrated the nurse assesses the patient's ability to use each device, corrects the technique when needed, or suggests an alternate device if proficiency is not achieved. They should also assess the number of devices prescribed, as inhaler device technique proficiency decreases as the number of prescribed devices increase [22]; the nurse has a role in communicating with prescribers in an effort to simplify inhaler regimen. A mnemonic to aid in the education of patients with their inhalers is described in Box 14.1. The nurse should reassess inhaler technique regularly during the pulmonary rehabilitation program and at follow-up, as inhaler device technique wanes with time.

Box 14.1: Mnemonic to Aid Inhaler Device Education

Tailor—Individualize the device to the patient's needs

Educate—Demonstrate the correct technique and need for correct use

Assess—Assess the patient's ability to use the device

Correct—Correct any errors

Have another go—After correction of technique, then reassess

Evaluate—Is this the correct device for this patient?

Reduce—Minimize the number of devices prescribed

Box 14.1 modified from [23], permissions pending.

Oxygen Therapy

In hypoxemic patients with COPD, long-term oxygen therapy has a demonstrated effect on reducing all cause mortality [24]. Long-term oxygen therapy is also known to increase exercise tolerance and decrease dyspnea, polycythaemia, sleep disorders, pulmonary artery pressures, and nocturnal arrhythmias in patients with a PaO_2 of less than 55 mm/Hg [25]. In order to achieve these benefits of long-term oxygen therapy, patients should ideally use their treatment for 18 h/day [26]. This will often require a negotiation with patients to optimize their adherence, and education regarding the use of their oxygen therapy and equipment. The respiratory nurse can work with individuals at assessment and during the program to do this. Specifically, the respiratory nurse will help individuals: understand how oxygen helps, or does not help in the case of normoxic patients; they can provide information regarding the range of oxygen equipment available and what might be best suited for individual patients; understand risks associated with oxygen therapy, such as continuing to smoke, and provide advice for travelling with oxygen, what to do in emergencies, such as power outages, and how to maintain the best health status whist using oxygen.

14.3.2.2 Exacerbation Management

Exacerbations of COPD are important events that lead to accelerated decline in lung function, higher hospitalization rates, lower exercise capacity, more severe health status impairment, and higher rates of mortality [27, 28]. Exacerbations of lung disease usually occur over a period of days or weeks rather than having a sudden onset, so essentially patients should be able to recognize deterioration and act accordingly to reduce the severity and duration; qualitative data however suggests that this often not the case [29]. A multinational, cross-sectional, interview-based study of 125 moderate-to-very severe COPD patients with a history of two or more exacerbations in the prior year reported that over one-third of COPD patients said that there were no recognizable signs or symptoms of a pending flare up of their disease [29]. Not only do exacerbations go unrecognized by patients they are also commonly undertreated. In a multicenter Canadian study 421 COPD patients were asked to complete daily diaries to document exacerbations and to contact the study center if the symptoms of the exacerbations were sustained [30]. The overall incidence of diary exacerbations was 2.7 per person per year, but in terms of the exacerbations reported to the clinic the rate was only 0.8 per person per year [30]. These data highlight the importance of patient education and behavioral change strategies directed at recognizing the signs and symptoms of exacerbations or flare ups and ensuring both patients and clinicians understand the impact of exacerbations and the importance of minimization or avoidance.

The respiratory nurse plays an important role in educating the patient about strategies to recognize and treat disease exacerbations. This starts during the initial assessment of the patient, by assessing how many exacerbations the patient has experienced in the past year, as one exacerbation is a predictor of future exacerbation [31], by assessing other risk factors for exacerbations, the symptoms experienced during previous exacerbations and whether or not they possess the required skills to act on these increased symptoms in a timely manner, or have a written action plan.

A written action plan facilitates the early detection and treatment of an exacerbation. It is a set of instructions prescribed to a person with COPD or asthma for use in the self-management of deteriorating symptoms. They are prescribed by physicians and usually form a component of a broader self-management or disease management program. A 2016 Cochrane review evaluated the use of action plans with brief education for exacerbations of COPD. The review, which included seven parallel-group randomized controlled trials and 1550 participants concluded that the use of COPD action plans with a single short educational component along with ongoing support directed at use of the action plan, but without a comprehensive self-management program, reduced in-hospital health care utilization and increased treatment of COPD exacerbations with corticosteroids and antibiotics [32].

The ingredients of a written action plan usually include the steps to identify when the action plan should be implemented, that is what are the action points (symptoms or peak flow in asthma), what treatment should be initiated, for how long should the escalation of treatment continue, and when should additional treatment be sought [33]. An essential element to these plans is the patient engagement and education. At all time-points the respiratory nurse can ensure the patient understands the symptoms, the treatment, has access to the prescribed management, and understands and accepts what is being asked of them. These elements should be reviewed and reinforced throughout the pulmonary rehabilitation program and again following each exacerbation.

14.3.2.3 Adherence

Nonadherence to therapy is frequently high in COPD with rates of adherence to inhaled and oral medicines reported to be between 30% and 57%

[34]. This is significantly lower than adherence rates in other chronic diseases, for example, a study that recruited US military veterans, reported that the proportion of patients adherent to COPD treatments (defined as proportion of days covered equal to or greater than 0.80), was approximately 30% versus 40–63% for other chronic diseases including coronary artery disease, diabetes, heart failure, and hyperlipidemia [34]. This may be related to intentional nonadherence, that is making a deliberate choice not to use the treatment or non-intentional nonadherence which may result from reasons that are not within the patient's locus of control, for example, they may have cognitive impairments or a physical disability like impaired vision or musculoskeletal problems that inhibit their ability to use the treatment correctly or as prescribed. The respiratory nurse can firstly assess the degree of adherence in each individual, determine the reasons for nonadherence, correct any erroneous understanding of therapeutic interventions, and implement strategies that promote behavioral change. A systematic review that examined effectiveness of interventions designed to improve medication adherence for individuals with COPD reported that the strategies associated with positive effects included brief counseling; monitoring and feedback about inhaler use through electronic medication delivery devices; and multicomponent interventions consisting of self-management and care coordination delivered by health professionals [35]. The respiratory nurse is ideally suited to these roles.

14.3.3 Symptom Management

Chronic respiratory diseases are associated with increased symptom burden. These symptoms may be caused by the index disease such as breathlessness, wheezing, coughing, chest tightness, or may be related to one of the multiple comorbidities that people with respiratory disease, particularly COPD, experience [14, 36], such as fatigue, anxiety, depression, chest pain, and poor sleep quality [37]. The symptom burden is chronic and most patients experience symptoms everyday [38]. The severity differs among patients, and individuals often under-report the severity of their symptoms, for example, in one study of 3265 participants that used an objective measurement scale (mMMRC dyspnea scale), a third of patients who were classified as "too breathless to leave the house" also subjectively reported their symptoms as mild to moderate [39]. The rating of symptom frequency and severity is also often discordant between patients and clinicians [8, 38].

Improving patients' assessment and management of symptoms is important and in the context of pulmonary rehabilitation is multifactorial. Patients will experience their day-to-day symptom burden as a consequence of their lung disease, but may also experience an increase in symptoms subsequent to their exercise intervention. These symptoms again may be related to the index respiratory disease or the comorbidity.

In terms of aiding patients in managing their chronic respiratory symptoms, during the assessment and throughout the program, respiratory nurses will encourage patients to use their medications as prescribed with the correct technique. They will also work in partnership with the individual to tailor non-pharmacological interventions, such as breathing control and pursed lip breathing and recommend other interventions for control of breathlessness such as the use of handheld fans, or a combination of these interventions [40]. The nurses may also assess symptoms and symptom clusters related to other comorbidities and address these accordingly.

During the program, individuals may experience increased symptoms for a variety of different reasons, be it increased respiratory symptoms such as wheeze, chest tightness, dyspnea, cough, and oxygen desaturation, or symptoms related to their comorbidities such as episodes of: hypo or hyperglycemia; or hypo or hypertension; episodes of chest pain; panic; anxiety or skin tears and falls. Nurses are trained in the acute management of these events and will be able to conduct a nursing assessment and intervene appropriately with non-pharmacological management strategies, nurse initiated medication management, wound management where needed and escalation of management as appropriate.

14.3.4 Comorbidity Management

We have briefly discussed comorbidities and these may impact the outcomes of pulmonary rehabilitation [41]. As stated, the respiratory nurse is in an ideal position to educate patients regarding comorbidity management, the recognition of deterioration or destabilization of disease (such as angina, cardiac arrhythmia, hypo/hyperglycemia) and ways to minimize the risk of such events occurring during exercise. The respiratory nurse can also provide education regarding the long-term management of such conditions [40].

14.3.5 Smoking Cessation

Smoking cessation is one of the most important treatment interventions for people with respiratory disease [42, 43], as it is the most effective intervention at reducing symptoms, and the progression of COPD and lung function impairment [44]. Pulmonary rehabilitation should be offered to all eligible patients despite their smoking status, and in those that continue to smoke their enrolment in the program is an opportunistic time to address the issue of smoking cessation [45].

The evidence for smoking cessation is unquestionable and the most effective treatment methods have been summarized in Cochrane systematic reviews [46–48]. One review was performed to determine the effectiveness of nursing interventions for smoking cessation. In this review 35 RCTs, involving over 17,000 participants comparing nursing interventions with usual care were assessed. The results of the analysis demonstrated that the nursing intervention increased the likelihood of quitting smoking by almost one-third (RR 1.29; 95% CI 1.20 to 1.39) [47]. The authors also concluded that the effect was weaker when the interventions were provided by nurses whose main role was not smoking cessation [47], highlighting the importance of respiratory nurses who consider this an integral part of their practice.

A further review assessed smoking cessation interventions for COPD, they included RCTs (16 studies involving 13,123 participants) that assessed the effectiveness of any behavioral or pharmacological treatment, or both, in smokers with COPD reporting at least 6 months of follow-up abstinence rates [46]. The authors of this review found evidence that a combination of psychosocial interventions and pharmacological interventions was superior to no treatment or to psychosocial interventions alone.

In countries such as Australia, Nicotine Replacement Therapy (NRT) is available over the counter and nurses are able to recommend NRT and combination NRT to patients. Respiratory nurses are also usually well equipped to provide behavioral interventions including smoking cessation counseling and motivational interviewing, and the combination of these skills within a pulmonary rehabilitation program is of great value to those patients that are attempting to quit during their program and after completion.

14.3.6 Other Risk Factors

In addition to smoking and physical inactivity, the largest preventable causes of chronic diseases [49, 50], other major risk factors include environmental factors and infection [51]. Environmental factors include outdoor allergens, weather phenomena, and air pollutants such as pollen and ambient air pollution. Weather phenomena referred to as thunderstorm asthma is where there is an epidemic of asthma exacerbations following a severe storm [52]. Inhaling occupational irritants including fumes, vapors, gases, dusts, fibers, biological enzymes and certain particles from textiles, grains, wood or latex can cause or exacerbate chronic respiratory diseases such as asthma and COPD, especially among smokers. Predisposing factors include atopy, alpha-1-antitrypsin deficiency, sex, and ethnicity. Other risk factors include overweight and obesity; these factors may increase the risk of developing or exacerbating chronic respiratory disease [51].

While chronic respiratory diseases share a number of common risk factors, the level of risk varies according to the individual disease. It is frequently the role of respiratory nurses to discuss these factors as part of the educational component of the pulmonary rehabilitation program in order to improve a patient's understanding of their disease and importantly to help minimize exacerbations. Most acute exacerbations of COPD are attributable to viral or bacterial respiratory tract infections [51].

14.3.7 Psychological Function

Anxiety and depression are common comorbidities associated with chronic respiratory disease, particularly COPD. These comorbid conditions cause significant symptom burden and are associated with increased exacerbations, frequent hospital admissions, poorer health status, and increased mortality compared to COPD patients without anxiety and depression [53–57]. Depression is also known to impact on patients' attendance at pulmonary rehabilitation [58]. While anxiety and depression in COPD has been reported to be as high as 26% and 58%, respectively [18, 53, 59], it is also acknowledged that psychological dysfunction is under-recognized and undertreated in this population. A study by Yohannes and colleagues reported that in a COPD population, one-quarter had unrecognized subclinical depression [60]. Other studies have demonstrated that less than one-third of patients with COPD and anxiety or depression were appropriately treated for their mood disorders [61, 62].

During the respiratory nurse's pulmonary rehabilitation assessment, they will usually assess those at risk or those experiencing symptoms of anxiety and depression, this is most often done with the use of a screening questionnaire, for example, the Hospital Anxiety and Depression Scale (HADS) [63]. Once identified, the nurse can then establish a rapport with the individuals to help bring about behavior change in terms of unhelpful or unhealthy habits of thinking, feeling, and behaving. An RCT evaluated the effectiveness of a nurse-led Minimal Psychological Intervention (MPI) in reducing depression and anxiety in patients with COPD [64]. MPI was compared to usual care in 187 COPD patients recruited from primary care. The intervention was based on the principles of cognitive behavioral therapy and self-management. Those in the intervention group reported significantly fewer depressive symptoms (mean Beck Depression Inventory difference 2.92, $p = 0.04$) and fewer symptoms of anxiety (mean Symptom Check List difference 3.69, $p = 0.003$) at 9 months compared with the usual care participants. The authors concluded that the nurse-led MPI appears to be a valuable addition to existing COPD disease-management programs [64].

14.3.8 End of Life and Advanced Care Directives

End of life planning is an important but underperformed initiative in the care of patients with chronic respiratory disease [65]. The reasons for this are multifactorial, it may be related to both a reluctance on the part of the patients and their family, but also the health care team. The disease trajectory associated with COPD may also play a role, whereby there are acute deteriorations of the disease followed by partial recovery, which may give patients, families, and clinicians an often erroneous belief that there will be a better time [65]. Patient knowledge of disease and its prognosis and ambiguity around wanting to know more may also be contributing factors.

A study by Jones et al. [66], who interviewed patients with COPD within their last year of life, found that most patients were aware of the name of their condition; however, even at this late stage of their disease half of the participants expressed a desire for more information about their disease and their prognosis. The other half however did not, either because they did not think that this knowledge would help them or because they feared what the information might be [66]. Furthermore in a study comparing quality of life and palliative care of COPD in comparison to lung cancer patients, similar themes were reported [67]. In that study patients were dissatisfied with the amount of information provided to them regarding their illness, its management, and the type of social help available. Among the COPD patients 30% reported a lack of diagnostic information and thought that information had been given insensitively. Most (78%) said that they did not receive enough information regarding their prognosis or future management from their doctors and the patients' awareness of their prognosis was often gained through their own experiences, via emergency department attendances or through interaction with other health care professionals such as nurses [67]. Another qualitative study of participants with COPD and asthma reported that the information needs identified by patients varied; some participants expressed a desire to know more while others were afraid to ask the questions [68]. Similarly in the study by Gore et al., many patients with COPD suggested they wanted more information regarding their illness and future management, however few wanted detailed information and implied that an accurate description of their prognosis would be distressing [67].

Advanced care directives which involve discussions about prognosis and end of life care are recommended but these are often neglected in the day-to-day management of chronic disease [69]. From the patients' perspective future expectation is a common and troubling issue. The expectations of different patients are often diverse and their expressed needs are ambiguous.

Pulmonary rehabilitation is an opportunistic time to introduce end of life care discussions, however clinicians need to be suitably skilled to do so. Studies have shown that non-physician clinicians can be effective in these end of life discussions and advance care planning [65]. The respiratory nurses can facilitate a partnership with the patient which allows their fears, concerns and expectations to be elicited. These can then be discussed with the patient, family, and multidisciplinary team to develop a plan that identifies their values, goals, and medical treatment preference for the future.

14.3.9 Summary

Throughout this chapter we have discussed the significant role that respiratory nurses play in the assessment and management of patients within pulmonary rehabilitation programs. Their training and skills prepares respiratory nurses with the competency and expertise to contribute significantly to patient education, disease management, self-management, and case management.

References

1. Spruit MA, Singh SJ, Garvey C, Zuwallack R, Nici L, Rochester C, et al. An official american thoracic society/european respiratory society statement: key concepts and advances in pulmonary rehabilitation. Am J Respir Crit Care Med. 2013;188(8):e13–64.
2. Watson J. Caring science as sacred science. Philadelphia, PA: FA Davis Company; 2005.
3. Hunter DJ, Fairfield G. Disease management. Br Med J. 1997;315(7099):50–3.
4. Hunter DJ. Disease management: has it a future? It has a compelling logic, but needs to be tested in practice. Br Med J. 2000;320(7234):530.
5. Case Management Society of America. What is a case manager? 2013. http://www.cmsa.org/Home/CMSA/WhatisaCaseManager/tabid/224/Default.aspx.
6. Bourbeau J, Lavoie KL, Sedeno M. Comprehensive self-management strategies. Semin Respir Crit Care Med. 2015;36(4):630–8.
7. McDonald VM, Higgins I, Wood LG, Gibson PG. Multidimensional assessment and tailored interventions for COPD: respiratory utopia or common sense? Thorax. 2013;68(7):691–4.
8. McDonald VM, Higgins I, Simpson JL, Gibson PG. The importance of clinical management problems in older people with COPD and asthma; do patients and physicians agree? Prim Care Respir J. 2011;20(4):389–95.
9. Gibson PG, McDonald VM, Marks GB. Asthma in the Older Adult. Lancet. 2010;374(9743):803–13.
10. McDonald VM, Higgins I, Gibson PG. Managing older patients with coexistent asthma and COPD: diagnostic and therapeutic challenges. Drugs Aging. 2013;30(1):1–17.
11. From the Global Strategy for the Diagnosis, Management and Prevention of COPD. Global Initiative for Chronic Obstructive Lung Disease (GOLD). 2016 [Internet]. http://goldcopd.org/. Accessed 11 Oct 2016.
12. Vanfleteren LEGW, Spruit MA, Groenen M, Gaffron S, Van Empel VPM, Bruijnzeel PLB, et al. Clusters of comorbidities based on validated objective measurements and systemic inflammation in patients with chronic obstructive pulmonary disease. Am J Respir Crit Care Med. 2013;187(7):728–35.
13. Barr RG, Celli BR, Mannino DM, Petty T, Rennard SI, Sciurba FC, et al. Comorbidities, patient knowledge, and disease management in a national sample of patients with COPD. Am J Med. 2009;122(4):348–55.
14. Negewo NA, Gibson PG, McDonald VM. COPD and its comorbidities: Impact, measurement and mechanisms. Respirology. 2015;20(8):1160–71.

15. George J, Phun YT, Bailey MJ, Kong DC, Stewart K. Development and validation of the medication regimen complexity index. Ann Pharmacother. 2004;38(9):1369–76.
16. Claxton AJ, Cramer J, Pierce C. A systematic review of the associations between dose regimens and medication compliance. Clin Ther. 2001;23(8):1296–310.
17. Willson MN, Greer CL, Weeks DL. Medication regimen complexity and hospital readmission for an adverse drug event. Ann Pharmacother. 2014;48(1):26–32.
18. McDonald VM, Simpson JL, Higgins I, Gibson PG. Multidimensional assessment of older people with asthma & copd: clinical management and health status. Age Ageing. 2011;40(1):42–9.
19. Lareau SC, Hodder R. Teaching inhaler use in chronic obstructive pulmonary disease patients. J Am Acad Nurse Pract. 2012;24(2):113–20.
20. Basheti IA, Armour CL, Bosnic-Anticevich SZ, Reddel HK. Evaluation of a novel educational strategy, including inhaler-based reminder labels, to improve asthma inhaler technique. Patient Educ Couns. 2008;72(1):26–33.
21. Bosnic-Anticevich SZ, Sinha H, So S, Reddel HK. Metered-dose inhaler technique: the effect of two educational interventions delivered in community pharmacy over time. J Asthma. 2010;47(3):251–6.
22. McDonald VM, Gibson PG. Inhalation device polypharmacy in asthma. Med J Aust. 2005;182(5):250–1.
23. McDonald VM, Gibson PG. Asthma education. In: Bernstein JA, Levy ML, editors. Clinical asthma: theory and practice, vol. 1. Bosa Roca, USA: CRC Press; 2014.
24. Medical Research Council Working Party. Long term domiciliary oxygen therapy in chronic hypoxic cor pulmonale complicating chronic bronchitis and emphysema: report of the Medical Research Council Working Party. Lancet. 1981;317:681–6.
25. Kim V, Benditt JO, Wise RA, Sharafkhaneh A. Oxygen therapy in chronic obstructive pulmonary disease. Proc Am Thorac Soc. 2001;5(4):513–8.
26. McDonald CF, Whyte K, Jenkins S, Serginson J, Frith P. Clinical practice guideline on adult domiciliary oxygen therapy: executive summary from the thoracic society of Australia and New Zealand. Respirology. 2016;21(1):76–8.
27. Pavord ID, Jones PW, Burgel PR, Rabe KF. Exacerbations of COPD. Int J Chron Obstruct Pulmon Dis. 2016;11(Spec Iss):21–30.
28. Hillas G, Perlikos F, Tzanakis N. Acute exacerbation of COPD: is it the "stroke of the lungs"? Int J Chron Obstruct Pulmon Dis. 2016;11:1579–86.
29. Kessler R, Stahl E, Vogelmeier C, Haughney J, Trudeau E, Lofdahl CG, et al. Patient understanding, detection, and experience of COPD exacerbations: an observational, interview-based study. Chest. 2006;130(1):133–42.
30. Langsetmo L, Platt RW, Ernst P, Bourbeau J. Underreporting exacerbation of chronic obstructive pulmonary disease in a longitudinal cohort. Am J Respir Crit Care Med. 2008;177(4):396–401.
31. Hurst JR, Donaldson GC, Quint JK, Goldring JJ, Baghai-Ravary R, Wedzicha JA. Temporal clustering of exacerbations in chronic obstructive pulmonary disease. Am J Respir Crit Care Med. 2009;179(5):369–74.
32. Howcroft M, Walters EH, Wood-Baker R, Walters JA. Action plans with brief patient education for exacerbations in chronic obstructive pulmonary disease. Cochrane Database Syst Rev. 2016;12:CD005074.
33. Gibson PG, Powell H. Written action plans for asthma: an evidence-based review of the key components. Thorax. 2004;59:94–9.
34. Neugaard BI, Priest JL, Burch SP, Cantrell CR, Foulis PR. Quality of care for veterans with chronic diseases: performance on quality indicators, medication use and adherence, and health care utilization. Popul Health Manag. 2011;14(2):99–106.
35. Bryant J, McDonald VM, Boyes A, Sanson-Fisher R, Paul C, Melville J. Improving medication adherence in chronic obstructive pulmonary disease: a systematic review. Respir Res. 2013;14:109.
36. Negewo NA, McDonald VM, Gibson PG. Comorbidity in COPD. Respir Investig. 2015;53(6):249–58.
37. Singh D, Miravitlles M, Vogelmeier C. Chronic obstructive pulmonary disease individualized therapy: tailored approach to symptom management. Adv Ther. 2017;34(2):281–99.
38. Kessler R, Partridge MR, Miravitlles M, Cazzola M, Vogelmeier C, Leynaud D, et al. Symptom variability in patients with severe COPD: a pan-European cross-sectional study. Eur Respir J. 2011;37(2):264–72.
39. Rennard S, Decramer M, Calverley PM, Pride NB, Soriano JB, Vermeire PA, et al. Impact of COPD in North America and Europe in 2000: subjects' perspective of Confronting COPD International Survey. Eur Respir J. 2002;20(4):799–805.
40. Johnson M, Carlo B, Currow D, Maddocks M, McDonald V, Mahadeva R, et al. Management of chronic breathlessness: non-pharmacological and pharmacological interventions. ERS Monogr. 2016;73:153–71.
41. Franssen FM, Rochester CL. Comorbidities in patients with COPD and pulmonary rehabilitation: do they matter? Eur Respir Rev. 2014;23(131):131–41.
42. Pauwels RA, Buist AS, Calverley PM, Jenkins CR, Hurd SSNHLBI. WHO Global initiative for chronic obstructive lung disease (GOLD) Workshop summary. Am J Respir Crit Care Med. 2001;163(5):1256–76.
43. National Collaborating Centre for Chronic Conditions. Chronic obstructive pulmonary disease: national clinical guideline on management of chronic obstructive pulmonary disease in adults in primary and secondary care. Thorax. 2004;59(1 Suppl):1S–232S.
44. Willemse BW, Postma DS, Timens W, ten Hacken NH. The impact of smoking cessation on respiratory symptoms, lung function, airway hyperresponsiveness and inflammation. Eur Respir J. 2004;23(3):464–76.
45. Hill K, Vogiatzis I, Burtin C. The importance of components of pulmonary rehabilitation, other

than exercise training, in COPD. Eur Respir Rev. 2013;22(129):405–13.
46. van Eerd EA, van der Meer RM, van Schayck OC, Kotz D. Smoking cessation for people with chronic obstructive pulmonary disease. Cochrane Database Syst Rev. 2016;8:CD010744.
47. Rice VH, Hartmann-Boyce J, Stead LF. Nursing interventions for smoking cessation. Cochrane Database Syst Rev. 2013;8:CD001188.
48. Stead LF, Perera R, Bullen C, Mant D, Lancaster T. Nicotine replacement therapy for smoking cessation. Cochrane Database Syst Rev. 2008;1:CD000146. doi:10.1002/14651858.CD000146.pub3.
49. Vozoris NT, Stanbrook MB. Smoking prevalence, behaviours, and cessation among individuals with COPD or asthma. Respir Med. 2011;105(3):477–84.
50. Lee IM, Shiroma EJ, Lobelo F, Puska P, Blair SN, Katzmarzyk PT. Effect of physical inactivity on major non-communicable diseases worldwide: an analysis of burden of disease and life expectancy. Lancet. 2012;380(9838):219–29.
51. Welfare AIoHa. Chronic respiratory diseases in Australia: their prevalence, consequences and prevention. Canberra; 2005.
52. D'Amato G, Vitale C, D'Amato M, Cecchi L, Liccardi G, Molino A, et al. Thunderstorm-related asthma: what happens and why. Clin Exp Allergy. 2016;46(3):390–6.
53. Cafarella PA, Effing TW, Usmani ZA, Frith PA. Treatments for anxiety and depression in patients with chronic obstructive pulmonary disease: a literature review. Respirology. 2012;17(4):627–38.
54. Jennings JH, Digiovine B, Obeid D, Frank C. The association between depressive symptoms and acute exacerbations of COPD. Lung. 2009;187(2):128–35.
55. Ng TP, Niti M, Tan WC, Cao Z, Ong KC, Eng P. Depressive symptoms and chronic obstructive pulmonary disease: effect on mortality, hospital readmission, symptom burden, functional status, and quality of life. Arch Intern Med. 2007;167(1):60–7.
56. Laurin C, Moullec G, Bacon SL, Lavoie KL. Impact of anxiety and depression on chronic obstructive pulmonary disease exacerbation risk. Am J Respir Crit Care Med. 2012;185(9):918–23.
57. Abrams TE, Vaughan-Sarrazin M, Van der Weg MW. Acute exacerbations of chronic obstructive pulmonary disease and the effect of existing psychiatric comorbidity on subsequent mortality. Psychosomatics. 2011;52(5):441–9.
58. Keating A, Lee A, Holland AE. What prevents people with chronic obstructive pulmonary disease from attending pulmonary rehabilitation? A systematic review. Chron Respir Dis. 2011;8(2): 89–99.
59. Zhang MW, Ho RC, Cheung MW, Fu E, Mak A. Prevalence of depressive symptoms in patients with chronic obstructive pulmonary disease: a systematic review, meta-analysis and meta-regression. Gen Hosp Psychiatry. 2011;33(3):217–23.
60. Yohannes AM, Baldwin RC, Connolly MJ. Prevalence of sub-threshold depression in elderly patients with chronic obstructive pulmonary disease. Int J Geriatr Psychiatry. 2003;18(5):412–6.
61. Kim HF, Kunik ME, Molinari VA, Hillman SL, Lalani S, Orengo CA, et al. Functional impairment in COPD patients: the impact of anxiety and depression. Psychosomatics. 2000;41(6):465–71.
62. Kunik ME, Roundy K, Veazey C, Souchek J, Richardson P, Wray NP, et al. Surprisingly high prevalence of anxiety and depression in chronic breathing disorders. Chest. 2005;127(4):1205–11.
63. Zigmond AS, Snaith RP. The Hospital Anxiety and Depression Scale. Acta Psychiatr Scand. 1983;67(6):361–70.
64. Lamers F, Jonkers CC, Bosma H, Chavannes NH, Knottnerus JA, van Eijk JT. Improving quality of life in depressed COPD patients: effectiveness of a minimal psychological intervention. COPD. 2010;7(5): 315–22.
65. Detering KM, Sutton EA, CF M. Recognising advanced disease, advance care planning and recognition of dying for people with COPD. ERS Monogr. 2016;73:204–20.
66. Jones I, Kirby A, Ormiston P, Loomba Y, Chan KK, Rout J, et al. The needs of patients dying of chronic obstructive pulmonary disease in the community. Fam Pract. 2004;21(3):310–3.
67. Gore JM, Brophy CJ, Greenstone MA. How well do we care for patients with end stage chronic obstructive pulmonary disease (COPD)? A comparison of palliative care and quality of life in COPD and lung cancer. Thorax. 2000;55(12):1000–6.
68. McDonald VM, HigginsI, Gibson PG. Gaining Insight into Older Australians' health care experiences with managing COPD and Asthma. J Asthma. 2013;50(5):497–504.
69. Haras MS. Planning for a good death: a neglected but essential part of ESRD care. Nephrol Nurs J. 2008;35(5):451–8.

15 The Physical Activity Coach in Pulmonary Rehabilitation

Fabio Pitta and Chris Burtin

15.1 Physical Activity Coaching

Although no clear consensus exists on the definition of "health coaching" [1], it can be considered as "a patient-centered approach wherein patients at least partially determine their goals, use self-discovery or active learning processes together with content education to work toward their goals, and self-monitor behaviors to increase accountability, all within the context of an interpersonal relationship with a coach" [2]. Others have defined health coaching as "any individual, one-on-one intervention that facilitates healthy behavior change through such techniques as motivational interviewing, stage-based motivational counseling and facilitative counseling approaches" [3]. These characteristics differentiate health coaching from traditional approaches. In this context, physical activity (PA) coaching may be understood as the use of strategies to stimulate patients toward higher levels of daily activities by modifying their behavior [4].

The objectives of PA coaching may be summarized as: helping patients progress with their PA goals; reinforcing COPD self-care skills; supporting patients' efforts to monitor their activities and symptoms; assisting with problems, solving PA barriers and troubleshooting any device or technology issues [5].

Using accurate assessment and feedback of levels of physical activity in daily life (PADL), individualized PA goals and/or tailored motivational messages, patients are able to learn from successes and failures to develop an effective behavioral strategy to achieve their goal [4].

Development of a new habit such as PA requires regular practice, collaborative monitoring, and ongoing reinforcement and support from credible peer models [5]. PA coaching is based on social cognitive [6] and self-regulation theories [7–9] and core principles of motivational interviewing [10] (e.g., expressing empathy, rolling with resistance, and supporting self-efficacy). In self-efficacy theory, the impetus for change resides in the individual's efficacy expectations or one's "confidence in one's ability to take and persist in action." These expectations reflect a person's beliefs about how capable he or she is in performing a task. Efficacy can also be increased by external environmental supports, such as professional, peer and family modeling and engagement in similar behaviors [5].

PA coaching (with activity monitoring, e.g. use of a pedometer) is a very successful intervention for increasing daily activity levels of patients with COPD [4, 11–19]. Olsen and Nesbitt (2010) [20] stated that four specific interventions were

The original version of this chapter was revised. An erratum to this chapter can be found at https://doi.org/10.1007/978-3-319-65888-9_30

F. Pitta (✉) • C. Burtin
Faculty of Medicine and Life Sciences, Rehabilitation Research Centre, Biomedical Research Institute, Hasselt University, Diepenbeek, Belgium
e-mail: chris.burtin@uhasselt.be

© Springer International Publishing AG 2018
E. Clini et al. (eds.), *Textbook of Pulmonary Rehabilitation*, https://doi.org/10.1007/978-3-319-65888-9_15

Table 15.1 Walk On! intervention mapping

Target concept (source)	Walk On! strategy
Enhancing self-efficacy for increasing physical activity	
• Performance or enactive accomplishments	Guiding patients to set achievable walking goals each week to increase their mastery of walking gradually
• Re-interpretation of signs and symptoms	Practicing breathing strategies to cope with dyspnea during walking, and, over time, developing a recognition that one can do more with the same level of dyspnea (desensitization to dyspnea)
	Tracking and reporting symptoms every week increased awareness of changes in symptoms that might interfere with walking and daily activities to facilitate earlier treatment and reduce disease-specific barriers to walking
• Vicarious experience	Social modeling allowed patients to be positively influenced by the achievement of other participants initially during the orientation session and during the ongoing monthly group meetings
• Social persuasion	Encouragement from coaches and peers during orientation session; ongoing reinforcement from coaches via phone/secure messaging; and peer interactions during monthly meetings
Exercise specific social support	Identification of family or friends to support efforts at increasing physical activity, including attendance at Walk On! activities
Iterative rational behavior change	
• Accurate self-monitoring	Study-issued step counting devices allowed patients to track their daily progress accurately
• Incremental goal setting	Dynamic individualized incremental goals suggested by the interactive voice response and internet-based intervention platforms
• Motivational feedback	Patients received real-time feedback from the step counting devices and personalized motivational feedback and guidance as needed from the coaches

From: Nguyen et al., Contemp Clin Trials 2016; 46: 18–29 [5]

the effective components of health coaching programs: (1) goal setting, (2) selected components of motivational interviewing, (3) collaborations with healthcare providers, and (4) program durations of 6–12 months. Elements from these interventions will be described in more detail further ahead in this chapter.

As an example, a very comprehensive intervention model designed to provide PA coaching was the one published by Nguyen and coworkers as part of the Walk on! program (Table 15.1) [5].

15.2 The Physical Activity Coach

The National Consortium for Credentialing Health and Wellness Coaches (NCCHWC) proposed the following definition of health and wellness coaches, which delineates core elements of the practice of coaching: Health and wellness coaches are professionals from diverse backgrounds and education who work with individuals and groups in a client-centered process to facilitate and empower the client to achieve self-determined goals related to health and wellness. Successful coaching takes place when coaches apply clearly defined knowledge and skills so that clients mobilize internal strengths and external resources for sustainable change [2, 21].

In the context of pulmonary rehabilitation, health coaches may provide patient support in several dimensions, such as adherence to medications, building collaborative plans on how to respond to exacerbations of COPD, and coordinating care between the patient and providers [22]. Physical activity coaches aim more specifically at promoting the engagement in activities (including exercise). Therefore, while a health coach encompasses a wider range of strategies and activities regarding general health, the PA coach generally involves a professional with background on physical activity and specific training on coaching.

Wolever and coworkers described that 93% (217 of 234) of the studies included in their systematic review about health coaching used professionals, while only 7% (17 of 234) used lay individuals [2]. In light of the current understanding of what health coaching represents, those authors extrapolated coaches' necessary core competencies as follows:

First, coaches must have training in a model of change that is patient-centered, and based on facilitating the patient's personal change process, rather than dictating it. Coaches must also have the interpersonal skills to understand the unique values, motivations resources, and obstacles that the patient brings to the change process and the ability to express their understanding effectively. Second, and along similar lines, the coach must be able to help patients identify their own goals for change that are personally important and achievable. Third, coaches must be trained in the use of a self-discovery process that facilitates patients working toward their goals through exploration and an active learning process rather than by dictating what should be done. Fourth, coaches must understand how to help patients be accountable to themselves and monitor their progress. Finally, coaches must have the relevant content knowledge to help their patients with the above four processes in the arena of change. Coaches also must have the interpersonal skill to integrate the content information into the patient's change process rather than dictating it [2].

It is important to understand that the approach of coaches directly involves patients' empowerment, in which it differs from most of the conventional medicine.

15.3 Motivational Interviewing During Activity Counseling

Counseling programs which are based on techniques of motivational interviewing are effective in inducing lifestyle changes in terms of smoking behavior [23], dietary habits [24], substance abuse [25], and physical activity [26]. Motivational interviewing has been described as a client-centered counseling style for eliciting behavioral change by helping clients to explore and resolve ambivalence [27]. In light of PA coaching, this patient-centered approach aims to identify personal barriers that preclude patients from being physically active and stimulates patients to find personal solutions to overcome the identified barriers. Enhancing motivation to be physically active and self-efficacy to perform sufficient activities plays a central role in this behavior change process. The communication style associated with motivational interviewing should create a collaborative, empathic, non-judgmental atmosphere. Patients should be doing the talking, while the activity coach is guiding the conversation using open questions and techniques of reflective listening. It is crucial that the activity coach does not show expert behavior, e.g., just asking questions and giving advice ("you should be more active, this is important for you").

During a counseling session using motivational interviewing it might be interesting to assess motivation to change using a simple Numeric Rating Scale. When patients report high scores on motivation to change (≥8/10), the focus of the counseling intervention can be moved to action planning, goal setting, facilitating barrier identification, and relapse prevention [28]. In the case of low scores on motivation (<8/10) it is necessary to initially enhance motivation using motivational interviewing. The activity coach supports the patient in the exploration process of their ambivalence towards change and to express their intrinsic attitude towards change. A decisional balance exercise asking patients to list benefits and costs of changing and not changing behavior can potentially assist this process.

Several trials investigating the effectiveness of PA coaching interventions throughout this chapter have used motivational interviewing techniques during the counseling sessions [16, 18, 29, 30].

15.4 Feedback from a Pedometer

The use of pedometers not only as method to assess PADL but also as a motivational tool to increase it has gained recent interest. The rationale for using these devices with such objective is that setting daily goals of PA and involving the patient in achieving these goals by monitoring his/her own activity may be an interesting option to increase adherence to an enhanced PADL level.

De Blok and coworkers [29] studied patients with COPD who were randomized into a group receiving PR plus physical activity counseling and feedback with pedometers, and another group who underwent PR only. The group with the pedometers improved their number of steps/day by 69% in comparison to baseline, versus 19% in the group that received PR only. This was one of the first studies to describe pedometers as useful tools to increase PADL. Several others have confirmed these findings, even though effects were typically more modest [11, 15, 16, 18, 31]. In the systematic review by Mantoani and coworkers [4] about interventions to modify PADL in COPD, the most common intervention was PA coaching plus feedback with a pedometer, and the majority of interventions increased PADL levels, especially those who implemented the use of feedback from an activity monitor.

Moy and coworkers have performed a series of studies involving the use of pedometers to increase PADL in COPD. The results can be summarized in view of the study published in 2016 [32]. They examined the effects of an Internet-mediated, pedometer-based walking intervention, called Taking Healthy Steps. During the first 4 months of this intervention, participants were instructed to wear the pedometer every day, upload daily step counts at least once a week, and were provided access to a website with four key components: individualized goal setting, iterative feedback, educational and motivational content, and an online community forum. Participants then entered a subsequent 8-month maintenance phase, with the same characteristics except that participants no longer received new educational content. Results showed that the intervention was efficacious at 4 months, however at 12 months the improvements obtained in daily step counts and quality of life were not maintained. This was possibly linked to the fact that adherence to the pedometer use and website engagement were progressively reduced [32], although another study showed that better long-term maintenance of benefits obtained with the pedometer were observed when only patients with low baseline PADL level were considered [18].

Along the same line, the PRO-Active consortium investigated the effectiveness of a telecoaching intervention using a smartphone application, that was specifically designed for the COPD population across the spectrum of illness severity and allowed human contact with healthcare providers when necessary [33]. They randomly allocated 343 patients from six centers across Europe into a semi-automated tele-coaching intervention group and a usual care group. During the 12-week intervention, patients were provided with an exercise booklet. A pedometer provided direct feedback and feedback via a smartphone application. This app provided an individual daily activity goal in terms of steps which was revised weekly. The patient received regular text messages and occasional telephone contacts with investigators were allowed if requested. At 12 weeks, the tele-coaching intervention group appeared more physically active than the usual care group (difference of about 1500 steps/day and 10 min spent at moderate intense activities per day). The intervention group also showed a favorable change in six-minute walking distance and subjective functional status compared to the usual care group [33].

The promising news of these innovative trials is that pedometers have proven to be a useful tool to increase PADL levels in the short-term, as also noted in other studies [13–16]; the challenge now lies in finding ways to use this tool to promote long-term behavior change and sustained engagement in PA for all patients.

In summary, the use of pedometers (or other activity monitors, in fact) as feedback tool by setting individualized PA goals, especially in combination with tailored motivational interventions, may be considered a successful intervention for increasing PADL of patients with COPD [4].

15.5 Barriers Toward Physical Activity

Disease-related problems have a central role among the barriers leading to the reduction of PADL in COPD, however they are not the only reason behind physical inactivity. These barriers can be categorized in three sub-items: barriers related to health, to motivation, and to external factors.

15.5.1 Barriers Related to Health

These include the abovementioned disease-related barriers (e.g., symptoms, anxiety, depression, comorbidities, and current smoking) as well as worsening of health status (e.g., exacerbations and consequently increased symptoms).

Breathlessness and fatigue are common symptoms in patients with chronic respiratory disease not only during exertion but also while performing ADL [34]. The fear of worsening symptoms is one of the reasons leading to the low adherence to pulmonary rehabilitation. The anxiety resulting from this fear may hinder patients in the initiative of performing any PA and may lead them to a lack of perspective of improvement, which increases the risk of depression [35].

The presence of comorbidities such as metabolic syndrome, cardiac, rheumatic, vascular, and osteomuscular diseases may induce further worsening of symptoms and functionality, impacting PADL. Furthermore, smoking by itself is associated to lower levels of PADL, even in subjects who did not develop COPD [35]. In subjects with impaired lung function such as those with COPD, smoking is related to poor diffusion capacity and consequently to low oxygen values, as well as to lower adherence and less pronounced improvements after PR in comparison to nonsmokers.

Exacerbations, especially those which require hospitalizations, are also an important barrier, since they further induce inactivity, muscle weakness, and even more fear of worsening symptoms [36]. A slow recovery may influence patient's self-confidence, in addition to the fact that they may feel discouraged to perform PA due to the comfort provided by the extra-oxygen they receive during the hospitalization. Interestingly, supplemental long-term oxygen delivered at home may induce physical inactivity when the oxygen source does not allow that the patient moves around [37].

15.5.2 Barriers Related to Motivation

These barriers are related to lack of motivation by the patient, relatives, and health professionals. Intuitively, patients who live alone (i.e., no relatives, partners, or carers) should be more active since they do not count on others for domestic tasks. However, no specific study was done yet to confirm this. Mesquita and coworkers have shown that despite subjects with COPD being less active than their loved ones, the patient's PADL level is directly related with that from his/her companion [38]. Further, patients who live with partner/relative were more motivated to attend PR sessions than those who live alone [39]. Therefore, regardless of the patient's exercise capacity and functional condition, personal and family-related motivation may play a role in PADL level.

Various studies showed that only a small proportion of patients with COPD are referred for PR programs (approximately 0.9–1.4% from patients assessed by their doctors [40–43]. Despite being alarming, these data show the importance that health professionals have in the care of these patients. The health professional can stimulate the patient to believe in his/her own potential, and the family and carers can be vectors of motivation to the patient. It is also a role from these professionals to educate the patient about the importance to perform PADL. The lack of knowledge about the benefits of PADL is an important factor leading to a low motivation to be more active and adhere to an exercise program [44].

15.5.3 Barriers Related to External Factors (or Environment)

These barriers are related to the difficulties to perform PADL due to factors such as climate, transportation, and accessibility, in addition to specific barriers from PA promotion programs.

Furlanetto and coworkers demonstrated that for each increase of 1 °C on average temperature during the day, patients with COPD increase an average of 6 min of PADL [45]. Furthermore, patients reduce their active time by an average of 20% during winter in comparison to summer. Besides temperature, the amount of daylight time, rain precipitation, and atmospheric pollution also interfere on PADL levels [46, 47].

Structured exercise training programs such as those in the scope of PR are a useful way to keep patients active. These programs are able to improve not only physiological outcomes but also psychological features such as self-management, motivation, and self-confidence to perform PA [34]. However, a potential problem is that these programs generally require a specialized center, and the reduced number of centers sometimes leads patients to the need to travel considerable distances many times per week in order to perform the training. In addition to the time consumed, there are also transportation issues to be solved.

The available structure may also be a barrier. For example, patients who cannot swim or bike will have difficulties in performing these kind of modalities. One can also believe that duration of the training session may be considered a barrier to the patient, since it must be long enough to include all required modalities, but not excessively long so that the patient does not perform any other PA after the session, compromising the performance of his/her activities of daily living.

15.5.4 How to Overcome These Barriers?

Overcoming these barriers is as important as identifying them. As observed in the literature, there is still scarce evidence on the most adequate way to achieve this goal. However, a potential way is by the means of personalized action (Table 15.2). That is, instead of the "one size fits all" recipe, the health professional must assess

Table 15.2 Suggestions on how to overcome barriers to physical activity

Barriers	Suggestions to overcome the barriers
Lack of time	• Identifying (with the patient) 30-min periods of available time during the day in which physical activity can be performed at least three (if possible five) times per week
	• Adding physical activity to his/her routine, e.g., including walks to work, supermarket, walking with a friend, relative, or dog; performing PA while watching television, etc.
	• Start with activities which require less time and effort
Social influence	• Ask him/her to explain to friends and relatives the interest in physical activity. Ask them to support the patient's effort
	• Ask him/her to invite friends and relatives to perform physical activity together. Plan social interactions which involve physical activity
	• Ask him/her to establish friendship with physically active persons
Lack of energy	• Organize moments of physical activity in periods in which the patient feels more energy
	• Convince the patient that if he/she gives him/herself a chance to try, physical activity can increase energy
Lack of motivation	• Plan the activity beforehand. Suggest that the patient turns the activity into something regular in his/her day-by-day and insert on the calendar/agenda the moments in which he/she should perform the activity
	• Suggest that the patient invites friends to perform physical activity and write in both calendars the date and time, in order to prevent them from giving up
	• Suggest that the patient takes part in groups of physical activity which follow pre-established frequency
Fear of injuries	• Instruct the patient to avoid injuries (e.g., warming up and stretching of the muscles to be worked)
	• Teach the patient to exercise adequately considering age, cardiorespiratory fitness, complexity of the exercise and general health status
	• Choose activities with minimal risk of injuries
Lack of resources	• Suggest activities which require minimal resources, such as walking or walking down/upstairs
	• Identify low-cost, convenient, and easily accessible resources (e.g., gym, community groups, recreational programs)
Climatic conditions	• Prepare a list of activities which the patient can perform in situations of bad weather (e.g., dancing, cycle-ergometer, active exercises, calisthenics, walking upstairs)

each patient individually and decide the most appropriate treatment plan.

After making clear to the patient and the involved professionals how important it is to perform PA, identifying the barriers and making sure that the appropriate measures to counteract them are taken, there is a final point to be considered in order to increase PADL. Patients and professionals must establish a strategy that both consider feasible, with goal setting and permanent assessment. This will make sure that new barriers are continuously identified and worked on, and new goals are proposed/adjusted whenever necessary.

15.6 Integration in Pulmonary Rehabilitation

Improvements in muscle function and exercise tolerance do not automatically translate into an increase of daily physical activity levels after pulmonary rehabilitation [48]. Enhanced physical activity levels reflect an effective change in the patient's physical activity behavior. Inducing such a behavioral change is much more complex than only improving the capacity to perform activities. Submaximal exercise tolerance, as assessed with whole-body constant work rate exercise tests, roughly doubles after pulmonary rehabilitation [34]. This increase in endurance capacity indicates that the ability to perform activities of daily life, which typically are submaximal efforts, is enhanced to a large extent. Unfortunately, comprehensive pulmonary rehabilitation only leads to modest improvements in daily physical activity levels of 15–20% [48].

Given the promising results of various PA coaching strategies, these approaches might be specifically interesting as a complement to exercise training and multidisciplinary rehabilitation. It can be assumed that optimization of physical activity behavior can further enhance long-term physiological effects obtained with exercise training. Furthermore, pulmonary rehabilitation programs allow intensive contact between patient and health coach.

Two studies in the same center have reported on the additional effect of a 3-month PA counseling program that was based on motivational interviewing techniques and pedometer feedback [18, 29]. The authors reported an improvement in amount of daily physical activity and daily amount of steps at 3 months [18, 29], which was preserved at 12 months in a subgroup of patients who were inactive at baseline [18]. Interestingly, these results could not be reproduced by Burtin et al. who investigated a similar 6-month intervention and found no additional effects on physical activities on top of pulmonary rehabilitation [30]. However, this intervention did not use direct feedback from a pedometer but only incorporated feedback on physical activity (as measured with an activity monitor) into the counseling sessions. This discrepancy in study results indicates that the patients' direct confrontation with their (in) activity might play a crucial role in the initial PA behavior change.

15.7 The Fun Factor Is Important

Successful PA coaching programs should not only focus on barriers toward physical activity but should also identify enablers that can facilitate behavioral change. Enabling factors that are typically reported by patients with COPD include sufficient social support, the opportunity to be active with others, the subjective feeling that one benefits from the physical activity, goal-setting to improve self-motivation, and the possibility to communicate with healthcare professionals [35]. One basic enabler that is too often forgotten is the fun factor: the chances of inducing a long-term PA behavior change increase if patients endorse physical activity as a hobby.

Austrian researchers have investigated to what extent a 3-month Nordic walking training program enhances exercise tolerance and physical activity behavior in patients with moderate to severe COPD [49]. This low-cost intervention consisted of three one-hour outdoor walking sessions per week at 75% of maximal heart rate. As expected, the Nordic Walkers improved their six-minute walking distance as compared to a control group. The Nordic Walkers also improved the daily time spent walking (+15 min/day) and standing (+129 min/day) as well as the intensity of walking, while daily sitting time decreased (−128 min/day). Interestingly, these positive effects were sustained at 3 and 6 months follow-up, making this one of few studies that are able to show long-term PA changes after a PA coaching or exercise intervention. This can be largely explained by the observation that 63% of patients in the Nordic Walking group reported to have adopted as regular physical exercise into weekly routine 6 months after the research period.

Pleguezuelos et al. developed 32 urban walking circuits in the city of Mataró, a Spanish city with 124,000 inhabitants, which were collected in a leaflet [50]. Each circuit had a different distance, slope, and general difficulty. The availability of cultural attractions and commercial areas along the track was also described. Patients received initial support in interpreting these circuits. The researchers conducted a randomized trial comparing patients that did or did not get access to these walking circuits after a short 2-week rehabilitation period. Nine months after the completion of rehabilitation, patients that had access to the walking circuits were significantly more active (+34 min/day of physical activity compared to the control group). The large variability in physical activity in the circuit group indicates that these urban walking circuits were a very successful enabler of long-term PA behavior change in some patients while they might not be the best PA coaching tool in others.

These successful examples illustrate that PA coaching strategies should always focus on triggering "the fun factor" in individual patients, regardless of the used approach.

References

1. Palmer S, Tubbs I, Whybrow A. Health coaching to facilitate the promotion of health behaviour and achievement of health-related goals. Int J Health Promot Educ. 2003;41:91–3.
2. Wolever RQ, Simmons LA, Sforzo GA, et al. A systematic review of the literature on health and wellness coaching: defining a key behavioral intervention in healthcare. Glob Adv Health Med. 2013;2(4):38–57.
3. Gale J. Health psychology meets coaching psychology in the practice of health coaching. InPsych. 2007;3:12–3.
4. Mantoani LC, Rubio N, McKinstry B, MacNee W, Rabinovich RA. Interventions to modify physical activity in patients with COPD: a systematic review. Eur Respir J. 2016;48(1):69–81.
5. Nguyen HQ, Bailey A, Coleman KJ, et al. Patient-centered physical activity coaching in COPD (Walk On!): a study protocol for a pragmatic randomized controlled trial. Contemp Clin Trials. 2016;46:18–29.
6. Bandura A. Social foundations of thought and action: a social cognitive theory. Englewood Cliffs: Prentice Hall; 1986.
7. Baumeister RF, Vohs KD, DeWall CN, Zhang L. How emotion shapes behavior: feedback, anticipation, and reflection, rather than direct causation. Personal Soc Psychol Rev. 2007;11(2):167–203.
8. Clarck NM, Zimmerman BJ. A social cognitive view of self-regulated learning about health. Health Educ Res. 1990;5(3):371–9.
9. Clark NM, Gong M, Kaciroti N. A model of self-regulation for control of chronic disease. Health Educ Behav. 2001;28(6):769–82.
10. Miller WR, Rollnick S. Motivational interviewing. 2nd ed. New York: Guilford Press; 2002.
11. Wewel AR, Gellermann I, Schwertfeger I, Morfeld M, Magnussen H, Jorres RA. Intervention by phone calls raises domiciliary activity and exercise capacity in patients with severe COPD. Respir Med. 2008;102(1):20–6.
12. Tabak M, Vollenbroek-Hutten MM, van der Valk PD, van der Palen J, Hermens HJ. A telerehabilitation intervention for patients with chronic obstructive pulmonary disease: a randomized controlled pilot trial. Clin Rehabil. 2014;28(6):582–91.
13. Moy ML, Weston NA, Wilson EJ, Hess ML, Richardson CR. A pilot study of an Internet walking program and pedometer in COPD. Respir Med. 2012;106(9):1342–50.
14. Moy ML, Janney AW, Nguyen HQ, et al. Use of pedometer and Internet-mediated walking program in patients with chronic obstructive pulmonary disease. J Rehabil Res Dev. 2010;47(5):485–96.
15. Mendoza L, Horta P, Espinoza J, et al. Pedometers to enhance physical activity in COPD: a randomised controlled trial. Eur Respir J. 2015;45(2):347–54.
16. Hospes G, Bossenbroek L, Ten Hacken NH, van Hengel P, de Greef MH. Enhancement of daily physical activity increases physical fitness of outclinic COPD patients: results of an exercise counseling program. Patient Educ Couns. 2009;75(2):274–8.

17. Barberan-Garcia A, Vogiatzis I, Solberg HS, et al. Effects and barriers to deployment of telehealth wellness programs for chronic patients across 3 European countries. Respir Med. 2014;108(4):628–37.
18. Altenburg WA, ten Hacken NH, Bossenbroek L, Kerstjens HA, de Greef MH, Wempe JB. Short- and long-term effects of a physical activity counselling programme in COPD: a randomized controlled trial. Respir Med. 2015;109(1):112–21.
19. Nguyen HQ, Gill DP, Wolpin S, Steele BG, Benditt JO. Pilot study of a cell phone-based exercise persistence intervention post-rehabilitation for COPD. Int J Chron Obstruct Pulmon Dis. 2009;4:301–13.
20. Olsen JM, Nesbitt BJ. Health coaching to improve healthy lifestyle behaviors: an integrative review. Am J Health Promot. 2010;25(1):e1–e12.
21. National Consortium for Credentialing of Health & Wellness Coaches. A call to action. 2013.; http://ncchwc.org/index.cfm?page=action. Accessed 31 May 2013.
22. Benzo R, Vickers K, Novotny PJ, et al. Health coaching and chronic obstructive pulmonary disease rehospitalization. a randomized study. Am J Respir Crit Care Med. 2016;194(6):672–80.
23. Heckman CJ, Egleston BL, Hofmann MT. Efficacy of motivational interviewing for smoking cessation: a systematic review and meta-analysis. Tob Control. 2010;19(5):410–6.
24. Brug J, Spikmans F, Aartsen C, Breedveld B, Bes R, Fereira I. Training dietitians in basic motivational interviewing skills results in changes in their counseling style and in lower saturated fat intakes in their patients. J Nutr Educ Behav. 2007;39(1):8–12.
25. Smedslund G, Berg RC, Hammerstrom KT, et al. Motivational interviewing for substance abuse. Cochrane Database Syst Rev. 2011;5:CD008063.
26. Bennett JA, Lyons KS, Winters-Stone K, Nail LM, Scherer J. Motivational interviewing to increase physical activity in long-term cancer survivors: a randomized controlled trial. Nurs Res. 2007;56(1):18–27.
27. Miller WR. Motivational interviewing with problem drinkers. Behav Psychother. 1983;11:147–72.
28. Michie S, Hyder N, Walia A, West R. Development of a taxonomy of behaviour change techniques used in individual behavioural support for smoking cessation. Addict Behav. 2011;36(4):315–9.
29. de Blok BM, de Greef MH, ten Hacken NH, Sprenger SR, Postema K, Wempe JB. The effects of a lifestyle physical activity counseling program with feedback of a pedometer during pulmonary rehabilitation in patients with COPD: a pilot study. Patient Educ Couns. 2006;61(1):48–55.
30. Burtin C, Langer D, van Remoortel H, et al. Physical activity counselling during pulmonary rehabilitation in patients with COPD: a randomised controlled trial. PLoS One. 2015;10(12):e0144989.
31. Kawagoshi A, Kiyokawa N, Sugawara K, et al. Effects of low-intensity exercise and home-based pulmonary rehabilitation with pedometer feedback on physical activity in elderly patients with chronic obstructive pulmonary disease. Respir Med. 2015;109(3):364–71.
32. Moy ML, Martinez CH, Kadri R, et al. Long-term effects of an internet-mediated pedometer-based walking program for chronic obstructive pulmonary disease: randomized controlled trial. J Med Internet Res. 2016;18(8):e215.
33. Demeyer H, Louvaris Z, Frei A, et al. Physical activity is increased by a 12-week semiautomated telecoaching programme in patients with COPD: a multicentre randomised controlled trial. Thorax. 2017;72(5):415–23.
34. Spruit MA, Singh SJ, Garvey C, et al. An official American Thoracic Society/European Respiratory Society statement: key concepts and advances in pulmonary rehabilitation. Am J Respir Crit Care Med. 2013;188(8):e13–64.
35. Thorpe O, Johnston K, Kumar S. Barriers and enablers to physical activity participation in patients with COPD: a systematic review. J Cardiopulm Rehabil Prev. 2012;32(6):359–69.
36. Thorpe O, Kumar S, Johnston K. Barriers to and enablers of physical activity in patients with COPD following a hospital admission: a qualitative study. Int J Chron Obstruct Pulmon Dis. 2014;9:115–28.
37. Gimeno-Santos E, Frei A, Steurer-Stey C, et al. Determinants and outcomes of physical activity in patients with COPD: a systematic review. Thorax. 2014;69(8):731–9.
38. Mesquita R, Nakken N, Janssen DJ, et al. Activity levels and exercise motivation in COPD patients and their resident loved ones. Chest. 2017;151(5):1028–38.
39. Fischer MJ, Scharloo M, Abbink JJ, et al. Drop-out and attendance in pulmonary rehabilitation: the role of clinical and psychosocial variables. Respir Med. 2009;103(10):1564–71.
40. Garvey C, Fullwood MD, Rigler J. Pulmonary rehabilitation exercise prescription in chronic obstructive lung disease: US survey and review of guidelines and clinical practices. J Cardiopulm Rehabil Prev. 2013;33(5):314–22.
41. Levack WM, Weatherall M, Reeve JC, Mans C, Mauro A. Uptake of pulmonary rehabilitation in New Zealand by people with chronic obstructive pulmonary disease in 2009. N Z Med J. 2012;125(1348):23–33.
42. Brooks D, Sottana R, Bell B, et al. Characterization of pulmonary rehabilitation programs in Canada in 2005. Can Respir J. 2007;14(2):87–92.
43. Yohannes AM, Connolly MJ. Pulmonary rehabilitation programmes in the UK: a national representative survey. Clin Rehabil. 2004;18(4):444–9.
44. Garrod R, Marshall J, Barley E, Jones PW. Predictors of success and failure in pulmonary rehabilitation. Eur Respir J. 2006;27(4):788–94.

45. Furlaneto KC, Demeyer H, Sant'Anna T, et al. Summer-winter variability of physical activity in daily life: comparison between Brazilian and Belgian patients with COPD. Eur Respir J. 2016;48(Suppl 60):A1886.
46. Demeyer H, Burtin C, Van Remoortel H, et al. Standardizing the analysis of physical activity in patients with COPD following a pulmonary rehabilitation program. Chest. 2014;146(2):318–27.
47. Alahmari AD, Mackay AJ, Patel AR, et al. Influence of weather and atmospheric pollution on physical activity in patients with COPD. Respir Res. 2015;16:71.
48. Troosters T, Gosselink R, Janssens W, Decramer M. Exercise training and pulmonary rehabilitation: new insights and remaining challenges. Eur Respir Rev. 2010;19(115):24–9.
49. Breyer MK, Breyer-Kohansal R, Funk GC, et al. Nordic walking improves daily physical activities in COPD: a randomised controlled trial. Respir Res. 2010;11:112.
50. Pleguezuelos E, Perez ME, Guirao L, et al. Improving physical activity in patients with COPD with urban walking circuits. Respir Med. 2013;107(12):1948–56.

16 Breathing Exercises and Mucus Clearance Techniques in Pulmonary Rehabilitation

Catherine J. Hill, Marta Lazzeri, and Francesco D'Abrosca

16.1 Introduction

One of the aims of pulmonary rehabilitation is to improve respiratory muscle function and reduce dyspnoea. This is generally achieved via systemic endurance training, such as walking or cycling, which increases the demand on the respiratory system resulting in either a physiological training effect, improved coordination and muscular or ventilator efficiency or a desensitization to the discomforting symptom of dyspnoea. Another aim is to reduce the frequency of exacerbations and hospitalization. In addition to whole body exercise, specific strategies may be employed within a pulmonary rehabilitation programme to address these aims. These include breathing exercises and mucus clearance techniques, both of which will be discussed in this chapter, or specific exercises to improve the strength and endurance of the respiratory muscles which will be discussed in Chap. 18.

C.J. Hill (✉)
Physiotherapy Department, Austin Health, Melbourne, Australia

Institute for Breathing and Sleep, Heidelberg, Australia
e-mail: catherine.hill@austin.org.au

M. Lazzeri
Cardio-Thoracic and Vascular Department, ASST Grande Ospedale Metropolitano Niguarda, Milan, Italy

ARIR—Associazione Riabilitatori dell'Insufficienza Respiratoria, Pavia, Italy

F. D'Abrosca
ARIR—Associazione Riabilitatori dell'Insufficienza Respiratoria, Pavia, Italy

SITRA—Fondazione IRCCS Ca' Granda, Ospedale Maggiore Policlinico, Milan, Italy

© Springer International Publishing AG 2018
E. Clini et al. (eds.), *Textbook of Pulmonary Rehabilitation*, https://doi.org/10.1007/978-3-319-65888-9_16

16.2 Breathing Exercises

The majority of the pulmonary rehabilitation literature discusses breathing exercises for people with COPD with little description of how to adapt these exercises for patients with other chronic respiratory conditions. Breathing exercises can be employed on an individual basis following identification of an abnormal breathing pattern or in a generalized sense. Individualized instruction in breathing exercises is generally referred to as breathing retraining, the most common technique being diaphragmatic breathing, also termed abdominal breathing or breathing control. Diaphragmatic breathing exercises are often prescribed in addition to whole body exercise during pulmonary rehabilitation or may be prescribed for patients who are unable to participate in the exercise component of pulmonary rehabilitation. Pursed lips breathing, achieved by exhaling through the mouth against the pressure of pursed lips, is a strategy that may be adopted by patients spontaneously or may be encouraged by the pulmonary rehabilitation clinician to reduce respiratory rate and dynamic hyperinflation during exercise training with the aim of an overall increase in endurance. Ventilation-feedback breathing or timed breathing during exercise training is another strategy that has been employed to increase endurance time. Other generalized breathing exercise strategies include coordination of breathing with movement such as pacing arm lifts during the inspiratory or expiratory phase or the use of body positioning to improve the pattern of breathing. Some alternative forms of pulmonary rehabilitation programmes include generalized breathing exercise strategies such as Yoga, particularly pranayama form (timed breathing with a focus on exhalation) and various inclusions of Tai Chi, singing or harmonica playing. This chapter will focus on the most commonly described breathing exercises in pulmonary rehabilitation, diaphragmatic breathing and pursed lips breathing for patients with COPD.

16.2.1 Description of Breathing Exercises

16.2.1.1 Diaphragmatic Breathing

There has been some inconsistency in the terminology and description of diaphragmatic breathing which is synonymous with breathing control, relaxed controlled breathing or abdominal breathing. Patients are encouraged to breathe predominantly with the diaphragm while minimizing the action of accessory muscles [1]. The technique is generally performed in a supported sitting position, with relaxation of the upper chest and shoulders, although several investigators have commenced instruction with patients in a supine position. Tactile feedback is given with one hand of the therapist or the patient on the abdomen, with or without the other hand on the chest. During inspiration, patients are instructed to move the abdominal wall outward, causing the hand on the abdomen to gently rise up and out ("breathe into my/your hand") with minimal movement palpable against the hand on the chest. Nasal inspiration is encouraged to facilitate recruitment of the diaphragm as well as enhancing natural humidification. Expiration is relaxed and passive with the hand on the abdomen returning gently to the resting position. Effective technique is evidenced by an increase in abdominal tidal excursion and a reduction in rib cage excursion or upper chest movement. Variations on this technique include combining diaphragmatic breathing on inspiration with pursed lips breathing on expiration or active abdominal expiration. Patients are encouraged to practice this technique daily, ranging from 10 min to an hour per session, two to three times per day, although the optimum dosage is not clear [2].

16.2.1.2 Pursed Lips Breathing

Pursed lips breathing is performed as a nasal inspiration followed by expiratory blowing against partially closed lips, avoiding forceful exhalation [3]. Some patients with COPD are observed to adopt a spontaneous pattern of pursed lips breathing at rest, during exercise or recovery from exercise or during acute illness. This observation has prompted many investigations into the physiological effects of pursed lips breathing and potential mechanisms of benefit in applying it as a training technique. Attempts have been made to train patients who do not naturally adopt pursed lips breathing, to use this technique to see if they will also benefit. Patients with COPD can be encouraged to trial pursed lips breathing during exercise training or recovery from exertion as well as during activities of daily living. Various instructions can be used to further illustrate the desired technique, "expiratory blowing through pursed lips to create a slight whistle" [4], "imagine a small candle, make the flame flicker but don't blow it out" [5]. In patients who do not adopt pursed lips breathing spontaneously, they are able to learn how to perform it using ear oximetry for feedback with a resultant significant increase in oxygen saturation and tidal volume and reduced respiratory rate, while maintaining minute ventilation [6]. Effective technique is evidenced by immediate reduction in respiratory rate with prolongation of expiration and improvement in symptoms.

16.2.2 Rationale for Breathing Exercises

People with COPD have an increased metabolic cost of breathing at rest compared with healthy people. The increase in airway resistance and loss of elastic recoil that occur in COPD lead to an increase in the work of the respiratory muscles during periods of increased ventilatory demand, evidenced by recruitment of rib cage and accessory muscles and abdominal muscle contraction [1, 2]. In addition to airflow limitation, some people with severe COPD have an increased functional residual capacity at rest, while others may develop dynamic hyperinflation during exertion which limits their exercise capacity. Hyperinflation alters the length–tension relationship of the respiratory muscles, in particular the diaphragm, reducing the force generation capacity of this muscle [1, 2]. Shortening of the costal diaphragmatic muscle fibres and resultant altered angle of contraction, in conjunction with increased use of upper chest accessory muscles for inspiration, can result in a paradoxical pattern of breathing with in-drawing of the lower ribs and abdomen on inspiration. Dyspnoea is more strongly associated with inspiratory muscle function than airflow limitation [2]. In addition, dyspnoea is positively associated with activity of accessory muscles and alterations in chest wall motion and negatively related to diaphragm activity. Consequently, breathing exercises for people with COPD aim to reduce dyspnoea by reducing exercise-induced hyperinflation, altering respiratory muscle recruitment, and improving respiratory muscle performance [7].

16.2.2.1 Diaphragmatic Breathing

The aim of diaphragmatic breathing exercises is to teach patients how to relieve and control dyspnoea by correcting breathing pattern abnormalities, thereby reducing the metabolic cost of breathing and improving distribution of ventilation with resultant improvements in gas exchange, exercise performance and symptoms. Patients are capable of voluntarily (temporarily) altering their pattern of breathing to slower, deeper inspirations with greater abdominal and less thoracic excursion [1]. In a systematic review of breathing control exercises, diaphragmatic breathing was shown to have a significant beneficial effect on abdominal and diaphragm excursion, respiratory rate, tidal volume, arterial oxygen saturation and percutaneous oxygen [8]. Most of these studies included patients with COPD and the findings were consistent when studies of other populations were removed. However diaphragmatic breathing was shown to have a significant detrimental effect on work of breathing and dyspnoea in people with severe COPD (FEV1% predicted 30–50%). There was no overall effect on physiological outcomes related to energy cost of breathing such as oxygen consumption and respiratory muscle efficiency, or outcomes related to gas exchange such as distribution of ventilation [8]. Diaphragmatic breathing has been associated with an increase in dyssynchronous and paradoxical rib cage motion in a number of studies [9, 10]. This may account for the detrimental effect on work of breathing and dyspnoea although there have been very few studies actually investigating the effect of diaphragmatic breathing on dyspnoea as a primary end point.

16.2.2.2 Pursed Lips Breathing

Most investigation into pursed lips breathing has been done in patients with stable COPD either at rest or during a single exercise session. In this setting, pursed lips breathing has been repeatedly shown to reduce respiratory rate and increase tidal volume [11]. This slower, deeper breathing pattern has been associated with an improvement in gas exchange [12] and a reduction in oxygen consumption compared with quiet breathing [13]. In some patients these presumably desirable sequelae are associated with an improvement in symptoms and exercise capacity, and yet in others there is no consequent improvement. The source of symptom relief from pursed lips breathing may be related to decreasing airway collapse and limiting increases in end expiratory lung volume and hyperinflation [14–16]. For patients with COPD who do not demonstrate large airway collapse, the added expiratory resistance of pursed lips breathing and increased tidal volume would result in an increase in the work of breathing and worsening of symptoms. It therefore appears that within the heterogeneous population of patients with COPD there is variable response to pursed lips breathing. Subsequently, further investigations have attempted to identify which patients are more likely to benefit from being trained in this technique and indeed if there are some patients in which this breathing pattern may be detrimental.

16.2.2.3 Other Considerations

Body positioning during breathing exercises aims to improve the length–tension relationship of the respiratory muscles. Positions that increase abdominal pressure, such as forward leaning, can increase diaphragm recruitment, improve chest wall movement, and decrease accessory muscle recruitment, reducing the development of paradoxical breathing and dyspnoea. Bracing the arms in this position, either on a table or arm supports while seated or using a rollator while walking, allows the accessory muscles to contribute to inspiration without the added work of unsupported arm activity. Active abdominal muscle contraction at the end of expiration increases abdominal pressure pushing the diaphragm up to a more favourable operating length and increases elastic recoil pressure of the diaphragm and rib cage, with benefits on hyperinflation and inspiratory muscle function [17].

Coordinating breathing with arm activity may improve arm exercise capacity. Arm elevation is associated with an increase in lung volume and a dyssynchronous pattern of breathing. Recommendations as to pace arm lifts with inspiration or expiration have been contradictory. More recently, Dolmage and colleagues demonstrated that expiration timed with arm lifts improved task performance with a significant increase in endurance time compared to inspiration or sham in hyperinflated patients [18].

16.2.3 Evidence for Breathing Exercises in Pulmonary Rehabilitation

A systematic review of breathing exercises in COPD, including 16 studies involving 1233 participants, did not demonstrate consistent effects of breathing exercises across outcomes of exercise capacity, dyspnoea and health-related quality of life [7]. Only two of these studies were designed to examine the additional contribution of breathing exercises to a pulmonary rehabilitation programme [19, 20]. Collins and colleagues demonstrated that patients with COPD could effectively prolong expiration with a reduction in respiratory rate and increase in expiratory time using ventilation-feedback by means of a heated pneumotachometer attached to a mouthpiece and interfaced to a computer providing visual expiration targets on a screen [19]. Ventilation-feedback was performed during exercise endurance training on a cycle ergometer (18 sessions) and treadmill walking (18 sessions). In a three-group comparison over 36 training sessions, ventilation-feedback breathing retraining plus exercise training reduced dynamic hyperinflation more than exercise training alone or ventilation-feedback alone and increased exercise duration more than ventilation-feedback alone. Exercise duration on a constant work-rate treadmill test was greater for the ventilation-feedback group than exercise alone, however failed to reach statistical significance on preset criteria ($p = 0.022$). Van Gestel and colleagues randomized 40 patients with COPD to exercise training versus exercise training plus 30 min of breathing control with combined inspiratory diaphragmatic breathing and pursed lips expiration over 10 sessions [20]. Breathing retraining used respiratory biofeedback with respiration sensors at the umbilical and abdominal level connected to an amplifier and converted into acoustical (earphone) and visual outputs (graphics on an overhead screen). The authors note that a number of patients found it difficult to change their breathing pattern and while both groups improved in key outcomes, there was no added benefit of breathing exercises on lung function, 6-min walk distance, health-related quality of life or cardiac autonomic function compared to exercise training alone.

There is currently insufficient evidence to suggest that including breathing exercises as a separate training component in addition to conventional exercise training in pulmonary rehabilitation is of additional benefit. While many pulmonary rehabilitation programmes include education on breathing exercises [21], it is not possible to discriminate the benefits of breathing exercises from those of whole body endurance exercise. However, a group education session on breathing exercises as part of a suite of education topics in pulmonary rehabilitation has not demonstrated any additional benefits in exercise capacity, dyspnoea or health-related quality of life over exercise training alone [22]. The role of breathing exercises in pulmonary rehabilitation for chronic respiratory disease populations other than COPD has not been investigated.

16.2.3.1 Diaphragmatic Breathing

Despite inconsistency in the reported acute effects of diaphragmatic breathing on symptoms, one randomized controlled trial in people with COPD reported that after 4 weeks of a diaphragmatic breathing programme, there was an increase in diaphragm participation in natural breathing and an improvement in functional capacity [23]. The mean difference between the diaphragmatic breathing group and usual care control group exceeded the minimum important difference for both 6-min walk distance (34.7 m) and the total score of the St Georges Respiratory Questionnaire (−10.5 points).

16.2.3.2 Pursed Lips Breathing

Four weeks of daily progressive training in pursed lips breathing for people with COPD resulted in a significant reduction in end 6-min walk test dyspnoea (−0.9 units, Borg scale) at 12-week follow-up compared with a control group and expiratory muscle training group [5]. While there was a significant improvement on the SF-36 physical function score for the pursed lips breathing group only, there was no difference between groups in 6-min walk distance. Several studies have looked at the acute effects of pursed lips breathing on exercise capacity in patients with COPD. For people who do not naturally use pursed lips breathing, end-exercise respiratory rate is significantly reduced by using pursed lips breathing compared with natural breathing [24, 25]. Exercise capacity using 6-min walk distance was increased with pursed lips breathing in one small study (mean 34.9 m, [25]) with no difference in incremental shuttle walk distance in the other [24]. There was, however, a significant improvement in recovery time following incremental shuttle walk test when pursed lips breathing was used (mean −24.9 s, [24]). There was a significant correlation between increased 6-min walk distance and increased diaphragmatic excursion during forced breathing measured via ultrasound in supine [25]. For patients who spontaneously use pursed lips breathing during exertion, crossover trials have compared exercise tests while breathing spontaneously, to inhibiting pursed lips breathing by the use of a mouthpiece. Using this method, Faager demonstrated that patients walked a mean 37 s longer and desaturated by 1.2% less on the endurance shuttle walk test when spontaneous pursed lips breathing was used than when it was prevented [26]. Inhibition of pursed lips breathing did not affect 6-min walk distance or functional performance in a multiple-task activity of daily living test (Glittre-ADL, [27]). However pursed lips breathing improved dynamic hyperinflation induced by the Glittre-ADL test (mean difference 0.12 L).

16.2.4 Clinical Practice Implications for Breathing Exercises in Pulmonary Rehabilitation

There is no current evidence that breathing exercises confer greater or additional benefits to a whole body training programme for people with COPD [7]. However, people attend pulmonary rehabilitation programmes to improve their breathing, often with the preconceived idea that the focus will be on teaching them breathing exercises. For people who instinctively use pursed lips breathing during exercise or recovery, they should be encouraged to continue this practice with reinforcement of when it may be useful. For people who do not adopt this pattern naturally, being able to identify responders by spirometry (more severe airflow obstruction) lung volumes (worse hyperinflation) or lower peak expiratory flow rate would be helpful [14, 15, 28]. Alternatively trialling the technique during exercise, recovery or functional activity, while monitoring breathing pattern, dyspnoea and oxygen saturation may be the easiest way to identify responders. Pursed lips breathing should be quick and simple to learn, and in the context of a typical pulmonary rehabilitation programme, it would be expected that responders could be readily identified by subjective response of benefit or observed increase in exercise capacity associated with the adoption of a pursed lips breathing strategy. People who experience an increased work of breathing associated with pursed lips breathing and no symptomatic relief would likely not adopt the technique and would not benefit from further training in it. A recent qualitative study involving a focus group of 13 patients identified several common themes associated with continuation of pursed lips training for up to 24 months after instruction: being in control of breathlessness, relaxation, reduced panic and anxiety and decreased use of short-acting bronchodilators [29].

Diaphragmatic breathing is more difficult to teach and learn and may require daily practice for at least 4 weeks in order to achieve a muscle training effect with translation into improved functional exercise capacity. While symptomatic benefit is not immediate with this technique, patients with a rapid shallow pattern of breathing may be more likely to respond, provided that they are capable of slowing the respiratory rate and increasing tidal volume. Patients who demonstrate a paradoxical breathing pattern and experience worsening dyspnoea during or after diaphragmatic breathing exercises are likely to be non-responders and training should be modified or ceased. A paradoxical breathing pattern that is worsened by diaphragmatic breathing is more likely in people with severe airflow obstruction and hyperinflation who are unable to increase diaphragmatic descent [9].

Effective performance of breathing exercises involves getting the right balance in slowing expiration to allow greater emptying of the lungs and increase the depth of inspiration in order to reduce dynamic hyperinflation, without altering the natural mechanics of breathing so much as to increase the work of breathing. Despite more than six decades of study in this area, what constitutes a clinically meaningful reduction in respiratory rate, increase in tidal volume or improvement in oxygenation has not been identified. Long-term adherence to breathing exercises is more likely in people who experience symptomatic benefit and associated improvement in functional activities.

16.3 Mucus Clearance Techniques

16.3.1 Rationale for Mucus Clearance Techniques

Mucus and cough are the main physical defence mechanisms against inhaled irritants and chemical damage of the bronchial epithelium, as they protect the lower respiratory tract and clear secretions from the upper airways [30]. Respiratory health relies on a good balance between production and removal of airway secretions from the lungs [31]. The mucociliary escalator and expiratory airflow move secretions to the central airways and a combination of swallowing or coughing finally remove them from the lungs.

Environmental and pathophysiological conditions can alter normal mucus clearance: age, prolonged exposure to cigarette smoke and pollutants reduce the efficacy of bronchial ciliary beat. Excessive mucus production and/or retention, excessive or ineffective cough are associated with many respiratory complications: increased work of breathing, ventilation-perfusion mismatch, gas exchange abnormalities, lung infections and inflammation [32]. A number of diseases are characterized by this alterations: rheological proprieties of mucus are altered in cystic fibrosis [33]; ciliary escalator is damaged in primary ciliary dyskinesia (Kartagener syndrome) and in other bronchial structural alteration, such as bronchiectasis [34]; neuromuscular diseases and other form of respiratory muscle weakness alter the ability to cough [35]; COPD, asthma and acute respiratory tract infections cause acute or chronic augmented production of bronchial mucus [36].

Patients, clinicians and caregivers all over the world spend much effort and time to clear secretions, using different strategies and devices.

16.3.2 Description of Mucus Clearance Techniques

From the beginning of twentieth century posture and forced expiration were first described as methods to favour mucus mobilization and expectoration. Postural drainage (PD) was described in detail by Nelson in 1934 [37], and the author argued a direct effect of gravity on the displacement of mucus through the airways, keeping defined postures for a long time. PD was applied in association with manual chest vibration and percussion (conventional chest physiotherapy) to change mucus rheology and enhance expectoration.

More recent mucus clearance techniques are based on the observation of the physiology and pathophysiology of the respiratory system and use physical principles aiming to change rheological proprieties of mucus, to splint open (or re-open) airways to gain volume, to vary gas flow modulating pulmonary pressures, lung volumes and compressive forces. In fact, the rhythmic ciliary metachronism slowly moves the mucus in a cephalad direction and its action is higher in the peripheral airways, while expiratory airflow exerts shear forces on the air–liquid interface between airflow and the mucus layer (two-phase gas–liquid transport) resulting from the combination of the above factors promoting higher displacement of secretions in the central airways [38].

In general, each intervention to help airway clearance aims to collect and mobilize mucus in a cephalad direction and to facilitate elimination by cough, or forced expiration (huff) or suctioning. Depending on the aim of the study or review, authors classify mucus clearance techniques by principles of action (positive pressure, percussion, vibration…) or by the use of devices or not. However, a functional classification by "level of action" could be more useful to guide the selection of mucus clearance techniques in clinical practice: those promoting the recruitment of lung volume, those supporting the mobilization of mucus from peripheral to upper airways, and those facilitating the elimination of mucus from upper airways by expectoration or deglutition [39].

Many non-pharmacological techniques are described to clear airways and to limit or resolve effects of mucus encumbrance, such as the Active Cycle of Breathing Techniques (ACBT), that includes thoracic expansion exercises, controlled breathing and forced expirations, the "Expiration Lente Totale a Glotte Ouverte en infraLatéral" (ELTGoL) [40] and Autogenic Drainage (AD) [41], that modulate expiratory flows varying the starting lung volume and expiratory time with open glottis. Positive expiratory pressure (PEP) [42] is widely used to gain volume behind an obstruction and to prevent early collapse of airways during expiration: PEP can be generated by asking the patient to breathe through a passive expiratory resistance, simulating "pursed lips breathing", expiring into devices generating PEP with oscillation (Flutter, RC Cornet, Acapella) [43], active continuous positive pressure in the airways (CPAP) [44] or temporary PEP (T-PEP) [45, 46]. Mechanical devices are also used to apply compression/oscillation into the airways (intermittent percussive ventilation—IPV), on the rib cage (high-frequency chest wall oscillation or compression—HFCO/HFCC) [47] or to passively enhance expiratory flows in less co-operative patients (Vaküm Technology) [48]. Manually assisted thoracic-abdominal compression techniques, alone or in combination with rescue-bag insufflation or mechanical in-exsufflation (cough-machines), are used to support/substitute ineffective cough [49].

The forced expiratory technique (FET) or "huff" is recommended in association with and after other strategies aimed to promote displacement of mucus to the upper airways. The FET generates a higher expiratory and lower intrathoracic pressure compared to a cough, while it is similar or more effective in mucus expectoration in situations of airways instability [50].

Body positioning modifies the breathing pattern, volumes and regional ventilation, so that in the acute phase of respiratory disease and in critically ill patients the ability to clear secretions can be affected. In critical care, after major surgery and in many other settings, the protracted supine position is the main responsible for respiratory complication such as atelectasis, resulting in lung volume reduction and mucus retention in the gravity-dependent areas. Early mobilization, alternating postures in lateral, prone and semi-recumbent, a quick recovery of sitting position, are the first line lung expansion therapy, that help to effectively clear secretions and maintain lung health [51].

Physical exercise is a mandatory component of pulmonary rehabilitation programmes. It has also been shown to facilitate airway clearance by reducing mucus mechanical impedance, and is recommended as an adjunctive therapy to other mucus clearance techniques in all chronic hyper-secretory patients [52].

When volitional, device assisted or not, strategies are ineffective and the requested work of breathing worsens dyspnoea and symptoms, increasing the discomfort of therapy, intermittent positive pressure breathing (IPPB) and non-invasive mechanical ventilation (NIMV) can be used to assist some phases of mucus clearance sessions [53, 54]. Modern devices have been developed to guide patients during the session of mucus clearance and to facilitate autonomy and adherence to prescriptions: they include visual or auditory feedback, "on screen" information and recording systems to track and monitoring the compliance.

16.3.3 Evidence for Mucus Clearance Techniques in Pulmonary Rehabilitation

Despite a number of techniques and devices being available, the use of mucus clearance techniques is widely debated. Many of the above-mentioned are proven to improve clearance and expectoration in cystic fibrosis (CF) patients and in non-CF bronchiectasis [55]. In patients with CF no differences between conventional chest physiotherapy and other mucus clearance techniques in terms of respiratory function was found [56]. Some evidence shows that self-administered mucus clearance techniques are preferred by patients and their families. Studies also show that mucus clearance techniques lead to improvements in symptoms, lung function and in quality of life, but long-term effects are not clearly demonstrated, potentially due to the chronic and progressive nature of disease. For these reasons a periodic assessment of strategy, in terms of efficacy and appropriateness related to clinical (and psychological) conditions, is recommended, especially in chronic hyper-secretory patients [57].

Clinical practice guidelines of the American Association for Respiratory Care do not recommend the routine use of mucus clearance techniques patients with COPD. They may be considered in cases of symptomatic secretion retention, taking into account patient preference, tolerance, and individual effectiveness related to shared therapeutic goals [58]. Mucus clearance techniques are not recommended for patients able to mobilize secretions with a cough, but education in effective cough or expiratory airflow modulation (i.e. FET) may be useful. For patients with COPD and a weak cough, thoracic-abdominal compression, alone or in association with mechanically assisted coughing, is also not recommended [59], except in some rare and carefully assessed cases of respiratory muscle weakness [60].

Even in the acute phase of chronic respiratory disease, evidence does not support the routine use of mucus clearance techniques, while single cases and clinical experience demonstrate that a tailored strategy targeted to patients with symptomatic retention of mucus and an inability to clear the airways can be useful. During acute exacerbations of COPD, application of mucus clearance techniques can significantly reduce the need for ventilatory support, days of mechanical ventilation and hospitalization, making the cost-benefit of this intervention favourable for these patients [61–63]. It is important to note that during an acute exacerbation, early mobilization programmes and physical re-conditioning are safer and more effective than mucus clearance techniques alone [64]. Available evidence also shows that only selected patients with COPD may have some adjunctive benefit from the use of PEP strategies during exacerbations [61]. Non-invasive ventilation (NIV) and CPAP have been shown to potentially promote mucus clearance and have been proposed as adjunctive therapies for mucus clearance alone or in combination with other techniques [53, 65]; however their use as a mucus clearance technique is controversial and more investigation is warranted [66, 67].

Evidence is lacking for the prophylactic systematic application of ACTs in patients undergoing major surgery, while studies show that early post-operative interventions to manage cough, early recover standing position and deambulation associated to a correct management of pain are mandatory to reduce respiratory complications. Moreover, CPAP, NIV and assisted cough shows to reduce the impact of complications in patients with high risk of respiratory fail [68, 69].

All scientific societies recommend the routine application of manually or mechanically assisted cough augmentation techniques for patients with neuromuscular diseases (NMD) and a weak cough. In fact, respiratory muscle weakness causes a dramatic increase in morbidity and mortality due to respiratory complications. Retention of secretions due to an inability to cough is the main cause of pneumonia and acute respiratory failure leading to intubation in NMD patients. A cough peak flow between 160 and 270 L/min is normally considered effective, but potentially inadequate to protect airways when secretions increase during acute illness. Therefore, assisted coughing is first aimed to maximally inflate the lungs by glossopharyngeal breathing, an ambu-bag or a mechanical ventilation device, and then to enhance spontaneous expulsive phase with manual thoracic and/or abdominal compression or assisted by a mechanical device (mechanical in-exsufflator). The best efficacy is reached with the combination of assisted inspiratory and expiratory manoeuvres [70]. Correct use of NIV and assisted coughing is associated with less hospitalization due to lung complications, a better survival and can prevent tracheostomy, at all or for a longer time compared to no respiratory management [50]. Evidence does not support the exclusive application of "usual" techniques to mobilize bronchial secretions from peripheral to the upper airways without an adequate competence to cough or to support expectoration [71].

Despite a number of studies comparing mucus clearance techniques to each other, no one technique demonstrated its superiority in terms of efficacy. Probably the lack of simple, shared and defined outcome measures contributes to the difficulty in designing studies on mucus clearance techniques [72]. No minimal clinical important differences (MCID) are defined in functional and measurable parameters (lung function tests and measures of bronchial obstruction, blood gases, mucus volume and/or weight, …) as strictly linked to the minimal detectable difference for the individual. Moreover, it has not been demonstrated if any difference can be related to other factors such as comfort in the use of technique and personal perception of quality of life.

16.3.4 Clinical Practice Implications for Mucus Clearance Techniques in Pulmonary Rehabilitation

Lacking strong evidence for mucus clearance techniques, it would be better to consider all "therapeutic options" for secretion removal, choosing according to an accurate assessment of underlying pathophysiological alterations, characteristics of mucus, patient collaboration, availability of equipment and materials, cost-benefit and preference of the individual patient/caregiver. The selection of the techniques/devices can be influenced by the clinical experience and confidence of the pulmonary rehabilitation clinician, so a trial can be performed to identify the best strategy for an individual patient, considering subjective and objective improvements. In general, a number of questions should guide the selection of patients who might benefit from intervention and related strategies: Is there a pathophysiologic rationale—hyper-secretory condition and trouble in clearing secretions—for the use of the therapy? Can it potentially harm and are retained secretions affecting lung function, such as gas exchange or lung mechanics? What is the potential for adverse effects from the therapy? What are the patient's preferences, including subjective perception of benefit?

Are the direct and indirect costs of the therapy sustainable? Is the patient able to manage the strategy independently to maintain airway clearance in the long-term? The last question is a key component especially when the treatment needs to be continued at home or for a long time. In these circumstances, patient preference, tolerance, locus of control, economy (time and resources) and self-perceived efficacy of the treatment will be predictive of good adherence and perseverance with the prescription [32].

Despite this lack of evidence, mucus clearance techniques are a fundamental component of real-life rehabilitation programmes for people with chronic respiratory disease, both in the acute (also in the critical care) and in the outpatient settings for hyper-secretory patients with ineffective management of secretions. As above-mentioned, mucus clearance techniques can play a role to reduce exacerbations and hospitalization, encouraging more support from governments and financial stakeholders to enable well-powered multi-centre high quality research, to give new sustainable solutions for patients troubled with secretions and to better address the daily work of thousands of respiratory physiotherapists and caregivers all over the world [73, 74].

References

1. Gosselink R. Breathing techniques in patients with chronic obstructive pulmonary disease (COPD). Chron Respir Dis. 2004;1(3):163–72.
2. Breslin EH. Breathing retraining in chronic obstructive pulmonary disease. J Cardiopulm Rehabil. 1995;15(1):25–33.
3. Pulmonary rehabilitation-1999. American Thoracic Society. Am J Respir Crit Care Med. 1999;159(5 Pt 1):1666–82.
4. Breslin EH. The pattern of respiratory muscle recruitment during pursed-lip breathing. Chest. 1992; 101(1):75–8.
5. Nield MA, Soo Hoo GW, Roper JM, Santiago S. Efficacy of pursed-lips breathing: a breathing pattern retraining strategy for dyspnea reduction. J Cardiopulm Rehabil Prev. 2007;27(4):237–44.
6. Tiep BL, Burns M, Kao D, Madison R, Herrera J. Pursed lips breathing training using ear oximetry. Chest. 1986;90(2):218–21.
7. Holland AE, Hill CJ, Jones AY, McDonald CF. Breathing exercises for chronic obstructive pulmonary disease. Cochrane Database Syst Rev. 2012;10:CD008250. doi:10.1002/14651858.CD008250.pub2.
8. Lewis LK, Williams MT, Olds T. Short-term effects on outcomes related to the mechanism of intervention and physiological outcomes but insufficient evidence of clinical benefits for breathing control: a systematic review. Aust J Physiother. 2007;53(4):219–27.
9. Cahalin LP, Braga M, Matsuo Y, Hernandez ED. Efficacy of diaphragmatic breathing in persons with chronic obstructive pulmonary disease: a review of the literature. J Cardiopulm Rehabil. 2002;22(1):7–21.
10. Fernandes M, Cukier A, Feltrim MIZ. Efficacy of diaphragmatic breathing in patients with chronic obstructive pulmonary disease. Chron Respir Dis. 2011;8(4):237–44.
11. Roberts SE, Stern M, Schreuder FM, Watson T. The use of pursed lips breathing in stable chronic obstructive pulmonary disease: a systematic review of the evidence. Phys Therapy Rev. 2009;14(4):240–6.
12. Mueller RE, Petty TL, Filley GF. Ventilation and arterial blood gas changes induced by pursed lips breathing. J Appl Physiol. 1970;28(6):784–9.
13. Jones AY, Dean E, Chow CC. Comparison of the oxygen cost of breathing exercises and spontaneous breathing in patients with stable chronic obstructive pulmonary disease. Phys Ther. 2003;83(5):424–31.
14. Spahija J, de Marchie M, Grassino A. Effects of imposed pursed-lips breathing on respiratory mechanics and dyspnea at rest and during exercise in COPD. Chest. 2005;128(2):640–50.
15. Bianchi R, Gigliotti F, Romagnoli I, Lanini B, Castellani C, Binazzi B, Stendardi L, Grazzini M, Scano G. Patterns of chest wall kinematics during volitional pursed-lip breathing in COPD at rest. Respir Med. 2007;101(7):1412–8.
16. Visser FJ, Ramlal S, Dekhuijzen PN, Heijdra YF. Pursed-lips breathing improves inspiratory capacity in chronic obstructive pulmonary disease. Respiration. 2011;81(5):372–8.
17. Casciari RJ, Fairshter RD, Harrison A, Morrison JT, Blackburn C, Wilson AF. Effects of breathing retraining in patients with chronic obstructive pulmonary disease. Chest. 1981;79(4):393–8.
18. Dolmage TE, Janaudis-Ferreira T, Hill K, Price S, Brooks D, Goldstein RS. Arm elevation and coordinated breathing strategies in patients with COPD. Chest. 2013;144(1):128–35.
19. Collins EG, Langbein WE, Fehr L, O'Connell S, Jelinek C, Hagarty E, Edwards L, Reda D, Tobin MJ, Laghi F. Can ventilation-feedback training augment exercise tolerance in patients with chronic obstructive pulmonary disease? Am J Respir Crit Care Med. 2008;177(8):844–52.
20. van Gestel AJ, Kohler M, Steier J, Teschler S, Russi EW, Teschler H. The effects of controlled breathing during pulmonary rehabilitation in patients with COPD. Respiration. 2012;83(2):115–24.

21. McCarthy B, Casey D, Devane D, Murphy K, Murphy E, Lacasse Y. Pulmonary rehabilitation for chronic obstructive pulmonary disease. Cochrane Database Syst Rev. 2015;2:CD003793. doi:10.1002/14651858.CD003793.pub3.
22. Blackstock FC, Webster KE, McDonald CF, Hill CJ. Comparable improvements achieved in chronic obstructive pulmonary disease through pulmonary rehabilitation with and without a structured educational intervention: a randomized controlled trial. Respirology. 2014;19(2):193–202.
23. Yamaguti WP, Claudino RC, Neto AP, Chammas MC, Gomes AC, Salge JM, Moriya HT, Cukier A, Carvalho C. Diaphragmatic breathing training program improves abdominal motion during natural breathing in patients with chronic obstructive pulmonary disease: a randomized controlled trial. Arch Phys Med Rehabil. 2012;93(4):571–7.
24. Garrod R, Dallimore K, Cook J, Davies V, Quade K. An evaluation of the acute impact of pursed lips breathing on walking distance in nonspontaneous pursed lips breathing chronic obstructive pulmonary disease patients. Chron Respir Dis. 2005;2(2):67–72.
25. Bhatt SP, Luqman-Arafath TK, Gupta AK, Mohan A, Stoltzfus JC, Dey T, Nanda S, Guleria R. Volitional pursed lips breathing in patients with stable chronic obstructive pulmonary disease improves exercise capacity. Chron Respir Dis. 2013;10(1):5–10.
26. Faager G, Stahle A, Larsen FF. Influence of spontaneous pursed lips breathing on walking endurance and oxygen saturation in patients with moderate to severe chronic obstructive pulmonary disease. Clin Rehabil. 2008;22(8):675–83.
27. de Araujo CLP, Karloh M, Dos Reis CM, Palú M, Mayer AF. Pursed-lips breathing reduces dynamic hyperinflation induced by activities of daily living test in patients with chronic obstructive pulmonary disease: A randomized cross-over study. J Rehabil Med. 2016;47(10):957–62.
28. Cabral LF, D'Elia TDC, Marins DDS, Zin WA, Guimarães FS. Pursed lip breathing improves exercise tolerance in COPD: a randomized crossover study. Eur J Phys Rehabil Med. 2015;51(1):79–88.
29. Roberts SE, Schreuder FM, Watson T, Stern M. Do COPD patients taught pursed lips breathing (PLB) for dyspnoea management continue to use the technique long-term? A mixed methodological study. Physiotherapy. 2016; doi:10.1016/j.physio.2016.05.006.
30. Rubin BK. Physiology of airway mucus clearance. Respir Care. 2002;47:761–8.
31. Houtmeyers E, Gosselink R, Gayan-Ramirez G, Decramer M. Regulation of mucociliary clearance in health and disease. Eur Respir J. 1999;13:1177–88.
32. Hess DR. Airway clearance: physiology, pharmacology, techniques, and practice. Respir Care. 2007;52(10):1392–6.
33. Zach MS. Lung disease in cystic fibrosis—an updated concept. Pediatr Pulmonol. 1990;8(3):188–202.
34. Hernandez ML, Harris B, Lay JC, Bromberg PA, Diaz-Sanchez D, Devlin RB, Kleeberger SR, Alexis NE, Peden DB. Comparative airway inflammatory response of normal volunteers to ozone and lipopolysaccharide challenge. Inhal Toxicol. 2010;22:648–56.
35. Rubin BK. Mucus, phlegm, and sputum in cystic fibrosis. Respir Care. 2009;54:726–32. Discussion 732
36. Fahy JV, Dickey BF. Airway mucus function and dysfunction. N Engl J Med. 2010;363:2233–47.
37. Nelson HP. Postural drainage of the lungs. Br Med J. 1934;2:251–5.
38. Kim CS, Iglesias AJ, Sackner MA. Mucus clearance by two-phase gas-liquid flow mechanism: asymmetric periodic flow model. J Appl Physiol. 1987;62:959–71.
39. Postiaux G. Chest physical therapy of the distal lung. Mechanical basis of a new paradigm. Rev Mal Respir. 2014;31:552–67.
40. Martins JA, Dornelas de Andrade A, Britto RR, Lara R, Parreira VF. Effect of slow expiration with glottis opened in lateral posture (ELTGOL) on mucus clearance in stable patients with chronic bronchitis. Respir Care. 2012;57:420–6.
41. Agostini P, Knowles N. Autogenic drainage: the technique, physiological basis and evidence. Physiotherapy. 2007;93:157–63.
42. Osadnik CR, McDonald CF, Miller BR, Hill CJ, Tarrant B, Steward R, Chao C, Stodden N, Oliveira CC, Gagliardi N, Holland AE. The effect of positive expiratory pressure (PEP) therapy on symptoms, quality of life and incidence of re-exacerbation in patients with acute exacerbations of chronic obstructive pulmonary disease: a multicentre, randomised controlled trial. Thorax. 2014;69:137–43.
43. Volsko TA, DiFiore J, Chatburn RL. Performance comparison of two oscillating positive expiratory pressure devices: Acapella versus Flutter. Respir Care. 2003;48:124–30.
44. Armstrong D. The use of continuous positive airway pressure or non-invasive ventilation as forms of respiratory support in children with cystic fibrosis. Paediatr Respir Rev. 2013;14(1):19–21.
45. Venturelli E, Crisafulli E, DeBiase A, Righi D, Berrighi D, Cavicchioli PP, Vagheggini G, Dabrosca F, Balbi B, Paneroni M, Bianchi L, Vitacca M, Galimberti V, Zaurino M, Schiavoni G, Iattoni A, Ambrosino N, Clini EM. Efficacy of temporary positive expiratory pressure (TPEP) in patients with lung diseases and chronic mucus hypersecretion. The UNIKO(R) project: a multicentre randomized controlled trial. Clin Rehabil. 2013;27:336–46.
46. Snijders D, Fernandez Dominguez B, Calgaro S, Bertozzi I, Escribano Montaner A, Perilongo G, Barbato A. Mucociliary clearance techniques for treating non-cystic fibrosis bronchiectasis: is there evidence? Int J Immunopathol Pharmacol. 2015;28:150–9.
47. Toussaint M, Guillet MC, Paternotte S, Soudon P, Haan J. Intrapulmonary effects of setting, parameters in portable intrapulmonary percussive ventilation devices. Respir Care. 2012;57:735–42.

48. Garuti G, Verucchi E, Fanelli I, Giovannini M, Winck JC, Lusuardi M. Management of bronchial secretions with Free Aspire in children with cerebral palsy: impact on clinical outcomes and healthcare resources. Ital J Pediatr. 2016;42:7.
49. Bach JR, Goncalves MR, Hon A, Ishikawa Y, De Vito EL, Prado F, Dominguez ME. Changing trends in the management of end-stage neuromuscular respiratory muscle failure. Am J Phys Med Rehabil. 2013;92:267–77.
50. McCool FD. Nonpharmacologic airway clearance therapies. Chest. 2006;129:250S–12.
51. Fink JB. Forced expiratory technique, directed cough, and autogenic drainage. Respir Care. 2007;52:1210–21. discussion1221–3
52. Dwyer TJ, Alison JA, McKeough ZJ, Daviskas E, Bye PTP. Effects of exercise on respiratory flow and sputum properties in patients with cystic fibrosis. Chest. 2011;139:870–7.
53. Rodriguez Hortal MC, Nygren-Bonnier M, Hjelte L. Non-invasive ventilation as airway clearance technique in cystic fibrosis. Physiotherapy. 2016; doi:10.1002/pri.1667.
54. Osadnik CR, McDonald CF, Holland AE. Advances in airway clearance technologies for chronic obstructive pulmonary disease. Expert Rev Respir Med. 2013;7:673–85.
55. Chalmers JD, Aliberti S, Blasi F. Management of bronchiectasis in adults. Eur Respir J. 2015;45:1446–62.
56. Warnock L, Gates A. Chest physiotherapy compared to no chest physiotherapy for cystic fibrosis. Cochrane Database Syst Rev. 2015;12:CD001401.
57. Flume PA. Mogayzel PJ Jr., Robinson KA, Goss CH, Rosenblatt RL, Kuhn RJ, Marshall BC, and the Clinical Practice Guidelines for Pulmonary Therapies Committee*. Cystic Fibrosis Pulmonary Guidelines. Am J Respir Crit Care Med. 2009;180:802–8.
58. Lee AL, Burge AT, Holland AE. Airway clearance techniques for bronchiectasis. Cochrane Database Syst Rev. 2015;11:CD008351.
59. Sivasothy P, Brown L, Smith IE, Shneerson JM. Effect of manually assisted cough and mechanical insufflation on cough flow of normal subjects, patients with chronic obstructive pulmonary disease (COPD), and patients with respiratory muscle weakness. Thorax. 2001 Jun;56(6):438–44.
60. Winck JC, Goncalves MR, Lourenço C, Viana P, Almeida J, Bach JR. Effects of mechanical insufflation-exsufflation on respiratory parameters for patients with chronic airway secretion encumbrance. Chest. 2004;126:774–80.
61. Osadnik CR, McDonald CF, Jones AP, Holland AE. Airway clearance techniques for chronic obstructive pulmonary disease. Cochrane Database Syst Rev. 2012;3:CD008328.
62. Andrews J, Sathe NA, Krishnaswami S, McPheeters ML. Nonpharmacologic airway clearance techniques in hospitalized Patients: a systematic review. Respir Care. 2013;58(12):2160–86.
63. Yang M, Yan Y, Yin X, Wang BY, Wu T, Liu GJ, Dong BR. Chest physiotherapy for pneumonia in adults. Cochrane Database Syst Rev. 2013;2:CD006338.
64. Tang CY, Taylor NF, Blackstock FC. Chest physiotherapy for patients admitted to hospital with an acute exacerbation of chronic obstructive pulmonary disease (COPD): a systematic review. Physiotherapy. 2010;96:1–13.
65. Stanford G, Parrott H, Bilton D, Agent P. Positive pressure—analysing the effect of the addition of non-invasive ventilation (NIV) to home airway clearance techniques (ACT) in adult cystic fibrosis (CF) patients. Physiother Theory Pract. 2014;31:270–4.
66. Aquino ES, Shimura F, Santos AS, Goto DM, Coelho CC, de Fuccio MB, Saldiva PHN, Lorenzi-Filho G, Rubin BK, Nakagawa NK. CPAP has no effect on clearance, sputum properties, or expectorated volume in cystic fibrosis. Respir Care. 2012;57:1914–9.
67. Gambazza S, Zuffo S. CPAP in cystic fibrosis: is it time to surrender yet? Respir Care. 2013;58:e116–7.
68. Ireland CJ, Chapman TM, Mathew SF, Herbison GP, Zacharias M. Continuous positive airway pressure (CPAP) during the postoperative period for prevention of postoperative morbidity and mortality following major abdominal surgery. Cochrane Database Syst Rev. 2014;8:CD008930.
69. Faria DAS, da Silva EMK, Atallah ÁN, Vital FMR. Noninvasive positive pressure ventilation for acute respiratory failure following upper abdominal surgery. Cochrane Database Syst Rev. 2015;10:CD009134.
70. LoMauro A, D'Angelo MG, Aliverti A. Assessment and management of respiratory function in patients with Duchenne muscular dystrophy: current and emerging options. Ther Clin Risk Manag. 2015;11:1475–88.
71. Finder JD, Birnkrant D, Carl J, Farber HJ, Gozal D, Iannaccone ST, Kovesi T, Kravitz RM, Panitch H, Schramm C, Schroth M, Sharma G, Sievers L, Silvestri JM, Sterni L. Respiratory care of the patient with Duchenne muscular dystrophy: ATS consensus statement. Am J Respir Crit Care Med. 2004;170(4):456–65.
72. Rubin BK. Designing clinical trials to evaluate mucus clearance therapy. Respir Care. 2007;52:1348–58. discussion1358–61
73. Ides K, Vissers D, De Backer L, Leemans G, De Backer W. Airway clearance in COPD: need for a breath of fresh air? A systematic review. COPD. 2011;8(3):196–205.
74. Volsko TA. Airway clearance therapy: finding the evidence. Respir Care. 2013;58:1669–78.

17 Self-Management in Pulmonary Rehabilitation

Jean Bourbeau, Waleed Alsowayan, and Joshua Wald

Pulmonary rehabilitation programmes have long recognized that, while exercise training is vitally important for patients with lung disease, equally important is the opportunity provided by a rehabilitation programme to deliver education to patients with chronic respiratory disease and help them to develop the skills and confidence they need to adopt a healthier lifestyle [1]. Patient education whether individually or in groups has always been an important component of pulmonary rehabilitation. The content and delivery of this education has gradually evolved from a traditional, didactic approach to one informed by an understanding of human psychology, which promotes adaptive behaviour change through the inclusion of collaborative self-management [2, 3].

Under the traditional didactic model "education" often takes the form of providers giving information and advice, and assuming that knowledge will lead to behaviour changes. This approach has often resulted in what has been termed the "knowledge behaviour gap", i.e. patients have the knowledge required to engage in healthier behaviours but fail to adopt or maintain these behaviours despite clear health benefits. The goal of self-management interventions is to narrow this gap between the knowledge of what "should" be done and individual's actual behaviour by targeting not only knowledge but also motivation to engage in behaviour change. Thus, by integrating collaborative self-management intervention into a standardized pulmonary rehabilitation programme there is the potential to not only improve traditional outcomes such as exercise capacity and health-related quality of life, but also to affect a sustainable change in patient behaviours such as physical activity, breathing management, medication adherence, and the recognition and management of exacerbations with an action plan.

This chapter will present (1) the definition of self-management and its role in pulmonary rehabilitation; (2) the evidence for the effectiveness of self-management in respiratory disease and what this evidence reveals about potential risks and challenges; (3) an approach for designing and implementing self-management

J. Bourbeau, M.D., M.Sc., F.R.C.P.C (✉)
Montreal Chest Institute,
McGill University Health Centre,
Montréal, QC, Canada

Center for Innovative Medicine (CIM),
McGill University Health Centre (MUHC),
1001 Decarie Blvd., Room C047371.5,
Montreal, QC, Canada, H4A 3J1
e-mail: jean.bourbeau@mcgill.ca

W. Alsowayan • J. Wald
Montreal Chest Institute,
McGill University Health Centre,
Montréal, QC, Canada

© Springer International Publishing AG 2018
E. Clini et al. (eds.), *Textbook of Pulmonary Rehabilitation*,
https://doi.org/10.1007/978-3-319-65888-9_17

intervention as a component of a pulmonary rehabilitation programme.

17.1 Definition of Self-Management and Its Role in Pulmonary Rehabilitation

Chronic respiratory disease is associated with a significant burden of disability, morbidity and mortality. It impacts quality of life, causes functional limitation, and leads to frequent use of healthcare resources including hospitalizations [4, 5]. The impact of chronic respiratory diseases is not simply a consequence of the physiological disorder [6], but of a combination of the disease itself and the individuals adaptation to the illness, its comorbidities, and its treatments [7]. As such, improving coping and disease management skills can lead to significant improvement even when the underlying disease physiology remains unchanged.

Traditional pulmonary rehabilitation improves exercise capacity and quality of life in the short term but has often failed to affect long-term changes in behaviours such as physical activity leading to a diminution of benefits over time [8, 9]. In order for patients to obtain long-lasting benefits from pulmonary rehabilitation they must be actively engaged and motivated to achieve a durable change in their health behaviour. Achieving successful behaviour change for patients requires that physician and healthcare professionals change their own behaviour and approach to education. Traditionally, physicians and healthcare professionals have viewed themselves as experts whose job is to get patients to behave in ways that reflect that expertise. In retrospect, it is no surprise that this approach has often brought disappointment and frustration for both patients and healthcare professionals. It is only by recognizing patients as experts on their own lives, and then adding their medical expertise to what they know about themselves that healthcare providers can work in collaboration with patient to help them achieve their goals [10]. This is the core insight of the self-management approach.

Increasingly, it has been recognized worldwide and endorsed the need for self-management interventions within national standards of care of chronic respiratory diseases [10–14]. However, the reality remains that often self-management intervention occur during brief clinical visits or through referral to limited-time education classes. Pulmonary rehabilitation is an ideal setting for self-management education, offering repeated interactions over many weeks, individual and/or group sessions, and the chance for self-management to be integrated into the medical treatment provided to the patient. Features that have been found to support self-management include: involving patient in decision making, assessment of patient specific needs and barriers, goal setting, enhancing skills, problem solving, follow-up and support and increasing access to resources [15]. This process requires a patient-centred communication style (motivational communication) in which healthcare practitioners work with patients to elicit the patient's own motivation for making changes in pursuit of the health goals which are important to them [16].

In addition to addressing behavioural risk factors, self-management also involves helping patients to monitor and manage the signs and symptoms of their disease, adhere to their agreed upon treatment plan, maintain regular contact with healthcare providers and manage the psychosocial impact of their condition [16]. In this way people with chronic health conditions and their families are aware, informed, engaged, activated, empowered, and confident they can self-manage their disease in partnership with healthcare providers.

A consensus <conceptual> definition of self-management interventions has recently been agreed upon, to clarify what should be considered under the heading of a self-management intervention [3]:

> *"A COPD self-management intervention is structured but personalised and often multi-component, with goals of motivating, engaging and supporting the patients to positively adapt their health behaviour(s) and develop skills to better manage their disease".*

The ultimate goals of self-management are: (a) optimising and preserving physical health; (b) reducing symptoms and functional impairments in daily life and increasing emotional well-being, social well-being and quality of life; and (c) establishing effective alliances with healthcare professionals, family, friends and community.

"The process requires iterative interactions between patients and healthcare professionals who are competent in delivering self-management interventions. These patient-centred interactions focus on: (1) identifying needs, health beliefs and enhancing intrinsic motivations; (2) eliciting personalised goals; (3) formulating appropriate strategies (e.g. exacerbation management) to achieve these goals; and if required (4) evaluating and re-adjusting strategies. Behaviour change techniques are used to elicit patient motivation, confidence and competence. Literacy sensitive approaches are used to enhance comprehensibility."

This multi-component approach fits well with the model of care used in pulmonary rehabilitation [17]; however, many of the education components of traditional pulmonary rehabilitation programmes would not be considered self-management interventions under this definition. It is important to keep in mind that the goal is to motivate, engage and support patients to positively adapt their health behaviour(s) and develop skills to better manage their disease.

17.2 Evidence for the Effectiveness of Self-Management in Respiratory Disease and Potential Risks and Challenges

17.2.1 Evidence for Effectiveness of Self-Management

Education as a component of treatment for patients with COPD has been a topic of study for decades [18–20]. However, results from early studies that focused on didactic education rather than collaborative self-management were disappointing [21, 22]. Over time the focus on didactic education was replaced with a more nuanced view of human psychology, motivation, and behaviour. Concepts such as social cognitive theory [23] were incorporated into the design of education programmes and interventions were developed with feedback and collaboration from patients and caregivers. These interventions resonate with patient's specific motivations and goals and targeted predisposing factors to behaviour change. Older studies of didactic education alone should not be confused with later studies of more comprehensive self-management and, for this reason, all studies published prior to 1995, when didactic interventions were the norm, were excluded from the most recent Cochrane analysis [17].

One of the first studies to show a significant benefit of self-management was an RCT by Bourbeau et al. published in 2003 [24]. The intervention tested in this trial employed self-management principles and was designed using both education theory and feedback from patients and health professionals. Patients in the intervention arm received self-management oriented educational materials, a personally tailored action plan, and case management patient coaching by a well-trained healthcare professional. The result was an impressive 39.8% reduction in hospital admissions for COPD in the self-management group compared to usual care at 12 months, as well as a reduction in other causes of hospitalization and emergency room visits [24]; to a lesser degree, reduction in hospital admission was maintained at 2 years [25] and the self-management intervention had the potential of being cost saving [26].

Since that initial success multiple systematic reviews have shown a benefit to self-management interventions. A Cochrane review on self-management in COPD was first published in 2007 and updated in 2014 [17]. This update identified 29 controlled or randomized control trials of self-management in COPD involving 3189 patients. Twenty-three trials compared self-management to usual care while six compared different self-management interventions to one another. Compared to usual care, patients receiving self-management showed a significant improvement in quality of life (SGRQ MD −3.51, 95% CI −5.37 to −1.65) as well as respiratory-related and all cause hospitalization (OR 0.57, 95% CI 0.43–0.75 and OR 0.60 95% CI 0.40–0.89, respectively) and dyspnoea (MRC score MD −0.83, 95% CI −1.36 to −0.30). No significant effect was seen for exercise capacity or mortality (OR 0.79, 95% CI 0.58–1.07).

17.2.1.1 Potential Problems with Self-Management Intervention

Despite these encouraging findings, inconsistent results of seemingly similar interventions have led some to question the utility and generalizability of self-management interventions. The safety of self-management in COPD was also called into question after the publication by Fan et al. [27] in 2012 of a trial that was stopped early due to an increased mortality in the group receiving the self-management intervention (HR 3.00 95% CI 1.46–6.17).

A number of factors may explain this heterogeneity. Firstly, unlike a drug trial where the dose, timing, and duration of the intervention can be standardized and controlled, self-management trials involve complex interventions with multiple components delivered by different healthcare professionals. This means that the success or failure of an intervention is determined not only by the content of the intervention but also by the process and fidelity with which the content is delivered. Thus, it is possible for a well-designed intervention to fail, not due to an intrinsic lack of efficacy, but rather because the components of the intervention were not delivered as intended. Failure to adequately assess and monitor the delivery of the intervention may account for some of some of the heterogeneity between trials of similar interventions.

Another possible explanation for the failure of some large trials of self-management interventions to show a difference in outcomes may be that they did not successful change the behaviours they sought to modify. This can be considered as a "failure to intervene" rather than a "failure of the intervention" i.e.: the goal of self-management is to encourage the long-term adoption of healthy behaviours by affecting the predisposing and enabling factors which lead to behaviour change. If the intervention fails to change these predisposing factors, and patients do not change their behaviour then the intervention will not improve health outcomes. Evidence for this "failure to intervene" comes from a number of sources including a secondary analysis of the Bucknall trial, which classified patients in the intervention arm into those who successfully learned to self-manage and those who did not. Only 42% of patients in the intervention group learned to successfully self-manage but those who did had a significant reduction in hospital admission compared to those in the intervention group who did not (HR 0.44 95% CI 0.44–0.22 $P = 0.003$). Likewise, a study by Bischoff et al. [28] examined adherence to an action plan in patients with COPD given a written action plan as part of a self-management intervention. Patients were judged to have adhered to their action plan in only 40.1% of recorded exacerbations. When comparing exacerbations in which patients had adhered to their action plan to those where they had not, recovery time was reduced by 5.8 days when the action plan was used appropriately ($P = > 0.0001$).

Although the publication of the Fan study [29] led to concerns regarding the safety of self-management interventions in severe COPD, a meta-analysis of 25 trials of COPD integrated care including the trial by Fan et al. looking specifically at mortality showed no impact of these programmes on mortality (pooled OR 1.00 95% CI 0.79–1.28) [30]. Although these results are reassuring, it is important to keep in mind that, for patient with severe disease, behavioural interventions do have the potential to cause harm and must be designed, implemented and evaluated carefully. Close follow-up needs to be provided to patients with advanced disease and those with important co-morbidities.

17.2.2 Self-Management Effectiveness in the Context of Pulmonary Rehabilitation

Pulmonary rehabilitation provides clinicians with an opportunity to deliver education and self-management skills to patients with chronic respiratory disease. Self-management as a component of pulmonary rehabilitation is now recommended in the joint Statement of the American Thoracic Society and European Respiratory Society [1]. However, surveys from different countries have reported variations in the content and delivery of education sessions between programmes [31–33].

Few studies have actually tested the effectiveness of self-management included into traditional pulmonary rehabilitation programmes. Studies done in the context of pulmonary rehabilitation were excluded from the 2014 Cochrane review of self-management in COPD [17]. One study by Blackstock et al. [34] reported a trial of 267 patients followed for one year which showed no difference in exercise capacity, quality of life, dyspnoea, or respiratory-related hospitalization between patients receiving supervised exercise alone compared to those who received exercise plus a self-management education intervention. No difference was found in health-directed behaviour between the groups suggesting that the self-management intervention failed to change patient behaviour or in other words a "failure to intervene". However, in a trial by Norweg et al. [35] it was shown that exercise training combined with a structured behaviour intervention focusing on dyspnoea management strategies, and using activities identified by participants as causing dyspnoea, resulted in significantly reduced dyspnoea and improved quality of life compared to either exercise alone or exercise and didactic education. This last study suggests that to be successful, patients must participate in treatment decisions, challenges and goals must be elicited from the patient, and then specific problem-solving skills to address those challenges should be taught and practiced.

Only one study has described the successful adaptation of a self-management programme (Living well with COPD) for use in pulmonary rehabilitation, and conducted a comprehensive process evaluation of the adapted programme [36]. Table 17.1 presents the self-management programme <Living well with COPD > adapted to pulmonary rehabilitation with the key topics and patient feedback. The results of this study indicated that the self-management programme had good reach, and patients attendance during the programme was high; dose delivery and dose received were good, the programme could feasibly be delivered across a range of pulmonary rehabilitation settings (community and hospital); and the programme was accepted by health professionals and patients, who identified areas of the programme that worked well. Health professionals' delivery of the programme was not directly observed so the fidelity of the delivery could not be confirmed; however, patients showed improved knowledge, understanding and self-efficacy after the programme.

Despite the increasing body of evidence supporting the effectiveness of self-management interventions in COPD there remain significant gaps in our knowledge of how to design and best use self-management interventions in pulmonary rehabilitation. The heterogeneity of self-management interventions as well as patient populations studied leaves many questions still to be answered. However, what we do know is that to design and implement self-management interventions that are integrated, coherent, and have a strong likelihood of success, we must address issues related to the healthcare professionals involved (the case managers or health coach), the patient (patient evaluation), and the fidelity of the programme as a whole (quality assurance). The next section will discuss an approach to some of these practical issues.

17.3 Designing and Implementing a Self-Management Programme

17.3.1 From Traditional Patient Education to Patient Self-Management

Education is a central part of pulmonary rehabilitation, however to be effective, it must be modified from traditional didactic patient education, to patient self-management [2] (Table 17.2). Knowledge change alone is unlikely to lead to the behaviour changes that will improve health outcomes (e.g. smoking cessation, physical activity) or to effective self-management skills

Table 17.1 Facilitating education in pulmonary rehabilitation using the self-management programme <Living well with COPD>

Self-management education	Session/component	Activity/feedback
Education	1. Management and breathlessness 2. Energy conservation 3. Overview of the Action plan and Exacerbation 4. COPD medication and appropriate use of devices 5. Management of stress, anxiety and depression 6. Continuing exercise and self-management strategies	• 30–45 min/session • Educational material • Guide to the case manager/health coach • Posters • Cue cards booklet, written action plan for patients
Patient feedbacks	Improved knowledge and self efficacy	Managing COPD, breathlessness, psychosocial issues and exacerbations Conserving energy Taking medications, Taking part in exercise
	Peer support	Meeting other people with COPD Sharing of information
	Staff/Atmosphere	Friendly, approachable and helpful Fun/enjoyable
	Content	Clear, understandable and useful information Interactive and practical demonstrations Visual reinforcement
	Suggestions for improvement	Delivery, content, location, length of sessions, facilitators, supplementary materials, inclusion of family

Adapted from Cosgrove D, Macmahon J, Bourbeau J et al. [36]

Table 17.2 Important differences between traditional "patient education" and "self management"

Patient education	Collaborative self-management
Compliance-driven	Adherence-driven
Goals/problems/challenges identified by healthcare providers	Goals/problems/challenges identified by the patient
Information/advice is disease-specific	Information/skills are problem-specific
Theory: knowledge = behaviour change	Theory: confidence = behaviour change

Adapted from Bourbeau JS, Sedeno M.F., Lavoie K [2]

(e.g. medication adherence, inhaler technique, being able to recognize an exacerbation and use an action plan appropriately). Self-management, unlike traditional education, is patient-centric, and encourages patients to effectively incorporate disease knowledge, use self-management skills, and develop problem-solving strategies, in order to more fully participate in treatment decisions and better cope with their disease. If done well this approach can lead to greater patient motivation and confidence in their own ability to manage the day-to-day challenges of living with COPD.

17.3.2 Beyond the Self-Management Programme, Team Members and Their Roles

Programme factors beyond the educational content such as provider expertise and programme delivery, can have a profound impact on outcomes. Issues that must be considered when designing and implementing a programme include: coordination of multiple inter-related components, standardization of content and training, and consistent delivery using motivational communication techniques. Special attention must also be paid to quality control. Key points for monitoring should include how the implementation (content and process, i.e. coaching) is carried out by the members of the pulmonary rehabilitation team, and whether or not patients are adherent (attended sessions, follow-up, etc).

Self-management programmes have been proposed as the best way to assist patients in acquiring and practicing the necessary skills to control their disease symptoms on a daily basis and to implement healthy behaviours [37, 38]. A healthcare professional team should encourage and support patients to participate in the self-management intervention as part of the pulmonary rehabilitation programme. The specific members of the pulmonary rehabilitation team who deliver the programme can vary depending on the availability of professional resources. Duties of the healthcare professionals who deliver the self-management programme should include (a) leading individual and group education; (b) coaching patients in specific self-management skills and behaviours; (c) assessing patients during the course of the intervention and evaluating each individual patient needs and progress, and (d) making adaptations to the intervention(s) as needed over time.

A model for a self-management programme that has been shown to be effective has been to provide patients with a designated healthcare professional who acts as the case manager or health coach [17]. Importantly in the context of a pulmonary rehabilitation programme, this case manager must work closely with the rest of the pulmonary rehabilitation and exercise staff. Recently, it has been demonstrated that a behaviour-change self-management programme along with a case manager acting as a health coach, the use of long-acting bronchodilators, and pulmonary rehabilitation, not only influence exercise capacity but also improves the amount and ease of physical-activity performance in patients with COPD [39].

17.3.3 Expertise and Experience of the Case Manager

This healthcare professional should be selected based on defined expertise and experience and should undergo formal training specific to this role. Programme specific process measures using questionnaires to monitor patients' motivation, confidence, and movement throughout the stages of change, should be periodically assessed so that the case manager and pulmonary rehabilitation team members can intervene with the patient if these measures fail to respond to the intervention. The role of the case manager can be vital to the efficacy of a programme; however, there are currently no agreed upon qualifications or criteria for the selection of a health professional to fill the case manager role. The case manager should be selected based on their expertise and experience and ideally should undergo formal training before taking on the role. Experience working with patients with chronic respiratory diseases will definitively be an important foundation. Other areas of expertise which are relevant to the role include: (a) experience with patient education and in motivating and engaging patients; (b) excellent communication skills; (c) working well with an interdisciplinary team; and (d) being knowledgeable about local health and community resources. In addition to this, individuals selected as case-managers must be willing to learn on the job and be open to constructive criticism.

17.3.3.1 Role and Training of the Case Manager

The role of the case manager on the team and the importance of training have not previously been addressed in much detail. There is no accepted gold standard for the training required, and no evidence that specific training is effective. Table 17.3 presents suggestions of the role and training of the case manager based on recent trials [39, 40]. It is generally accepted that training in behaviour change and self-management skills is needed; however, the details of the training required and proof of its effectiveness remains to be shown. Case managers and members of the pulmonary rehabilitation team would benefit from having at least basic training in the principles of behaviour change, as well as basic training in motivational communication skills (how to engage, motivate, and build patient confidence). These brief interventions borrowing from

Table 17.3 Suggestions of the role of the case manager/health coach and training requirement for the self-management as part of the pulmonary rehabilitation programme

Role of the case manager	1. Lead with the other team members the individual and group education sessions; 2. Guide/coach the patient in self-management behaviours that aid in achieving physical activity and other self-management goals (medication adherence, exacerbations), while improving daily COPD management; 3. Assess/record the patient's progress throughout the study using patient worksheets for measures of stage of change, motivation and self-efficacy tailored to the patient needs and make adaptations to the programme as needed over time; 4. Use motivational enhanced communication strategies, goal setting, reinforcement; 5. Work with exercise staff to discuss patient goals and establish stage of change. 6. Provide direction to exercise staff for providing consistent message to the patient, evaluate barriers for a coordinated approach to the patient. 7. Reinforce skills during the exercise programme such as the ability of the patient to use their inhaler properly, using oxygen appropriately, and discussing changes that should generate or consider using the Action Plan.
Training[a] of the case manager	1. Training can be based on a self-management programme such as 'Living Well with COPD' which is designed to help patients with COPD and their families cope with their disease on a daily basis; 2. Reference guides 'Living Well with COPD' should be provided to assist the case manager/health coach in engaging with their patients and facilitating improved disease self-management; 3. Basic training in motivational communication skills should be provided as an important component of the training and includes: • using open questions and building motivation to engage patients in more physical activity and other behaviours, • using reflective listening to manage and overcome resistance, and • providing information by offering, sharing and asking patients for feedback.

[a]Training should be delivered to the other members of the pulmonary rehabilitation team

principles of motivational interviewing are not strictly speaking motivational interviewing and are better described as motivational enhancement. Additional studies are needed to better define the necessary expertise and validate the training required by the COPD case managers.

17.3.4 Standardizing Self-Management Content

Table 17.4 presents examples of specific skills that patients with COPD may need to master and specific health behaviours they may need to adopt and maintain in order to effectively self-manage, as part of the pulmonary rehabilitation programme. The number of sessions and content can vary but it is important to keep sessions short (no more than 1 h), ensure that the environment remains collaborative and friendly and that patients are encouraged to participate (see patient feedbacks Table 17.1). A written action plan would be an asset both to help the patient identify threats to their health, and to guide the case manager in monitoring and reinforcing the plan. The written action plan should focus on increasing physical activity and prompt recognition and decision making in the event of a COPD exacerbation. Patients are taught to recognize an exacerbation by the presence of a change (beyond usual the daily symptom variation) for at least 24 h in any of the following three major symptoms: dyspnoea, sputum volume and sputum colour. In this case, the recommended actions would include: (1) to make prompt decisions around the use of rescue medication; (2) to contact their healthcare provider for additional treatment such as antibiotics and/or prednisone prescription. Healthcare professionals and patients can register online in the Living well with COPD online platform (www.livingwellwithcopd.com) to access an example of patient educational materials (modules, brochures), reference guides and other tools for the healthcare professional (slides, posters, flipchart and a written action plan template, among others).

Table 17.4 Self-management skills and healthy behaviours for COPD self-management as part of the pulmonary rehabilitation programme

Healthy behaviour	Self-management skill (strategy)
Live in a smoke-free environment	Quit smoking, remain non-smoker, and avoid second-hand smoke
Comply with your medication	Take medication as prescribed on a regular basis and use proper inhalation techniques
Manage to maintain comfortable breathing	Use according to directives: • The pursed-lip breathing technique • The forward body positions
Conserve your energy	Prioritize your activities, plan your schedule, and pace yourself
Manage your stress and anxiety	Use your relaxation and breathing techniques, try to solve one problem at a time, talk about your problems and do not hesitate to ask for help, and maintain a positive attitude
Prevent and seek early treatment of COPD exacerbations	Get your flu shot every year and your vaccine for pneumonia Identify and avoid factors that can make your symptoms worse Use your plan of action according to the directives (recognition of symptom deterioration and actions to perform) Contact your resource person when needed
Maintain an active lifestyle	Maintain physical activities (activities of daily living, walking, climbing stairs, etc.) Exercise regularly (according to a prescribed home exercise programme)
Keep a healthy diet	Maintain a healthy weight, eat food high in protein and eat smaller meals more often (5–6 meals/day)
Have good sleep habits	Maintain a routine, avoid heavy meals and stimulants before bedtime, and relax before bedtime
Maintain a satisfying sex life	Use positions that require less energy Share your feelings with your partner Do not limit yourself to intercourse, create a romantic atmosphere Use your breathing, relaxation, and coughing techniques
Get involved in leisure activities	Choose leisure activities that you enjoy Choose environments where your symptoms will not be aggravated Pace yourself through the activities while using your breathing techniques Respect your strengths and limitations

Adapted from Bourbeau J, Nault D [41]

17.3.5 Standardizing Self-Management Delivery

17.3.5.1 Initial Individualized Self-Management Session

Usually, an individualized session by the case manager/health coach will be performed as part of the initial assessment of each patient, to determine their current knowledge, beliefs, skills and behaviours with the primary focus of defining with the patient what their personal goal(s) will be. This assessment includes the current level of physical activity, functional limitations and clinical barriers (including motivation). The patient's ultimate goal is defined at this stage as their desired achievements in work, home and/or leisure by the end of the programme. The case manager/health coach will guide the patient in defining and reaching their ultimate goals (e.g. what they will be able to do at the end of the programme, such as being able to play in the park with grandchildren). In some programmes, patients select and review their own personal goals and can sign a "learning contract" as a symbolic gesture to formalize these goals.

The exercise trainer, assisted by the case manager/health coach should give specific instructions to the patient throughout the exercise programme and provide guidance for the patient to perform exercise at home. Some may use an activity monitor, which can subsequently be used during the programme for setting intermediate goals (e.g. number of daily steps before the next session). An example of goal can be: *"Your first objective will be to add 1000 steps to your daily average. Maintain this level over a 1-month period. If you reach your goal, add another 1000 steps and maintain this for 1 month. Keep increasing your objective in this way, until you have reached 5000 to 6000 steps per day. If your condition allows it, you can keep increasing up to 10,000 steps per day."* The patient's progress can be recorded using a patient worksheet.

At the beginning of each education session, the case manager/health coach should use questionnaires, in order to assess and tailor the intervention to increase the likelihood of behaviour change: "Stage of change" (Fig. 17.1) for specific behaviours including also physical activity (which gauges readiness to engage in physical activity). At the end of each session, the case manager/health coach should ask a set of self-efficacy and motivation questions (0–10 Likert-type scales) tailored to specific behaviours, including physical activity (Figs. 17.2 and 17.3). Patient worksheets and patient-evaluation/programme-evaluation questionnaires should remain with the case manager/health coach and be accessible to other members of the pulmonary rehabilitation team throughout the programme in order to track each patient's progress.

Choose the number in this picture (1-5) that best describes where you are today with respect to your physical activity program: ________

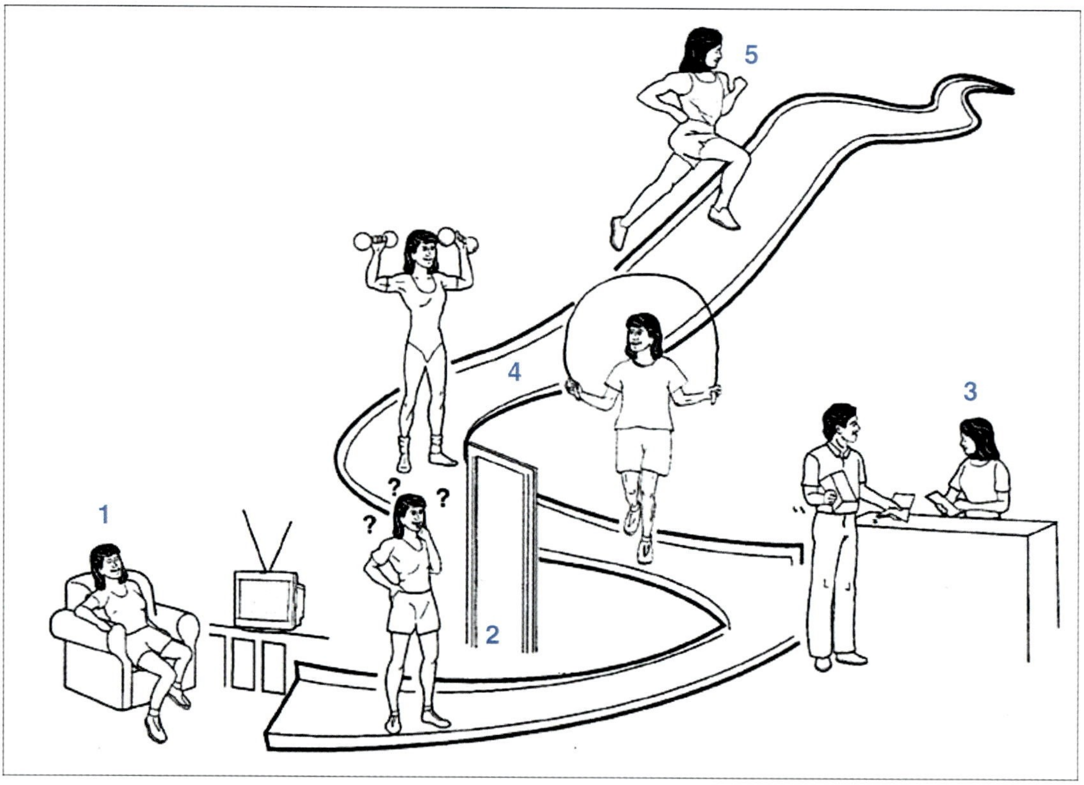

1 - I am not thinking about being more physically active
2 - I am thinking about becoming more physically active
3 - I am preparing to become more physically active
4 - I have started being more physically active
5 - I have been more physically active for a while

Fig. 17.1 Stage of Change Scale. Questionnaire (scale) "Stage of change" to be administered at the beginning of each education session in order to assess and tailor the intervention to increase the likelihood of behaviour change: for example specific behaviours such as physical activity to help the case manager/health coach gauging readiness to engage patient in physical activity

1	2	3	4	5	6	7	8	9	10
not at all important								very important	

	On a scale from **1 to 10**(1-not at all important, 10-very important), **how important do you think it is to...**	**Answer**
1	... maintain regular physical activity, at least 30 min per day or ______ number of steps?	
2	... avoid/reduce your exposure to factors in the environment that make your symptoms worse?	
3	... take your medications as prescribed (proper dose, right timing)?	
4	... use your medication inhalation devices properly?	
5	... use the breathing techniques and body positions to help you better manage your shortness of breath?	
6	... use the energy conservation principles to help you accomplish your daily life activities?	
7	... use the strategies discussed to break the anxiety-breathlessness cycle?	
8	... use relaxation techniques to better manage your stress and anxiety?	

Fig. 17.2 Motivation. Questionnaire (scale) to be administered at the end of each session; the case manager/health coach should ask a set of motivation questions (0–10 Likert-type scales) tailored to specific behaviours, including physical activity

17.3.5.2 Group/individual Self-Management Education Sessions as Part of the Pulmonary Rehabilitation Programme

In order to respond to the changing needs of individual patients with COPD as they progress through the pulmonary rehabilitation programme, self-management intervention should be flexible enough to allow for adjustments. These adjustments are based on feedback from the participants to the case management/health coach and other team members who participate in the sessions (individual and group). At the beginning of each individual session, the case management/health coach or the other healthcare professionals from the pulmonary rehabilitation team will: (a) welcome the participant to the session; (b) review with the participant his/her motivation to continue to pursue their physical activity goals and any other goals defined earlier by the patient(s); (c) discuss barriers and facilitators to continuing physical activity and other health behaviours, and possible solutions; (d) encourage patient(s) to set new personal goals (e.g. 30-min of physical activity per day or the number of steps as recorded by their activity monitor, whatever is determined to be a reasonable); and v) finally, thank patients for their participation and encourage them to continue to apply the skills learned throughout the programme. These sessions can be supplemented with the self-management focused patient materials. An example of such materials is the "Living Well with COPD" programme, which contains a variety of learning booklets on a comprehensive set of topics such as promotion of physical activity, COPD and medication, breathing and energy-conservation techniques, stress and anxiety management, and improving health behaviours. Patients can be assigned sections to read after each session, and each topic concludes with a series of questions to test understanding.

Comprehension, attitudes and skills should be assessed throughout the programme to determine if the patient(s) has met their pre-established goals and objectives. Several methods can be

Fig. 17.3 Self-efficacy/confidence. Questionnaire (scale) to be administered at the end of each session; the case manager/health coach should ask a set of self-efficacy questions (0–10 Likert-type scales) tailored to specific behaviours, including physical activity

1	2	3	4	5	6	7	8	9	10
not at all confident									very confident

	On a scale from **1 to 10** (1-not at all confident, 10-very confident), **how confident are you in your ability to...**	**Answer**
1	... use your pedometer to track your progress?	
2	... maintain regular physical activity, at least 30 min per day or ___ number of steps?	
3	... avoid/reduce your exposure to factors in the environment that make your symptoms worse?	
4	... take your medications as prescribed (proper dose, right timing)?	
5	... use your medication inhalation devices properly?	
6	... use your pursed-lip breathing technique with your daily activities?	
7	... adopt body positions to reduce shortness of breath?	
8	... manage your breathing during an acute attack of shortness of breath?	
9	... use coughing techniques to clear sputum from your airways?	
10	... use energy conservation principles in your daily life?	
11	... identify stressors in your life?	
12	... control your reactions when facing stressful situations?	
13	... using stress management strategies (e.g. relaxation techniques such as deep breathing)?	

used to supplement information and correct misunderstandings in a constructive way, as well as reinforce newly acquired skills and behaviours. These methods include direct open questioning, problem-solving exercises, simulations (patients demonstrate a proposed technique, such as using an inhaler) and direct observation. Throughout the session, patients should be asked to repeat key instructions and summarize in their own words what they have learned and understood.

17.3.5.3 Group Empowerment Self-Management Sessions in Post Rehabilitation

These sessions could be used to empower self-management and increase long-term maintenance of the learned skills and behaviours. The frequency of these sessions can vary depending on the resources available after the completion of the pulmonary rehabilitation programme. Topics could include a review of what has been done in the pulmonary rehabilitation. Short presentations (15 min segments) can be used to allow time for patients to review the content, interact with others in the group, and ask questions about topics important to them. These group sessions are also used (a) to identify any barriers that may have prevented patients from maintaining their physical activity goals and; (b) to allow the sharing of knowledge, ideas and experience between the participants. Peer learning is an important concept in education theory and is being increasingly employed in pulmonary rehabilitation with positive feedback from many of the patients involved.

17.3.6 Quality-Assurance for Self-Management

Quality assurance is the activities intending to improve the quality of care in either a defined medical setting or a programme. The concept includes the assessment or evaluation of the quality of care; identification of problems or shortcomings in the delivery of care; implementing changes to overcome these deficiencies; and follow-up monitoring to ensure the effectiveness of the corrective steps.

As part of a self-management intervention in a pulmonary rehabilitation programme, quality assurance is rarely considered or carried out. In real-life practice, we may have to prioritize assessing the most important components of the self-management programme based on the resources available for quality assurance:

(a) The required expertise of the case manager is crucial if not the most important.
(b) The standardization of the self-management intervention can be done by using existing and recognized self-management interventions such as Living well with COPD (www.livingwellwithcopd.com). This programme already includes all aspects already presented and a reference guide to self direct the healthcare professional in his/her specific interventions.
(c) The last and most challenging, it is to evaluate whether the programme has been delivered and the follow-up has been done as required, to provide any feedback to healthcare professionals and a continuous feedback loop.

Different approaches to implementing this quality assurance programme are possible, and the specifics will depend on each organization. Based on the self-management intervention content, standard forms can be used to monitor each of the points described above.

17.4 Conclusion and Implications

In this chapter, we have tried to provide a picture of what a comprehensive, well-defined behavioural self-management intervention programme looks like, and how it can be designed and delivered to increase the likelihood of effecting a change in patients' behaviours, including physical activity. Although there are studies of self-management intervention that have shown promising results, more work is needed to better understand how these programme can best be structured to benefits our patients across all care settings in real-life practice. We have given special attention to discussion of the healthcare professionals on the rehabilitation team, the case manager/health coach, the patient (including patient evaluation), and quality-assurance activities.

Pulmonary rehabilitation cannot stand-alone nor can its goal be only to improve exercise and functional capacity. Self-management interventions that go beyond education have been proposed as the best way to assist patients in acquiring and practising the necessary skills to control their disease symptoms on a daily basis and to implement healthy behaviours. Pulmonary rehabilitation is an optimal setting to initiate, support and empower self-management, and help patient to optimally manage and cope with their disease, to improve many of the poor outcomes often related to chronic disease.

The effectiveness of any complex intervention, such as self-management in patients with chronic respiratory diseases, crucially depends on the health-care professionals and the delivery of the intervention to the patient. There is still no accepted best practice for the level of qualification and training required, and no evidence that training is effective. However, it is generally accepted that training in behaviour-change and self-management skills are required. Another very important aspect of the self-management programme is the attention given to relevant "enablers" for behaviour modification in attempting to effect change in patients' behaviour, including levels of physical activity. It is well known that it is important to equip patients with the proper techniques and skills (e.g. knowledge and confidence) required to effectively self-manage their condition. Furthermore, enhancing patients' motivation to change and helping them overcome ambivalence is crucial. This is best achieved using patient-centred, motivational communication techniques that encourage participants to express their intrinsic motivations to adopt certain health behaviours (e.g. consistent with their values or life goals). Questionnaires to assess the process of change can be used by the case manager and healthcare professionals on the rehabilitation team. The use of these questionnaires (scales) at multiple time points allows the case manager and healthcare professionals of the rehabilitation team to evaluate the patient's progress and to help direct and individualize the self-management intervention. The results of these questionnaires inform the personalized delivery of the behavioural intervention to patients based on their readiness to change and progress through the programme.

Finally, we emphasized that in order to ensure the effectiveness of any self-management interventions not only must the behavioural intervention be clearly defined but also quality assurance must be carried out on a continuing basis. We recognize that this is often not planned nor done in many pulmonary rehabilitation programmes. It is often perceived as too challenging to do outside of formal trials due to resource limitations. However, without quality assurance we cannot know if the intervention is being delivered as intended. Quality assurance can start with a simple assessment of the programme delivered and can be developed over time from this initial foundation. This will require a change in the assumption that evaluation is only part of research towards an understanding that evaluation is an essential component of any intervention if we want to improve the way our interventions are delivered in real-life clinical practice settings.

References

1. Spruit MA, Singh SJ, Garvey C, ZuWallack R, Nici L, Rochester C, Hill K, Holland AE, Lareau SC, Man WD, Pitta F, Sewell L, Raskin J, Bourbeau J, Crouch R, Franssen FM, Casaburi R, Vercoulen JH, Vogiatzis I, Gosselink R, Clini EM, Effing TW, Maltais F, van der Palen J, Troosters T, Janssen DJ, Collins E, Garcia-Aymerich J, Brooks D, Fahy BF, Puhan MA, Hoogendoorn M, Garrod R, Schols AM, Carlin B, Benzo R, Meek P, Morgan M, Rutten-van Molken MP, Ries AL, Make B, Goldstein RS, Dowson CA, Brozek JL, Donner CF, Wouters EF. Rehabilitation AETFoP: an official american thoracic society/european respiratory society statement: key concepts and advances in pulmonary rehabilitation. Am J Respir Crit Care Med. 2013;188:e13–64.
2. Bourbeau J, Lavoie KL, Sedeno M. Comprehensive self-management strategies. Semin Respir Crit Care Med. 2015;36:630–8.
3. Effing TW, Vercoulen JH, Bourbeau J, Trappenburg J, Lenferink A, Cafarella P, Coultas D, Meek P, van der Valk P, Bischoff EW, Bucknall C, Dewan NA, Early F, Fan V, Frith P, Janssen DJ, Mitchell K, Morgan M, Nici L, Patel I, Walters H, Rice KL, Singh S, Zuwallack R, Benzo R, Goldstein R, Partridge MR, van der Palen J. Definition of a copd self-management intervention: international expert group consensus. Eur Respir J. 2016;48:46–54.
4. Colak Y, Afzal S, Nordestgaard BG, Vestbo J, Lange P. Prognosis of asymptomatic and symptomatic, undiagnosed copd in the general population in denmark: a prospective cohort study. Lancet Respir Med. 2017; 5(5):426–34.
5. Janson C, Marks G, Buist S, Gnatiuc L, Gislason T, McBurnie MA, Nielsen R, Studnicka M, Toelle B, Benediktsdottir B, Burney P. The impact of copd on health status: findings from the bold study. Eur Respir J. 2013;42:1472–83.
6. Huijsmans RJ, de Haan A, ten Hacken NN, Straver RV, van't Hul AJ. The clinical utility of the gold classification of copd disease severity in pulmonary rehabilitation. Respir Med. 2008;102:162–71.
7. Effing TW, Bourbeau J, Vercoulen J, Apter AJ, Coultas D, Meek P, Valk P, Partridge MR, Palen J. Self-management programmes for copd: moving forward. Chron Respir Dis. 2012;9:27–35.
8. Ries AL, Kaplan RM, Limberg TM, Prewitt LM. Effects of pulmonary rehabilitation on physiologic and psychosocial outcomes in patients with chronic obstructive pulmonary disease. Ann Intern Med. 1995;122:823–32.
9. Soicher JE, Mayo NE, Gauvin L, Hanley JA, Bernard S, Maltais F, Bourbeau J. Trajectories of endurance activity following pulmonary rehabilitation in copd patients. Eur Respir J. 2012;39:272–8.
10. Alison JA, McKeough ZJ, Johnston K, McNamara RJ, Spencer LM, Jenkins SC, Hill CJ, McDonald VM, Frith P, Cafarella P, Brooke M, Cameron-Tucker HL, Candy S, Cecins N, Chan AS, Dale MT, Dowman LM, Granger C, Halloran S, Jung P, Lee AL, Leung R, Matulick T, Osadnik C, Roberts M, Walsh J, Wootton S, Holland AE, Lung Foundation A, the Thoracic Society of A. New Z: Australian and new zealand pulmonary rehabilitation guidelines. Respirology. 2017;22:800–19.
11. Bolton CE, Bevan-Smith EF, Blakey JD, Crowe P, Elkin SL, Garrod R, Greening NJ, Heslop K, Hull JH, Man WD, Morgan MD, Proud D, Roberts CM,

Sewell L, Singh SJ, Walker PP, Walmsley S, British Thoracic Society Pulmonary Rehabilitation Guideline Development G, British Thoracic Society Standards of Care C. British thoracic society guideline on pulmonary rehabilitation in adults. Thorax. 2013;68(Suppl 2):ii1–30.

12. O'Donnell DE, Aaron S, Bourbeau J, Hernandez P, Marciniuk D, Balter M, Ford G, Gervais A, Goldstein R, Hodder R, Maltais F, Road J, Canadian Thoracic S. Canadian thoracic society recommendations for management of chronic obstructive pulmonary disease--2003. Can Respir J. 2003;10 Suppl A:11A–65A.
13. O'Donnell DE, Aaron S, Bourbeau J, Hernandez P, Marciniuk DD, Balter M, Ford G, Gervais A, Goldstein R, Hodder R, Kaplan A, Keenan S, Lacasse Y, Maltais F, Road J, Rocker G, Sin D, Sinuff T, Voduc N. Canadian thoracic society recommendations for management of chronic obstructive pulmonary disease—2007 update. Can Respir J. 2007;14 Suppl B:5B–32B.
14. Vogelmeier CF, Criner GJ, Martinez FJ, Anzueto A, Barnes PJ, Bourbeau J, Celli BR, Chen R, Decramer M, Fabbri LM, Frith P, Halpin DM, Lopez Varela MV, Nishimura M, Roche N, Rodriguez-Roisin R, Sin DD, Singh D, Stockley R, Vestbo J, Wedzicha JA, Agusti A. Global strategy for the diagnosis, management, and prevention of chronic obstructive lung disease 2017 report: gold executive summary. Eur Respir J. 2017;49
15. Bodenheimer T, Lorig K, Holman H, Grumbach K. Patient self-management of chronic disease in primary care. JAMA. 2002;288:2469–75.
16. Bourbeau J, Nault D, Dang-Tan T. Self-management and behaviour modification in copd. Patient Educ Couns. 2004;52:271–7.
17. Zwerink M, Brusse-Keizer M, van der Valk PD, Zielhuis GA, Monninkhof EM, van der Palen J, Frith PA. Effing T: self management for patients with chronic obstructive pulmonary disease. Cochrane Database Syst Rev. 2014:CD002990.
18. Agle DP, Baum GL, Chester EH, Wendt M. Multidiscipline treatment of chronic pulmonary insufficiency. 1. Psychologic aspects of rehabilitation. Psychosom Med. 1973;35:41–9.
19. Cockcroft A, Bagnall P, Heslop A, Andersson N, Heaton R, Batstone J, Allen J, Spencer P, Guz A. Controlled trial of respiratory health worker visiting patients with chronic respiratory disability. Br Med J. 1987;294:225–8.
20. Howland J, Nelson EC, Barlow PB, McHugo G, Meier FA, Brent P, Laser-Wolston N, Parker HW. Chronic obstructive airway disease. Impact of health education. Chest. 1986;90:233–8.
21. Kaptein AA, Fischer MJ, Scharloo M. Self-management in patients with copd: theoretical context, content, outcomes, and integration into clinical care. Int J Chron Obstruct Pulmon Dis. 2014;9:907–17.
22. Monninkhof E, van der Valk P, van der Palen J, van Herwaarden C, Partridge MR, Zielhuis G. Self-management education for patients with chronic obstructive pulmonary disease: a systematic review. Thorax. 2003;58:394–8.
23. Bandura A. Self-efficacy: toward a unifying theory of behavioral change. Psychol Rev. 1977;84:191–215.
24. Bourbeau J, Julien M, Maltais F, Rouleau M, Beaupre A, Begin R, Renzi P, Nault D, Borycki E, Schwartzman K, Singh R, Collet JP. Chronic Obstructive Pulmonary Disease axis of the Respiratory Network Fonds de la Recherche en Sante du Q: Reduction of hospital utilization in patients with chronic obstructive pulmonary disease: a disease-specific self-management intervention. Arch Intern Med. 2003;163:585–91.
25. Gadoury MA, Schwartzman K, Rouleau M, Maltais F, Julien M, Beaupre A, Renzi P, Begin R, Nault D, Bourbeau J, Chronic Obstructive Pulmonary Disease axis of the Respiratory Health Network, FdlresdQ. Self-management reduces both short- and long-term hospitalisation in COPD. Eur Respir J. 2005;26:853–7.
26. Bourbeau J, Collet JP, Schwartzman K, Ducruet T, Nault D, Bradley C. Economic benefits of self-management education in COPD. Chest. 2006;130:1704–11.
27. Fan VS, Gaziano JM, Lew R, Bourbeau J, Adams SG, Leatherman S, Thwin SS, Huang GD, Robbins R, Sriram PS, Sharafkhaneh A, Mador MJ, Sarosi G, Panos RJ, Rastogi P, Wagner TH, Mazzuca SA, Shannon C, Colling C, Liang MH, Stoller JK, Fiore L, Niewoehner DE. A comprehensive care management program to prevent chronic obstructive pulmonary disease hospitalizations: a randomized, controlled trial. Ann Intern Med. 2012;156:673–83.
28. Bischoff EW, Hamd DH, Sedeno M, Benedetti A, Schermer TR, Bernard S, Maltais F, Bourbeau J. Effects of written action plan adherence on copd exacerbation recovery. Thorax. 2011;66:26–31.
29. Bucknall CE, Miller G, Lloyd SM, Cleland J, McCluskey S, Cotton M, Stevenson RD, Cotton P, McConnachie A. Glasgow supported self-management trial (gsust) for patients with moderate to severe copd: randomised controlled trial. BMJ. 2012;344:e1060.
30. Peytremann-Bridevaux I, Taffe P, Burnand B, Bridevaux PO, Puhan MA. Mortality of patients with copd participating in chronic disease management programmes: a happy end? Thorax. 2014;69:865–6.
31. Camp PG, Hernandez P, Bourbeau J, Kirkham A, Debigare R, Stickland MK, Goodridge D, Marciniuk DD, Road JD, Bhutani M, Dechman G. Pulmonary rehabilitation in canada: a report from the canadian thoracic society copd clinical assembly. Can Respir J. 2015;22:147–52.
32. O'Neill B, Elborn J, MacMahon J, Bradley JM. Pulmonary rehabilitation and follow-on services: a northern ireland survey. Chron Respir Dis. 2008;5:149–54.
33. Yohannes AM, Connolly MJ. Pulmonary rehabilitation programmes in the uk: A national representative survey. Clin Rehabil. 2004;18:444–9.
34. Blackstock FC, Webster KE, McDonald CF, Hill CJ. Comparable improvements achieved in chronic obstructive pulmonary disease through pulmonary rehabilitation with and without a structured

educational intervention: a randomized controlled trial. Respirology. 2014;19:193–202.

35. Norweg AM, Whiteson J, Malgady R, Mola A, Rey M. The effectiveness of different combinations of pulmonary rehabilitation program components: a randomized controlled trial. Chest. 2005;128:663–72.
36. Cosgrove D, Macmahon J, Bourbeau J, Bradley JM, O'Neill B. Facilitating education in pulmonary rehabilitation using the living well with copd programme for pulmonary rehabilitation: a process evaluation. BMC Pulm Med. 2013;13:50.
37. Bourbeau J. The role of collaborative self-management in pulmonary rehabilitation. Semin Respir Crit Care Med. 2009;30:700–7.
38. Bourbeau J. Making pulmonary rehabilitation a success in copd. Swiss Med Wkly. 2010;140:w13067.
39. Bourbeau J, Lavoie KL, Sedeno M, De Sousa D, Erzen D, Hamilton A, Maltais F, Troosters T, Leidy N. Behaviour-change intervention in a multicentre, randomised, placebo-controlled copd study: methodological considerations and implementation. BMJ Open. 2016;6:e010109.
40. Bourbeau J, Casan P, Tognella S, Haidl P, Texereau JB, Kessler R. An international randomized study of a home-based self-management program for severe copd: the comet. Int J Chron Obstruct Pulmon Dis. 2016;11:1447–51.
41. Bourbeau J, Nault D. Self-management strategies in chronic obstructive pulmonary disease. Clin Chest Med. 2007;28:617–28. vii

Inspiratory Muscle Training 18

Daniel Langer

18.1 Rationale and Background

Notably, the most prominent exercise-limiting symptom of patients with chronic respiratory conditions is dyspnea [1] which is associated with avoidance of activities, with subsequent deconditioning [2]. Dyspnea is defined as an uncomfortable sensation of breathing [3]. The respiratory muscles play a key role in the perception of dyspnea [4–6] and in limiting exercise tolerance in patients [6–8]. Respiratory muscle dysfunction is moreover frequently observed in patients with chronic lung diseases [9, 10]. Several factors contribute to respiratory muscle dysfunction in these patients, including lung hyperinflation, hypoxemia, hypercapnia, inflammation, malnutrition, long-term use of corticosteroids, physical inactivity, and changes in the fiber type distribution in the respiratory muscles (Fig. 18.1a) [6–8, 11–13]. Lung hyperinflation is a major cause of respiratory muscle dysfunction in patients with obstructive lung disease since it places the inspiratory muscles at a mechanical disadvantage. In addition, many shared risk factors contribute to both respiratory and limb muscle dysfunction (Fig. 18.1a). Lung hyperinflation causes shortening of the diaphragm, so that the muscle is able to generate less pressure during contraction [14]. At the same time, the inspiratory muscles have to overcome higher elastic and resistive loads, especially during exercise. There are compensatory mechanisms present by which the respiratory muscles of patients adapt to these mechanical disadvantages and increased chronic loading (Fig. 18.1b). With these adaptations the diaphragm partially preserves its ability to generate pressure during normal breathing despite its shortened operating length and becomes more fatigue resistant [2, 15–17]. In response to chronic hyperinflation, for example, the inspiratory muscles adapt by shortening of sarcomeres, such that, at a given lung volume, pressure generation is well preserved or even increased (Fig. 18.1b) [18]. This is however not effective to adapt to acute changes induced by dynamic hyperinflation during physical activities. Other adaptations (e.g., changes in fiber type distribution) are generally believed to be responses to chronic overload (Fig. 18.1b).

D. Langer
KU Leuven-University of Leuven, Faculty of Kinesiology and Rehabilitation Sciences, Leuven, Belgium

Laboratory of Respiratory Diseases, KU Leuven—Campus Gasthuisberg—O&N1, Herestraat 49 Box 706, B-3000 Leuven, Belgium

Respiratory Rehabilitation and Respiratory Division, University Hospitals Leuven, Leuven, Belgium
e-mail: daniel.langer@kuleuven.be

© Springer International Publishing AG 2018
E. Clini et al. (eds.), *Textbook of Pulmonary Rehabilitation*,
https://doi.org/10.1007/978-3-319-65888-9_18

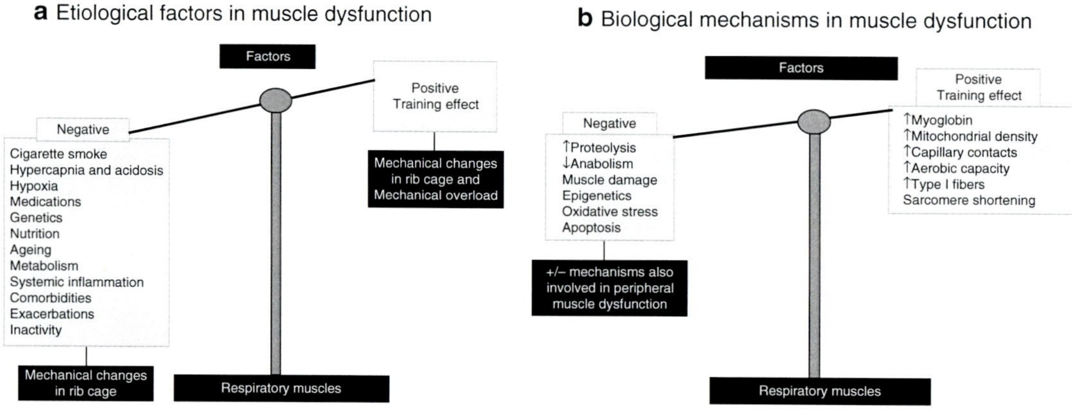

Fig. 18.1 Respiratory muscle adaptations in patients with COPD

In the respiratory muscles, etiologic factors such as alterations in the chest geometry and mechanical overload can to some extent counteract (training effect, right tray of the scales) the deleterious effects of the other etiologic factors of a more systematic nature (left tray of the scales). The factors mentioned on the left tray of the scales also contribute to limb muscle dysfunction in these patients. (b) In the respiratory muscles, several structural adaptation have beneficial effects (adaptive mechanisms, right tray of the scales), which partly counteract the deleterious effects of the other biological mechanisms (left tray of the scales). Reproduced with permission from: Arch Bronconeumol 2015;51:384–95 – Vol. 51(8). doi: 10.1016/j.arbr.2015.04.027 Recommendations of SEPAR Guidelines for the Evaluation and Treatment of Muscle Dysfunction in Patients With Chronic Obstructive Pulmonary Disease.

The compensatory mechanisms present are believed to not fully compensate for the deleterious effects on the respiratory muscles, especially in patients with severe COPD (Fig. 18.1a, b) [19]. Moreover they can quickly become overwhelmed when the ventilation requirements are acutely increased during physical activities. Not only are inspiratory muscle training not able to adapt to length changes brought about by this acute hyperinflation but they are also not trained to operate at shorter lengths and higher contraction velocities. The resulting imbalances between load and capacity of the respiratory muscles are closely related to the perception of dyspnea in patients with lung disease especially during exercise (Fig. 18.2) [20].

While highlighting these specific mechanisms that contribute to exercise limitation it is however also important to stress that in patients with lung disease, other factors besides dyspnea, mechanical constraints, and ventilatory limitation are relevant. These factors include peripheral muscle dysfunction and inappropriate increase in energy demands due to recruitment of abdominal muscles [21, 22].

Several pharmacological and non-pharmacological treatment options are available to enable the respiratory muscles of patients to better cope with these high loads, either by attempting to decrease the load on the respiratory muscles (e.g., bronchodilation or ventilatory support) or by improving respiratory muscle function [23, 24]. IMT has been frequently applied in the last decades to improve inspiratory muscle function (both pressure generating capacity and endurance) in patients in order to reduce dyspnea and improve exercise capacity [25].

18.2 Evidence

Different methods for respiratory muscle training have been applied in the past during pulmonary rehabilitation (PR). These include methods that predominantly aim to increase muscle strength, such as targeted resistive breathing [26], and

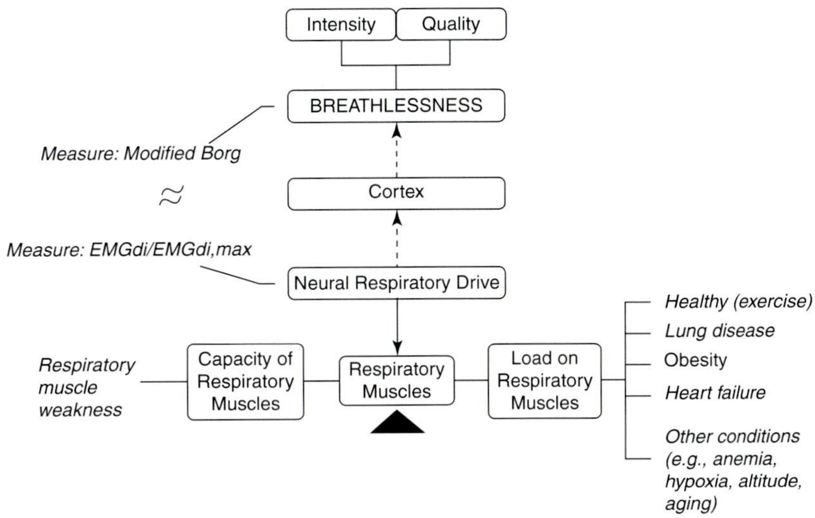

Fig. 18.2 The ventilatory load-capacity balance and dyspnea in COPD (Reprinted with permission of the American Thoracic Society. Copyright© 2016 American Thoracic Society. Jolley CJ, Moxham J. 2016. Dyspnea Intensity: A Patient-reported Measure of Respiratory Drive and Disease Severity. Am J Respir Crit Care Med; 193(3):236–8

threshold loading [27], as well as methods that predominantly aim at increasing muscle endurance, such as isocapnic hyperpnea [28]. Recently a hybrid between threshold loading and targeted resistive loading (tapered flow resistive loading) has gained more popularity [29]. We will discuss the different methodologies in more detail in the following paragraph. In general, the role of the respiratory muscle training in respiratory rehabilitation remains controversial, even after more than 40 years of research [30]. The available evidence in patients with COPD will be reviewed first. After that the (more limited) evidence available in other obstructive and nonobstructive respiratory disorders will also be discussed.

18.2.1 COPD

In terms of the demonstrated functional responses to IMT, three meta-analyses have been of key importance in patients with COPD [25, 31, 32]. The first meta-analysis by Smith et al. from 1992 has been very influential and has shaped the perception about effectiveness of this intervention for several years. The review included 17 randomized trials [32]. Across included studies small and non-significant effect sizes were reported: maximal inspiratory mouth pressure (Pimax): 0.12, $p = 0.38$; inspiratory muscle endurance 0.21, $p = 0.14$; exercise capacity −0.01, $p = 0.43$; functional exercise capacity 0.20, $p = 0.15$; and functional status 0.06, $p = 0.72$. This meta-analysis, however, took all studies into account, regardless of whether or not training load was controlled. A subgroup analysis indicated more consistent improvements in inspiratory muscle strength and endurance in those studies where targeted resistive loading with adequate loads was applied [32].

A second meta-analysis by Lötters et al. from 2002 more carefully selected only randomized controlled studies in which training load was adequately controlled during training, restricting intake to 15 studies employing loads of at least 30% of Pimax in comparison with either sham or no IMT intervention [31]. This meta-analysis was subsequently updated by Gosselink et al. in 2011 to include 32 randomized controlled trials (total $n = 830$; IMT: $n = 430$, control: $n = 400$) based on similar selection criteria [25]. On the basis of a methodological framework, a critical review was performed, and summary effect sizes were calculated by applying both fixed and random effect models. This approach more clearly demonstrated the effects of IMT. Indeed, both IMT alone and IMT combined with general exercise reconditioning significantly increased inspiratory muscle function (strength and endurance) in comparison with control groups. Dyspnea symptoms were also reduced. A trend for improved functional exercise capacity after IMT which did not reach statistical significance in the 2002 meta-analysis was found to be statistically significant after inclusion of more studies in the 2011 meta-analysis [25]. An overview of overall results from the 2011 meta-analysis including effect sizes and transformation of observed effects into natural units improvements is provided in Table 18.1. IMT studied in addition to a general exercise program improved Pimax significantly, while additional improvements in functional exercise capacity could not be demonstrated. However, subgroup analysis in studies combining IMT with exercise training demonstrated that patients with inspiratory muscle weakness improved significantly more than patients with preserved muscle function [25]. This observation may be of more general interest. Indeed, so far, most studies in this area have included all COPD patients, instead of selecting COPD patients whose outcomes are more likely related to inspiratory muscle function. Some phenotypes defined by stage of COPD, presence of inspiratory muscle weakness, degree of hyperinflation, severity of dyspnea, level of exercise intolerance, and reduced health status may be other important determinants of the response to IMT [30]. Due to absence of conclusive data it is however still unclear how to best identify patients that are most likely to benefit from the intervention.

A word of caution is required in relation to the interpretation of results from these meta-analyses. Pooling of results is associated with a number of methodological problems. These include differences in populations, study design, training interventions, duration of trials, collection of data, drop out, and other inconsistencies between the studies. A large prospective randomized study is currently ongoing which addresses most of these issues and should facilitate interpretation of outcomes [33].

Most current guidelines are not undisputedly positive on the application of IMT during PR. The most recent ERS/ATS statement on respiratory rehabilitation acknowledges that "current evidence indicates that IMT used in isolation does confer benefits across several outcome areas." [34] It stresses however also the lack of proven added benefit of this intervention as an adjunct to general exercise training in COPD. Based on this (lack of convincing) data the recommendation was formulated that "IMT might be useful when added to whole-body exercise training in individuals with marked inspiratory muscle weakness" [34]. In this context it is worth mentioning that many other add-on treatments to general exercise training, including, for example, lower limb strength training, have also failed to result in additional

Table 18.1 Overall results of the meta-analysis (Gosselink et al. [25])

Outcome	SES	95% CI	*p*-Value	Natural units
$P_{i,max}$	0.73	0.53 to 0.93	0.001	+13 cmH_2O
RMET	1.05	0.62 to 1.49	0.001	+261 s
ITL	0.98	0.72 to 1.25	0.001	+13 cmH_2O
MVV	0.23	−0.27 to 0.72	0.373	+3 L min^{-1}
Functional exercise capacity	0.28	0.12 to 0.44	0.001	6MWD: +32 m
Endurance exercise capacity	0.72	−0.12 to 1.55	0.087	+198 s
$V'_{O2,max}$ mL min^{-1} kg^{-1}	0.3	−0.02 to 0.63	0.067	+1.3 mL min^{-1} kg^{-1}
$V'_{E,max}$	−0.04	−0.3 to 0.2	0.696	−0.7 L min^{-1}
W_{max}	0.07	−0.16 to 0.3	0.562	+1.7 W
Dyspnoea Borg score	−0.45	−0.66 to −0.24	0.001	−0.9
Dyspnoea TDI	1.58	0.86 to 2.3	0.001	+2.8
Dyspnoea CRQ-Dyspnoea	0.34	−0.03 to 0.71	0.068	+1.1

SES summary effect size, $P_{i,max}$ maximal inspiratory mouth pressure, *RMET* respiratory muscle endurance test, *ITL* incremental threshold loading, *MVV* maximal voluntary ventilation, $V'_{O2,max}$ maximal oxygen uptake, $V'_{E,max}$ maximal minute ventilation, W_{max} maximal power output, *TDI* transition dyspnoea index, *CRQ* chronic respiratory questionnaire

improvements in functional exercise capacity or quality of life in similar study designs. This evidence has recently been summarized in a systematic literature review [35]. Quite in contrast to the similarities in available data the addition of lower limb strength training to PR is however generally encouraged [34]. It has been argued that priority during PR programs in the context of limited resources and time available should be given to the most effective components of the program (i.e., general exercise training) instead of spending too much time on add-on interventions with unproven additional benefit [36]. In the following paragraph innovations in training methods and equipment will be reviewed that might contribute to facilitate implementing well-controlled respiratory muscle training as add-on interventions during PR. Based on the currently available evidence, the recent GOLD guidelines acknowledge the potential benefits of respiratory muscle training especially when combined with general exercise training with evidence level C [37]. To provide additional evidence in support of more clinically relevant effects of IMT as an add-on treatment to PR carefully designed studies implemented in highly selective patient groups using the most appropriate outcomes will be needed [35]. A challenge in conducting these studies will be the considerable sample sizes needed to demonstrate additional effects on functional exercise capacity or quality of life on top of the large effects that will already be obtained in the active control groups (patients participating in general exercise training). It will therefore be necessary to selectively identify and include patients in these studies who are not able to benefit to the fullest from a standard rehabilitation program.

Two additional lines of evidence further support the beneficial effect on inspiratory muscle function with properly controlled IMT. First, Gayan-Ramirez et al. demonstrated in an elegantly designed animal model in rats that intermittent resistive loading resulted in type II fiber hypertrophy in the diaphragm [38]. Second, Ramirez-Sarmiento et al. observed an increase in external intercostal muscle fiber cross-sectional area and an increase in proportion of type I fibers in COPD patients following 5 week of resistive loading [39]. These studies both demonstrated that structural remodeling of the inspiratory muscles occurred with IMT. An effect of IMT on dyspnea is also expected on the basis of the pathophysiological observations made by Redline and colleagues [40]. They demonstrated in normal subjects that the sensation of respiratory force was related to the fraction of Pimax used in breathing maneuvers. Hence, increasing Pimax would be expected to reduce the sensation of respiratory force. Whether these concepts truly apply to patients with COPD has not been convincingly demonstrated. Recent data collected in patients with COPD has provided initial evidence on possible beneficial effects on breathing pattern and operating lung volumes during exercise in response to IMT [41, 42]. The adoption of a more efficient breathing pattern in combination with reduced neural activation of the respiratory muscles should improve neuromechanical coupling and might be related to improvements in exertional breathlessness in these patients in response to IMT [43]. More research on possible mechanisms explaining the reduction in dyspnea after IMT and on identifying the most suitable candidates for this intervention is warranted in the coming years.

The general conclusion for patients with COPD appears to be that, if properly applied, IMT improves inspiratory muscle function. Particularly in patients with compromised inspiratory muscle function these improvements also seem to translate into functional and symptomatic benefits. Based on clinical experience and the available evidence it can therefore at this moment be recommended to select motivated patients with impaired respiratory muscle function in whom dyspnea is an important contributor to activity limitation to participate in add-on IMT interventions during their PR program.

18.2.2 IMT in Other Obstructive Lung Diseases

The consequences of expiratory flow limitation and dynamic hyperinflation on the load/capacity balance of the respiratory muscles in patients with other obstructive lung diseases (e.g., asthma, cystic fibrosis, or non-CF bronchiectasis) are similar to those observed in patients with COPD. Differences exist concerning the prevalence and severity of respiratory muscle dysfunction between those patient populations. Volume and quality of available data are moreover not comparable to the literature available in COPD. In the following paragraphs the available evidence and applied training protocols in these patient groups will be summarized.

18.2.2.1 Asthma

Improving respiratory muscle function in these patients could help to prevent overload of respiratory muscles during asthma attacks and should relieve acute symptoms of breathlessness due to dynamic hyperinflation. Respiratory muscle function in non-steroid dependent asthmatics however seems to be on average less impaired than in patients with COPD [44–47]. The available data in terms of randomized controlled trials is less comprehensive and results are less conclusive than in patients with COPD. The results of 5 randomized controlled trials (total n = 113) were summarized in a 2013 Cochrane meta-analysis [48]. Except for a statistically significant improvement in Pimax no significant improvements in symptoms or dependency on medical treatment could be demonstrated. All studies applied either flow resistive or mechanical threshold loading with controlled training intensities (40–60% $P_{i,max}$). Vast differences were however present concerning training frequency and duration of IMT programs. With exception of a study by Sampaio and colleagues all subjects were categorized as having mild to moderate persisting asthma [48]. A further study by Turner and colleagues (2011) which was not included in the meta-analysis investigated the effects of 6 weeks of mechanical threshold loading IMT in patients with mild to moderate persisting asthma [49]. Patients trained twice daily at 50% of their $P_{i,max}$ (n = 7) or at 15% $P_{i,max}$ (sham-control-group, n = 8). The IMT group achieved significant increases in $P_{i,max}$ (+28%), endurance cycling time (+16%), and symptoms of dyspnea on exertion (−16%). No significant changes were observed in the control group. Due to the small number of participants, the between group comparisons did however not reach statistical significance. Larger (multicenter) studies performed in patients with more severe and persisting forms of asthma are needed to find out whether IMT can result in functional and symptomatic benefits in these patients.

18.2.2.2 Cystic Fibrosis

In analogy to patients with COPD ventilatory needs during exercise are increased for a given workrate in these patients. Airway resistance, increases in intrinsic positive end expiratory pressure, and decreased lung compliance with increasing breathing frequencies increase the load on these muscles [50]. Moreover in patients with CF insufficient uptake of nutrients in combination with a persisting catabolic metabolism due to chronic inflammation can contribute to peripheral and respiratory muscle dysfunction [51, 52]. In analogy to patients with COPD the higher load on the respiratory muscles is thus combined with a reduced capacity [51, 52].

Despite this solid physiological rationale for the application of IMT in these patients, the available database is limited. Only one further study has investigated the effects of IMT in patients with CF following a meta-analysis by Reid and colleagues performed in 2008 [50, 53]. Since this study investigated the effects of a combined general exercise and IMT intervention with a control intervention, it is however less relevant in the current context [54]. In neither of the two randomized controlled studies that were included in the meta-analysis (total n = 36) improvements in symptoms or quality of life were observed [55, 56]. Further studies would therefore be needed to find out whether IMT can result in symptomatic benefits in patients cystic fibrosis.

18.2.2.3 Non-CF Bronchiectasis

In analogy with COPD patients Koulouris and colleagues demonstrated a relationship between negative consequences of expiratory flow limitation on loading of the respiratory muscles, dyspnea, and reductions in exercise capacity [57]. Moran and colleagues observed reductions in respiratory muscle strength in most patients with Non CF-Bronchiectasis (NCFB) [58]. Owing to these similarities in pathophysiology between COPD and NCFB comparable rehabilitative strategies, including respiratory muscle training, are recommended for both patient groups [59]. The available evidence is however, similar to the situation in asthma and patients with cystic fibrosis, far less comprehensive than in patients with COPD.

Only two studies have so far investigated the effects of IMT in NCFB. Newall and colleagues compared general exercise training in combination with either IMT (twice daily training for 15 min each, starting at 30% $P_{i,max}$ weekly increase of resistance of ~5%, $n = 12$) or "Sham" MTL-Training (fixed resistance of 7cmH2O, $n = 11$) with a control group (usual care, $n = 9$) [60]. Patients were not selected for having respiratory muscle weakness. The larger increase in exercise capacity and respiratory muscle function in the combined exercise training/IMT group in comparison with exercise training /Sham-IMT did not reach statistical significance due to small group sizes. Only differences of both groups with the usual care group could be demonstrated. Liaw et al. investigated the effects of "stand-alone" IMT in comparison with a control group ("usual care") [61]. Patient characteristics and training program were very similar to the study of Newall and colleagues. Statistically significant improvements in respiratory muscle function were observed. Due to the limited group sizes (both $n = 13$) clinically relevant larger increase in 6-min walking distance (42 m) did however not reach statistical significance. These preliminary results found in very small studies are promising. Larger studies will however be needed to investigate whether IMT can truly result in functional benefits in these patients.

18.2.3 Restrictive Respiratory Disorders: Interstitial Lung Disease

Patients with ILD have to cope with higher elastic loads during breathing. In the ILD group, respiratory muscles, and in particular the diaphragm, are however less disadvantaged compared with patients with COPD, probably owing to the relatively lower EELV and more favorable length–tension characteristics [62–64]. Accordingly, resting MIP and MVV are greater, together with a greater diaphragmatic contribution to increasing ventilation [63]. Specific studies on the effects of IMT in ILD are currently not available. Only the combination of IMT and general exercise training in comparison to a control group has been studied so far [65]. There are however indications that improvements in peak tidal volumes after general exercise training programs in patients with ILD are significantly correlated ($r = 0.78$, $p = 0.001$) with improvements in V′O2peak values [66]. This has been attributed to the repetitive stimulus of high ventilatory demand during exercise sessions in combination with chest expansion during deep-breathing exercises and stretching of the thoracic muscles. This is consistent with a review paper that suggested a beneficial effect of thoracic expansion and stretching on pulmonary restriction in IPF [67]. It is likely that specific inspiratory muscle resistance will have a larger impact on these variables than general exercise training or normocapnic hyperpnea. It might therefore be worthwhile to study additional effects of IMT in this population despite the relatively well-preserved respiratory muscle function.

18.3 Implementation of IMT in Clinical Practice

18.3.1 Patient Assessment

Assessment prior to IMT requires measurements of inspiratory muscle function (strength and endurance) in addition to outcome measures such as dyspnea, exercise capacity, and HRQOL. Both maximum static inspiratory pressure that a subject can generate at the mouth (Pimax) and muscle endurance are often measured in specialized respiratory medicine laboratories [54]. Small handheld devices have however become commercially available for these purposes [68]. These devices have made it easier to perform these tests in less specialized centers or even in the home setting.

18.3.2 Strength

Measurement of Pimax is a simple way to measure inspiratory muscle strength in a clinical setting. Practice attempts are required because Pimax improves significantly with familiarization [69]. To standardize the measurement, it has been recommended to measure Pimax at or close to RV [54]. The test should be performed by a trained operator who should strongly encourage subjects to make maximum inspiratory efforts. Subjects are normally seated and noseclips are required. Because this is an unfamiliar maneuver, careful instruction and encouraged motivation are essential. Subjects also often need coaching to prevent air leaks around the mouthpiece. Once the operator is satisfied, the maximum value of three maneuvers that vary by less than 10% is recorded. The system requires a small leak to prevent glottic closure during the Pimax maneuver. The inspiratory pressure should be maintained, ideally for at least 2 s, so that the maximum pressure sustained for 1 s can be recorded. The peak pressure is on average higher than the 1 s of sustained pressure but is believed to be less reproducible [54, 70]. The pressure transducers should ideally be connected with a screen in order to display pressure-time curves and computations of the 1-sec plateau pressure. Flanged mouthpieces are readily available in pulmonary function laboratories and although they give values somewhat lower than those obtained with rubber tube mouthpieces, the differences are not usually considered important in a clinical setting [54]. In spite of many assumptions, the recorded pressure is believed to usefully reflect global respiratory muscle strength for clinical evaluation [54]. Sources of variation include type of mouthpiece, presence of a small leak, evaluated pressure (peak or plateau), number of trials performed, and lung volume from which the test is performed. Increases in $P_{i,max}$ have been found in response to specific training in comparison to control groups which indicates that the test is responsive to IMT interventions [25]. Twenty-two studies have been identified that provide reference values for MIP measurements collected in accordance with the abovementioned ATS/ERS measurement guidelines [71]. These data have recently been synthesized to provide age-specific reference values (Table 18.2) [71].

Comparison of $P_{i,max}$ before and after IMT allows clinicians to determine whether the training load was adequate to induce a training-related improvement in inspiratory muscle strength. A lack of change in $P_{i,max}$ is likely to indicate inadequate training loads. Improvements in muscle endurance have also been demonstrated after high flow, low pressure endurance training methods (e.g., isocapnic hyperpnea, for description of technique see next paragraph). There are however indications that higher training resistances tolerated during training result in larger improvements in endurance parameters [29].

18.3.3 Endurance

External loading protocols are frequently used to measure respiratory muscle endurance. These tests are characterized by the imposition of either incremental or constant submaximal inspiratory loads, sustained until symptom limitation [72]. Loads that have typically been applied in these tests include threshold loads [54, 72], or a hybrid between flow resistive loads and threshold loads (tapered flow resistive loading) [73]. Since performance during these

Table 18.2 Age-specific reference values for maximal respiratory pressure (average peak plateau pressure (95% CI) over 1 s measured from RV and expressed in cmH_2O)

Pi,max	18–29	30–39	40–49	50–59	60–69	70–83
Male	128 (116–140)	129 (118–139)	117 (105–129)	108 (99–118)	93 (85–101)	76 (66–86)
Female	97 (89–105)	89 (85–94)	93 (78–107)	80 (75–85)	75 (67–83)	65 (58–73)

Sclauser Pessoa et al. Can Respir J 2014;21(1):43–50

tests is influenced by breathing pattern (both timing components and inspiratory volumes), it has been recommended that these parameters should be controlled during tests [72, 74]. Since this adds complexity to the procedure, measurements of inspiratory muscle endurance have until recently been regarded as being beyond the scope of usual clinical practice [75]. It has been argued that these problems might be overcome to some extent by registering mouth pressure, flow, and inspiratory volumes during the test [54]. External work performed during the test has been put forward as the most dominant determinant of endurance time (t_{lim}), regardless of the pattern of breathing [54]. With the advance of new handheld devices capable of continuously registering flow, volume, and pressure responses, it has become feasible to monitor breathing pattern and external work of breathing during these tests [29, 73]. This has created an opportunity to implement well-controlled endurance tests into the standard clinical evaluation of IMT interventions. The protocol that will be presented here has recently been successfully implemented into a large multicenter trial evaluation of respiratory muscle function [33]. In short, during this constant load test patients are asked to breathe against a submaximal inspiratory load until task failure due to symptom limitation. It has been proposed that inspiratory loads should be selected that result in a t_{lim} of less than 7 min at baseline [72, 73]. In this way maximal post-intervention test durations can be limited to 15 min without important ceiling effects [72, 73]. Longer baseline t_{lim} data have previously been shown to result in ceiling effects. This lowered effect sizes of a constant load test (small to medium effect size of 0.44) in comparison to an incremental threshold endurance test (medium to large effect size of 0.68) in response to IMT [76]. Based on these data it was concluded that the threshold test might be more responsive to IMT interventions. Data from a large multicenter RCT however demonstrated a large effect size in endurance time (0.77) measured with the constant load protocol ensuring shorter baseline t_{lim} (less than 7 min) in response to IMT (Fig. 18.3) [33].

Standardized breathing instructions should be provided and post-intervention tests should be repeated using an identical load. Improvements in t_{lim} and total external work performed during the tests can be recorded as main outcomes of the test. Typical changes in breathing parameters observed during this test after IMT include [1] higher inspiratory flow resulting in shorter inspiratory time (Ti) and [2] increased inspiratory volume and work per breath [29]. While a shorter Ti could be interpreted as a breathing pattern adaptation that reduces the load on the muscles it also reflects the ability of the muscle to perform faster contractions against high resistances (i.e., improvements in muscle power). The observed increases in inspiratory volume and external work (both total and work per breath) are clearly not in favor of adopting a breathing pattern that would reduce load on the muscles. These changes are rather in support of the presence of true improvements in inspiratory muscle endurance capacity after IMT. They also reflect the standardized instructions given to patients on both occasions (pre- and post-intervention) to perform inspirations as fast, forceful, and as deep as possible. The same instructions are provided during training sessions. In summary, this constant load endurance protocol with standardized breathing instructions and registration of breathing parameters offers a feasible technique for implementing measures of respiratory muscle endurance into clinical practice.

18.3.4 Training Modalities

At this moment, there are few studies available comparing different training devices or training protocols head to head. Recommendations on preferred devices and training protocols for different purposes are therefore not supported by firm evidence. General characteristics along with potential benefits and disadvantages of the different methods will be discussed in the following sections. Three different types of loading have been used in most respiratory muscle training programs over the last decades. These approaches are either primarily aimed at improving muscle strength (intermediate

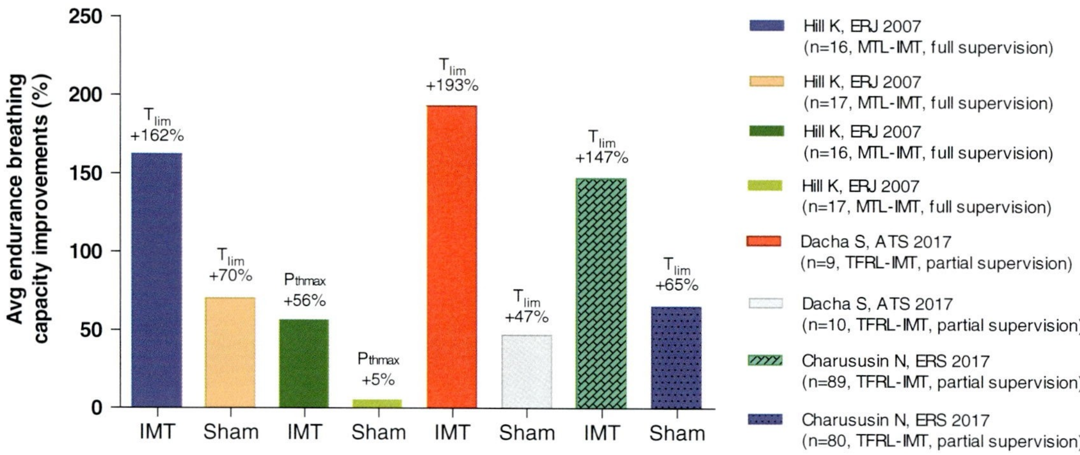

Fig. 18.3 Improvements in endurance breathing time from incremental (Pthmax) or constant load (t_{lim}) tests in response to high intensity IMT protocols in patients with COPD

flow/high pressure approach: targeted resistive loading and threshold loading) or muscle endurance (high flow/low pressure approach: normocapnic hyperpnea). For all these training modalities devices are commercially available that allow to offer controlled home-based training interventions. A fourth type of loading has gained popularity in recent years. This so-called tapered flow resistive loading can be regarded as a hybrid between threshold loading and targeted flow resistive loading. More recently developed electronic devices offer the availability to store data in an internal memory. These recent developments might help to facilitate better monitoring and control of home-based training interventions. A summary of the characteristics of available methods and devices is provided in the paragraphs below and in Table 18.3.

18.3.5 Targeted Flow Resistive Loading

In order to generate a sufficient training resistance of at least 30% of the maximal inspiratory mouth pressure patients are instructed to generate high inspiratory flows while breathing through small holes with varying diameters. The smaller the diameter, the larger the resistance that needs to be overcome. Since resistance will be flow dependent devices should be able to register inspiratory flow and to provide feedback on the achieved flow and pressure response ("targeted resistive breathing").

18.3.6 Mechanical Threshold Loading

During this method a known and fixed resistance generated by a spring loaded valve (isotonic threshold load) needs to be overcome before inspiratory airflow can be generated. After overcoming the threshold load an inspiration against this constant load is possible. This resistance, which should also be set at least at 30% of patients $P_{\text{i,max}}$ is not dependent on the inspiratory flow rate of the patient. A feedback-system is therefore less necessary. A disadvantage of this method (as with any isotonic limb muscle training) is the fact that the inspiratory muscles will only receive an optimal resistance (relative to their maximal pressure generating capacity) over a short fragment of their full contraction range. As an example let's assume that the $P_{\text{i,max}}$ measured at RV is taken as a reference to determine training intensity (e.g., training at 50% $P_{\text{i,max}}$ RV). On initiation of the inspiration at RV the training load will be optimal according to this target intensity. With increasing lung volume, however the constant load will represent an increasingly larger fraction of the maximal pressure generating capacity. This will prematurely lead to an isometric contraction which will eventu-

Table 18.3 Overview of different training methods and available devices

Training method	Focus	Costs	Feedback-system	Storage training data	Devices
Mechanical threshold loading	Strength and endurance	Low	NA	NA	Threshold IMT®; POWERbreathe Medic®
Controlled targeted flow resistive loading	Strength and endurance	High	Visual	Yes	Respifit S®
Tapered flow resistive loading	Strength and endurance	Moderate	Visual/accoustical	Yes	Powerbreathe (K-Series)®
Normocapnic hyperpnea	Endurance	High	Visual/accoustical	Yes	Spirotiger®

ally limit the ability of the muscle to perform further shortening. This will limit volume response and the ability to perform full vital capacity inhalations, especially at higher training intensities (50% $P_{i,max}$ and more) (Fig. 18.4). This has implications for the lengths at which the respiratory muscles can be stimulated during training. It is likely to also impact on the perception of inspiratory effort against a given load [29].

18.3.7 Tapered Flow Resistive Loading

This recently developed type of loading combines the beneficial characteristics of the two aforementioned loading approaches. After flow-independently overcoming a threshold load the resistance is subsequently flow dependently tapered down during inspiration. This accommodates the pressure volume relationship of the respiratory system and allows full vital capacity inspirations even at higher training resistances. This has been shown to result in higher inspiratory volumes achieved during training at comparable resistances in comparison with mechanical threshold loading (Fig. 18.4).

The training intensities during an IMT program that could be tolerated by patients with COPD in comparison with mechanical threshold loading were higher with this loading approach in comparison with mechanical threshold loading with comparable perceived respiratory effort scores [29].

18.3.7.1 Normocapnic Hyperpnea

In contrast to the three previously mentioned techniques, this type of training does not apply additional resistances to breathing that need to be overcome. In contrast, by stimulating hyperpnea at around 60% of the subject's maximal voluntary ventilation over a large range of the subject's vital capacity (deep in- and expirations) for longer durations (typical training durations of about 30 min) it stimulates the generation of high inspiratory and expiratory flow rates. This approach is supposed to mainly improve endurance and not strength of the respiratory muscles. To prevent hyperventilation resulting in hypocapnia home training devices have been developed which ensure normocapnia by partial rebreathing of the expired air. The execution of the training is technically challenging and coordination of breathing has to be practiced thoroughly [76]. It is moreover challenging to perform for patients with severe expiratory flow limitation. Based on principles of training specificity, this type of training is not expected to increase maximal pressure generating capacity. This was confirmed in the latest meta-analysis in patients with COPD [25]. Moreover the method did also not result in significant effects on dyspnea symptoms and functional exercise capacity [25]. Finally, advanced and rather expensive home training devices providing both optical and acoustical feedback seem mandatory to efficiently execute this type of training in the home setting.

18.3.7.2 Training Parameters

We recommend the use of either mechanical threshold loading, targeted flow resistive loading, or tapered flow resistive loading to train the inspiratory muscles during PR. Based on available evidence and the complexity of the normocapnic hyperpnea method, this training modality seems

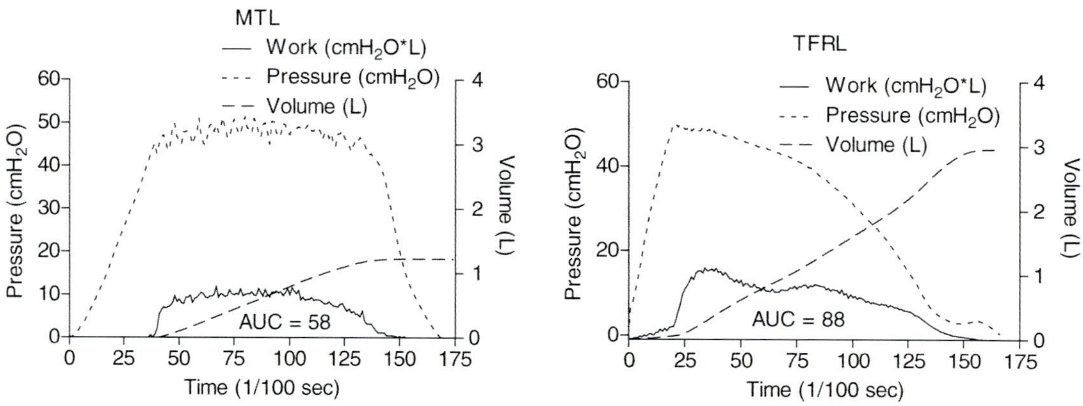

Fig. 18.4 Comparison between two training devices during a typical inhalation against a resistance corresponding to 60% of baseline $P_{i,max}$ (50 cmH$_2$O). *TFRL* tapered flow resistive loading, *MTL* mechanical threshold loading, *AUC* area under the curve for total external inspiratory work as integrated from mouth pressure (cmH$_2$O) and volume (L) signals over time

less ideal in this specific setting. Previously many programs were applied using mechanical threshold loading that consisted of 30 min of daily strength training at a resistance of at least 30% of the individuals PI,max. Recently, shorter, high intensity programs have been shown to be feasible and effective [29, 77, 78]. These programs reduce daily training time to less than 10 min and use intensities of at least 40% (mechanical threshold loading) or even 50% $P_{i,max}$ (tapered flow resistive loading). They have been studied under both fully and partly supervised conditions (supervision of one training session per week). Since the aim of the intervention is to facilitate breathing during periods of increased ventilatory needs (i.e., during daily physical activities), these shorter training durations should be well adapted to the functional requirements of patients during daily life. Activity monitoring of these patients has revealed that most daily activities of patients are carried out in bouts of less than 10 min [79, 80]. Training durations of 15 or 30 min seem to be less adequate in this context. Moreover these high intensity programs have been proven to result in large changes in $P_{i,max}$ (Fig. 18.5) and comparable improvements in respiratory muscle endurance (Fig. 18.3) in comparison to programs applying longer training durations [29, 77, 78].

One training session typically consists of 30 full vital capacity breaths against resistance and takes an average of 4–5 min to complete. Training takes place with the patient seated. Wearing a noseclip is not obligated. Patients are permitted to lean forward and fix their upper limbs on the arms of a chair or a table if desired. It is recommended that during the rehabilitation period at least one training session per week is supervised in order to permit the training load to be increased and to monitor compliance and progress. In case devices are used with an internal storage for data these supervised sessions offer an ideal opportunity to compare the quality of home-based sessions with supervised sessions. This will enable health care providers to provide patients with specific instructions. It is important to stress the importance of fast and forceful inspirations and the need to achieve the largest possible volume response with every breath. This will maximize gains in muscle power and increase total work performed during training sessions. As with other skeletal muscles, improvements in strength are likely to be dose-dependent [81]. Progression of training intensity by increasing loads over time is therefore mandatory. An initial training load should be selected equivalent to at least 30% of a patient's Pi,max. Loads of less than 30% of $P_{i,max}$ are insufficient to induce improvement in inspiratory muscle strength [25, 32]. A typical example of progression in training loads during IMT in patients with COPD is provided in Fig. 18.6.

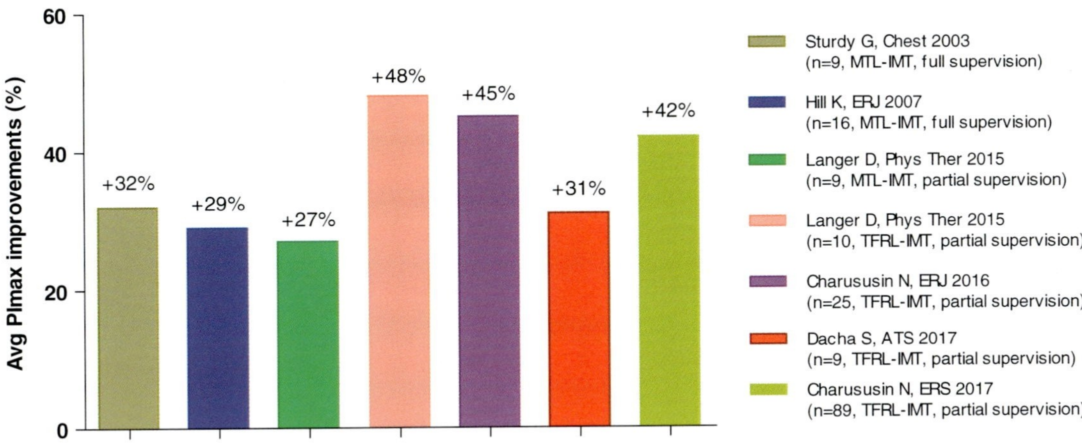

Fig. 18.5 Comparison of improvements in maximum inspiratory mouth pressure (Pi,max) in intervention groups in studies applying short, high intensity IMT protocols

Fig. 18.6 Progression of training intensity expressed as a percentage of baseline Pi, max. *TFRL* tapered flow resistive loading; *MTL* mechanical threshold loading. *$p < 0.05$ between groups. *Dotted lines* represent the highest average training intensities reached in the TFRL and the MTL group, respectively

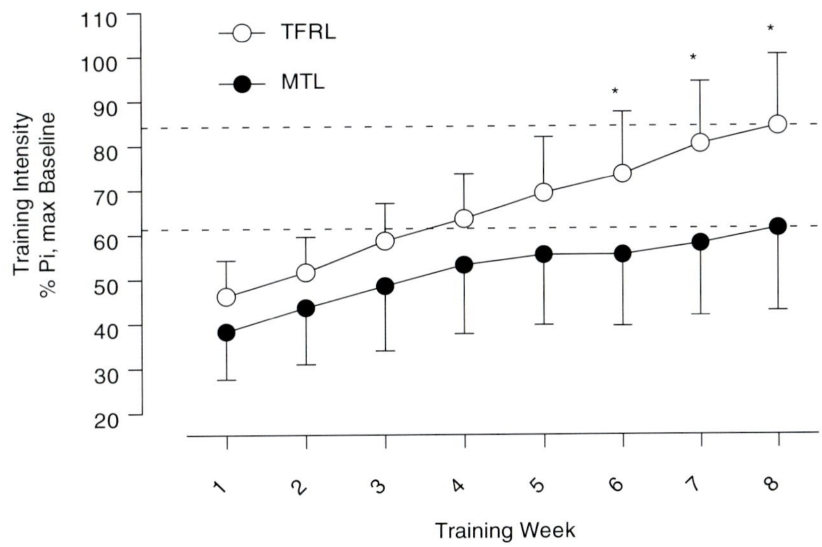

A symptom-limited approach is recommended to guide the progression of training loads. Selecting loads during which patients describe their respiratory effort at the end of a training session (after 30 breaths) as somewhat hard—that is, between 4–5 on the modified Borg Scale (0–10), seems appropriate. Patients can train at loads corresponding to a higher perceived effort if tolerated. One should aim for the highest tolerable load that still enables full volume expansion (full vital capacity inspiration). On completion of the first training week, patients are often training at loads equal to approximately 40% of $P_{i,max}$ with the mechanical threshold loading or 50% with tapered flow resistive loading (Fig. 18.6). The inspiratory load usually needs to be increased rapidly during the first 4 weeks of training, largely because of neural adaptations to training [81, 82]. Weekly adaptation and supervision is therefore strongly recommended during this initial period in order to optimize training response. Thereafter, the rate of increase often slows, and further increments in muscle function are likely to reflect gains resulting from muscular hypertrophy [39].

In the beginning of the program patients should be informed about the physiological rationale underlying the training (i.e., facilitating exercise breathing and reducing perceived breathing discomfort during endurance exercise training sessions and daily physical activities). They should also be informed about the expected training effects and physiological adaptations that take place in response to the training. When initiating the training the patients should not only receive information about the correct technical execution of the exercises, but also about hygienic measures that should be taken to maintain the equipment. Daily cleaning of mouthpieces and breathing valves by flushing these parts with tap water and regular disinfection of these parts are recommended to ensure hygienic training circumstances and optimal functioning of the breathing devices.

18.4 General Conclusions and Recommendations

Until recently well-controlled respiratory muscle training interventions were mostly restricted to the laboratory setting or specialized hospital environment and required extensive supervision in order to be performed effectively. Technical progress in training equipment and modifications in training regimens have however been made in recent years. These developments have been shown to result in effective and well-controlled training programs that can be offered largely unsupervised. These recent developments have the potential to reduce time investment for both health care providers and patients and are believed to contribute to facilitate implementation of respiratory muscle training interventions into PR programs in the coming years. Current guidelines acknowledge the potential added value of respiratory muscle training within the framework of PR mainly for selected patients with more pronounced respiratory muscle weakness. The additional effects on outcomes beyond improvements in respiratory muscle function when IMT was studied as an add-on intervention to general exercise training have mostly been reported in this selected group of patients. Better identifying those patients who are most likely to benefit from the intervention will be the most important challenge in the years to come.

References

1. Rennard S, Decramer M, Calverley PM, et al. Impact of COPD in North America and Europe in 2000: subjects' perspective of confronting COPD International Survey. Eur Respir J. 2002;20(4):799–805.
2. O'Donnell DE. Hyperinflation, dyspnea, and exercise intolerance in chronic obstructive pulmonary disease. Proc Am Thorac Soc. 2006;3(2):180–4.
3. Manning HL, Schwartzstein RM. Pathophysiology of dyspnea. N Engl J Med. 1995;333(23):1547–53.
4. Killian KJ, Jones NL. Respiratory muscles and dyspnea. Clin Chest Med. 1988;9:237–48.
5. Hamilton N, Killian KJ, Summers E, Jones NL. Muscle strength, symptom intensity, and exercise capacity in patients with cardiorespiratory disorders. Am J Respir Crit Care Med. 1995;152:2021–31.
6. Gosselink R, Troosters T, Decramer M. Peripheral muscle weakness contributes to exercise limitation in COPD. Am J Respir Crit Care Med. 1996;153(3):976–80.
7. Laghi F, Tobin MJ. Disorders of the respiratory muscles. AmJ Respir Crit Care Med. 2003;168(1):10–48.
8. Begin P, Grassino A. Inspiratory muscle dysfunction and chronic hypercapnia in chronic obstructive pulmonary disease. Am Rev Respir Dis. 1991;143:905–12.
9. Decramer M, Demedts M, Rochette F, Billiet L. Maximal transrespiratory pressures in obstructive lung disease. Bull Eur Physiopathol Respir. 1980;16(4):479–90.
10. Polkey MI, Kyroussis D, Hamnegard CH, Mills GH, Green M, Moxham J. Diaphragm strength in chronic obstructive pulmonary disease. Am J Respir Crit Care Med. 1996;154(5):1310–7.
11. Satta A, Migliori GB, Spanevello A, et al. Fibre types in skeletal muscles of chronic obstructive pulmonary disease patients related to respiratory function and exercise tolerance. Eur Respir J. 1997;10(12):2853–60.
12. Levine S, Kaiser L, Leferovich J, Tikunov B. Cellular adaptations in the diaphragm in chronic obstructive pulmonary disease. N Engl J Med. 1997;337(25):1799–806.
13. Testelmans D, Crul T, Maes K, et al. Atrophy and hypertrophy signalling in the diaphragm of patients with COPD. Eur Respir J. 2010;35(3):549–56.
14. De Troyer A, Wilson TA. Effect of acute inflation on the mechanics of the inspiratory muscles. J Appl Physiol (1985). 2009;107(1):315–23.
15. Similowski T, Yan S, Gauthier AP, Macklem PT, Bellemare F. Contractile properties of the human diaphragm during chronic hyperinflation. N Engl J Med. 1991;325(13):917–23.

16. Gorman RB, McKenzie DK, Pride NB, Tolman JF, Gandevia SC. Diaphragm length during tidal breathing in patients with chronic obstructive pulmonary disease. Am J Respir Crit Care Med. 2002;166(11):1461–9.
17. Rochester DF. The diaphragm in COPD. Better than expected, but not good enough. N Engl J Med. 1991;325(13):961–2.
18. Clanton TL, Levine S. Respiratory muscle fiber remodeling in chronic hyperinflation: dysfunction or adaptation? J Appl Physiol (1985). 2009;107(1):324–35.
19. Barreiro E, Bustamante V, Cejudo P, et al. Guidelines for the evaluation and treatment of muscle dysfunction in patients with chronic obstructive pulmonary disease. Arch Bronconeumol. 2015;51(8):384–95.
20. Jolley CJ, Moxham J. Dyspnea intensity: a patient-reported measure of respiratory drive and disease severity. Am J Respir Crit Care Med. 2016;193(3):236–8.
21. Aliverti A, Macklem PT. The major limitation to exercise performance in COPD is inadequate energy supply to the respiratory and locomotor muscles. J Appl Physiol (1985). 2008;105(2):749–51. discussion 755–747
22. Debigare R, Maltais F. The major limitation to exercise performance in COPD is lower limb muscle dysfunction. J Appl Physiol (1985). 2008;105(2):751–3. discussion 755-757
23. Marchand E, Decramer M. Respiratory muscle function and drive in chronic obstructive pulmonary disease. Clin Chest Med. 2000;21(4):679–92.
24. Langer D. Non-pharmacological treatment options for hyperinflation. In: Siafakas N, O'Donnell D, editors. Hyperinflation of the lung and its management. p. 90–100.
25. Gosselink R, De Vos J, van den Heuvel SP, Segers J, Decramer M, Kwakkel G. Impact of inspiratory muscle training in patients with COPD: what is the evidence? Eur Respir J. 2011;37(2):416–25.
26. Belman MJ, Shadmehr R. Targeted resistive ventilatory muscle training in chronic obstructive pulmonary disease. J Appl Physiol. 1988;65(6):2726–35.
27. Larson JL, Kim MJ, Sharp JT, Larson DA. Inspiratory muscle training with a pressure threshold breathing device in patients with chronic obstructive pulmonary disease. Am Rev Respir Dis. 1988;138(3):689–96.
28. Scherer TA, Spengler CM, Owassapian D, Imhof E, Boutellier U. Respiratory muscle endurance training in chronic obstructive pulmonary disease: impact on exercise capacity, dyspnea, and quality of life. Am J Respir Crit Care Med. 2000;162(5):1709–14.
29. Langer D, Charususin N, Jacome C, et al. Efficacy of a novel method for inspiratory muscle training in people with chronic obstructive pulmonary disease. Phys Ther. 2015;95(9):1264–73.
30. Decramer M. Response of the respiratory muscles to rehabilitation in COPD. J Appl Physiol. 2009;107(3):971–6.
31. Lötters F, van TB KG, Gosselink R. Effects of controlled inspiratory muscle training in patients with COPD: a meta-analysis. J Eur Respir. 2002;20(3):570–6.
32. Smith K, Cook D, Guyatt GH, Madhavan J, Oxman AD. Respiratory muscle training in chronic airflow limitation: a meta-analysis. Am Rev Respir Dis. 1992;145:533–9.
33. Charususin N, Gosselink R, Decramer M, et al. Inspiratory muscle training protocol for patients with chronic obstructive pulmonary disease (IMTCO study): a multicentre randomised controlled trial. BMJ Open. 2013;3(8):e003101.
34. Spruit MA, Singh SJ, Garvey C, et al. An official American Thoracic Society/European Respiratory Society statement: key concepts and advances in pulmonary rehabilitation. Am J Respir Crit Care Med. 2013;188(8):e13–64.
35. Camillo CA, Osadnik CR, van Remoortel H, Burtin C, Janssens W, Troosters T. Effect of "add-on" interventions on exercise training in individuals with COPD: a systematic review. ERJ Open Res. 2016;2(1). pii: 00078-2015.
36. Polkey MI, Moxham J, Green M. The case against inspiratory muscle training in COPD. Eur Respir J. 2011;37(2):236–7.
37. Vogelmeier CF, Criner GJ, Martinez FJ, et al. Global strategy for the diagnosis, management, and prevention of chronic obstructive lung disease 2017 report: GOLD executive summary. Eur Respir J. 2017;49(3).
38. Gayan-Ramirez G, Rollier H, Vanderhoydonc F, Verhoeven G, Gosselink R, Decramer M. Nandrolone decanoate does not enhance training effects but increases IGF-I mRNA in rat diaphragm. J Appl Physiol (1985). 2000;88(1):26–34.
39. Ramirez-Sarmiento A, Orozco-Levi M, Guell R, et al. Inspiratory muscle training in patients with chronic obstructive pulmonary disease: structural adaptation and physiologic outcomes. Am J Respir Crit Care Med. 2002;166(11):1491–7.
40. Redline S, Gottfried SB, Altose MD. Effects of changes in inspiratory muscle strength on the sensation of respiratory force. J Appl Physiol (1985). 1991;70(1):240–5.
41. Charususin N, Gosselink R, McConnell A, et al. Inspiratory muscle training improves breathing pattern during exercise in COPD patients. Eur Respir J. 2016;47(4):1261–4.
42. Petrovic M, Reiter M, Zipko H, Pohl W, Wanke T. Effects of inspiratory muscle training on dynamic hyperinflation in patients with COPD. Int J Chron Obstruct Pulmon Dis. 2012;7:797–805.
43. Langer D, Ciavaglia C, Webb K, et al. Inspiratory muscle training reduces respiratory neural drive in patients with COPD. Eur Respir J. 2014;44(Suppl 58):1912.
44. Perez T, Becquart LA, Stach B, Wallaert B, Tonnel AB. Inspiratory muscle strength and endurance in steroid-dependent asthma. Am J Respir Crit Care Med. 1996;153:610–5.
45. Stell IM, Polkey MI, Rees PJ, Green M, Moxham J. Inspiratory muscle strength in acute asthma. Chest. 2001;120(3):757–64.

46. Lavietes MH, Grocela JA, Maniatis T, Potulski F, Ritter AB, Sunderam G. Inspiratory muscle strength in asthma. Chest. 1988;93(5):1043–8.
47. McKenzie DK, Gandevia SC. Strength and endurance of inspiratory, expiratory, and limb muscles in asthma. Am Rev Respir Dis. 1986;134(5):999–1004.
48. Silva IS, Fregonezi GA, Dias FA, Ribeiro CT, Guerra RO, Ferreira GM. Inspiratory muscle training for asthma. Cochrane Database Syst Rev. 2013;9:CD003792.
49. Turner LA, Mickleborough TD, McConnell AK, Stager JM, Tecklenburg-Lund S, Lindley MR. Effect of inspiratory muscle training on exercise tolerance in asthmatic individuals. Med Sci Sports Exerc. 2011;43(11):2031–8.
50. Reid WD, Geddes EL, O'Brien K, Brooks D, Crowe J. Effects of inspiratory muscle training in cystic fibrosis: a systematic review. Clin Rehabil. 2008;22(10–11):1003–13.
51. Pinet C, Cassart M, Scillia P, et al. Function and bulk of respiratory and limb muscles in patients with cystic fibrosis. Am J Respir Crit Care Med. 2003;168(8):989–94.
52. Ionescu AA, Chatham K, Davies CA, Nixon LS, Enright S, Shale DJ. Inspiratory muscle function and body composition in cystic fibrosis. Am J Respir Crit Care Med. 1998;158(4):1271–6.
53. Santana-Sosa E, Gonzalez-Saiz L, Groeneveld IF, et al. Benefits of combining inspiratory muscle with 'whole muscle' training in children with cystic fibrosis: a randomised controlled trial. Br J Sports Med. 2014;48(20):1513–7.
54. American Thoracic Society. ERS ATS/ERS Statement on respiratory muscle testing. Am J Respir Crit Care Med. 2002;166(4):518–624.
55. Enright S, Chatham K, Ionescu AA, Unnithan VB, Shale DJ. Inspiratory muscle training improves lung function and exercise capacity in adults with cystic fibrosis. Chest. 2004;126(2):405–11.
56. de Jong W, van Aalderen WM, Kraan J, Koeter GH, van der Schans CP. Inspiratory muscle training in patients with cystic fibrosis. Respir Med. 2001;95(1):31–6.
57. Koulouris NG, Retsou S, Kosmas E, et al. Tidal expiratory flow limitation, dyspnoea and exercise capacity in patients with bilateral bronchiectasis. Eur Respir J. 2003;21(5):743–8.
58. Moran F, Piper A, Elborn JS, Bradley JM. Respiratory muscle pressures in non-CF bronchiectasis: repeatability and reliability. Chron Respir Dis. 2010;7(3):165–71.
59. Rochester CL, Fairburn C, Crouch RH. Pulmonary rehabilitation for respiratory disorders other than chronic obstructive pulmonary disease. Clin Chest Med. 2014;35(2):369–89.
60. Newall C, Stockley RA, Hill SL. Exercise training and inspiratory muscle training in patients with bronchiectasis. Thorax. 2005;60(11):943–8.
61. Liaw MY, Wang YH, Tsai YC, et al. Inspiratory muscle training in bronchiectasis patients: a prospective randomized controlled study. Clin Rehabil. 2011;25(6):524–36.
62. de Troyer A, Yernault JC. Inspiratory muscle force in normal subjects and patients with interstitial lung disease. Thorax. 1980;35(2):92–100.
63. Faisal A, Alghamdi BJ, Ciavaglia CE, et al. Common mechanisms of dyspnea in chronic interstitial and obstructive lung disorders. Am J Respir Crit Care Med. 2016;193(3):299–309.
64. O'Donnell DE, Chau LK, Webb KA. Qualitative aspects of exertional dyspnea in patients with interstitial lung disease. J Appl Physiol (1985). 1998;84(6):2000–9.
65. Jastrzebski D, Kozielski J, Zebrowska A. Pulmonary rehabilitation in patients with idiopathic pulmonary fibrosis with inspiratory muscle training. Pneumonol Alergol Pol. 2008;76(3):131–41.
66. Vainshelboim B, Oliveira J, Yehoshua L, et al. Exercise training-based pulmonary rehabilitation program is clinically beneficial for idiopathic pulmonary fibrosis. Respiration. 2014;88(5):378–88.
67. Kenn K, Gloeckl R, Behr J. Pulmonary rehabilitation in patients with idiopathic pulmonary fibrosis—a review. Respiration. 2013;86(2):89–99.
68. Hamnegard CH, Wragg S, Kyroussis D, Aquilina R, Moxham J, Green M. Portable measurement of maximum mouth pressures. Eur Respir J. 1994;7(2):398–401.
69. Larson JL, Covey MK, Vitalo CA, Alex CG, Patel M, Kim MJ. Maximal inspiratory pressure. Learning effect and test-retest reliability in patients with chronic obstructive pulmonary disease. Chest. 1993;104(2):448–53.
70. Windisch W, Hennings E, Sorichter S, Hamm H, Criee CP. Peak or plateau maximal inspiratory mouth pressure: which is best? Eur Respir J. 2004;23(5):708–13.
71. Sclauser Pessoa IM, Franco Parreira V, Fregonezi GA, Sheel AW, Chung F, Reid WD. Reference values for maximal inspiratory pressure: a systematic review. Can Respir J. 2014;21(1):43–50.
72. Hill K, Jenkins SC, Philippe DL, Shepherd KL, Hillman DR, Eastwood PR. Comparison of incremental and constant load tests of inspiratory muscle endurance in COPD. Eur Respir J. 2007;30(3):479–86.
73. Langer D, Jacome C, Charususin N, et al. Measurement validity of an electronic inspiratory loading device during a loaded breathing task in patients with COPD. Respir Med. 2013;107(4):633–5.
74. Hart N, Hawkins P, Hamnegard CH, Green M, Moxham J, Polkey MI. A novel clinical test of respiratory muscle endurance. Eur Respir J. 2002;19(2):232–9.
75. Hill K, Cecins NM, Eastwood PR, Jenkins SC. Inspiratory muscle training for patients with chronic obstructive pulmonary disease: a practical guide for clinicians. Arch Phys Med Rehabil. 2010;91(9):1466–70.

76. Göhl O, Walker DJ, Walterspacher S, et al. Respiratory muscle training: state of the art. Pneumologie. 2016;70(1):37–48.
77. Hill K, Jenkins SC, Philippe DL, et al. High-intensity inspiratory muscle training in COPD. Eur Respir J. 2006;27(6):1119–28.
78. Sturdy G, Hillman D, Green D, Jenkins S, Cecins N, Eastwood P. Feasibility of high-intensity, interval-based respiratory muscle training in COPD. Chest. 2003;123(1):142–50.
79. Donaire-Gonzalez D, Gimeno-Santos E, Balcells E, et al. Physical activity in COPD patients: patterns and bouts. Eur Respir J. 2013;42(4):993–1002.
80. van Remoortel H, Camillo CA, Langer D, et al. Moderate intense physical activity depends on selected metabolic equivalent of task (MET) cut-off and type of data analysis. PLoS One. 2013;8(12):e84365.
81. Kraemer WJ, Fleck SJ, Evans WJ. Strength and power training: physiological mechanisms of adaptation. Exerc Sport Sci Rev. 1996;24:363–97.
82. Huang CH, Martin AD, Davenport PW. Effect of inspiratory muscle strength training on inspiratory motor drive and RREP early peak components. J Appl Physiol (1985). 2003;94(2):462–8.

Part V

Outcomes and Expected Results

Patient-Centered Outcomes 19

Karina C. Furlanetto, Nidia A. Hernandes,
and Fabio Pitta

19.1 Introduction

As common sense, the term "patient-centered outcomes" can be understood as outcomes from healthcare that are important to patients. Patient-centered outcomes involve both physiological and psychological outcomes which are usually quantified by a variety of assessment tools. These key measures are applied for patient assessment and measurement of change or impact of interventions (e.g., pulmonary rehabilitation [PR]) in patients with chronic respiratory disease.

This chapter describes different outcomes involving the following assessment domains: lung function and respiratory muscle force, symptoms, exercise capacity, peripheral muscle force, balance, body composition, quality of life, anxiety, depression, functional status, physical activity in daily life, and self-efficacy. Each of these assessment domains has its own characteristics and interpretation. In common, the authors aimed to identify the most widely used tests to assess that outcome, providing an overview of its use and its minimal important difference (MID), when available. The MID is the smallest difference in a measurable clinical parameter that indicates a meaningful change in the condition for better or for worse, as perceived by the patient, clinician, or investigator. It is advisable to avoid using group MIDs in the context of individual patients, since they rather reflect group responses.

In the context of PR, patient-centered outcomes are useful to characterize individuals and populations, assess the impact of programs, and follow the course of the treatment, as well as the course of the disease itself. Most of the tools which measure these outcomes, as described in this chapter, pertain predominantly to patients with chronic obstructive pulmonary disease (COPD), although most of these items can be directly indicated for use in other populations with chronic respiratory diseases as well.

19.2 Lung Function

Although lung function, specially the forced expiratory volume in the first second (FEV_1), is essential to diagnose and to determine disease severity in COPD, it is clear in the literature that PR does not generate an important effect on measures of pulmonary function. Since the first studies in this field, results showed that short- or long-term PR programs were effective for improving exercise capacity, quality of life, and symptoms, but with no clinically relevant changes in lung function [1, 2]. The American Thoracic Society–European Respiratory Society

K.C. Furlanetto • N.A. Hernandes • F. Pitta (✉)
Departamento de Fisioterapia,
Universidade Estadual de Londrina,
Londrina, Parana, Brazil
e-mail: karinafurlanetto@gmail.com;
nyhernandes@gmail.com; fabiopitta@uol.com.br

© Springer International Publishing AG 2018
E. Clini et al. (eds.), *Textbook of Pulmonary Rehabilitation*,
https://doi.org/10.1007/978-3-319-65888-9_19

(ATS-ERS) statement on pulmonary rehabilitation [3] is also clear when affirming that "improvements in skeletal muscle function after exercise training lead to gains in exercise capacity despite the absence of changes in lung function." Hence, it is not advisable to use parameters of lung function, such as forced vital capacity (FVC) and FEV_1, as outcomes of PR, albeit their assessment is very important to diagnose the disease and follow its progression over time.

Despite the absence of effects of PR on lung function, a recent study [4] has raised an important point of discussion: the influence of PR associated to optimal pharmacotherapy in the decline of FEV_1 over time. Data published about the FIRST study [4], a prospective observational study conducted in Italy, showed that a group of patients with COPD receiving only pharmacotherapy (inhaled corticosteroids and/or long-acting beta 2 agonist and/or tiotropium) (control group), in comparison to patients undergoing PR (repeated programs of 6 weeks of duration over 3 years) and pharmacotherapy, presented a larger decline in FEV_1 over 3 years. In addition, the authors observed that among patients who received PR there was no difference in FEV1 decline comparing current smokers with never smoker patients, and comparing those with at least one acute exacerbation with no exacerbation during the follow-up period. Thus, it appears that rehabilitation should not aim at improving lung function, but at controlling its progression. Certainly, more studies are necessary to reinforce these findings.

19.3 Symptoms

Symptoms frequently reported by patients with chronic respiratory disease are dyspnea, cough, sputum production, weakness, fatigue, and psychological distress. Among them, dyspnea (at rest and/or during exertion) is considered the more disabling symptom; thus, reducing dyspnea is one of the principal goals of PR. In recent years, studies consistently showed positive effects of this intervention in reducing intensity of breathlessness (Evidence A) [3, 5].

There are several instruments available to evaluate symptoms in PR. In general, these instruments are questionnaires which assess presence, severity, and impact of symptoms. Some specific questionnaires validated for patients with COPD are: Chronic Respiratory Disease Questionnaire (CRQ) (fatigue and dyspnea subscales), Modified Pulmonary Functional Status and Dyspnea Questionnaire (PFSDQ-M) (dyspnea and fatigue domains), Saint George Respiratory Questionnaire (SGRQ) (symptoms domain), Baseline and Transitional Dyspnea Indexes (BDI and TDI), and COPD Assessment Test (CAT), among others [3]. All of the abovementioned instruments had its MID published and they are listed in the Box 19.1. Although the Medical Research Council (MRC) scale is largely used to assess dyspnea in pulmonary rehabilitation settings due to its good capacity to categorize patients according to the severity of their breathlessness, it is limited to evaluate the effect of intervention due to its reduced number of options. Since the scale has only five levels of limitation due to dyspnea, this may not be enough to detect moderate changes after PR [6].

CAT COPD assessment test; *CRQ* chronic respiratory disease questionnaire; *MDI* minimal important difference; *PFSD-Q* modified pulmonary functional status and dyspnea questionnaire; *SGRQ* saint george respiratory questionnaire; *TDI* transitional dyspnea index

The benefits of PR in terms of reduction of symptoms are well reported in the literature. In the recent update of their Cochrane Review about effects of pulmonary rehabilitation, McCarthy and colleagues demonstrated that at least 4 weeks of rehabilitation based on exercise therapy associated or not with educational or psychological support induce the reduction of COPD symptoms. The review showed effect sizes of 0.68

Box 19.1 Minimal important difference for instruments used to assess symptoms in COPD

Instrument	MID
CAT [7]	2 units
CRQ [8]	0.5 unit (per subscale)
PFSDQ-M [9]	5 units (per domain)
SGRQ [10]	4 units (per domain)
TDI [11]	1 unit

[95% CI: 0.45; 0.92] and 0.79 [0.56; 1.03] for the CRQ fatigue and dyspnea subscales, respectively; and −5.09 [−7.69; −2.49] for the SGRQ symptoms domain. In addition, it was shown that all these effect sizes exceed the instruments' MID, demonstrating that the effects of PR are not only statistically significant but also clinically relevant for the patients [12].

Although reduction of symptoms after rehabilitation is well documented, it is important to be aware that not all patients enrolled in a PR program will respond to the intervention by reducing their symptoms. Troosters and colleagues [13] showed that less than half of COPD patients (44%) were "responders" to a 12-week rehabilitation program, based upon a 10-point improvement in the CRQ. Similar results were found by de Torres and colleagues [14] in a study which approximately 50% of patients presented improvement exceeding the MID of 0.5 unit in the CRQ dyspnea domain.

Some authors consider that multidimensional instruments such as the TDI might be more responsive to intervention. An increase of about 4 units in the TDI has been reported in previous studies [15, 16]; in addition, approximately half of the patients improve more than the MID (i.e., 1 unit) [14]. Interestingly, von Leopoldt and colleagues found that reduction of dyspnea evidenced by increase in the TDI was the most important predictor of improvement in quality of life of patients with moderate to severe COPD enrolled in an intensive 3-week outpatient PR program [15].

Furthermore, it is import to consider that the reduction of symptoms achieved with PR can be maintained after its completion, especially in long-lasting programs. Troosters and colleagues [2] showed that the improvement of 14 units in the CRQ dyspnea domain observed in patients with COPD after a 6-month rehabilitation program was sustained during a follow-up period of 12 months.

19.4 Exercise Capacity

Exercise training has been considered the cornerstone of PR [17] and improvement in exercise capacity has very strong evidence level in individuals with COPD submitted to PR [1, 3, 12]. The term "exercise" means a structured, planned, and repetitive way of performing activities. It is a subset of "physical activity" and is commonly assessed by tests of exercise capacity [18].

A large number of randomized controlled trials (RTCs) comparing conventional care and PR in COPD are available in the current literature. They suggest that positive effects on exercise capacity are expected after PR [12]; therefore, exercise capacity improvement has been commonly used as a parameter to identify whether PR program was effective. Patients may improve maximal or submaximal exercise capacity by modifying different parameters such as the distance walked (m), the time cycled (s), and the maximal work rate (W), among others. Because of this, standardized recommendations must be taken into account when exercise capacity tests are performed. Furthermore, there are many examples of exercise tests used for this purpose in patients with COPD which include laboratory or field walking tests.

The most common laboratory cycle ergometer tests are the cardiopulmonary exercise testing (CPET) and the cycling endurance test. During the former, patients achieve maximum exercise capacity by an incremental protocol, whereas the latest test allows the assessment of submaximum exercise capacity by the endurance time resulted from a constant-load cycle ergometer test (i.e., constant work rate cycle endurance test [CET]). Incremental exercise tests present an excellent ability for identifying abnormalities during the test as well as characterizing the patient's profile. On the other hand, endurance cycle ergometer tests seems to be more sensitive to change and better discriminate intervention results in terms of improved exercise capacity, such as those observed after PR [19, 20].

Field tests are commonly used in the clinical practice to evaluate exercise capacity since they are easier to perform and require inexpensive equipment. Holland et al. have described the standard procedures for some increasingly used field walking tests in the official ATS/ERS statement published in 2014, which includes the 6 min walk test (6MWT), the incremental and enduwrance shuttle walk tests (ISWT and ESWT, respectively). A growing based-evidence confirms that the 6MWT, ISWT, and ESWT are valid, reliable, and responsive to detect changes after some interventions [3]. However, Laviolette et al. have shown that CET was more sensitive to detect short- and long-term changes after PR than the 6MWT [21].

Moreover, there are other available tests to evaluate patients with COPD which require less time and space to be performed when compared to the 6MWT. These tests are commonly called "functional tests" because they are performed with functional activities such as walking, sit-down, and stand-up, among others. Due to their simplicity and low requirement in terms of equipment, these lower limb functional tests have been increasingly used in home settings. These simple tests include gait speed (GS), timed Up and Go (TUG), sit-to-stand (STS) test, and step test, which were not included in the official statement of field tests but had their properties described in detail in a systematic review by Bisca et al. including 42 studies involving patients with COPD [22]. In these tests, patients perform pre-established activities as fast as possible. Other recommendations for using these simple tests in clinical practice to evaluate lower limb exercise capacity are provided elsewhere [22].

Numerous methods to assess exercise capacity in patients with COPD are currently available and chapter five has discussed this topic in detail. Knowledge about assessment methods of exercise capacity is essential to understand how to quantify the improvements obtained with PR. Patients should be assessed before the PR program begins and after the program is finished. In general, patients present significant exercise capacity impairments at the entry, but fortunately, PR may attenuate this clinical condition; on the other hand, the response to change may vary according to each population characteristics and training protocol.

Complementary information about the effects of PR on exercise capacity is given by the MID values. MID reflects the smallest difference in exercise capacity (or any other clinical measurable parameter) according to the amount of change for better or for worse, as perceived by the investigator, clinician, or patients when the intervention finishes [23]. Despite the MID not being particularly relevant for interpretation of individual results, it provides guidance to identify whether changes achieved by patients reflect substantial improvement associated with clinical outcomes [20]. MID values available for different exercise tests are described in Box 19.2.

Data from 16 RCT (779 participants) included in a systematic review by McCarthy et al. have shown that Wmax (W) increases after PR with a Mean Difference (MD) of 6.77 [95% CI: 1.89; 11.65] in the incremental cycle ergometer when compared to usual care [12]. This value exceed the MID of 4 watts proposed by Puhan et al. [24]. On the other hand, CET may increase at least 80% from baseline assessment [1]. Cambach et al. have shown an increase in CET of 421 s after 3 months of PR in comparison to a control group [34]. This difference exemplifies why endurance tests are considered more responsive than incremental tests.

The responsiveness of various exercise testing protocols have been investigated in a review study from Borel et al. [20]. Figure 19.1 summarizes the responsiveness of six different exercise tests after interventions.

Box 19.2 Minimal important differences (MID) of some exercise tests commonly used in patients with COPD

	MID
Laboratory tests	
Incremental cycle ergometer tests [24, 25]	4–10 W
Endurance cycle ergometer test [21, 26]	100–200 s
Field walking tests	
6MWT [24, 27, 28]	25–35 m
ISWT [29]	47.5 m
ESWT [30]	65 s[a] or 180 s[b]
Simple functional tests	
4MGS [31]	(−) 0.11 m/s
TUG [32]	(−) 1.4 s (14%)
5STS [33]	(−) 1.7 s

MID minimal important difference; *ISWT* incremental shuttle walk test; *ESWT* endurance shuttle walk test; *6MWT* 6-min walk test; *4MGS* 4-m gait speed; *TUG* timed up and go; *5STS* five repetition sit-to-stand test

[a]ESWT MID after bronchodilator

[b]Approximate ESWT MID after pulmonary rehabilitation

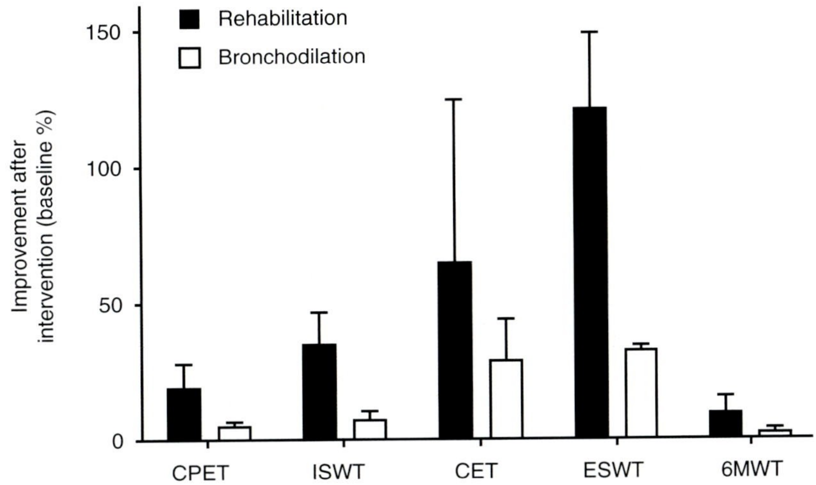

Fig. 19.1 The impact of interventions on the exercise performance following testing methodologies in COPD population. *CPET* cardiopulmonary exercise test, *ISWT* incremental shuttle walking test, *CET* cycle endurance test, *ESWT* endurance shuttle walking test and 6MWT: 6 min walking test **Source:** Borel et al., *Pulm Med*, 2013. [20]

In case of assessing exercise capacity with field tests before and after PR, the meta-analysis from McCarthy et al. based on data from 1879 participants showed that 6MWT presents an average improvement of 43.93 m [CI95% 32.64; 55.21] after PR compared with usual care [12]. This significant 6MWT improvement easily exceed the MID of 30 m [35]. Furthermore, McCarthy et al. also reported a significant increase of 39.77 m [CI 95% 22.38; 57.15] in the ISWT after PR compared with usual care [12]. Although statistically significant, this result based on eight trials (694 participants) does not exceed the MID of 47.5 m [29].

Regarding the ESWT, there is no meta-analysis available due to the limited number of trials providing data from this test. However, Singh et al. have investigated the responsiveness of this test in the official ATS/ERS systematic review about measurement properties of field walking tests for chronic respiratory disease [36]. Seven studies which examined the responsiveness of the ESWT (three using bronchodilator, two using oxygen therapy and two after PR) showed a moderate to high responsiveness of the test. The average change of walked distance (302 ± 387 m) or time (439 ± 346 s) based on those two studies comparing the ESWT before and after PR indicated large variability in exercise capacity [36]. More studies investigating the effects of PR on the ESWT are necessary to understand its response in more depth.

In summary, the message from the current statement of the field walking tests in chronic pulmonary disease reaffirm that ISWT, 6MWT, and ESWT are all responsive [35] and show large variability on average change values. On the other hand, if simple functional tests are performed before and after PR, changes are in a smaller scale expected, since these tests' duration are considerably lower than laboratory and field tests previously discussed in this chapter. For instance, the 4-m gait speed test improved in average 0.08 m/s after PR [31]; the TUG test improved 0.9 s [32]; and the sit-to-stand test (five repetitions protocol) improved 1.4 s [33]. Note that all these simple functional tests improvement occurred due to an increased speed and consequently reduced average values, which reflects performance of patients with COPD after PR.

Another important point of discussion is that, high intensity exercise should be prescribed to obtain significant physiologic improvements [37]. Exercise capacity improvement occurs after PR due to important muscular adaptations, which includes changes in peripheral muscle structure and function. Furthermore, larger training effects on exercise capacity and reduction of symptoms were generally achieved by programs eliciting more pronounced skeletal muscle fatigue [38]. Despite the physiological benefits obtained with exercise training, non-physiologic factors, such as desensitization to dyspnea, improvement on mechanical body efficiency to perform work, and reduction of anxiety and depression, also contribute to the improved exercise capacity in patients with COPD after PR [39].

Finally, nonconventional strategies of PR have also shown positive results in exercise capacity, which means that professionals may opt for prescribing high intensity exercises of different forms aiming to enhance exercise capacity. Interval training, one-legged exercise training, and downhill walking protocols, among others, can be chosen as training protocols. Furthermore, home-based and community-based exercise training, as well as the technology-assisted exercise training by telehealth (telemonitoring and telephone support) are promising treatment options for patients with COPD [3].

19.5 Peripheral Muscle Strength

Skeletal muscle dysfunction in patients with COPD has been increasingly studied in the last two decades [40]. Nowadays, some structural changes of the limb muscles, such as poor oxidative capacity, atrophy, weakness, mitochondrial dysfunction, and shift in fiber type are well recognized and described [41]. These muscle dysfunctions seem to be associated with morbidities and, moreover, may impact on the ability to perform daily activities. The body of knowledge on this topic was recently updated and is now available in the official ATS/ERS statement on limb muscle dysfunction in COPD [41].

The assessment of limb muscle function is strongly encouraged. Patients with COPD present reduced quadriceps force as well as reduced quadriceps endurance when compared with healthy individuals [42, 43]. Experts from the ATS and ERS suggest that assessing peripheral muscle strength and body composition, two important clinical outcomes which are directly related to each other, allows the identification of patients at increased risk of mortality and exercise intolerance. Body composition will be discussed in the next topic.

Peripheral muscle strength can be assessed by volitional and non-volitional techniques. Volitional tests, such as manual muscle testing, handheld dynamometry, one-repetition measurement, or maximal voluntary contraction (MVC), are more familiar to clinicians. In fact, the methodology of MVC is considered highly reliable and reproducible [44]. Furthermore, aiming to provide more clinical context for clinicians and patients, Canavan et al. recently determined and validated MVC cut points of 5.99 kg/m^2 for women and 8.30 kg/m^2 for men for predicting failure to stand up [45]. Moreover, the handgrip strength, a simple measure of upper limb muscle function, is associated with mortality in patients with COPD [46]. Normative values and specific cutoff points providing prognostic information (i.e., 10th centile of normative values) are available to define handgrip weakness in patients with COPD [47, 48].

As another important feature, peripheral muscle strength assessment also allows for prescribing adequate loads for resistance training since improving skeletal muscle function is an important goal of exercise training programs [3]. In general, PR leads to increased peripheral muscle strength in patients with COPD. However, intensity and duration of exercise programs are considered very important factors when developing a training program. Following the exercise training principles, the total training load must be prescribed individually; furthermore, it must exceed the load achieved in activities of daily living and a progression (or increase) in load must occur for physical training to be effective [3].

De Brandt and colleagues have recently published a systematic review which helps to understand the changes in metabolic and structural muscle characteristics in patients with COPD following exercise-based training [49]. Very positive results after high intensity interval training were found. Furthermore, after combined aerobic and resistance training, improvements in muscle structure outcomes such as fiber proportion, fiber size, and capillarity-to-fiber ratio are observed. Moreover, in general, improvements in inflammation, mitochondrial enzyme activity, muscle protein turnover regulation, and oxidative and nitrosative stress were also detected as results after exercise training-based interventions [49].

In fact, further evidence confirms that the positive impact of PR on muscle strength occurs in different modalities of exercise training. Both endurance training and resistance training increases strength or muscle mass in patients with COPD [50–52]. However, resistance training has a greater potential of improvement in strength or muscle mass when compared to endurance exercise [50, 51, 53]. In this line, Liao and colleagues have shown in a systematic review including eighteen trials with 750 patients with COPD that skeletal muscle function of leg press strength assessed in patients who performed resistance training improves with a weighted mean difference (WMD) of 16.67 [95% CI: 2.87; 30.47] kg *versus* a non-exercise group($P = 0.02$) [52]. Furthermore, combined resistance and endurance-training group showed significant improvements in leg press strength (WMD: 12.34 [5.96; 18.72] kg) in comparison to the endurance-training alone ($P = 0.001$). In these studies, there were no reports of adverse events related to exercise training, which suggests that resistance exercise training or combined endurance and resistance exercise training can be successfully performed and do not generate adverse events during PR in COPD [52].

19.6 Body Composition

Among the recognized extrapulmonary manifestations of patients with COPD, abnormalities in body composition such as nutritional depletion are commonly observed [54]. Low values of body mass index (BMI, body weight in kilograms divided by height in squared meters) as well as the fat-free mass (FFM) depletion leads to important clinical impacts since these factors are associated with increased mortality risk in patients with COPD [54–56]. Interestingly, weight gain in those patients with a BMI below 25 kg m^{-2} is associated with decreased mortality; additionally, the "obesity paradox" acts as a protecting factor and patients with advanced stages of the disease may benefit of being obese, reducing mortality [54, 57, 58].

A study indicated that FFM depletion occurred in approximately 37% of male and 59% of female patients with moderate-severe COPD and it was associated with worse quality of life, reduced muscle strength and exercise capacity [59]. FFM and other variables of body composition are commonly measured either by bio-electrical impedance analysis (BIA), using a validated prediction equation, or by dual energy X-ray absorptiometry (DEXA), which quantifies body composition.

Another characteristic associated with malnutrition and chronic diseases which reflects loss of skeletal muscle mass is sarcopenia, with approximately 15% of prevalence in patients with COPD [60]. Sarcopenia increases with age and severity of airway obstruction (GOLD classification); however, it does not differ between gender and presence of quadriceps weakness [60].

Since patients with COPD in general should be referred to PR [3, 5], previous studies have investigated the effects of PR on patients with different abnormalities in body composition. Obese patients present worse performance in walking (but not cycling) [61]; however, the magnitude of improvement after PR seems to be similar despite obesity degree [61, 62], BMI value [63], presence of FFM depletion [64], or sarcopenia [60].

As previously discussed in this chapter, PR leads to some muscle adaptations [41]. Muscle mass constitutes the major part of FFM; therefore, improvements in exercise performance and muscle changes, such as increased FFM with consequent weight gain, are expected as benefits of PR on normal-weight patients [65]. On the other hand, obese patients who respond to PR present weight reduction with maintenance of skeletal muscle mass, among other benefits [66]. Despite the fact that positive effects of PR on body composition are described in the current scientific literature, difficulties in increasing FFM in patients with COPD following PR have been previously reported and seem associated with worse dyspnea in daily life and more impaired lung function [67].

19.7 Balance

A growing body of scientific evidence suggests that patients with COPD present important impairments in balance control when compared with age-matched subjects without the disease [68–70]. The association between balance and fall risk reinforces the importance of correctly identifying balance disturbances as well as treating and improving balance control in patients with COPD [71].

The Berg Balance Scale (BBS), Balance Evaluation Systems Test (BESTest), Mini-BESTest, and the Brief-BESTest were described as useful tools to assess balance in this population. Jácome and colleges have shown that these four balance tests are valid, reliable, and valuable to identify fall status in patients with COPD [72]. Moreover, the force platform provides detailed and reliable information about static balance, for example, by performing the one-legged stance on it [69]. However, so far its use is generally restricted to research purposes since it is an expensive equipment.

As an additional option to assess balance, the TUG test has been used. It is quick and simple to perform, has been validated for this population, and can be easily implemented in clinical practice [32, 69].

Due to the recognized balance impairments in patients with COPD, some strategies aiming to reduce fall risk have been proposed. PR seems to be effective in improving balance in patients with COPD, especially when specific programs to improve balance were implemented and longer PR programs were performed, i.e., above 6 months [73–75]. However, a recent systematic review investigating the effects of PR on balance and risk of fall in patients with COPD suggested that further studies involving this outcome are still required [76]. Only seven studies were included and none have focused only on falls. The authors concluded that there are still inconsistent results and inconclusive evidence to properly ascertain the significant effects of PR on balance [76].

19.8 Quality of Life

Health status is a general concept that includes physiological functioning, functional impairment, symptoms, and quality of life. The concept of quality of life is also subdivided, including the term health-related quality of life which is defined as satisfaction with health [3], and constitutes the focus of this section. Improvement of quality of life is one of the main objectives of PR; thus, ideally the treatment should be tailored to individual patient's needs. According to the GOLD report, increase in quality of life in one of the benefits of PR with level of evidence A [5].

There are several instruments which evaluate quality of life. Among them, there are the generic questionnaires that are less discriminative and consequently less sensitive to change after intervention. Despite the Medical Outcomes Survey Short Form 36-item (SF-36) being a generic instrument, it has been used in studies which evaluated the effects of PR and showed to be sensitive to detect improvement after the treatment. Benzo and colleagues [77] demonstrated that quality of life improved after a PR program in all dimensions of the SF-36.

Disease-specific instruments are more sensitive to detect changes after treatment since they approach specific limitations experienced by patients with chronic respiratory disease. The most widely used disease-specific questionnaires used in the PR context are the Saint George's Respiratory Questionnaire (SGRQ) and the Chronic Respiratory Disease Questionnaire (CRQ or CRDQ). More recently, the COPD Assessment Test (CAT) was developed to be a simple and short instrument to assess quality of life. These questionnaires have defined MID, which allows better interpretation of rehabilitation results in the clinical practice (Box 19.1). Although the MID for the SGRQ was previously determined, Welling and colleagues [78] more recently proposed new values of MID for this instrument when used to assess quality of life in patients with severe COPD. The authors found a MID of −8.3 units (or −13.4%) after 1 month of intervention, and −7.1 units (or −11.1%) after 6 months of intervention.

The Cochrane Review about the benefits of PR, which was updated in 2015, confirmed that 4 weeks of rehabilitation are able to improve quality of life in patients with COPD. The effect sizes of the CRQ subscales varied from 0.56 to

0.79, all exceeding the MID. The SGRQ total score also exceeded the MID of 4 units presenting an effect size of −6.89 (95%CI: -9.26; −4.52) [12]. The CAT was also shown to be responsive to rehabilitation. The first study which showed its responsiveness was published by Jones and colleagues [79]; after 6 weeks of PR patients with COPD had a median reduction of −2.2 ± 5.3 units ($P = 0.002$) in the instrument.

It seems that severity of the disease interferes in the effectiveness of PR in improving quality of life. Bratas and colleagues [80] found a reduction of −3.1 units (95% CI: −5.1; −1.1) ($P = 0.003$) in the SGRQ total score of patients with COPD enrolled in a 4-week inpatient PR program. However, they also found that patients with a FEV1 ≥ 50% of predicted, i.e., those patients with mild to moderate disease, were approximately four times more likely to achieve a clinically important improvement (change SGRQ ≥ 4 units) than patients with severe or very severe disease. Recently, Alfarroba and colleagues [81] demonstrated that there was reduction in the SGRQ total score in all GOLD categories (A to D), however with more pronounced decrease in the scores of patients classified as categories A, B, and C.

Although the most recent ATS-ERS statement on PR reiterates that there is no consensus on the optimal duration of PR, some data have demonstrated that 8 weeks of outpatient rehabilitation with 3 sessions per week are sufficient for most patients with COPD to reach a plateau in terms of quality of life improvement [82]. On the other hand, some studies showed that quality of life can progressively increase during a longer-term PR program [83, 84]. When repeated PR programs (5 programs along 7 years) were used as a strategy to treat patients with COPD, Foglio and colleagues [85] showed that quality of life achieve a plateau. The greatest reduction in the SGRQ total score (−9 ± 10 units) was seen after the first program and in the four remaining programs the reductions were around 4 units ($P = 0.067$ among post-rehabilitation changes).

Other point of discussion in PR is the long-term maintenance of its benefits. In general, when patients finish the intervention and remain without any maintenance strategy, quality of life was better maintained than exercise capacity, and the benefits appear to reduce over 6–12 months [3]. However, there is evidence otherwise: for example, Godoy and colleagues [86] reported that the reduction in the SGRQ total score observed immediately after a 12-week rehabilitation program was statistically sustained during 24 months. Future research regarding this issue is welcome.

19.9 Anxiety and Depression

Symptoms of anxiety and depression are commonly observed in patients who attend PR programs. Approximately 40% of patients with COPD refer symptoms of anxiety or depression, although it does not necessarily mean that they have a depressive or anxiety disorder. Additionally, it is known that the prevalence of those symptoms is higher in patients with advanced disease especially those in use of long-term oxygen therapy (LTOT) [3].

The most recent ATS/ERS statement on PR recommends that supervised exercise combined with psychological support in rehabilitation programs should offer management strategies for patients who present anxiety and/or depression symptoms [3], since studies have shown the positive effects of this intervention on mood symptoms. Coventry and Hind [87] in a systematic review with meta-analysis showed the effects of comprehensive rehabilitation in comparison to usual care. In this review, three randomized controlled trials demonstrated reduction in anxiety and depression after intervention with effect sizes for anxiety and depression of −0.33 [95% CI: −0.57; −0.09] and −0.58 [−0.93; −0.23], respectively. Thus, it is important to include an instrument to evaluate anxiety and depression in the initial and posttreatment assessments of PR programs.

Although the diagnosis of depression or anxiety must be based on the Diagnostic and Statistical Manual of Mental Disorders criteria, screening tools were developed and can be used to assess mental symptoms. Among the instruments validated for patients with COPD, the Hospital Anxiety and Depression Scale (HADS) [88] is widely used in rehabilitation settings. The MID of this scale is 1.5 units [89].

Bhandari and colleagues [90] studied 366 patients with COPD submitted to PR and found that abnormal scores on HADS for anxiety or depression were predictors of no completion of the program. In addition, those patients who completed the treatment had reduction of symptoms of anxiety and depression, and approximately 40% reached the MID in the HADS. Another interesting finding was that those patients with abnormal HADS score at the beginning of the rehabilitation program were those with better response to intervention in terms of mood symptoms (around 90% reached the MID in the HADS). Similar results were observed by Harrison and colleagues [91]. In this clinical trial, the authors found that patients without evidence of symptoms, i.e., HADS anxiety and/or depression $\leq$ 7 units, did not present significant change in the HADS after a 7-week outpatient PR program. On the other hand, those patients with higher baseline HADS score ($\geq$ 8 units for anxiety or depression) had improved (i.e., reduced) scores after rehabilitation with better results on those with scores between 11 and 21 units (change in the HADS for anxiety and depression of -3.11 ± 0.35 and -3.19 ± 0.47, respectively).

Despite the relationship of mood symptoms with other outcomes in chronic respiratory disease such as poor quality of life, mortality, and hospitalization [92], presence of anxiety and depression symptoms does not limit the effects of PR. Trappenburg and colleagues [93] studied the effects of a 12-week PR program on 65 patients with COPD who previously presented mood symptoms (average HADS anxiety and depression of 8±4 units for both; approximately 40% with scores $\geq$ 10 units). The authors observed that the group of patients had improvement on functional and maximal exercise capacity, health-related quality of life, functional status, and also on anxiety and depression symptoms (change in the HADS for anxiety and depression of -2 ± 3 and -3 ± 3 units, respectively).

19.10 Functional Status and Activities of Daily Living

Functional status refers to the capacity of an individual to undertake normally his/her activities of daily living in the physiological, psychological, and social domains [94]. Activities of daily living (ADL) are all activities or tasks undertaken for daily functioning. They are usually divided in three types: basic (required for basic survival, such as feeding, personal hygiene, and dressing); instrumental (more complex, such as working and shopping); and advanced (e.g., social and recreational activities) [95]. Therefore, as a general concept, functional status is a wide term which concerns the capacity to undertake different ADL to maintain functioning, and the subject's perception about the limitations to undertake them.

Assessment of patients' performance concerning their ADL should be part of PR programs since lung diseases are closely related to the occurrence of dyspnea, fatigue, functional limitation, muscle dysfunction, physical inactivity, anxiety, and depression [5]. There are basically two ways to assess functional status: self-reported instruments (questionnaires, scales, indexes), i.e., tools in which patients report their perception on difficulties and limitations to perform given ADLs; and standardized ADL tests, which require patients to perform a set routine of tasks.

19.10.1 Self-Reported Instruments

The most widely used questionnaires and scales which are specific to assess functional status in patients with chronic respiratory disease are the following:

19.10.1.1 Pulmonary Functional Status and Dyspnea Questionnaire—Modified Version (PFSDQ-M) [96]

This questionnaire was modified from a previous and longer version [97] which was developed by the same authors. It is self-administered and evaluates the intensity of dyspnea and fatigue in ten ADLs. The questionnaire is valid and reliable for the evaluation of dyspnea, fatigue, and changes in

ADL in COPD [96]. A MID of 5 points (range −3 to −6) for each component has been described in patients with severe COPD [9], and the PFSDQ-M's 'change in activity' domain showed responsiveness to detect changes in functional status after 3 months of high-intensity exercise training in patients with COPD [98].

19.10.1.2 London Chest Activity of Daily Living Scale (LCADL) [99]

This scale evaluates the degree of functional status impairment in patients with COPD concerning 15 ADL divided in four domains (physical activities, domestic activities, self–care, and leisure), whereas a total score is calculated based on the sum of the four domains. The subject rates his/her difficulties in performing these activities in a 0-to-5 scale, where 5 means higher impairment. The scale is reliable and was validated through evidence of correlations with other self-reported instruments such as the Saint George's Respiratory Questionnaire [99]. A change of 4 points in the total score can be interpreted as a meaningful change [100], and the LCADL has been shown to be more responsive to PR than other functional status tools in patients with COPD [98].

19.10.1.3 Manchester Respiratory Activities of Daily Living Questionnaire (MRADL) [101]

The MRADL is a 21-item questionnaire which evaluates four domains of functional incapacity in elderly with COPD: mobility, kitchen, domestic tasks, and leisure. The questionnaire is valid, reliable (including its postal version) [102], and responsive to PR [103]. No minimal important difference has been established, although a score <12 has been described as an univariate predictor of 1-year mortality in patients discharged from hospital due to an acute exacerbation of COPD [103].

19.10.1.4 Pulmonary Functional Status Scale-Short Form (PFSS-11) [104]

The PFSS-11 is a short form derived from a previous and longer scale, the 35-item PFSS [105]. It is a valid instrument, although some of its psychometric properties have not been properly addressed, such as its responsiveness. No minimal important difference has been established.

19.10.1.5 Functional Performance Inventory-Short Form (FPI-SF) [106]

The FPI-SF is a self-administered questionnaire developed based on an analytical framework of functional status. It aims to assess the level of difficulty that respondents have with physical activities across six domains or subscales, namely body care, maintaining the household, physical exercise, recreation, spiritual activities, and social interaction. It was reduced from a 65-item tool [107] to a 32-item short form [106] through a systematic process of qualitative and quantitative item reduction, as well as it was formatted for greater clarity and ease of use.

19.10.1.6 Canadian Occupational Performance Measure (COPM) [108]

The COPM is an individualized measure of functional performance which aims to identify self-perceived difficulties in ADL. It was shown to be reliable and sensitive to change after PR [108].

19.10.1.7 Other Instruments

Certain health status questionnaires contain domains which also evaluate various aspects of functional status, mainly the disease impact on daily life. These include (but are not limited to) the Medical Outcomes Study (MOS/SF-36) [109], the SGRQ [110], the CRQ [111], and the Seattle Obstructive Lung Questionnaire (SOLQ) [112].

19.10.1.8 Improvement of Self-Reported Instruments of Functional Status After PR

Functional status assessed by self-reported methods has been generally shown to be responsive to PR, reflecting the fact that patients rate themselves as having less difficulties to perform their ADL after undergoing the program [101, 113]. There is preliminary evidence suggesting that some instruments may be more responsive than others (e.g., the LCADL) [98], but self-reported functional status is generally regarded as one of the outcomes which are prone for improvement after rehabilitation.

19.10.2 Standardized ADL Tests

In standardized ADL tests, patients perform a set of routine ADL tasks while being assessed in their performance. Differently than the self-reported methods, these tests reflect patients' capacity rather than their perception. Among those available, two examples used in patients with COPD may be described:

19.10.2.1 Glittre ADL Test

To date, the most widely used standardized ADL test in patients with COPD is the Glittre ADL test [114]. In this test, subjects are instructed to rise from a chair, walk, ascend and descend stairs, and move cartons up and down in a shelf (Fig. 19.2). The sequence is then reversed so that the subject walks back and returns to the starting position sitting on the chair, and immediately rises to begin the next lap. Subjects are told to perform the test as quickly as possible, and the primary outcome is the time taken to complete 5 laps. During the test, patients wear a backpack filled with a 2.5 (women) or 5 kg (men) weight. The additional weight simulates the weight of a supplemental oxygen unit, which can be exchanged for the weight when appropriate. The differential backpack weight appears to be a way to normalize for differences in muscle mass between men and women. Alternatively, an extra-weight of 10% of the patient's body weight can also be used.

The Glittre ADL test induces slightly higher oxygen uptake than the 6MWT, with similar cardiovascular and ventilatory demand [115]. Furthermore, the test duration and ventilatory parameters are reproducible, although a 6–7% learning effect was shown, leading to the recommendation to perform two tests [116]. Evidence on the test's responsiveness to PR is still lacking.

19.10.2.2 Londrina ADL Protocol (LAP)

A new standardized ADL test has been proposed, the Londrina ADL protocol, or LAP [117] in order to counteract some limitations of the Glittre ADL test (i.e., it does not comprise an in-depth and objective assessment of problematic activities involving the upper limbs; and it is performed as quickly as possible instead of at a usual pace) [117]. It is composed by five activities representing ADL involving upper limbs, lower limbs, and trunk movements. The LAP showed to be a valid and reliable test, even when subjects were using a mask for gas analysis [117]. Normal values are already available [118], but responsiveness of the LAP to PR has not been investigated to date.

Regardless of the outcome chosen in order to reflect functional status, reassessment is crucial in understanding whether the patient has reduced his/her limitation and improved ADL performance, so that behavioral change was achieved and improvements in exercise capacity obtained after rehabilitation translate into meaningful improvements in the patient's real life.

19.10.3 Physical Activity in Daily Life

Due to the pronounced deleterious effects of inactivity, it is imperative that PR programs aim at enhancing physical activity in daily life (PADL), interrupting the disease "vicious circle" of deconditioning and inactivity. In order to properly assess the achievement of this goal, the use of accurate and valid instruments to quantify PADL is advisable.

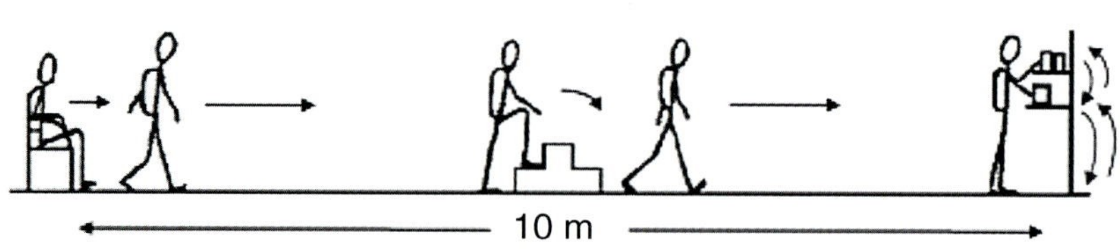

Fig. 19.2 Glittre ADL test. Source: Skumlien et al., *Respir Med*, 2006 [114]

The quantification of PADL is generally performed by three different means: questionnaires, measures of energy expenditure, and motion sensors.

19.10.3.1 Questionnaires (or Self-Reported Methods)

The main advantages of questionnaires are the fact that they are simple and easy to apply, what favors their use for epidemiological purposes. However, since they rely on patients' memory, reliability of the information decreases as the recall period increases. Additionally, the lighter the physical activity performed, the more difficult it is for the patient to recall it adequately. Questionnaires better reflect activities performed at high intensity than those at light-to-moderate intensity, what does not favor their use in chronically ill subjects. Furthermore, reliability of the information may also vary according to patient characteristics such as age, cultural aspects, and cognitive capacity. The instrument's design may also play a role in the quality of the assessment, so that simple questionnaires have higher chance of adequately assessing PADL. Moreover, specific questions (e.g., how many days per week are you physically active?) lead to overestimation of PADL in comparison to "open" questions. For all these reasons, it is worthwhile to remember that despite their usefulness in population-based studies, their capacity to reflect individual estimations is questionable [119]. In general, individual patients with COPD are unable to report accurately the amount of PADL performed in a day and even in 1 h [120].

There is a variety of questionnaires which aim at quantifying PADL. However, not many were adapted and/or validated to patients with respiratory diseases. A brief list of self-reported instruments previously used in patients with COPD is found below. They have different designs, length, and recall period, as well as varying levels of validity, reliability, and responsiveness.

Stanford Seven-Day Physical Activity Recall (7D–PAR or Simply PAR)

This is a semi-structured questionnaire which estimates the time spent in physical activity and resistance/flexibility exercises in the 7 days prior to its application. It is considered valid for utilization in patients with cystic fibrosis and COPD [121, 122].

Baecke Physical Activity Questionnaire

The objective of this questionnaire is to classify individuals as having low, moderate, or high level of PADL according to the duration and energy spent in the activities performed in the last year. This questionnaire has been used in studies involving patients with COPD, presenting correlation with important disease outcomes such as muscle function [123].

Yale Physical Activity Survey (YPAS)

The YPAS was specifically developed for the assessment of PADL in elderly. It encompasses a wide variety of activities related to domestic care, recreational activities, and exercise, including light, moderate, and high intensity activities. This instrument was not found to be valid to quantify PADL in COPD, however it is valid to classify this population's PADL profile, since its final score was able to identify sedentary patients [124].

It is worthwhile to highlight that questionnaires should undergo the process of cultural adaptation prior to their use in population based on a different country or region than the original one.

19.10.3.2 Measures of Energy Expenditure

Calorimetry (direct and indirect) and doubly labelled water are considered as gold standard methods for the quantification of energy expenditure [125]. However, these methods are relatively expensive and demand specific training for its complex handling, hindering its applicability. Moreover, estimation of energy expenditure does not provide data on duration and frequency of physical activity, which are key components for the characterization and quantification of PADL [119]. For these reasons, measures of energy expenditure will not be described in further detail in this chapter.

The Physical Activity Level (PAL) index, which is based on energy expenditure, has been commonly used in the scientific literature, including in patients with COPD [126]. It consists of dividing total energy expenditure by the basal metabolic rate. A PAL index ≥ 1.70 defines a physically active person; between 1.40 and 1.69 defines a predominantly sedentary person; and <1.40 defines a very inactive person.

19.10.3.3 Motion Sensors

Due to the limitations which characterize the previously mentioned methods, there is growing interest in motion sensors by researchers and clinicians. These instruments detect body movement, objectively quantifying PADL. They are basically divided into pedometers and accelerometers [119].

Pedometers

These are simple, small, and financially accessible devices which detect the number of steps performed by the subject in a given period of time. The majority of models is worn on the waist and the outcomes generally are number of steps/day and eventually also distance walked and energy expenditure. The higher the number of steps/day, the higher the level of PADL. Disadvantages of these devices include the absence of information on type, pattern, and intensity of physical activity performed, and its inaccuracy in slow walking speeds, such as in the case of patients with COPD [127].

Accelerometers

These are technologically more advanced devices which are capable of registering the amount and intensity of movement in daily life for long periods of time. They can be uniaxial or multiaxial. Multiaxial devices detect movements in two or more axis of movement and allow a more detailed data analysis. Some multiaxial accelerometers can even detect specific activities and postures, functioning as physical activity monitors and allowing to assess the profile of PADL in a very detailed and accurate way [119]. Disadvantages of accelerometers include their inability to assess activities performed by the upper limbs (in the majority of the devices) and their higher cost in comparison to pedometers.

Two studies investigated the accuracy of a number of motion sensors in patients with COPD. The first study evaluated the validity of 6 motion sensors against indirect calorimetry in a 1-h standardized protocol. It showed that the DynaPort MiniMod (McRoberts, the Netherlands), the Actigraph GT3X (Actigraph, United States of America), and the SenseWear armband (BodyMedia, United States of America) were the most valid devices, whereas the former two showed the best capacity to discriminate different walking speeds [128]. The second study also evaluated the validity of 6 motion sensors, but this time against doubly labeled water in real-life PADL assessment in patients with COPD. It showed that the DynaPort MoveMonitor and the Actigraph GT3X better reflected activity and total energy expenditure in this population [129]. One must consider that there is a growing variety of motion sensor devices available, and technology advances quickly, so that models may rapidly become outdated.

Commonly used variables for motion sensors include (but are not limited to) time spent per day in activities above a certain intensity threshold (i.e., "active" time); time spent per day in activities below a certain intensity threshold (i.e., "inactive" [or sedentary] time); activity counts; and vector magnitude units, movement intensity, and number of steps/day. Some motion sensors are able to provide an estimation of energy expenditure, calculated based mainly on the quantification of movements detected by the device. However, evidence seems to point out that motion sensors are more accurate for the quantification of movement (their original purpose) than for the estimation of energy expenditure [119].

Regardless of the outcome used to reflect PADL, results may be highly dependent on some characteristics such as number of assessment days, sensitivity and usability of each device, outcome of interest, daylight length, and environmental-climatic-social factors, among others [130, 131].

Whether PADL is improved after PR has been the object of great debate. This depends on the content and duration of the rehabilitation program, sensitivity of the chosen motion sensor, and other factors. Some studies have found positive results, and others have not [132]. Furthermore, an increase of 600–1100 steps/day after PR has been suggested as a MID for PADL since it reflects a reduced risk for hospital admission in patients with COPD [133].

19.10.4 A Hybrid Outcome: The PROactive Tool

PROactive is a consortium consisting of 18 partners, including academic institutions, pharmaceutical companies, and a small to medium-sized enterprise (SME). This consortium developed a hybrid instrument which aims to capture all dimensions of physical activity, the PROactive tool [134]. It is composed by a questionnaire (two versions: daily and clinical visit) combined with outcomes obtained from an activity monitor. This combination allows not only to quantify the "amount" of PADL but also the patient's experience of "difficulty" related to physical activity during day-by-day functioning. It provides simple, valid, and reliable measures of physical activity in patients with COPD.

19.11 Self-Efficacy

Self-efficacy can be considered as the belief that one can successfully execute particular behaviors to produce certain outcomes [135]. It is currently recognized as a crucial concept in understanding to translate an improved exercise capacity into greater functional performance and increased self-management skills [3].

The Pulmonary Rehabilitation Adapted Index of Self-Efficacy (PRAISE) tool is an example of a reliable instrument capable of detecting improvements in self-efficacy after PR [136]. Another instrument, the COPD Self-Efficacy Scale (CSES) has also been used [137, 138]. Further studies involving these tools are welcome.

Acknowledgements The authors would like to thank Hindawi Publishing Corporation for granting permission to reproduce material from the article by Borel B, Provencher S, Saey D, Maltais F: Responsiveness of Various Exercise-Testing Protocols to Therapeutic Interventions in COPD. Pulmonary Medicine 2013, 2013:410748; and Elsevier for granting permission to reproduce material from the article by Skumlien S, Hagelund T, Bjortuft O, Ryg MS: A field test of functional status as performance of activities of daily living in COPD patients. Respiratory Medicine 2006, 100:316-323.

References

1. Ries AL, Kaplan RM, Limberg TM, Prewitt LM. Effects of pulmonary rehabilitation on physiologic and psychosocial outcomes in patients with chronic obstructive pulmonary disease. Ann Intern Med. 1995;122:823–32.
2. Troosters T, Gosselink R, Decramer M. Short- and long-term effects of outpatient rehabilitation in patients with chronic obstructive pulmonary disease: a randomized trial. Am J Med. 2000;109:207–12.
3. Spruit MA, Singh SJ, Garvey C, ZuWallack R, Nici L, Rochester C, Hill K, Holland AE, Lareau SC, Man WD, et al. An official American Thoracic Society/European Respiratory Society statement: key concepts and advances in pulmonary rehabilitation. Am J Respir Crit Care Med. 2013;188:e13–64.
4. Incorvaia C, Russo A, Foresi A, Berra D, Elia R, Passalacqua G, Riario-Sforza GG, Ridolo E. Effects of pulmonary rehabilitation on lung function in chronic obstructive pulmonary disease: the FIRST study. Eur J Phys Rehabil Med. 2014;50:419–26.
5. Global strategy for the diagnosis, management, and prevention of chronic obstructive pulmonary disease. 2016. www.goldcopd.org
6. Crisafulli E, Clini EM. Measures of dyspnea in pulmonary rehabilitation. Multidiscip Respir Med. 2010;5:202–10.
7. Kon SS, Canavan JL, Jones SE, Nolan CM, Clark AL, Dickson MJ, Haselden BM, Polkey MI, Man WD. Minimum clinically important difference for the COPD assessment test: a prospective analysis. Lancet Respir Med. 2014;2:195–203.
8. Redelmeier DA, Guyatt GH, Goldstein RS. Assessing the minimal important difference in symptoms: a comparison of two techniques. J Clin Epidemiol. 1996;49:1215–9.
9. Regueiro EM, Burtin C, Baten P, Langer D, van Remoortel H, Di Lorenzo VA, Costa D, Janssens W, Decramer M, Gosselink R, Troosters T. The minimal important difference of the pulmonary functional status and dyspnea questionnaire in patients with severe chronic obstructive pulmonary disease. Respir Res. 2013;14:58.
10. Jones PW. St. George's respiratory questionnaire: MCID. COPD. 2005;2:75–9.
11. Witek TJ Jr, Mahler DA. Minimal important difference of the transition dyspnoea index in a multinational clinical trial. Eur Respir J. 2003;21:267–72.

12. McCarthy B, Casey D, Devane D, Murphy K, Murphy E, Lacasse Y. Pulmonary rehabilitation for chronic obstructive pulmonary disease. Cochrane Database Syst Rev. 2015;2:CD003793.
13. Troosters T, Gosselink R, Decramer M. Exercise training in COPD: how to distinguish responders from nonresponders. J Cardiopulm Rehabil. 2001;21:10–7.
14. de Torres JP, Pinto-Plata V, Ingenito E, Bagley P, Gray A, Berger R, Celli B. Power of outcome measurements to detect clinically significant changes in pulmonary rehabilitation of patients with COPD. Chest. 2002;121:1092–8.
15. von Leupoldt A, Hahn E, Taube K, Schubert-Heukeshoven S, Magnussen H, Dahme B. Effects of 3-week outpatient pulmonary rehabilitation on exercise capacity, dyspnea, and quality of life in COPD. Lung. 2008;186:387–91.
16. Wadell K, Webb KA, Preston ME, Amornputtisathaporn N, Samis L, Patelli J, Guenette JA, O'Donnell DE. Impact of pulmonary rehabilitation on the major dimensions of dyspnea in COPD. COPD. 2013;10:425–35.
17. Nici L, Donner C, Wouters E, Zuwallack R, Ambrosino N, Bourbeau J, Carone M, Celli B, Engelen M, Fahy B, et al. American Thoracic Society/European Respiratory Society statement on pulmonary rehabilitation. Am J Respir Crit Care Med. 2006;173:1390–413.
18. Caspersen CJ, Powell KE, Christenson GM. Physical activity, exercise, and physical fitness: definitions and distinctions for health-related research. Public Health Rep. 1985;100:126–31.
19. Palange P, Ward SA, Carlsen KH, Casaburi R, Gallagher CG, Gosselink R, O'Donnell DE, Puente-Maestu L, Schols AM, Singh S, Whipp BJ. Recommendations on the use of exercise testing in clinical practice. Eur Respir J. 2007;29:185–209.
20. Borel B, Provencher S, Saey D, Maltais F. Responsiveness of various exercise-testing protocols to therapeutic interventions in COPD. Pulm Med. 2013;2013:410748.
21. Laviolette L, Bourbeau J, Bernard S, Lacasse Y, Pepin V, Breton MJ, Baltzan M, Rouleau M, Maltais F. Assessing the impact of pulmonary rehabilitation on functional status in COPD. Thorax. 2008;63:115–21.
22. Bisca GW, Morita AA, Hernandes NA, Probst VS, Pitta F. Simple lower limb functional tests in patients with chronic obstructive pulmonary disease: a systematic review. Arch Phys Med Rehabil. 2015;96:2221–30.
23. Kiley JP, Sri Ram J, Croxton TL, Weinmann GG. Challenges associated with estimating minimal clinically important differences in COPD-the NHLBI perspective. COPD. 2005;2:43–6.
24. Puhan MA, Chandra D, Mosenifar Z, Ries A, Make B, Hansel NN, Wise RA, Sciurba F. The minimal important difference of exercise tests in severe COPD. Eur Respir J. 2011;37:784–90.
25. Sutherland ER, Make BJ. Maximum exercise as an outcome in COPD: minimal clinically important difference. COPD. 2005;2:137–41.
26. Casaburi R. Factors determining constant work rate exercise tolerance in COPD and their role in dictating the minimal clinically important difference in response to interventions. COPD. 2005;2:131–6.
27. Holland AE, Hill CJ, Rasekaba T, Lee A, Naughton MT, McDonald CF. Updating the minimal important difference for six-minute walk distance in patients with chronic obstructive pulmonary disease. Arch Phys Med Rehabil. 2010;91:221–5.
28. Puhan MA, Mador MJ, Held U, Goldstein R, Guyatt GH, Schunemann HJ. Interpretation of treatment changes in 6-minute walk distance in patients with COPD. Eur Respir J. 2008;32:637–43.
29. Singh SJ, Jones PW, Evans R, Morgan MD. Minimum clinically important improvement for the incremental shuttle walking test. Thorax. 2008;63:775–7.
30. Pepin V, Laviolette L, Brouillard C, Sewell L, Singh SJ, Revill SM, Lacasse Y, Maltais F. Significance of changes in endurance shuttle walking performance. Thorax. 2011;66:115–20.
31. Kon SS, Canavan JL, Nolan CM, Clark AL, Jones SE, Cullinan P, Polkey MI, Man WD. The 4-metre gait speed in COPD: responsiveness and minimal clinically important difference. Eur Respir J. 2014;43:1298–305.
32. Mesquita R, Wilke S, Smid DE, Janssen DJ, Franssen FM, Probst VS, Wouters EF, Muris JW, Pitta F, Spruit MA. Measurement properties of the Timed Up & Go test in patients with COPD. Chron Respir Dis. 2016. pii: 1479972316647178.
33. Jones SE, Kon SS, Canavan JL, Patel MS, Clark AL, Nolan CM, Polkey MI, Man WD. The five-repetition sit-to-stand test as a functional outcome measure in COPD. Thorax. 2013;68:1015–20.
34. Cambach W, Chadwick-Straver RV, Wagenaar RC, van Keimpema AR, Kemper HC. The effects of a community-based pulmonary rehabilitation programme on exercise tolerance and quality of life: a randomized controlled trial. Eur Respir J. 1997;10:104–13.
35. Holland AE, Spruit MA, Troosters T, Puhan MA, Pepin V, Saey D, McCormack MC, Carlin BW, Sciurba FC, Pitta F, et al. An official European Respiratory Society/American Thoracic Society technical standard: field walking tests in chronic respiratory disease. Eur Respir J. 2014;44:1428–46.
36. Singh SJ, Puhan MA, Andrianopoulos V, Hernandes NA, Mitchell KE, Hill CJ, Lee AL, Camillo CA, Troosters T, Spruit MA, et al. An official systematic review of the European Respiratory Society/American Thoracic Society: measurement properties of field walking tests in chronic respiratory disease. Eur Respir J. 2014;44:1447–78.

37. Garber CE, Blissmer B, Deschenes MR, Franklin BA, Lamonte MJ, Lee IM, Nieman DC, Swain DP, American College of Sports Medicine position stand. Quantity and quality of exercise for developing and maintaining cardiorespiratory, musculoskeletal, and neuromotor fitness in apparently healthy adults: guidance for prescribing exercise. Med Sci Sports Exerc. 2011;43:1334–59.
38. Burtin C, Saey D, Saglam M, Langer D, Gosselink R, Janssens W, Decramer M, Maltais F, Troosters T. Effectiveness of exercise training in patients with COPD: the role of muscle fatigue. Eur Respir J. 2012;40:338–44.
39. Vogiatzis I, Zakynthinos S. The physiological basis of rehabilitation in chronic heart and lung disease. J Appl Physiol (1985). 2013;115:16–21.
40. Skeletal muscle dysfunction in chronic obstructive pulmonary disease. A statement of the American Thoracic Society and European Respiratory Society. Am J Respir Crit Care Med. 1999;159:S1–40.
41. Maltais F, Decramer M, Casaburi R, Barreiro E, Burelle Y, Debigare R, Dekhuijzen PN, Franssen F, Gayan-Ramirez G, Gea J, et al. An official American Thoracic Society/European Respiratory Society statement: update on limb muscle dysfunction in chronic obstructive pulmonary disease. Am J Respir Crit Care Med. 2014;189:e15–62.
42. Evans RA, Kaplovitch E, Beauchamp MK, Dolmage TE, Goldstein RS, Gillies CL, Brooks D, Mathur S. Is quadriceps endurance reduced in COPD? A systematic review. Chest. 2015;147:673–84.
43. Bernard S, LeBlanc P, Whittom F, Carrier G, Jobin J, Belleau R, Maltais F. Peripheral muscle weakness in patients with chronic obstructive pulmonary disease. Am J Respir Crit Care Med. 1998;158:629–34.
44. Maffiuletti NA, Bizzini M, Desbrosses K, Babault N, Munzinger U. Reliability of knee extension and flexion measurements using the Con-Trex isokinetic dynamometer. Clin Physiol Funct Imaging. 2007;27:346–53.
45. Canavan JL, Maddocks M, Nolan CM, Jones SE, Kon SS, Clark AL, Polkey MI, Man WD. Functionally relevant cut point for isometric quadriceps muscle strength in chronic respiratory disease. Am J Respir Crit Care Med. 2015;192:395–7.
46. Puhan MA, Siebeling L, Zoller M, Muggensturm P, ter Riet G. Simple functional performance tests and mortality in COPD. Eur Respir J. 2013;42:956–63.
47. Spruit MA, Sillen MJ, Groenen MT, Wouters EF, Franssen FM. New normative values for handgrip strength: results from the UK Biobank. J Am Med Dir Assoc. 2013;14:775 e775–11.
48. Burtin C, Ter Riet G, Puhan MA, Waschki B, Garcia-Aymerich J, Pinto-Plata V, Celli B, Watz H, Spruit MA. Handgrip weakness and mortality risk in COPD: a multicentre analysis. Thorax. 2016;71:86–7.
49. De Brandt J, Spruit MA, Derave W, Hansen D, Vanfleteren LE, Burtin C. Changes in structural and metabolic muscle characteristics following exercise-based interventions in patients with COPD: a systematic review. Expert Rev Respir Med. 2016;10:521–45.
50. Spruit MA, Gosselink R, Troosters T, De PK, Decramer M. Resistance versus endurance training in patients with COPD and peripheral muscle weakness. Eur Respir J. 2002;19:1072–8.
51. O'Shea SD, Taylor NF, Paratz J. Peripheral muscle strength training in COPD: a systematic review. Chest. 2004;126:903–14.
52. Liao WH, Chen JW, Chen X, Lin L, Yan HY, Zhou YQ, Chen R. Impact of resistance training in subjects with COPD: a systematic review and meta-analysis. Respir Care. 2015;60:1130–45.
53. Ortega F, Toral J, Cejudo P, Villagomez R, Sanchez H, Castillo J, Montemayor T. Comparison of effects of strength and endurance training in patients with chronic obstructive pulmonary disease. Am J Respir Crit Care Med. 2002;166:669–74.
54. Vestbo J, Prescott E, Almdal T, Dahl M, Nordestgaard BG, Andersen T, Sorensen TI, Lange P. Body mass, fat-free body mass, and prognosis in patients with chronic obstructive pulmonary disease from a random population sample: findings from the Copenhagen City Heart Study. Am J Respir Crit Care Med. 2006;173:79–83.
55. Lainscak M, von Haehling S, Doehner W, Sarc I, Jeric T, Ziherl K, Kosnik M, Anker SD, Suskovic S. Body mass index and prognosis in patients hospitalized with acute exacerbation of chronic obstructive pulmonary disease. J Cachexia Sarcopenia Muscle. 2011;2:81–6.
56. Schols AM, Broekhuizen R, Weling-Scheepers CA, Wouters EF. Body composition and mortality in chronic obstructive pulmonary disease. Am J Clin Nutr. 2005;82:53–9.
57. Schols AM, Slangen J, Volovics L, Wouters EF. Weight loss is a reversible factor in the prognosis of chronic obstructive pulmonary disease. Am J Respir Crit Care Med. 1998;157:1791–7.
58. Prescott E, Almdal T, Mikkelsen KL, Tofteng CL, Vestbo J, Lange P. Prognostic value of weight change in chronic obstructive pulmonary disease: results from the Copenhagen City Heart Study. Eur Respir J. 2002;20:539–44.
59. Rutten EP, Spruit MA, Wouters EF. Critical view on diagnosing muscle wasting by single-frequency bio-electrical impedance in COPD. Respir Med. 2010;104:91–8.
60. Jones SE, Maddocks M, Kon SS, Canavan JL, Nolan CM, Clark AL, Polkey MI, Man WD. Sarcopenia in COPD: prevalence, clinical correlates and response to pulmonary rehabilitation. Thorax. 2015;70:213–8.
61. Sava F, Laviolette L, Bernard S, Breton MJ, Bourbeau J, Maltais F. The impact of obesity on walking and cycling performance and response to pulmonary rehabilitation in COPD. BMC Pulm Med. 2010;6:10–55.

62. Ramachandran K, McCusker C, Connors M, Zuwallack R, Lahiri B. The influence of obesity on pulmonary rehabilitation outcomes in patients with COPD. Chron Respir Dis. 2008;5:205–9.
63. Greening NJ, Evans RA, Williams JE, Green RH, Singh SJ, Steiner MC. Does body mass index influence the outcomes of a Waking-based pulmonary rehabilitation programme in COPD? Chron Respir Dis. 2012;9:99–106.
64. Berton DC, Silveira L, Da Costa CC, De Souza RM, Winter CD, Zimermann Teixeira PJ. Effectiveness of pulmonary rehabilitation in exercise capacity and quality of life in chronic obstructive pulmonary disease patients with and without global fat-free mass depletion. Arch Phys Med Rehabil. 2013;94:1607–14.
65. Franssen FM, Broekhuizen R, Janssen PP, Wouters EF, Schols AM. Effects of whole-body exercise training on body composition and functional capacity in normal-weight patients with COPD. Chest. 2004;125:2021–8.
66. McDonald VM, Gibson PG, Scott HA, Baines PJ, Hensley MJ, Pretto JJ, Wood LG. Should we treat obesity in COPD? The effects of diet and resistance exercise training. Respirology. 2016;21:875–82.
67. Emtner M, Hallin R, Arnardottir RH, Janson C. Effect of physical training on fat-free mass in patients with chronic obstructive pulmonary disease (COPD). Ups J Med Sci. 2015;120:52–8.
68. Beauchamp MK, Sibley KM, Lakhani B, Romano J, Mathur S, Goldstein RS, Brooks D. Impairments in systems underlying control of balance in COPD. Chest. 2012;141:1496–503.
69. de Castro LA, Ribeiro LR, Mesquita R, de Carvalho DR, Felcar JM, Merli MF, Fernandes KB, da Silva RA, Teixeira DC, Spruit MA, et al. Static and functional balance in individuals with COPD: comparison with healthy controls and differences according to sex and disease severity. Respir Care. 2016;61:1488–96.
70. Butcher SJ, Meshke JM, Sheppard MS. Reductions in functional balance, coordination, and mobility measures among patients with stable chronic obstructive pulmonary disease. J Cardiopulm Rehabil. 2004;24:274–80.
71. Beauchamp MK, Hill K, Goldstein RS, Janaudis-Ferreira T, Brooks D. Impairments in balance discriminate fallers from non-fallers in COPD. Respir Med. 2009;103:1885–91.
72. Jacome C, Cruz J, Oliveira A, Marques A. Validity, reliability, and ability to identify fall status of the berg balance scale, BESTest, Mini-BESTest, and Brief-BESTest in patients with COPD. Phys Ther. 2016;96:1807–15.
73. Mkacher W, Mekki M, Tabka Z, Trabelsi Y. Effect of 6 months of balance training during pulmonary rehabilitation in patients with COPD. J Cardiopulm Rehabil Prev. 2015;35:207–13.
74. Beauchamp MK, Janaudis-Ferreira T, Parreira V, Romano JM, Woon L, Goldstein RS, Brooks D. A randomized controlled trial of balance training during pulmonary rehabilitation for individuals with COPD. Chest. 2013;144:1803–10.
75. Marques A, Jacome C, Cruz J, Gabriel R, Figueiredo D. Effects of a pulmonary rehabilitation program with balance training on patients with COPD. J Cardiopulm Rehabil Prev. 2015;35:154–8.
76. Hakamy A, Bolton CE, McKeever TM. The effect of pulmonary rehabilitation on mortality, balance, and risk of fall in stable patients with chronic obstructive pulmonary disease: a systematic review. Chron Respir Dis. 2017;14(1):54–62.
77. Benzo R, Flume PA, Turner D, Tempest M. Effect of pulmonary rehabilitation on quality of life in patients with COPD: the use of SF-36 summary scores as outcomes measures. J Cardiopulm Rehabil. 2000;20:231–4.
78. Welling JB, Hartman JE, Ten Hacken NH, Klooster K, Slebos DJ. The minimal important difference for the St George's respiratory questionnaire in patients with severe COPD. Eur Respir J. 2015;46:1598–604.
79. Jones PW, Harding G, Wiklund I, Berry P, Tabberer M, Yu R, Leidy NK. Tests of the responsiveness of the COPD assessment test following acute exacerbation and pulmonary rehabilitation. Chest. 2012;142:134–40.
80. Bratas O, Espnes GA, Rannestad T, Walstad R. Pulmonary rehabilitation reduces depression and enhances health-related quality of life in COPD patients—especially in patients with mild or moderate disease. Chron Respir Dis. 2010;7:229–37.
81. Alfarroba S, Rodrigues F, Papoila AL, Santos AF, Morais L. Pulmonary rehabilitation in COPD according to global initiative for chronic obstructive lung disease categories. Respir Care. 2016;61:1331–40.
82. Solanes I, Guell R, Casan P, Sotomayor C, Gonzalez A, Feixas T, Gonzalez M, Guyatt G. Duration of pulmonary rehabilitation to achieve a plateau in quality of life and walk test in COPD. Respir Med. 2009;103:722–8.
83. Reis LF, Guimaraes FS, Fernandes SJ, Cantanhede LA, Dias CM, Lopes AJ, De Menezes SL. A long-term pulmonary rehabilitation program progressively improves exercise tolerance, quality of life and cardiovascular risk factors in patients with COPD. Eur J Phys Rehabil Med. 2013;49:491–7.
84. Pitta F, Troosters T, Probst VS, Langer D, Decramer M, Gosselink R. Are patients with COPD more active after pulmonary rehabilitation? Chest. 2008;134:273–80.
85. Foglio K, Bianchi L, Bruletti G, Porta R, Vitacca M, Balbi B, Ambrosino N. Seven-year time course of lung function, symptoms, health-related quality of life, and exercise tolerance in COPD patients undergoing pulmonary rehabilitation programs. Respir Med. 2007;101:1961–70.
86. Godoy RF, Teixeira PJ, Becker Junior B, Michelli M, Godoy DV. Long-term repercussions of a pulmonary rehabilitation program on the indices of anxiety, depression, quality of life and physical per-

formance in patients with COPD. J Bras Pneumol. 2009;35:129–36.
87. Coventry PA, Hind D. Comprehensive pulmonary rehabilitation for anxiety and depression in adults with chronic obstructive pulmonary disease: systematic review and meta-analysis. J Psychosom Res. 2007;63:551–65.
88. Zigmond AS, Snaith RP. The hospital anxiety and depression scale. Acta Psychiatr Scand. 1983;67:361–70.
89. Puhan MA, Frey M, Buchi S, Schunemann HJ. The minimal important difference of the hospital anxiety and depression scale in patients with chronic obstructive pulmonary disease. Health Qual Life Outcomes. 2008;6:46.
90. Bhandari NJ, Jain T, Marolda C, ZuWallack RL. Comprehensive pulmonary rehabilitation results in clinically meaningful improvements in anxiety and depression in patients with chronic obstructive pulmonary disease. J Cardiopulm Rehabil Prev. 2013;33:123–7.
91. Harrison SL, Greening NJ, Williams JE, Morgan MD, Steiner MC, Singh SJ. Have we underestimated the efficacy of pulmonary rehabilitation in improving mood? Respir Med. 2012;106:838–44.
92. Pumar MI, Gray CR, Walsh JR, Yang IA, Rolls TA, Ward DL. Anxiety and depression-important psychological comorbidities of COPD. J Thorac Dis. 2014;6:1615–31.
93. Trappenburg JC, Troosters T, Spruit MA, Vandebrouck N, Decramer M, Gosselink R. Psychosocial conditions do not affect short-term outcome of multidisciplinary rehabilitation in chronic obstructive pulmonary disease. Arch Phys Med Rehabil. 2005;86:1788–92.
94. Liu Y, Li H, Ding N, Wang N, Wen D. Functional status assessment of patients with COPD: a systematic review of performance-based measures and patient-reported measures. Medicine (Baltimore). 2016;95:e3672.
95. De Vriendt P, Gorus E, Cornelis E, Velghe A, Petrovic M, Mets T. The process of decline in advanced activities of daily living: a qualitative explorative study in mild cognitive impairment. Int Psychogeriatr. 2012;24:974–86.
96. Lareau SC, Meek PM, Roos PJ. Development and testing of the modified version of the pulmonary functional status and dyspnea questionnaire (PFSDQ-M). Heart Lung. 1998;27:159–68.
97. Lareau SC, Carrieri-Kohlman V, Janson-Bjerklie S, Roos PJ. Development and testing of the pulmonary functional status and dyspnea questionnaire (PFSDQ). Heart Lung. 1994;23:242–50.
98. Kovelis D, Zabatiero J, Oldemberg N, Colange AL, Barzon D, Nascimento CH, Probst VS, Pitta F. Responsiveness of three instruments to assess self-reported functional status in patients with COPD. COPD. 2011;8:334–9.
99. Garrod R, Bestall JC, Paul EA, Wedzicha JA, Jones PW. Development and validation of a standardized measure of activity of daily living in patients with severe COPD: the London chest activity of daily living scale (LCADL). Respir Med. 2000;94:589–96.
100. Bisca GW, Proenca M, Salomao A, Hernandes NA, Pitta F. Minimal detectable change of the London chest activity of daily living scale in patients with COPD. J Cardiopulm Rehabil Prev. 2014;34:213–6.
101. Yohannes AM, Roomi J, Winn S, Connolly MJ. The manchester respiratory activities of daily living questionnaire: development, reliability, validity, and responsiveness to pulmonary rehabilitation. J Am Geriatr Soc. 2000;48:1496–500.
102. Yohannes AM, Greenwood YA, Connolly MJ. Reliability of the manchester respiratory activities of daily living questionnaire as a postal questionnaire. Age Ageing. 2002;31:355–8.
103. Yohannes AM, Baldwin RC, Connolly MJ. Predictors of 1-year mortality in patients discharged from hospital following acute exacerbation of chronic obstructive pulmonary disease. Age Ageing. 2005;34:491–6.
104. Chen YJ, Narsavage GL, Culp SL, Weaver TE. The development and psychometric analysis of the short-form Pulmonary Functional Status Scale (PFSS-11). Res Nurs Health. 2010;33:477–85.
105. Weaver TE, Narsavage GL, Guilfoyle MJ. The development and psychometric evaluation of the Pulmonary Functional Status Scale: an instrument to assess functional status in pulmonary disease. J Cardiopulm Rehabil. 1998;18:105–11.
106. Leidy NK, Hamilton A, Becker K. Assessing patient report of function: content validity of the functional performance inventory-short form (FPI-SF) in patients with chronic obstructive pulmonary disease (COPD). Int J Chron Obstruct Pulmon Dis. 2012;7:543–54.
107. Larson JL, Kapella MC, Wirtz S, Covey MK, Berry J. Reliability and validity of the functional performance inventory in patients with moderate to severe chronic obstructive pulmonary disease. J Nurs Meas. 1998;6:55–73.
108. Sewell L, Singh SJ, Williams JE, Collier R, Morgan MD. Can individualized rehabilitation improve functional independence in elderly patients with COPD? Chest. 2005;128:1194–200.
109. Ware JE Jr, Sherbourne CD. The MOS 36-item short-form health survey (SF-36). I. Conceptual framework and item selection. Med Care. 1992;30:473–83.
110. Jones PW, Quirk FH, Baveystock CM. The St George's respiratory questionnaire. Respir Med. 1991;85(Suppl B):25–31. discussion 33-27
111. Guyatt GH, Berman LB, Townsend M, Pugsley SO, Chambers LW. A measure of quality of life for clinical trials in chronic lung disease. Thorax. 1987;42:773–8.
112. Tu SP, McDonell MB, Spertus JA, Steele BG, Fihn SD. A new self-administered questionnaire to monitor health-related quality of life in patients with COPD. Ambulatory Care Quality Improvement Project (ACQUIP) Investigators. Chest. 1997;112:614–22.

113. Probst VS, Kovelis D, Hernandes NA, Camillo CA, Cavalheri V, Pitta F. Effects of 2 exercise training programs on physical activity in daily life in patients with COPD. Respir Care. 2011;56:1799–807.
114. Skumlien S, Hagelund T, Bjortuft O, Ryg MS. A field test of functional status as performance of activities of daily living in COPD patients. Respir Med. 2006;100:316–23.
115. Karloh M, Karsten M, Pissaia FV, de Araujo CL, Mayer AF. Physiological responses to the Glittre-ADL test in patients with chronic obstructive pulmonary disease. J Rehabil Med. 2014;46:88–94.
116. Dos Santos K, Gulart AA, Munari AB, Cani KC, Mayer AF. Reproducibility of ventilatory parameters, dynamic hyperinflation, and performance in the Glittre-ADL TEST in COPD patients. COPD. 2016;13:700–5.
117. Sant'Anna T, Donaria L, Furlanetto KC, Morakami F, Rodrigues A, Grosskreutz T, Hernandes NA, Gosselink R, Pitta F. Development, validity and reliability of the Londrina activities of daily living (ADL) protocol for patients with COPD. Respir Care. 2017;62(3):288–97.
118. Paes T, Belo LF, Silva DR, Morita AA, Donaria L, Furlanetto KC, Sant'Anna T, Pitta F, Hernandes NA. Londrina ADL Protocol: reproducibility, validity and reference values in physically independent adults aged 50 and older. Respir Care. 2017;62(3):298–306.
119. Pitta F, Troosters T, Probst VS, Spruit MA, Decramer M, Gosselink R. Quantifying physical activity in daily life with questionnaires and motion sensors in COPD. Eur Respir J. 2006;27:1040–55.
120. Pitta F, Troosters T, Spruit MA, Decramer M, Gosselink R. Activity monitoring for assessment of physical activities in daily life in patients with chronic obstructive pulmonary disease. Arch Phys Med Rehabil. 2005;86:1979–85.
121. Ruf KC, Fehn S, Bachmann M, Moeller A, Roth K, Kriemler S, Hebestreit H. Validation of activity questionnaires in patients with cystic fibrosis by accelerometry and cycle ergometry. BMC Med Res Methodol. 2012;12:43.
122. Garfield BE, Canavan JL, Smith CJ, Ingram KA, Fowler RP, Clark AL, Polkey MI, Man WD. Stanford seven-day physical activity recall questionnaire in COPD. Eur Respir J. 2012;40:356–62.
123. Serres I, Gautier V, Varray A, Prefaut C. Impaired skeletal muscle endurance related to physical inactivity and altered lung function in COPD patients. Chest. 1998;113:900–5.
124. Donaire-Gonzalez D, Gimeno-Santos E, Serra I, Roca J, Balcells E, Rodriguez E, Farrero E, Anto JM, Garcia-Aymerich J; en representación del PAC-COPD Study Group. Validation of the yale physical activity survey in chronic obstructive pulmonary disease patients. Arch Bronconeumol. 2011;47:552–60.
125. Ainslie P, Reilly T, Westerterp K. Estimating human energy expenditure: a review of techniques with particular reference to doubly labelled water. Sports Med. 2003;33:683–98.
126. Watz H, Waschki B, Meyer T, Magnussen H. Physical activity in patients with COPD. Eur Respir J. 2009;33:262–72.
127. Turner LJ, Houchen L, Williams J, Singh SJ. Reliability of pedometers to measure step counts in patients with chronic respiratory disease. J Cardiopulm Rehabil Prev. 2012;32:284–91.
128. Van Remoortel H, Raste Y, Louvaris Z, Giavedoni S, Burtin C, Langer D, Wilson F, Rabinovich R, Vogiatzis I, Hopkinson NS, et al. Validity of six activity monitors in chronic obstructive pulmonary disease: a comparison with indirect calorimetry. PLoS One. 2012;7:e39198.
129. Rabinovich RA, Louvaris Z, Raste Y, Langer D, Van Remoortel H, Giavedoni S, Burtin C, Regueiro EM, Vogiatzis I, Hopkinson NS, et al. Validity of physical activity monitors during daily life in patients with COPD. Eur Respir J. 2013;42:1205–15.
130. Watz H, Pitta F, Rochester CL, Garcia-Aymerich J, ZuWallack R, Troosters T, Vaes AW, Puhan MA, Jehn M, Polkey MI, et al. An official European Respiratory Society statement on physical activity in COPD. Eur Respir J. 2014;44:1521–37.
131. Demeyer H, Burtin C, Van Remoortel H, Hornikx M, Langer D, Decramer M, Gosselink R, Janssens W, Troosters T. Standardizing the analysis of physical activity in patients with COPD following a pulmonary rehabilitation program. Chest. 2014;146:318–27.
132. Cindy Ng LW, Mackney J, Jenkins S, Hill K. Does exercise training change physical activity in people with COPD? A systematic review and meta-analysis. Chron Respir Dis. 2012;9:17–26.
133. Demeyer H, Burtin C, Hornikx M, Camillo CA, Van Remoortel H, Langer D, Janssens W, Troosters T. The minimal important difference in physical activity in patients with COPD. PLoS One. 2016;11:e0154587.
134. Gimeno-Santos E, Raste Y, Demeyer H, Louvaris Z, de Jong C, Rabinovich RA, Hopkinson NS, Polkey MI, Vogiatzis I, Tabberer M, et al. The PROactive instruments to measure physical activity in patients with chronic obstructive pulmonary disease. Eur Respir J. 2015;46:988–1000.
135. Bandura A. Self-efficacy: toward a unifying theory of behavioral change. Psychol Rev. 1977;84:191–215.
136. Vincent E, Sewell L, Wagg K, Deacon S, Williams J, Singh S. Measuring a change in self-efficacy following pulmonary rehabilitation: an evaluation of the PRAISE tool. Chest. 2011;140:1534–9.
137. Garrod R, Marshall J, Jones F. Self efficacy measurement and goal attainment after pulmonary rehabilitation. Int J Chron Obstruct Pulmon Dis. 2008;3:791–6.
138. Scherer YK, Schmieder LE. The effect of a pulmonary rehabilitation program on self-efficacy, perception of dyspnea, and physical endurance. Heart Lung. 1997;26:15–22.

COPD: Economical and Surrogate Outcomes—The Case of COPD

20

Roberto W. Dal Negro and Claudio F. Donner

We will discuss the overall economics in pulmonary rehabilitation by taking chronic obstructive pulmonary disease (COPD) as a model because it is the most prevalent and incident chronic respiratory pathology [1, 2] in both western and developing countries [3] which is provided by a large and consolidated literature. What is available specifically for pulmonary rehabilitation will be addressed in a devoted sub-section. In general, all countries, even those characterized by evolved health models, took their first operational steps quite recently in the field of the "respiratory chronicity", and of COPD in particular.

If we assume that the term "chronic disease" corresponds, as in COPD, to "*a disease or a pathological condition characterized by a slow course, and then by a poor tendency to achieving the outcome (namely, the complete recovery, or the death, or the adaptation to a novel balance in the life style)*, then the continuous and specific assessment of the resources consumption represents the irreplaceable instrument for checking the impact of COPD on the overall health system and the community, and also for choosing and programming the most convenient actions aimed to its containment.

As the overall impact of COPD recognizes different targets, some general assumptions are needed. Actually, there is "the *individual impact*", which is strictly limited to the patient conditions and perceptions, but also "the *social impact*", which involves the patient's family and the related microcosm where the patient is embedded (namely, his work environment, his care givers, his friends, etc.). Finally, there is "the *societal impact*", which depends on the multiple, integrated effects on the overall community to which all patients belong (Table 20.1).

As previously mentioned, COPD has a high prevalence and generate an important healthcare resource utilization together to a high societal impact. COPD is a major cause of chronic morbidity and mortality worldwide, and is projected to be the third leading cause of death in the world by 2030, and the seventh in terms of burden of disease [4, 5]. Moreover, while populations' mean age is also progressively raising, thus leading to a

Table 20.1 Different domains of COPD impact

Site of impact	Domain of impact
Individual	Humanistic (+ + +) & economic (+ − −)
Social	Humanistic (+ + −) & economic (+ + −)
Health system	Organizational (+ + +) & economic (+ + +)

R.W. Dal Negro
National Centre for Respiratory Pharmacoeconomics and Pharmacoepidemiology, CESFAR, Verona, Italy

C.F. Donner (✉)
Mondo Medico, Multidisciplinary and Rehabilitation Outpatient Clinic, Borgomanero, Novara, Italy
e-mail: cfdonner@mondomedico.it

© Springer International Publishing AG 2018
E. Clini et al. (eds.), *Textbook of Pulmonary Rehabilitation*,
https://doi.org/10.1007/978-3-319-65888-9_20

further increase of the prevalence and the incidence of chronic diseases, including COPD, the cost of pharmacological treatments is steadily increasing in all European countries.

Around the end of the last century, a growing interest in pharmacoeconomic issues corresponded to the overall need for "accountability", and the economic evaluation of operative strategies became the crucial point for decision makers in order to better allocate the decreasing healthcare resources.

Although pharmacoeconomic data are not easy to compare among the different national health systems, common stemming points were: the very high absolute and relative burden of COPD (despite its diffuse and substantial underdiagnosis); the increase of costs proportional to the disease severity (the major costs being due to disease exacerbations and hospitalizations); the high proportion of long-term oxygen therapy (LTOT) costs among overall therapy costs, and the inadequate coverage for drug expenses [6].

The restless progression of COPD burden is confirmed by some studies aimed to the periodic assessment of COPD impact in different countries, characterized by different public health systems. In the USA, the total cost of COPD was calculated in 24 billion $ in 2000; in particular, more than 60% was due to direct costs, 18% to loss of income, and 20% to related morbidity [7]. A few years later, this cost increased to 32 billion US$, and the proportion of direct costs was almost doubled [8]. A perspective study carried out in 2006 calculated that the total cost of COPD will increase from 32 to 176.8 billion US$ in the five following years, but to 389.2 billion US$ in the ten years, and to 832.9 billion US$ in the 20 following years [9]. In 2010, the estimated direct healthcare costs of COPD were $29.5 billion [10]. Of these, $13.2 billion were due to hospital care, $5.5 billion to physician costs, $5.8 billion to outpatient prescription drug costs, $1.3 billion to home healthcare costs, and $3 billion to nursing home care. LTOT Medicare costs were more than $2 billion per year for COPD and the cost is growing by an annual rate of 12–13% [11]. In addition, there were $20.4 billion in indirect costs due to lost productivity from death and disability.

In a corresponding period of time, the mean annual cost/patient in Italy ranged from 608.4 in mild to 2457.3€ in severe COPD, with a mean annual cost/patient of 1801€ [12]. This range changed to 1314.9–5451.1€ in 2007, with a mean annual cost/patient of 2724€ [13], and to 1161.0–6158.9€ in 2015, with a mean annual cost of 3291€ in 2015 [14].

The assessment of the economic burden of chronic disease should then represent a constant point of interest in the agenda of policy makers of healthcare systems. The economic crisis has worsened the context, with national healthcare budgets generally shrinking in many European and Non-European countries. In other words, the growing interest in health economic evolutions stems from the need of maximizing health benefits from increasingly limited resources [15].

Following the first episodic papers [12, 16, 17], epidemiologic studies had proceeded at the same pace of pharmacoeconomic studies, just to achieve a deeper understanding of the intrinsic dynamics leading to the most convenient and strategic choices in this field. Eventually, the impact of COPD became a critical topic and worth of continuous investigation starting from the beginning of the current century, being the production of specific literature dramatically increased in recent years, and particularly over the last decade (Fig. 20.1).

In general terms, COPD is a progressive condition which is characterized by a dramatic socioeconomic impact in all countries where the cost-of-illness of COPD had been calculated [18], particularly in active and income producing subjects [19]. It has also been assessed that the direct annual cost for COPD in primary care is higher than that of other respiratory diseases [17, 20, 21], being the annual cost due to hospitalizations and the cost for ambulatory services 2.5 and 1.6 times as high as those of other chronic patients, respectively. Furthermore, when COPD and bronchial asthma are coexisting (namely, in the asthma COPD overlap syndrome—ACOS) the healthcare resource utilization is even much higher [22]. Other comorbidities [23], racial disparities [24], and the obstructive sleep apnoea syndrome (OSAS) may add additional economic burden in COPD [25].

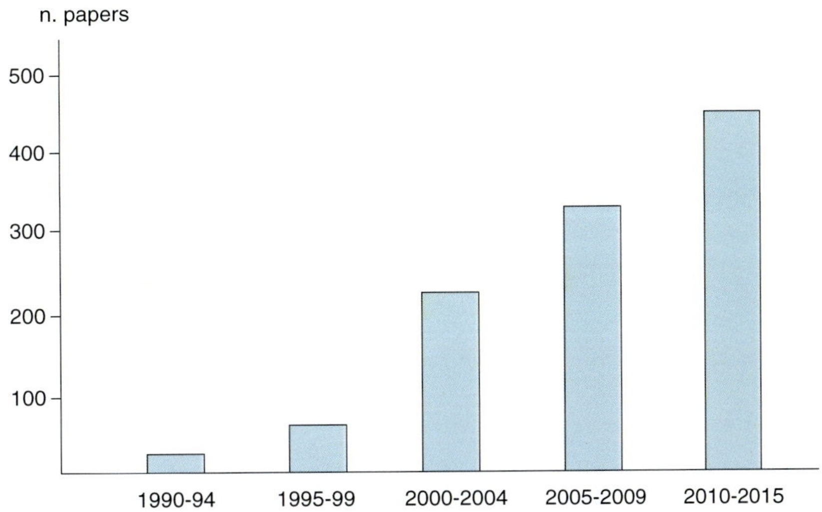

Fig. 20.1 Trend of literature on COPD Health Economics. Time interval 1990–2015

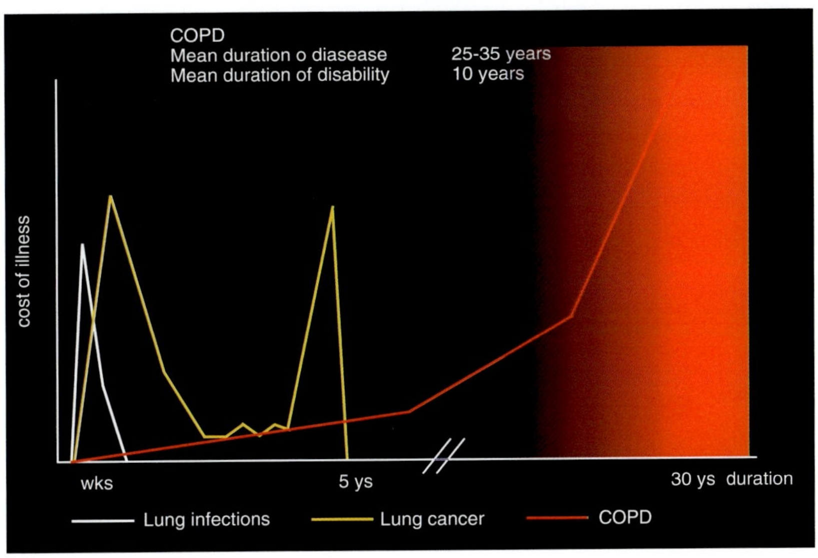

Fig. 20.2 Different duration and different patterns of cost-of-illness for respiratory infectious diseases, lung cancer, and COPD

When calculated, also the indirect burden of COPD proves substantial, and mainly related to work days off, loss of productivity, loss of opportunities, all conditions leading to loss of personal income [26].

From a general point of view, the long duration of COPD (20–30 years) should be recognized as the critical factor which is able to transform systematically this chronic and progressive pathological condition into one of the most costly diseases. Actually, much more costly than severe infectious and/or neoplastic diseases, which are usually characterized by a shorter duration, independently of their final outcome (such as, the complete recovery rather than the death) (Fig. 20.2).

All cost components vary according to the clinical severity of COPD. Whenever direct costs considered, around the 70% of COPD cost-of-illness is related to hospital admissions, independently of the COPD stage of severity [13, 14, 16, 27]. To pinpoint that this figure is likely partially under-esteemed because: (1) it is mainly derived from clinical trials, which are usually designed for regulatory purposes [15]; (2) data presently available are usually limited to situations where COPD

Table 20.2 Possible valuable actions oriented to the effective containment of COPD burden

A—Early diagnosis
B—Smoking cessation
C—Pharmacotherapy
D—Educational approach to treatment
E—Rehabilitation
F—Strategic policies

is reported as the main diagnosis in the patients' clinical files, thus excluding all those conditions where COPD is likely occurring as a relevant comorbidity (namely, chronic congestive heart failure, recurrent lower tract infections, etc.).

The great majority of studies indicate confirm that exacerbations are the main driver of COPD burden because they can affect morbidity, mortality, quality of life, and related healthcare expenditure during COPD [2, 28–33]. On the other hand, both the hospitalization and the exacerbation rates were described as strictly related to the length of survival, and the corresponding annual costs showed the same trend and showed a surprisingly high predicting value [34].

As previously reported, the healthcare burden of COPD is challenging major public health organizations and provoking vigorous efforts aimed to face and to contain the socio-economic effects of the disease. The attitude towards COPD governance is still largely insufficient and inadequate from the prevention to both diagnosis and treatment. The effective actions of proved economic value, and oriented to a more effective management of COPD, are summarized in Table 20.2.

20.1 A: Early diagnosis

Early diagnosis of COPD offers the best opportunity to identify subjects suffering from COPD in their first stages, when the structural lesions are at their beginning phase, but also when the risk of lung function decline is higher [35]. The undiagnosed or the delayed diagnosis of COPD lead to a substantial and progressive increase of cost, mainly due to direct (such as: scheduled and unscheduled GP and Specialist visits, ER visits, hospital admissions, use of healthcare resources, and drugs) and indirect (such as: absenteeism, loss of income, poor quality of life) cost components. Furthermore, if undiagnosed, COPD can progress rapidly according to its natural history, which frequently leads to significant lung function decline, severe dyspnoea, and disability, while the early diagnosis offers a good opportunity to slow the disease progression [36].

To emphasize that a not negligible proportion of COPD diagnosis still is missing even in severe patients [37], and that, unfortunately, only a small proportion of diagnostic tests which could consent to define the clinical and lung function stage of COPD are carried out extensively in clinical practice.

20.2 B: Smoking Cessation

The effect of smoking cessation on COPD burden has been already documented. The smoking cessation programme was proved as the dominant strategy when compared to usual care: the intervention led to an increase of 0.54 QALYs and was cost-saving in the lifetime Markow model [38]. In the probabilistic analysis, smoking cessation dominated in 95% of simulations, even if some uncertainty was found in terms of disease progression, particularly in early stages of COPD.

Various strategies have been adopted with encouraging results, and various models were adopted for assessing the possible benefits [39, 40]. In all these studies, funding and supporting smoking cessation were invariably confirmed as a cost-saving policy. In particular, to pinpoint that the introduction of Varenicline for smoking cessation changed dramatically and highly improved outcomes, also in terms economic convenience [41].

20.3 C: Pharmacotherapy

The pharmacological strategy is certainly the most frequently adopted in COPD, and the most widely studied in terms of possible cost-saving effects since long ago.

However, as the majority of pharmacological treatments are costly and healthcare resources are scarce, healthcare providers and decision makers are highly interested in data on whether treatments are really effective and/or offer significant improvements in terms of clinical governance and disease progression of COPD. Obviously, outcomes and perspectives of treatments vary with the different therapeutic options used for managing COPD.

Different classes of bronchodilators used alone [42–44], or combined to inhaled corticosteroids [45–47] represent the most investigated therapeutic options from this point of view. In general, independently of the particular molecule(s) used, the main message systematically emerging from this huge number of studies is that the strategy based on the regular, long-term treatment of COPD is the only approach which is able to consent a better control of symptoms, together to a better and long lasting quality of life to patients.

A number of studies have also been dedicated to the economic convenience of antimicrobial agents, with conflicting results. Actually, even if some studies are showing significant benefits [48, 49], the true economic value of antibiotic use still results highly influenced by different factors (namely, the difficulties in recognizing the role of infectious agents; their resistances; in defining the antimicrobial dose and duration of treatment) [50].

Some studies also investigated the possible economic benefits due to other pharmacological options, as the PDE_4 inhibitor Roflumilast (administered for 12 months to severe and very severe COPD in the societal perspective [51] and Erdosteine, (an anti-oxidant mucoactive drug, which reduced the exacerbation and the hospitalization rates over an 8-month daily treatment) [52], which proved cost-effective.

In emphysema patients with α1-antitrypsine deficiency, a significant prolongation of years of life was obtained with α1-antitrypsine supplementation, and at a cost/year gained which was comparable to that of other usual therapeutic intervention [53].

The pharmacoeconomics of both influenza vaccination and pneumococcal conjugate vaccination programmes were also investigated, and significant economic benefits were proved, particularly in risk groups of COPD subject [54, 55].

Finally, oxygen supplementation has been studied from this point of view with conflicting results. The main drivers for cost savings in severe COPD was the appropriateness of oxygen prescription, the quality of programmed interventions, the strict control of delivery systems, and the strict supervision of oxygen use. In this particular case, the programmes aimed to facilitate the home care use of oxygen and the programmes aimed to support tele-medicine surprisingly consented dramatic containment of costs and proved highly cost-effective [56].

20.4 D: Educational Approach to Treatment

The adherence to treatments is a very crucial topic in the governance of COPD. Actually, no molecule and no therapeutic intervention will be effective if patients do not follow their appropriate prescription sufficiently. As it has been documented that only an average of 40–60% of COPD patients adhere to their prescribed treatment [57], the non-adherence to medication regimens (namely, intentional or non-intentional under-use, but also the improper or the over-use) represent a substantial component of healthcare resources' absorption.

A systematic review which was carried out aimed to assess the impact of non-adherence in COPD patients on economic outcomes (such as: mortality, quality of life, work productivity, and costs) indicated a clear relationship between the degree of adherence and economic outcomes, making non-adherent subjects a priority for cost-effective interventions [58].

In particular, the use of inhalation devices substantially different in their technologies further emphasizes the consequences of adherence or non-adherence to therapeutic regimens, being only one out of ten patients who use metered dose inhalers who actuates all required manoeuvres appropriately [57, 59]. This is the reason why improving usability of devices may cause substantial cost savings in COPD treatment [60].

Usability and cost-of-usability of different dry-powder inhalers were recently assessed and compared in patients with COPD in terms of cost for their overall usability track. The number of manoeuvres for their actuation; the time for understanding their inhalation procedures; the time for overall training, and the time for proper usability represent the main characteristics which can vary substantially from each other, and may lead to a dramatically different patient's usability and a dramatically different impact in economic terms [61]. Obviously, the choice of the most appropriate inhaler device should be carefully considered before prescribing new therapies, even in terms of its possible economic impact.

20.5 E: Pulmonary rehabilitation

The non-pharmacological approach to COPD is mainly represented by pulmonary rehabilitation (PR), which is recommended by current guidelines in COPD.

The American Thoracic Society and the European Respiratory Society have published an official statement on pulmonary rehabilitation [62] aimed to favour implementation, use, and delivery of PR, as this therapeutic approach has demonstrated clinical and economic benefits in COPD patients [63]. Nevertheless, despite these consolidated evidence, only a negligible proportion of patients are included in rehabilitation programmes of at least 8-week duration in usual care.

Conflicting results only exist concerning the effectiveness of integrated programmes in lowering the exacerbation and hospitalization rates in severe COPD patients, being only a few studies available on the economic impact of PR in severe COPD.

The cost-effectiveness of an 8-week in-patient PR programme followed by 16 weeks of outpatient training in patients with severe stable COPD showed that the costs required for a single patient to achieve the minimal clinically important improvement in various components of the Chronic Respiratory Questionnaire were Can $28,993 for mastery; Can $38,270 for emotional function; Can $47,548 for dyspnoea, and Can $51,027 for fatigue [64].

More recently, some controlled studies were aimed to investigate the economic healthcare benefits of different intervention models for PR. A pneumologist-led disease management programme proved to be cost-effective, and decreased severe exacerbations, by an annual savings estimated at $1.17 million [65].

A further randomized trial of 12-month duration focused the economic convenience of a low-intensity maintenance programme in primary and secondary care setting. Patients who completed at least 60% of a standard PR programme were randomized to a 2-h maintenance session or to usual treatment. Outcomes were: changes in symptom score, EQ-5D QALYs, cost for UK social service (NHS), and incremental cost-effectiveness ratios (ICERs). PR maintenance for 12 months dominated treatment from the perspective of NHS in terms of cost per QALY gained, and there was a 72.9% probability that the ICER is below £20,000–30,000 per QALY [66].

Another study investigated the cost-utility at six months of a self-management programme in COPD carried out in 30 primary care settings. Results suggested that the intervention was more costly, but more effective than usual care, and that the probability of the intervention being cost-effective was 97% at a threshold of £ 20,000/QALY, thus suggesting the cost-effectiveness of the PR programme [67].

A systematic review of economic evaluation of health-related PR has been published a few months ago. Sixty-four systematic reviews were considered, and the great proportion of these reviews included economic data evaluations from randomized clinical trials. Data showed that some PR interventions are cost-effective, and consent some not negligible results in disabled patients, even though these results were clear in high income countries only [68]. Obviously, these data immediately stimulates the debate on the hot problem concerning opportunities, disparities, inequalities, and iniquities in healthcare.

To underline that the comparison of the various estimates of cost-effectiveness is frequently complicated by differences in the specific content and intensity of PR programme, outcome measures, target population, and comparators [62].

20.6 F: Strategic Policies

The containment of the "epidemic" trend of COPD is still causing huge epidemiological, medical and social problems, together to severe concerns to the health policy makers, independently of the healthcare model locally adopted and operating.

On the other hand, if the last century paid a great attention to health in general, nevertheless it bequeathed sanitary models which were almost uniquely oriented to face those acute diseases (mainly infectious in origin) which dramatically characterized its first decades by high mortality in all ages of life, and particularly in childhood.

Actually, little or nothing was done for preventing the incoming huge problems related to the ever increasing respiratory chronic diseases until the end of the twentieth century. Yet, the ever increasing industrialization, the progressive high production of environmental pollutants, the almost complete dependence on fossil fuels, the huge abuse of unnecessary toxic substances (in particular, cigarette smoke), and the substantial increase of people ageing and life expectancy should have easily advise the health policy makers that "respiratory chronicity" would have undermine in short time the consolidated public health system, absolutely "unripe" for facing this incoming challenge.

The role of the socio-economic condition of COPD still is scarcely valued, even if lower are the educational degree and the economic status of subjects, higher is their probability to suffer from COPD [69–71]. Actually, these two conditions tend to synergize and usually lead to a poorer housing and nutritional intake; a higher incidence of respiratory infections, particularly in childhood; a higher prevalence of smoking; a higher probability to accept disadvantaged jobs, etc. [72].

The present organization of health systems requires decisions of high value in terms of cost-effectiveness and cost-utility of strategic actions to adopt. Even if these decisions usually appear progressively distant from the old welfare model, they should however be aimed to the sustainability of choices in terms of their convenience, and would lead to the best possible outcomes and the most convenient allocation of resources. A much stronger empowerment of institutions is required also for these reasons.

It is time for decision makers to change their philosophy towards a new strategic vision for approaching the burden of COPD, just stemming from the huge amount of epidemiological, clinical, and economic data available: all systematically in favour of appropriate long-term medical and organizational interventions. In other words, the adoption of decision criteria still merely based on the sole annual cost cutting (namely, of the drugs used, of expenses for rehabilitation programmes, of expenses for educational programmes) have proven ineffective, because usually merely oriented to financial restrictions rather than to the effective containment of COPD, and of its dramatic long-term health-economic consequences [73].

Meanwhile, populations are getting older and older in all countries; pollutions are growing restless in industrialized and non-industrialized countries; the tobacco consumption is still high, and the proportion of people at low income is also growing: all these factors can be easily presumed as able to further drive the future burden of COPD.

Development of more appropriate socio-economic models of intervention in COPD and of more specific indices for predicting outcomes likely represent the most crucial and convenient actions in favour of the Health System and the Community.

References

1. Murray CJ, Lopez AD. Alternative projections of mortalità and disability by cause 1990–2020—Global Burden of Disease Study. Lancet. 1997;349:1498–504.
2. Global Initiative for Chronic Obstructive Lung Disease. Global strategy for the diagnosis, management, and prevention of chronic obstructive pulmonary disease (Updated February 2013), 2013.

Available from: http://www.goldcopd.org/Guidelines/guidelines-global-strategy-for-diagnosis-management-2013.html Accessed December 10, 2014
3. Yack D, Hawkes C, Gould CL, Hofman KJ. The global Burden of chronic diseases. Overcoming impediments of prevention and control. JAMA. 2004;291(21)
4. Mathers CD, Loncar D. Projections of global mortality and Burden of disease from 2002 to 2030. PLoS Med. 2006;3(11):e442.
5. Mannino DM, Higuchi K, Yu TC, Zhou H, Li Y, Tian H, Suh K. Economic burden of chronic obstructive pulmonary disease by presence of comorbidities. Chest. 2015;147:1199–201.
6. Donner CF, Virchow JC, Lusuardi M. Pharmacoeconomics in COPD and inappropriateness of diagnostics, management and treatment. Respir Med. 2011;105:828–37.
7. Sullivan SD, Ramsey SD, Lee TA. The economic burden of COPD. Chest. 2000;117(Suppl. 2):5–9s.
8. Sullivan SD, Buist AS, Weiss K. Health outcomes assessment and economic evaluation in COPD: challenges and opportunities. Eur Respir J Suppl. 2003;41:1–3s.
9. Lee TA, Sullivan SD, Buist AS, Vollmer W, Weiss KB. Estimating the future burden of COPD; 2006; ATS Abstract Issue, vol. 3: A598.
10. National Heart, Lung, and Blood Institute. Morbidity and mortality: 2009 chart book on cardiovascular, lung, and blood diseases. http://www.nhlbi.nih.gov/resources/docs/2009_ChartBook.pdf. accessed 18.01.2010.
11. Croxton TL, Bailey WC. Long-term oxygen treatment in chronic obstructive pulmonary disease: recommendations for future research: an NHLBI workshop report. Am J Respir Crit Care Med. 2006;174:373e8.
12. Dal NR, Berto P, Tognella S, Quareni L. Cost-of-illness of lung disease in the TriVeneto Region, Italy: the GOLD study. Monaldi Arch Chest Dis. 2002;57:1–7.
13. Dal Negro RW, Tognella S, Tosatto R, Dionisi M, Turco P, Donner CF. Costs of chronic obstructive pulmonary disease (COPD) in Italy: the SIRIO study. Respir Med. 2008;102:92–101.
14. Dal Negro RW, Bonadiman L, Turco P, Tognella S, Iannazzo S. Costs of illness analysis in Italian patients with chronic obstructive pulmonary disease (COPD): an update. Clinicoecon Outcomes Res. 2015;7:153–9.
15. Sculpher M. Using economic evaluations to reduce the burden of asthma and chronic obstructive pulmonary disease. Pharmacoeconomics. 2001;19(Suppl. 2):21–5.
16. Ruchlin HS, Dasbach AJ. An economic overview of chronic obstructive pulmonary disease. Pharmacoeconomics. 2001;19:623–42.
17. Rennard S, Decramer M, Calverley PMA, et al. Impact of COPD in North America and Europe in 2000: subjects' perspective of Confronting COPD International Survey. Eur Respir J. 2002;20:799–805.
18. Mathers CD, Loncar D. Projections of global mortality and burden of disease from 2002 to 2030. PLoS Med. 2006;3(11):e442.
19. van Boven JF, Vegter S, van der Molen T, Postma MJ. COPD in the working age population: the economic impact on both patients and government. COPD. 2013;10:629–39.
20. Grupo DAFNE- Direct costs to primary care of chronic bronchitis. Analysis of a prospective study. Aten Primaria. 2001;27:399–4.
21. Rutten van-Molken MP, Feenstra TL. The burden of asthma and chronic obstructive pulmonary disease: data from The Nederlands. Pharmacoeconomics. 2001;19 Suppl. 2:1–6.
22. Shaya FT, Dongyi D, Akazawa MO, Blanchette CM, Wang J, Mapel DW, Dalal A, Scharf SM. Burden of concomitant asthma and COPD in a Medical population. Chest. 2008;134:14–9.
23. Srivastava K, Thakur D, Sharma S, Punekar YS. Systematic review of humanistic and economic burden of symptomatic chronic obstructive pulmonary disease. Pharmacoeconomics. 2015;33:467–88.
24. Shaya FT, Maneval MS, Gbarayor CM, Sohn K, Dalal A, Du D, Scharf SM. Burden of COPD, asthma, and concomitant COPD and asthma among adults: racial disparities in a medical population. Chest. 2009;136:405–11.
25. Shaya FT, Lin PJ, Aljiawadi MH, Scharf SM. Elevated economic burden in obstructive lung disease patients with concomitant sleep apnea syndrome. Sleep Breath. 2009;13:317–23.
26. Patel JG, Nagar SP, Dala AA. Indirect costs in chronic obstructive pulmonary disease: e reiew of the economic burden on employers and individuals in the United states. Int J Chron Obstruct Pulmon Dis. 2014;19:289–300.
27. Hilleman DE, Dewan N, Malesker M, Friedman M. Pharmacoeconomic evalutation of COPD. Chest. 2000;118:1278–85.
28. Toy EL, Gallagher KF, Stanley EL, Swensen AR, Duh MS. The economic impact of exacerbations of chronic obstructive pulmonary disease and exacerbation definition: a review. COPD. 2010;7:214–28.
29. Jahnz-Rozyk K, Targowski T, From S. Costs of exacerbations of chronic obstructive pulmonary disease in primary ans secondary care in 2007—results of a multicenter Polish study. Pol Menkur Lekarski. 2009;26:208–14.
30. Seemungal TA, Donaldson GC, Bhowmik A, Jeffries DJ, Wedzicha JA. Time course and recovery of exacerbations in patients with chronic obstructive pulmonary disease. Am J Respir Crit Care Med. 2000;161(5):1608–13.
31. Soler-Cataluña JJ, Martínez-García MA, Román Sánchez P, Salcedo E, Navarro M, Ochando R. Severe acute exacerbations and mortality in patients with chronic obstructive pulmonary disease. Thorax. 2005;60(11):925–31.
32. Simoens S, Decramer M. Pharmacoeconomics of the management of acute exacerbations of chronic obstructive pulmonary disease. Expert Opin Pharmacother. 2007;8:633–48.
33. Mapel DW, Schum M, Lydick E, MArton JP. A new method for examining the cost savings of reduc-

ing COPD exacerbations. Pharmacoeconomics. 2010;28:733–49.
34. Dal Negro RW, Celli BR. The BODECOST Index (BCI): a composite index for assessing the impact of COPD in real life. Multidiscip Respir Med. 2016;11:10.
35. Tantucci C, Modina D. Lung function decline in COPD. Int J ChronObstruct Pulmon Dis. 2012;7:95–9.
36. Ramsey SD, Sullivan SD. Chronic obstructive pulmonary disease: is there a case for early intervention? Am J Med. 2004;117 Suppl 12A:3S–10S.
37. Zoia MC, Corsico AG, Beccaria M, Guarnone R, Cervio G, Testi R, Bressan MA, Pozzi E, Cerveri I. Exacerbations as a starting point of pro-active chronic obstructive pulmonary disease management. Respir Med. 2005;99(12):1568–75.
38. Menn P, Leidl R, Holle R. A lifetime Markov model for the economic evaluation of chronic obstructive pulmonary disease. Pharmacoeconomics. 2012;30(9):825–40.
39. Getsios D, Marton JP, Revankar N, Ward AJ, Willke RJ, Rublee D, Ishak KJ, Xenakis JG. Smoking cessation treatment and outcomes patterns simulation: a new framework for evaluating the potential health and economic impact of smoking cessation interventions. Pharmacoeconomics. 2013;31(9):767–80.
40. Jiménez-Ruiz CA, Solano-Reina S, Signes-Costa J, de Higes-Martinez E, Granda-Orive JI, Lorza-Blasco JJ, Riesco-Miranda JA, Altet-Gomez N, Barrueco M, Oyagüez I, Rejas J, SESEPARAR's Integrated Tobacco Research Program. Budgetary impact analysis on funding smoking-cessation drugs in patients with COPD in Spain. Int J Chron Obstruct Pulmon Dis. 2015;10:2027–36.
41. Howard P, Knight C, Boler A, Baker C. Cost-utility analysis of varenicline versus existing smoking cessation strategies using the BENESCO Simulation model: application to a population of US adult smokers. Pharmacoeconomics. 2008;26(6):497–511.
42. Lee KH, Phua J, Lim TK. Evaluating the pharmacoeconomic effect of adding tiotropium bromide to the management of chronic obstructive pulmonary disease patients in Singapore. Respir Med. 2006;100(12):2190–6.
43. Zaniolo O, Iannazzo S, Pradelli L, Miravitlles M. Pharmacoeconomic evaluation of tiotropium bromide in the long-term treatment of chronic obstructive pulmonary disease (COPD) in Italy. Eur J Health Econ. 2012;13(1):71–80.
44. Ferroni E, Belleudi V, Cascini S, Di Martino M, Kirchmayer U, Pistelli R, Patorno E, Formoso G, Fusco D, Perucci CA, Davoli M, Agabiti N, OUTPUL study group. Role of tiotropium in reducing exacerbations of chronic obstructive pulmonary disease when combined with long-acting B2-agonists and inhaled corticosteroids: the OUTPUL Study. J Clin Pharmacol. 2016; doi:10.1002/jcph.750. [Epub ahead of print]
45. Halpin DM. Symbicort: a pharmacoeconomic review. J Med Econ. 2008;11:345–62.
46. Najafzadeh M, Marra CA, Sadatsafavi M, Aaron SD, Sullivan SD, Vandemheen KL, Jones PW, Fitzgerald JM. Cost effectiveness of therapy with combinations of long acting bronchodilators and inhaled steroids for treatment of COPD. Thorax. 2008;63(11):962–7.
47. Dal Negro R, Bonadiman L, Tognella S, Micheletto C, Turco P. The impact of LABA+ICS fixed combinations on morbidity and economic burden of COPD in Italy: a six-year observational study. Ther Adv Respir Dis. 2011;5(2):83–90.
48. Simoens S, Decramer M. A pharmacoeconomic review of the management of respiratory tract infections with moxafloxacin. Expert Opin Pharmacother. 2008;9:1735–44.
49. Simoens S, Laekeman G, Decramer M. Preventing COPD exacerbations with macrolids; a review and budget impact analysis. Respir Med. 2013;107:637–48.
50. Simoens S, Decramer M, Laekeman G. Economic aspects of antimicrobial therapy of acute exacerbations of COPD. Respir Med. 2007;101(1):15–26.
51. Rutten-van Mölken MP, van Nooten FE, Lindemann M, Caeser M, Calverley PM. A 1-year prospective cost-effectiveness analysis of roflumilast for the treatment of patients with severe chronic obstructive pulmonary disease. Pharmacoeconomics. 2007;25(8):695–711.
52. Moretti M, Bottrighi P, Dallari R, Da Porto R, Dolcetti A, Grandi P, Garuti G, Guffanti E, Roversi P, De Gugliemo M, Potena A, EQUALIFE Study Group. The effect of long-term treatment with erdosteine on chronic obstructive pulmonary disease: the EQUALIFE Study. Drugs Exp Clin Res. 2004;30(4):143–52.
53. Sclar DA, Evans MA, Robison LM, Skaer TL. α1-Proteinase inhibitor (human) in the treatment of hereditary emphysema secondary to α1-antitrypsin deficiency: number and costs of years of life gained. Clin Drug Investig. 2012;32(5):353–60.
54. Słominski JM, Kubiak A. Pharmacoeconomics of vaccinations in chronic obstructive pulmonary disease. Pol Merkur Lekarski. 2004;16(Suppl 1):83–5.
55. Rodríguez González-Moro JM, Menéndez R, Campins M, Lwoff N, Oyagüez I, Echave M, Rejas J, Antoñanzas F. Cost effectiveness of the 13-valent pneumococcal conjugate vaccination program in chronic obstructive pulmonary disease patients aged 50+ years in Spain. Clin Drug Investig. 2016;36(1):41–53.
56. Dal Negro RW. The tele-control at home. In: Dal Negro RW, Hodder R, editors. Long-term oxygen therapy. New insights & perspectives. Milan: Springer Verlag; 2012. p. 171–84.
57. Restrepo RD, Alvarez MT, Wittnebel LD, Sorenson H, Wettstein R, Vines DL, Sikkema-Ortiz J, Gardner DD, Wilkins RL. Medication adherence issues in patients treated for COPD. Int J Chron Obstruct Pulmon Dis. 2008;3(3):371–84.
58. van Boven JF, Chavannes NH, van der Molen T, Rutten-van Mölken MP, Postma MJ, Vegter S. Clinical

and economic impact of non-adherence in COPD: a systematic review. Respir Med. 2014;108(1):103–13.
59. Virchow JC, Crompton GK, Dal Negro RW, Pedersen S, Magnan A, Seidemberg J, et al. Importance of inhaler devices in the management of airway diseases. Respir Med. 2008;102:10–9.
60. van Boven JF, Tommelein E, Boussery K, Mehuys E, Vegter S, Brusselle GG, Rutten-van Mölken MP, Postma MJ. Improving inhaler adherence in patients with chronic obstructive pulmonary disease: a cost-effectiveness analysis. Respir Res. 2014;15:66. doi:10.1186/1465-9921-15-66.
61. Dal Negro RW, Povero M. The economic impact of educational training assessed by the Handling Questionnaire with three inhalation devices in asthma and Chronic Obstructive Pulmonary Disease patients. Clinicoeconomics Outcomes Res. 2016;8:171–6.
62. Spruit MA, Singh SJ, Garvey C, Zuwallack R, Nici L, Rochester C, Hill K, Holland AE, Lareau SC, Man WD, Pitta F, Sewell L, Raskin J, Bourbeau J, Crouch R, Franssen FM, Casaburi R, Vercoulen JH, Vogiatzis I, Gosselink R, Clini EM, Effing TW, Maltais F, van der Palen J, Troosters T, Janssen DJ, Collins E, Garcia-Aymerich J, Brooks D, Fahy BF, Puhan MA, Hoogendoorn M, Garrod R, Schols AM, Carlin B, Benzo R, Meek P, Morgan M, Rutten-van Mölken MP, Ries AL, Make B, Goldstein RS, Dowson CA, Brozek JL, Donner CF, Wouters EF, ATS/ERS Task Force on Pulmonary Rehabilitation. An official American Thoracic Society/European Respiratory Society statement: Key concepts and advances in pulmonary rehabilitation. Am J Respir Crit Care Med. 2013;188(8):e13–64. doi:10.1164/rccm.201309-1634ST.
63. Rochester CL, Vogiatzis I, Holland AE, Lareau SC, Marciniuk DD, Puhan MA, Spruit MA, Masefield S, Casaburi R, Clini EM, Crouch R, Garcia-Aymerich J, Garvey C, Goldstein RS, Hill K, Morgan M, Nici L, Pitta F, Ries AL, Singh SJ, Troosters T, Wijkstra PJ, Yawn BP, RL ZW. ATS/ERS Task Force on Policy in Pulmonary Rehabilitation. Am J Respir Crit Care Med. 2015;192(11):1373–86.
64. Goldstein RS, Gort EH, Guyatt GH, Feeny D. Economic analysis of respiratory rehabilitation. Chest. 1997;112:370–9.
65. Jain VV, Allison R, Beck SJ, Jain R, Mills PK, McCurley JW, Van Gundy KP, Peterson MW. Impact of an integrated disease management program in reducing exacerbations in patients with severe asthma and COPD. Respir Med. 2014;108(12):1794–800.
66. Burns DK, Wilson EC, Browne P, Olive S, Clark A, Galey P, Dix E, Woodhouse H, Robinson S, Wilson A. The cost effectiveness of maintenance schedules following pulmonary rehabilitation in patients with chronic obstructive pulmonary disease: an economic evaluation alongside a randomised controlled trial. Appl Health Econ Health Policy. 2016;14(1):105–15.
67. Dritsaki M, Johnson-Warrington V, Mitchell K, Singh S, Rees K. An economic evaluation of a self-management programme of activity, coping and education for patients with chronic obstructive pulmonary disease. Chron Respir Dis. 2016;13(1):48–56.
68. Howard-Wilsher S, Irvine L, Fan H, Shakespeare T, Suhrcke M, Horton S, Poland F, Hooper L, Song F. Systematic overview of economic evaluations of health-related rehabilitation. Disabil Health J. 2016;9(1):11–25.
69. Prescott E, Lange P, Vestbo J. Socioeconomic status, lung function and admission to hospital for COPD: results from the Copenhagen City Health Study. Eur Respir J. 1999;13:1109–14.
70. Thorn J, Bjorkelund C, Bengtsson C, Guo X, Lissenr L, Sundh V. Low socio-economic status, smoking, mental stress and obesity predict obstructive symptoms in women, but only smoking also predicts subsequent experience of poor health. Int J Med Sci. 2006;4:7–12.
71. Kanervist M, Vasankari T, Laitinen T, Heliovaara M, Jpusilathi P, Saarelainen S. Low socioeconomic status is associated with chronic obstructive airway disease. Respir Med. 2011;105:1140–6.
72. Bousquet J, Dahl R, Khaltaev N. Global Alliance against chronic respiratory disease. Allergy. 2007;62:216–23.
73. Roberts MH, Borrego ME, Kharat AA, Marshik PL, Mapel DW. Economic evaluations of fluticasone-propionate/salmeterol combination therapy for chronic obstructive pulmonary disease: a review of published studies. Expert Rev Pharmacoecon Outcomes Res. 2016;16(2):167–92.

Part VI

Organization

21 Conventional Programs: Settings, Cost, Staffing, and Maintenance

Carolyn L. Rochester and Enrico Clini

21.1 Introduction

Pulmonary rehabilitation (PR) can be implemented and delivered successfully in a variety of settings [1, 2]. Inpatient, outpatient, and home-based programs exist. In these settings, PR can be delivered to medically stable individuals with chronic respiratory diseases, as well as to those with COPD early following COPD exacerbation. The location and composition of PR programs varies widely within and across countries [3–5]. Program settings, components, and staff depend principally on individual countries' health systems, as well as on locally available program funding and resources. To be considered PR, however, the core components including patient assessments [at least including exercise capacity, symptoms and health status/quality of life (QOL)], supervised multimodality exercise training of the upper and lower extremities, education geared towards health-enhancing behavior change, and outcomes measures must be included [1, 6, 7]. The severity of the patient's respiratory disease, complexity of comorbidities, patient preference, and availability of transportation also influence the optimal setting for PR. Maintenance of benefits achieved in PR is an important goal. While resources for maintenance PR programs are not universally available, several models of such programs have been investigated. The settings, staffing, and cost for conventional PR programs will be considered further below.

C.L. Rochester, M.D. (✉)
Section of Pulmonary, Critical Care and Sleep Medicine, Yale University School of Medicine, 333 Cedar Street, BLDG LCI-105, New Haven, CT 06520, USA
e-mail: carolyn.rochester@yale.edu

E. Clini
Department of Medical and Surgical Sciences, University of Modena, Azienda Ospedaliero Universitaria di Modena Policlinico, Modena, Italy

21.2 Outpatient Pulmonary Rehabilitation

A majority of the published studies on PR have been conducted in outpatient, hospital center-based or community-based programs [1, 6, 8–11]. Outpatient PR programs are the most commonly available setting for PR, yet models of outpatient PR program delivery vary [5]. Most typical outpatient PR programs hold sessions located at a hospital, specialty PR center or community-based rehabilitation facility two to three times per week. Many programs include 1 h for multimodality exercise training, and 1 h for education sessions, but some PR program sessions last up to 4 h [1]. Program duration usually ranges from 6 to 12 weeks, although longer programs may lead to greater more durable gains [1, 12–14]. The landmark randomized, controlled trial conducted by Ries and colleagues first demonstrated that 8 weeks of comprehensive outpatient PR led to significantly greater gains in exercise

© Springer International Publishing AG 2018
E. Clini et al. (eds.), *Textbook of Pulmonary Rehabilitation*,
https://doi.org/10.1007/978-3-319-65888-9_21

capacity (METS, maximal oxygen uptake, and exercise endurance), self-efficacy for walking, and reduction in dyspnea and leg fatigue as compared to education alone [15]. Recently, a systematic review and meta-analysis of 65 randomized controlled trials including a total of 3822 patients comparing various outcomes of PR compared to conventional care for patients with COPD was undertaken [16]. For this analysis, PR was defined as at least 4 weeks of exercise training, with or without education and/or other interventions. The PR programs in 41 of the studies were outpatient or inpatient hospital-based; the programs in 23 of the studies were community-based. The duration of the PR ranged from 4 to 52 weeks, with a majority of the programs of 8–12 weeks' duration. In this analysis, PR led to significant improvements in maximal exercise capacity, 6-min walk distance (mean effect size 43.93 m, greater than the recognized MCID; 95% CI 32.64–55.21), all domains of the Chronic Respiratory Disease Questionnaire (CRQ; dyspnea, fatigue, emotion and mastery) with effect sizes greater than the MCID of 0.5 for each component, as well as the St. Georges Respiratory Questionnaire (SGRQ; effect size > the MCID of 4 units change in score) [16]. A subgroup analysis comparing the findings of RCT involving hospital-based vs. community-based PR programs demonstrated a somewhat greater magnitude of effects of hospital-based programs on the CRQ but not the SGRQ [16]. The clinical significance of this finding is not fully clear. Importantly, benefits of outpatient PR demonstrated in randomized controlled clinical trials have been confirmed in the "real-world" clinical practice setting [17, 18]. The evidence demonstrating benefits of outpatient PR for patients with COPD is now considered unequivocal. Outpatient PR has demonstrated benefits also for several respiratory disorders other than COPD including individuals with asthma, cystic fibrosis, pulmonary hypertension, interstitial lung disease, and lung cancer [19].

A recent pilot study demonstrated feasibility and clinical benefits of physiotherapist-supervised community-based PR conducted in community gymnasium [20]. Participants referred to center-based rehabilitation were carefully screened for their suitability to participate; these individuals were considered "low risk", i.e., were without requirement for supplemental oxygen or wheelchair, lacked cognitive, hearing or visual impairments, had body weights < 150 kg and were felt not likely at risk of medical events requiring immediate medical care [20]. Notably, the wait time for entry into the center-based program (for individuals with higher complexity illness) decreased following implementation of the community-gymnasium-based supervised PR program. Implementation of this type of an outpatient PR program model may offer a means of increasing access to PR for patients with varying severity and complexity of illness and rehabilitation needs.

21.3 Inpatient Pulmonary Rehabilitation

In contrast to models of outpatient PR wherein patients travel to the PR program two to three times per week, patients who participate in inpatient PR programs are typically admitted to the rehabilitation program and undertake their rehabilitation as an inpatient up to 6 days per week for 2–4 weeks [1, 21–23]. Programs of longer duration are available in some countries such as Belgium [14]. Availability of inpatient PR programs, and thresholds of severity of medical illness and requirements for program admission varies across countries. In some countries, patients who would potentially be suitable to undertake outpatient PR based on severity of illness and functional status but who live at a distance from a PR center and/or who have complex comorbidities are able to undertake inpatient PR [22, 23]. In other countries such as the United States, however, inpatient PR is available only to individuals whose functional disability is such that they are not able to live at home and/or who require an inpatient rehabilitation stay due to their medical and/or nursing needs. In this context, inpatient PR is generally the preferred setting for individuals requiring rehabilitation following an acute illness requiring hospitalization who are still too disabled to return home to participate in home-based or outpatient PR. Thus, the content and goals of inpatient rehabilitation also varies across countries and health systems.

In general, the benefits of inpatient PR are comparable to those of outpatient PR with regard to gains in exercise tolerance and quality of life [1, 16, 23, 24], at least for individuals with COPD. Specialty inpatient respiratory care units can be effective environments in which patients can successfully both undergo general rehabilitation and management of acute on chronic respiratory failure [25, 26]. Depression can also be improved following inpatient PR [27]. Differential patient responses may be seen for varying outcomes measures [21]. Studies of PR for respiratory disorders other than COPD conducted in the inpatient setting have also demonstrated benefits across various outcomes [19, 28–30].

Typical advantages of inpatient PR are: (a) the presence and availability of a comprehensive multidisciplinary team of healthcare professionals to perform complex multifaceted assessments, address patients' complex multi-morbid conditions, and meet diverse patient rehabilitation needs [31], (b) availability of specialty nursing services (e.g., to enable management of issues such as complex wound care, etc.), (c) access to specialty rehabilitative equipment (such as bariatric exercise equipment and walkers, neuromuscular electrical stimulation machines, etc.), (d) assistance for patients with acclimation to noninvasive ventilation (NIV) and availability of exercise training using NIV, (e) regular on-site team meetings to discuss and review each patient's progress, formulate the rehabilitation plan, and set realistic goals, and (f) the presence of care coordinators to assist with managing the patient's transition from their inpatient stay back to their home and community.

21.4 Home-based Pulmonary Rehabilitation

Two definitions of "home-based PR" have been historically described. In one, patients are living at home but participate in a non-hospital-based PR program in their local community. In the other, patients undergo the PR in the home itself. While both models of home-based PR have been used successfully, true PR in the home itself has, to date, been conducted largely in the context of clinical research trials, and is not used widely in most countries—it is currently utilized in fewer than 5% of PR programs [5]. Also, research trials of home-based PR conducted to date have largely involved individuals with COPD. Studies comparing efficacy of home-based PR to other models of PR delivery for people with chronic respiratory diseases other than COPD are thus far lacking.

Two studies of "home-based" PR, wherein patients with stable severe COPD lived at home but initially underwent 3 months of twice weekly physiotherapist-supervised community-based exercise training followed by weekly or monthly physiotherapist-supervised exercise training, breathing and inspiratory muscle training, and relaxation exercises, and were visited at home by pulmonary specialty nurses and had monthly visits to a general practitioner demonstrated significant gains in QOL that were sustained over 12 months [32]. No clear gains in exercise tolerance were seen following the interventions, but individuals in a control group who received no PR had declines in exercise capacity over time [32, 33].

Several trials have demonstrated significant gains in 6 min walk distance (6MWD) and/or QOL following participation in at least partially supervised, home-based PR as compared with "usual care" in people with stable COPD [34–37]. Individuals with moderate to very severe COPD were included in these trials, but patients were assessed initially at hospital-based centers in each of these studies. One study comparing benefits of a 12-week home-based PR intervention (wherein patients received initial training from a healthcare professional at the rehabilitation center regarding the exercise training protocol and subsequent exercise training sessions were unsupervised but were followed by telephone calls) demonstrated comparable gains in 6MWD and BODE Index Scores to those made by patients in an outpatient, center-based PR program [38].

Another randomized trial comparing outpatient hospital-based vs. home-based rehabilitation demonstrated comparable benefits of the two programs immediately following and at 6 months following PR in cycle-based exercise capacity and Borg dyspnea and leg fatigue scores, but these gains were better maintained over the subsequent 12 months among persons who had completed the home-based PR program [39].

A randomized controlled trial by Maltais and colleagues [40] also demonstrated that an 8-week comprehensive self-monitored home-based exercise training program following an initial 4-week education program led to comparable gains in dyspnea (assessed by the CRQ dyspnea score) to those of an outpatient hospital-based exercise program. The home-based program was non-inferior to the outpatient intervention at the 3 month and 1 year follow-up time points. Cycling endurance time and health status (assessed by the SGRQ) were also significantly improved in both patient intervention groups. Of note, however, in this trial, patients were provided with portable cycle ergometers during the study to enable the home-based aerobic exercise training; hence this trial did not represent a "real-world" situation for home-based rehabilitation. Recently, however, another randomized, controlled trial wherein carefully structured home-based PR was provided for individuals with stable COPD using minimal resources, confirmed non-inferiority of home-based PR as compared to outpatient center-based PR for gains in 6MWD at 6 months after program completion [41]. Equivalent gains in QOL were also demonstrated following completion of PR and at the 12-month follow-up time point. Neither the home-based PR group nor the group who had undergone center-based outpatient PR maintained the gains achieved in the PR program at the 12-month follow-up time point. There were no significant differences in the number of hospitalizations or hospital days between the two groups, although a trend was seen for home-based participants to have a longer time to hospital admission following rehabilitation [41]. The program completion rate was higher among the participants of home-based rehabilitation. Notably, this trial, wherein no specialty exercise equipment was needed to perform the rehabilitation, demonstrates the potential feasibility of undertaking a similar low cost PR program in routine clinical practice. It must be emphasized however, that the success of this program depended on skills training in motivational interviewing for the physiotherapists, and careful structuring and monitoring of the home-based rehabilitation intervention. Moreover, the patients were medically stable, and few were either morbidly obese or required supplemental oxygen therapy. Thus, the true generalizability and safety of this type of PR intervention for a broader range of patients remains unknown. Other randomized controlled trials of PR, some of which have been home-based, have, however, also demonstrated efficacy of PR utilizing minimal exercise equipment in improving exercise capacity and QOL [42].

Home-based rehabilitation can also be successfully delivered via a variety of tele-rehabilitation interventions, including interactive step-wise progressive web-based exercise and education sessions [43, 44], or real-time video-conferencing, wherein one or more patients at home (or in a small group in another community setting) undertake rehabilitation while interacting live with a physiotherapist or other PR expert located at a specialty rehabilitation center [45–47]. To date, despite some demonstrated benefits of home-based tele-rehabilitation in improving performance on field walk tests and patient-reported QOL in these studies, and despite its potential to increase access to PR in areas where PR programs are lacking, the optimal criteria for patient candidacy for tele-rehabilitation remain unknown. It is likely best suited for individuals with lesser severity of respiratory illness, fewer medical comorbidities, and low levels of disability, who are at lower risk of adverse medical events. One recent study demonstrated the ability of tele-rehabilitation to reduce hospitalizations and urgent healthcare visits [48]. Tele-rehabilitation has, to date, largely been conducted in the context of clinical trials and is not yet available for widespread use in routine clinical settings, due to equipment, staffing, cost, and other logistic constraints. Its eventual role in the spectrum of PR services remains to be defined. Pros and cons related to tele-rehabilitation are extensively discussed in detail in Chap. 24.

Home-based PR has potential to increase access to PR for patients who live in areas wherein center-based PR programs are lacking, or for those who lack transportation or are unwilling to attend center-based programs. It also has potential to better engage patients to participate in and maintain health-enhancing behaviors such as exercise and physical activity long-term, by virtue of undertaking exercise training and education in a familiar environment without requirement for specialty equipment, disrupting patients' daily routine, or incurring significant extra costs. However, the optimal candidates and program structure for home-based PR in routine clinical practice remain unknown, and it is not yet clear that home-based PR is suitable for all patients in all health systems. Home-based rehabilitation may be less effective for severely disabled people [49]. Those with severe disease and complex multi-morbidity, those who require specialty rehabilitation equipment or training methods, and/or who need individualized psychosocial, occupational, or nutritional interventions may be better served in traditional center-based PR programs with multidisciplinary PR program teams [1]. Other potential disadvantages of home-based PR include lack of support from a peer group, limited availability of a multidisciplinary team, variable safety of the environment in which to undertake exercise training, and costs associated with required visits/support from healthcare professionals. Further research is needed to determine the feasibility, safety, and efficacy of home-based PR for people with non-COPD respiratory disorders. The ability of home-based PR to improve other outcomes such as physical activity levels, fatigue, anxiety, depression, ability to return to work, to reduce urgent healthcare utilization or hospitalizations, or prepare patients for thoracic surgery (including lung transplantation) also remains largely unexplored.

21.5 Early Rehabilitation Following Acute COPD Exacerbation

Acute exacerbations of COPD (AECOPD) result in worsening of lung function, symptoms, QOL, activity limitation, functional limitation and disability, and often result in hospitalization [50]. While historically delivered to medically stable patients with COPD, benefits of PR delivered early (within 30 days) of AECOPD have been recognized in recent years [1, 13]. A recent meta-analysis of 20 randomized controlled trials (including a total of 1477 participants) demonstrated that there was a moderate-to-large effect size of PR implemented early after AECOPD for improving exercise capacity (mean gains in 6MWD of 62 m, 95% CI 38–86) and health-related QOL [51]. Eight studies in the analysis (810 participants) showed that post-exacerbation PR reduced hospital readmissions (pooled odds ratio of 0.44; 95% CI 0.21–0.91). Pooled results of the six studies (670 participants) that evaluated the effect of post-exacerbation PR on mortality did not show a statistically significant effect [51]. Of note, the effects of post-exacerbation PR on hospitalizations and mortality in this analysis were heterogeneous, possibly as a result of varying PR program content and structure and health-care systems in which the RCT were conducted. Another meta-analysis of several RCT confirmed that participation in PR in the post-exacerbation period was associated with reduced hospitalization rates [52]. Combined results analyzed from observational cohort studies in this analysis did not demonstrate a clear reduction in hospitalizations, possibly as a result of heterogeneous study protocols.

Despite evidence of significant benefits of PR in the post-exacerbation period, fewer than 25–35% of patients are referred to PR on discharge from the hospital [53], and fewer than 10% of patients complete PR following hospital discharge [54]. Further work is needed to understand the health system, PR program and patient-related barriers to post-exacerbation PR for individuals with COPD.

The issue of whether to initiate PR during acute care hospitalizations for patients with COPD still remains controversial. To date professionals in pulmonary rehabilitation around the world have promoted pulmonary rehabilitation during AECOPD by using adapted programs [7] and found that this may provide clinically relevant improvements in exercise performance, peripheral muscle function, and quality of life compared to usual care. To date, more than 75% of the current pulmonary rehabilitation programs include those patients [5]. In addition, some evidence suggests that rehabilitation including interventions such as resistance training and/or neuromuscular electrical stimulation can be implemented successfully during hospitalizations and that early mobilization for critically ill patients can improve patient outcomes (as discussed in Chap. 27). Notwithstanding, some practitioners remain concerned about the safety of PR implemented during the acute care hospitalization. This concern largely stems from a recent randomized controlled trial wherein a rehabilitation intervention begun in-hospital followed by an unsupervised home-based exercise intervention was ineffective, and was accompanied by a slight increase in mortality 6 months after the intervention was completed [55]. Given the lack of efficacy of the particular intervention undertaken in this trial, it is unlikely that the mortality signal seen several months later related to the intervention. Nevertheless, caution is warranted pending further research regarding PR begun during AECOPD. Also, to date, studies evaluating effects of early PR following exacerbation of non-COPD respiratory disorders are lacking.

21.6 Maintenance Pulmonary Rehabilitation Programs

The benefits of pulmonary rehabilitation typically wane over 6–12 months following program participation [1, 15]. Therefore, efforts to maintain the gains made in PR are needed. Several studies have evaluated the efficacy and feasibility of various models for maintenance PR programs. Maintenance interventions following PR have been comprised of unsupervised or minimally supervised exercise training sessions in the community and/or at home, support groups, follow-up telephone calls from staff, and/or education sessions of varying frequency conducted over 6-month to 2 year follow-up periods [48, 56–59].

To date, results of these studies have been variable, with some demonstrating ability to prolong and maintain at least some of the short-term gains made in the initial PR program [60, 61], and others showing no clear benefit of the maintenance program [58, 59]. Recent systematic reviews of several RCT of maintenance interventions following PR suggest that supervised exercise programs after completion of a PR program help to preserve exercise endurance for 3–6 months but that benefits wane over 1 year [62, 63], and no clear benefits have been seen for maintenance of gains in HRQOL [62].

Recently, in a multicenter randomized controlled trial involving 143 patients with moderate-to-severe COPD, Guell and colleagues demonstrated that a 3-year exercise-based maintenance intervention after an initial 8-week outpatient PR program led to better maintenance of 6MWD and BODE Scores over 24 months as compared to the control group [64]. As was true in other studies, there was no clear benefit of the maintenance intervention on health-related QOL. No benefits of the PR intervention were sustained at the 3-year time point.

Thus, at present, the optimal method for maintaining benefits of PR is as of yet unknown, but will likely vary in different healthcare systems and for individual patients with widely varying needs over time [65]. Currently, drop-out rates from maintenance PR programs is high [66]. Many factors, including program structure and content, as well as patient motivation, learning, self-efficacy, and behavior change likely influence the success or failure of maintenance PR programs to improve patient outcomes [67, 68]. Further work is needed to determine how to best implement maintenance PR programs in differing healthcare environments while also accommodating individual patients' type and severity of respiratory disease, varying medical comorbidities, psychosocial issues and logistic problems such as transportation, work obligations, requirement for special adaptive equipment and other factors.

21.7 Pulmonary Rehabilitation Program Staffing

Pulmonary rehabilitation program staffing varies widely across programs in different countries [3–5], depending on program setting and available resources. Program staffing ranges from one or two providers to comprehensive multidisciplinary teams of PR specialists [69]. Staffing for conventional PR programs typically includes one or more physiotherapists (or exercise physiologist), nurses, respiratory therapist, a respiratory physician/medical director, and may also include a health psychologist, dietician, occupational therapist, pharmacist, social worker, and other staff [1, 3–5, 10, 70, 71]. Most programs in the United States have a designated program coordinator in addition to the medical director [71]. Pulmonary rehabilitation program staff must demonstrate core competencies in delivery of PR [70, 71]. Staff should also be skilled in cardiopulmonary resuscitation techniques and resuscitative equipment should be available on site. Requirements for staff-to-patient ratios vary across countries [6] and the optimal ratio is not known [1]. A ratio of 1:4 has been recommended for exercise training in the United States, whereas a ratio of 1:8 is used in the United Kingdom [1].

Opportunities for training in the discipline of PR vary across healthcare disciplines and countries. To date, training of most healthcare professionals regarding the core processes and benefits of PR is not universally required [7], and standardized curricula in PR for each type of healthcare professional who will likely provide care for people with chronic respiratory diseases are lacking. Training in PR must therefore largely be sought by interested persons. Post-graduate courses, symposia, on-line clinical practice guidelines, and video content regarding PR are available through several respiratory societies including the American Thoracic Society, European Respiratory Society, Canadian Thoracic Society, Australian Lung Foundation, British Thoracic Society, American Association for Cardiovascular and Pulmonary Rehabilitation, and others.

Pulmonary rehabilitation program staff must have knowledge of the pathophysiology, clinical manifestations, comorbidities, and available treatments of chronic respiratory diseases including chronic obstructive pulmonary disease, asthma, cystic fibrosis, pulmonary hypertension, interstitial lung disease, lung cancer, and neuromuscular disorders [70, 72]. The core competencies and roles for each aspect of PR program delivery have been reviewed recently [10, 70]. The role of the pulmonary physician is to review each patient's medical history and perform a physical examination to ensure that the patient can likely benefit from PR and is safe to participate. Based on this evaluation, patients may be referred for additional testing (such as pharmacologic cardiac stress testing) if needed prior to enrollment in PR. The pulmonologist also liaisons with the other PR program staff to monitor patients' medical stability, may recommend and/or implement changes to the patients' medical regimen (including supplemental oxygen prescription) and assists in managing any unanticipated medical issues that may arise during the course of the PR program as needed. In some countries, including the United States, the PR program physician must be immediately available on site during the times when the PR program sessions are ongoing. The physiotherapist and/or exercise physiologist typically performs the assessment of the patient's exercise capacity, formulates the patient's exercise prescription, implements and oversees the exercise training, and performs several of the outcomes measures. In some programs, this role is performed by a pulmonary specialty nurse and/or a respiratory therapist. Respiratory nurses and/or respiratory therapists provide disease-relevant education and assist in development of action plans for managing acute exacerbations of disease. The extent of the role of the other types of providers listed above depends on local PR program resources and availability. Where available, the health psychologist typically works with program participants on strategies to cope with their disease, manage anxiety and depression, and to facilitate specialty referrals to a psychologist or psychiatrist as needed. The pharmacist works with participants to understand the benefits, proper use technique and potential adverse effects of patients' pharmacotherapies. Respiratory therapists (where available) also play a role in patients' learning proper technique for inhaled medications, and assist patients in managing supplemental oxygen therapy and/or noninvasive ventilation, as well as use of pacing, proper breathing techniques and symptom management. Dieticians help patients learn how to eat a healthy diet and best manage their nutritional needs—underweight or cachectic individuals may be provided with meal plans to meet their caloric needs, whereas obese persons may be provided with an individualized weight loss plan. Occupational therapists work with patients to best manage their activities of daily living and/or devise strategies to help them manage their recreational and/or work-related tasks.

Table 21.1 resumes the roles that professionals should play in a multidisciplinary PR staff.

21.8 Pulmonary Rehabilitation Program Costs

The costs of providing pulmonary rehabilitation vary depending on the program setting and composition, as well as the health system in which PR is delivered. Much of the data evaluating costs of PR has been derived from outpatient PR programs. Where investigated, costs of PR interventions have ranged from $75.00 US for simple walking programs [73] to ~$2200.00 US for more comprehensive PR interventions [74]. In general, PR is one of the most cost-effective treatments for people with COPD [75, 76], on a par with bronchodilator therapies and immunizations [77]. No data are yet available on the cost-efficacy of PR relative to other treatments for disorders other than COPD. While some studies suggest inpatient PR is more costly than PR delivered in the outpatient setting [6, 78], others have demonstrated reduced total cost of a short intensive inpatient program as compared to a longer outpatient PR program [79]. To date, however, there is no definitive comparison of the costs of PR among PR conducted in different settings. Pulmonary rehabilitation has the potential to reduce healthcare costs by virtue of reducing hospitalizations [1, 17, 18] and urgent healthcare visits. However, these cost reductions must be weighed against the costs of administering the PR to patients. The per-person cost reduction in the year following PR as compared with the year before PR was estimated in one Canadian Study as ~$344 (Canadian dollars) per year [80]. Further work is needed to more fully detail the costs and cost effectiveness of PR in pragmatic real-world trials of PR in different healthcare systems for individuals with COPD and other forms of respiratory disease.

Conclusions

Pulmonary rehabilitation can be provided in several different settings. Published evidence demonstrates that patients can achieve benefits in each of these settings, as long as the core components of PR are included, a suitable number and intensity of exercise training sessions are provided, and relevant education sessions are incorporated.

The type of health system and local resources available currently dictate the precise composition of most PR programs. Efforts towards international benchmarking for optimal PR program settings and staff are needed.

Table 21.1 Main roles/actions of professionals within a pulmonary rehabilitation staff

	PR staff							
	Physician	Physio/exercise physiologist	Nurse	Health psychologist	Pharmacist	Respiratory therapist	Dieticians	Occupational therapist
Actions								
History & Examination	√							
Reference for additional test(s)	√							
Changes of drugs	√							
Exercise assessment		√						
Exercise prescription		√						
Training oversee		√						
Outcome(s) measurement		√						
Disease education			√					
Action plan(s)			√					
Copying strategies				√				
Manage anxiety/depression				√				
Referral to Psychiatrist				√				
Education on drug use/abuse					√			
Learning techniques					√	√		
Use of supplemental oxygen/NIV						√		
Nutritional assessment							√	
Diet plan							√	
Planning ADLs								√
Recreational/work task(s)								√

References

1. Spruit MA, et al. ATS/ERS Task Force on Pulmonary Rehabilitation. An official American Thoracic Society/European Respiratory Society statement: key concepts and advances in pulmonary rehabilitation. Am J Respir Crit Care Med. 2013;188:e13–64.
2. Troosters T, et al. Pulmonary rehabilitation in chronic obstructive pulmonary disease. Am J Respir Crit Care Med. 2005;172:19–38.
3. Brooks D, et al. Characterization of pulmonary rehabilitation programs in Canada in 2005. Can Respir J. 2007;14:87–92.
4. Garvey C, et al. Pulmonary rehabilitation exercise prescription in chronic obstructive lung disease; US Survey and review of guidelines and clinical practices. J Cardiopulm Rehabil Prev. 2013;33:314–22.
5. Spruit MA, et al. Differences in content and organizational aspects of pulmonary rehabilitation programmes. Eur Respir J. 2014;43:1326–37.
6. Nici L, et al. American Thoracic Society/European respiratory Society statement on pulmonary rehabilitation. Am J Respir Crit Care Med. 2006;173:1390–413.
7. Rochester CL, et al. An Official American Thoracic Society/European respiratory Society policy statement: enhancing implementation, use and delivery of pulmonary rehabilitation. Am J Respir Crit Care Med. 2015;192:1373–86.
8. Bolton CE, et al. British Thoracic Society guideline on pulmonary rehabilitation in adults. Thorax. 2013;68:ii1–ii30.
9. Casaburi R, et al. Pulmonary rehabilitation for management of chronic obstructive pulmonary disease. New Engl J Med. 2009;360(13):1329–35.
10. Jenkins S, et al. State of the art: how to set up a pulmonary rehabilitation program. Respirology. 2010;15:1157–73.
11. Ries A, et al. Pulmonary rehabilitation; Joint ACCP/AACVPR evidence-based clinical practice guidelines. Chest. 2007;131:4S–42S.
12. Berry MJ, et al. A randomized, controlled trial comparing long-term and short-term exercise in patients with chronic obstructive pulmonary disease. J Cardiopulm Rehabil. 2003;23(1):60–8.
13. Marciniuk D, et al. Optimizing pulmonary rehabilitation in chronic obstructive pulmonary disease—practical issues: a Canadian Thoracic Society Clinical Practice Guideline. Can Respir J. 2010;17(4):159–68.
14. Pitta F, et al. Are patients with COPD more active following pulmonary rehabilitation? Chest. 2008;134:273–80.
15. Ries A, et al. Effects of pulmonary rehabilitation on physiologic and psychosocial outcomes in patients with chronic obstructive pulmonary disease. Ann Intern Med. 1995;122:823–32.
16. McCarthy B, et al. Pulmonary rehabilitation for chronic obstructive pulmonary disease. Cochrane Database Syst Rev. 2015;2:CD003793. doi:10.1002/14651858.
17. California Pulmonary Rehabilitation Collaborative Group. Effects of pulmonary rehabilitation on dyspnea, quality of life and healthcare costs in California. J Cardiopulm Rehabil. 2004;24:52–62.
18. Raskin J, et al. The effect of pulmonary rehabilitation on healthcare utilization in chronic obstructive pulmonary disease: the Northeast Pulmonary Rehabilitation Consortium. J Cardiopulm Rehabil. 2006;26:231–6.
19. Rochester CL, et al. Pulmonary rehabilitation for respiratory disorders other than COPD. Clin Chest Med. 2014;35:369–89.
20. McNamara RJ, et al. Community-based exercise training for people with chronic respiratory and chronic cardiac disease, a mixed-methods evaluation. Int J COPD. 2016;11:2839–50.
21. Haave E, et al. Improvements in exercise capacity during a 4-weeks pulmonary rehabilitation program for COPD patients do not correspond with improvements in self-reported health status or quality of life. Int J COPD. 2007;2(3):355–9.
22. Kenn K, et al. Predictors of success for pulmonary rehabilitation in patients awaiting lung transplantation. Transplantation. 2015;99:1072–7.
23. Korczak D, et al. Outpatient pulmonary rehabilitation–rehabilitation models and shortcomings in outpatient aftercare. GMS Health Technol Assess. 2010;6 doi:10.3205/hta000089.
24. Clini E, et al. Inpatient pulmonary rehabilitation: does it make sense? Chron Respir Dis. 2005;2:43–6.
25. Confalonieri M, et al. Respiratory intensive care units in Italy: a national census and prospective cohort study. Thorax. 2001;56:373–8.
26. Nava S. Rehabilitation of patients admitted to a respiratory intensive care unit. Arch Phys Med Rehabil. 1998;79:849–54.
27. Alexopoulos GS, et al. Outcomes of depressed patients undergoing inpatient pulmonary rehabilitation. Am J Geriatr Psychiatry. 2006;14(5):466–75.
28. Jose A, et al. Inpatient rehabilitation improves functional capacity, peripheral muscle strength and quality of life in patients with community acquired pneumonia: a randomised trial. J Physiother. 2016;62(2):96–102.
29. Lai Y, et al. Systematic short-term pulmonary rehabilitation before lung cancer lobectomy: a randomized trial. Interact Cardiovasc Thorac Surg. 2017; doi:10.1093/icvts/ivx141.
30. Morris NR, et al. Exercise-based rehabilitation programmes for pulmonary hypertension. Cochrane Database Syst Rev. 2017;1:CD011285. doi:10.1002/14651858.
31. Vanfleteren L, et al. Tailoring the approach to multimorbidity in adults with respiratory disease: the NICE Guideline. Eur Respir J. 2017;49:1601696. doi:10.1183/13993003.01696-2016.
32. Wijkstra PJ, et al. Long term benefits of rehabilitation at home on quality of life and exercise tolerance in patients with chronic obstructive pulmonary disease. Thorax. 1995;50:824–8.

33. Wijkstra PJ, et al. Long-term effects of home rehabilitation on physical performance in chronic obstructive pulmonary disease. Am J Respir Crit Care Med. 1996;153:1234–41.
34. Alison J, et al. Australian and New Zealand Pulmonary rehabilitation guidelines. Respirology. 2017;22:800–19.
35. Boxall AM, et al. Managing chronic obstructive pulmonary disease in the community. A randomized controlled trial of home-based pulmonary rehabilitation for elderly housebound patients. J Cardiopulm Rehabil. 2005;25:378–85.
36. Hernandez MTE, et al. Results of a home-based training program for patients with COPD. Chest. 2000;118:106–14.
37. Munoz-Fernandez A, et al. Home-based pulmonary rehabilitation in very severe COPD: is it safe and useful? J Cardiopulm Rehabil Prev. 2009;29:325–31.
38. Mendes de Oliveira JC, et al. Outpatient vs. home-based pulmonary rehabilitation in COPD: a randomized controlled trial. Multidisciplinary Respiratory Medicine. 2010;5(6):401–8.
39. Strijbos JH, et al. A comparison between an outpatient hospital-based pulmonary rehabilitation program and a home-care pulmonary rehabilitation program in patients with COPD. Chest. 1996;109:366–72.
40. Maltais F, et al. Effects of home-based pulmonary rehabilitation in patients with chronic obstructive pulmonary disease. Ann Intern Med. 2008;149:869–78.
41. Holland AE, et al. Home-based rehabilitation for COPD using minimal resources: a randomised, controlled equivalence trial. Thorax. 2017;72:57–65.
42. Alison JA, et al. Pulmonary rehabilitation for COPD: are programs with minimal exercise equipment effective? J Thoracic Dis. 2014;6(11):1606–14.
43. Chaplin E, et al. The evaluation of an interactive web-based pulmonary rehabilitation programme: protocol for the WEB SPACE for COPD feasibility study. BMJ Open. 2015;5:3008055.
44. Chaplin E, et al. Interactive web-based pulmonary rehabilitation programme: a randomized controlled feasibility trial. BMJ Open. 2017;7:e013682.
45. Burkow TM, et al. Comprehensive pulmonary rehabilitation in home-based online groups: a mixed-method pilot study in COPD. BMC Res Notes. 2015;8:766–76.
46. Stickland M, et al. Using telehealth technology to deliver pulmonary rehabilitation in chronic obstructive pulmonary disease patients. Can Respir J. 2011;18(4):216–20.
47. Tsai LLY, et al. Home-based tele-rehabilitation via real-time videoconferencing improves endurance exercise capacity in patients with COPD: the randomized controlled TeleR Study. Respirology. 2017;22:699–707.
48. Vasilopoulou M, et al. Home-based maintenance tele-rehabilitation reduces the risk for acute exacerbations of COPD, hospitalisations and emergency department visits. Eur Respir J. 2017;49:1602129. (doi.org/10.1183/13993003.02129-2016)
49. Wedzicha JA, et al. Randomized controlled trial of pulmonary rehabilitation in severe chronic obstructive pulmonary disease patients, stratified with the MRC dyspnoea scale. Eur Respir J. 1998;12:363–9.
50. Goldstein R, et al. Pulmonary rehabilitation at the time of the COPD exacerbation. Clin Chest Med. 2014;35:391–8.
51. Puhan MA, et al. Pulmonary rehabilitation following exacerbations of chronic obstructive pulmonary disease. Cochrane Database Syst Rev. 2016;12:CD005305. doi:10.1002/14651858.
52. Moore E, et al. Pulmonary rehabilitation as a mechanism to reduce hospitalizations for acute exacerbations of COPD. Chest. 2016;150(4):837–59.
53. Harth L, et al. Physical therapy practice patterns in acute exacerbations of chronic obstructive pulmonary disease. Can Respir J. 2009;16(3):86–92.
54. Jones SE, et al. Pulmonary rehabilitation following hospitalization for acute exacerbation of COPD: referrals, uptake and adherence. Thorax. 2014;69(2):181–2.
55. Greening NJ, et al. An early rehabilitation intervention to enhance recovery during hospital admission for an exacerbation of chronic respiratory disease: a randomised controlled trial. BMJ. 2014;349:g4315. doi:10.1136/bmj.g4315.
56. Brooks D, et al. The effect of postrehabilitation programmes among individuals with chronic obstructive pulmonary disease. Eur Respir J. 2002;20:20–9.
57. Heppner PS, et al. Regular walking and long-term maintenance of outcomes after pulmonary rehabilitation. J Cardiopulm Rehabil. 2006;26:44–53.
58. Spencer LM, et al. Maintaining benefits following pulmonary rehabilitation: a randomised controlled trial. Eur Respir J. 2010;35:571–7.
59. Wilson AM, et al. The effects of maintenance schedules following pulmonary rehabilitation in patients with chronic obstructive pulmonary disease: a randomised controlled trial. BMJ Open. 2015;5:e005921.
60. Cockram J, et al. Maintaining exercise capacity and quality of life following pulmonary rehabilitation. Respirology. 2006;11:98–104.
61. Ries A, et al. Maintenance after pulmonary rehabilitationin chronic lung disease: a randomized trial. Am J Respir Crit Care Med. 2003;167:880–8.
62. Beauchamp MK, et al. Systematic review of supervised exercise programs after pulmonary rehabilitation in individuals with COPD. Chest. 2013;144(4):1124–33.
63. Busby AK, et al. Pulmonary rehabilitation maintenance interventions: a systematic review. Am J Health Behav. 2014;38(3):321–30.
64. Guell M-R, et al. Benefits of long-term pulmonary rehabilitation maintenance program in patients with severe chronic obstructive pulmonary disease; three-year follow-up. Am J Respir Crit Care Med. 2017;195(5):622–9.
65. Rochester CL, et al. Maintaining the benefits of pulmonary rehabilitation: the holy grail. Am J Respir Crit Care Med. 2017;195(5):548–51.

66. Heerema-Poelman A, et al. Adherence to a maintenance exercise program 1 year after pulmonary rehabilitation. J Cardiopulm Rehabil Prev. 2013;33:419–26.
67. Blackstock FC, et al. Why don't our patients with chronic obstructive pulmonary disease listen to us? The enigma of non-adherence. Ann Am Thorac Soc. 2016;13(3):317–23.
68. Stewart KF, et al. Maintenance of a physically active lifestyle after pulmonary rehabilitation in patients with COPD: a qualitative study toward motivational factors. J Am Med Dir Assoc. 2014;15(9):655–64.
69. Spruit MA, et al. Differential response to pulmonary rehabilitation in COPD: multidimensional profiling. Eur Respir J. 2015;46:1538–40.
70. Collins EG, et al. Clinical competency guidelines for pulmonary rehabilitation professionals. Position statement of the American Association of Cardiovascular and Pulmonary Rehabilitation. J Cardiopulm Rehabil Prev. 2014; doi:10.1097/HCR.0000000000000077.
71. Garvey C, et al. Program organization in pulmonary rehabilitation. Clin Chest Med. 2014;35:423–8.
72. Holland AE, et al. How to adapt the pulmonary rehabilitation programme to patients with chronic respiratory disease other than COPD. Eur Respir Rev. 2013;22:577–86.
73. Farias CC, et al. Costs and benefits of pulmonary rehabilitation in chronic obstructive pulmonary disease: a randomized controlled trial. Braz J Phys Ther. 2014;18(2):165–73.
74. Fan VS, et al. Costs of pulmonary rehabilitation and predictors of adherence in the national emphysema treatment trial. COPD: J COPD. 2008;5(2):105–16.
75. Atsou K, et al. Simulation-based estimates of the effectiveness and cost-effectiveness of pulmonary rehabilitation in patients with chronic obstructive pulmonary disease in France. PLoS One. 2016;11(6):e0156514.
76. Griffiths TL, et al. Cost effectiveness of an outpatient multidisciplinary pulmonary rehabilitation program. Thorax. 2001;56:779–84.
77. Zoumot Z, et al. Emphysema: time to say farewell to therapeutic nihilism. Thorax. 2014;69:973–5.
78. Goldstein RS, et al. Economic analysis of respiratory rehabilitation. Chest. 1997;112:370–9.
79. Clini E, et al. In-hospital short-term training program for patients with chronic airway obstruction. Chest. 2001;120:1500–5.
80. Golmohammadi K, et al. Economic evaluation of a community-based pulmonary rehabilitation program for chronic obstructive pulmonary disease. Lung. 2004;182(3):187–96.

22 Contemporary Alternative Settings

Anne E. Holland

22.1 Introduction

The benefits of centre-based, supervised pulmonary rehabilitation has been well described [1]. Programs that involve supervised whole body exercise training with education and instruction in self management have been successfully applied in inpatient and outpatient hospital settings around the world [2]. Despite this, a significant number of people who might benefit from pulmonary rehabilitation do not participate, with estimates suggesting that as few as 10% of potential candidates with COPD ever complete a program [3]. Barriers to uptake are well understood and include inadequate commissioning of programs, poor referral practices, patient expectation of benefit, travel, transport and disability [3, 4]. These barriers to uptake have ignited interest in alternative models that may broaden the application of pulmonary rehabilitation to individuals who do not currently take part.

Contemporary alternative settings for pulmonary rehabilitation may involve changing the location of the program (e.g. home- or community-based programs) or changing the modality of exercise (e.g. water-based exercise, tai chi or Nordic walking). Most of these new models have demonstrated clinically important benefits for patient outcomes such as exercise capacity (Fig. 22.1) and health-related quality of life (Fig. 22.2). Telehealth applications may also provide new opportunities to engage people with chronic lung disease in pulmonary rehabilitation, either through delivery of telerehabilitation into the home using videoconferencing and remote monitoring, or use of mobile applications. The role of telehealth in pulmonary rehabilitation will be addressed in Chap. 23. There may also be opportunities to expand the traditional centre-based model to provide more comprehensive care, including integration of advance care planning and expanding the successful model to include other chronic diseases such as heart failure. These emerging models for pulmonary rehabilitation will be addressed in this chapter.

22.2 Changing the Location of Pulmonary Rehabilitation

22.2.1 Home-Based Pulmonary Rehabilitation

The importance of travel and transport as access barriers to pulmonary rehabilitation for people with COPD [3] has led to widespread interest in delivery of pulmonary rehabilitation directly into the home, with growing numbers of randomized controlled trials conducted across the world. Outcomes of these trials have been largely favourable. A recent systematic review [5] reported on

A.E. Holland, B.App.Sc., Ph.D.
Alfred Health and Institute for Breathing and Sleep, La Trobe University, Melbourne, Australia
e-mail: a.holland@alfred.org.au

© Springer International Publishing AG 2018
E. Clini et al. (eds.), *Textbook of Pulmonary Rehabilitation*, https://doi.org/10.1007/978-3-319-65888-9_22

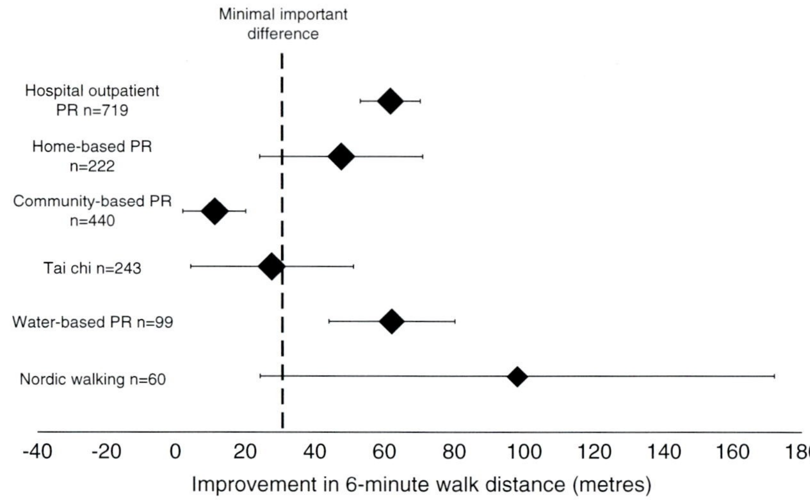

Fig. 22.1 Improvement in 6-min walk distance following traditional pulmonary rehabilitation and alternative programs in people with COPD. Data are means and 95% confidence intervals taken from systematic reviews [1, 5, 26, 31] and original studies [35]. *Dotted line* represents minimal important difference; *n* represent the number of participants

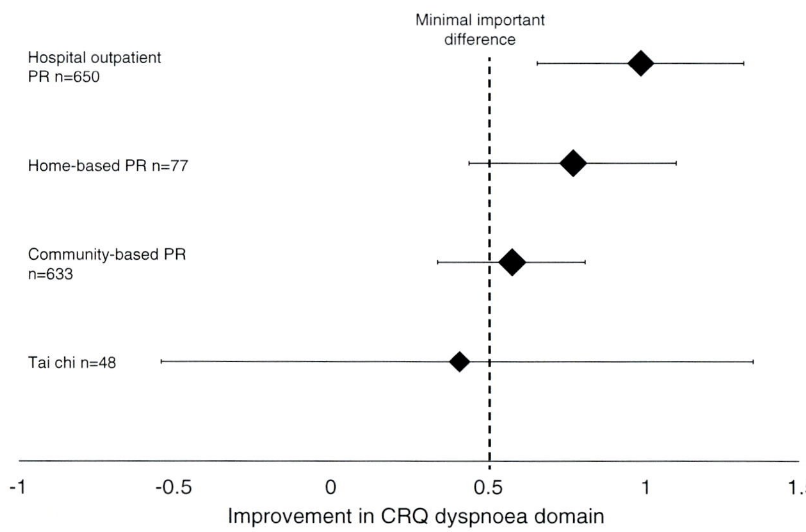

Fig. 22.2 Improvement in health-related quality of life following traditional pulmonary rehabilitation and alternative programs in people with COPD. Data are means and 95% confidence intervals for the Chronic Respiratory Questionnaire Dyspnoea domain, taken from systematic [1, 5, 31]. *Dotted line* represents minimal important difference; *n* represent the number of participants. CRQ—chronic respiratory questionnaire

11 RCTs that compared home-based pulmonary rehabilitation to usual care (no rehabilitation), most of which included participants with stable COPD. Large and clinically significant improvements in health-related quality of life were reported consistently across studies. The gains in 6MWD in stable COPD exceeded the minimal important difference (47 m, 95% confidence interval 24–71 m, Fig. 22.1). A direct comparison with centre-based pulmonary rehabilitation was examined in six RCTs, including two larger studies that were powered for equivalence [6, 7]. Similar improvements in health-related quality of life and exercise capacity were reported in both home-based and centre-based pulmonary rehabilitation programs, with changes that were clinically significant [5]. Limitations of this body of literature include few data on the impact of home-based rehabilitation in people with COPD who are recovering from an acute exacerbation; lack of assessor blinding in many studies; and the wide variety of home-based pulmonary rehabilitation models that were tested.

This variation in content and delivery of home-based pulmonary rehabilitation makes it difficult to decide on a 'best' model to implement in practice. Components of home-based pulmonary rehabilitation that have been tested in RCTs are in Fig. 22.3. Walking training is a commonly

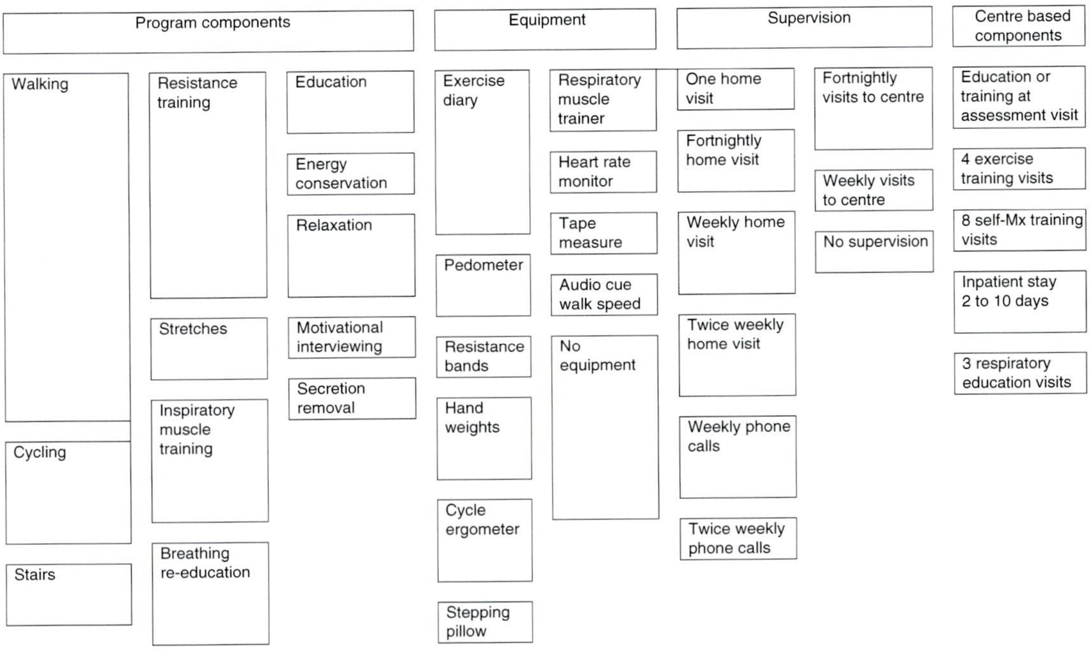

Fig. 22.3 Models of home-based pulmonary rehabilitation used in randomized controlled trials. Size of the rectangle is proportional to the number of studies that have used the modality in home-based rehabilitation. Data from 22 RCTs examining home-based rehabilitation [6–10, 12–14, 16, 17, 50–61]. Self Mx—self management

used form of endurance exercise, as it is easy to implement for most patients either inside the home or outdoors. However some programs have more closely mimicked the components of centre-based pulmonary rehabilitation, including the use of a cycle ergometer, allowing for greater control of exercise intensity and progression. In the majority of cases this equipment was provided to participants and removed from the home at the conclusion of the training period. Many programs use home diaries or exercise logs to record adherence, with some also providing a pedometer to monitor or progress step counts. Resistance training for the upper and lower limbs is frequently included, with some programs providing hand weights or resistance bands, whilst others use objects commonly available in the home such as cans of food, bottles of water or body weight.

Home-based pulmonary rehabilitation models vary in the degree of supervision provided. Earlier studies used frequent home visits by physiotherapists or nurses, to supervise exercise and enhance adherence [8–10]. These models allow for a similar degree of supervision to that provided in a centre-based program, however they may be more expensive to deliver and have not been widely adopted in clinical practice [11]. Other models have required home-based participants to make frequent visits to the hospital [12, 13], which is unlikely to overcome access barriers in debilitated patients. More recently, largely unsupervised models of home-based pulmonary rehabilitation have emerged that may include one home visit followed by regular telephone calls to set goals and progress the program [14, 15]. Whilst unsupervised, these models are highly structured with regular discussion and feedback to patients. Good outcomes have been reported and costs are likely to be low, but replication of outcomes by other groups is needed. It should be noted that in all but one study [16] patients had to attend the hospital for assessment, prior to commencing the program, where a robust exercise test could be performed. In the absence of a clear gold standard, the choice of home-based pulmonary rehabilitation model is likely to be determined by local resources and preferences.

Patient selection for home-based pulmonary rehabilitation requires careful consideration. Some trials of home-based rehabilitation focused on patients with severe COPD or those who were housebound, with variable outcomes [10, 17]. More recent studies have included patients with COPD across the spectrum of disease and have demonstrated convincing benefits [6, 15]. As a result there is no reason to restrict access to home-based pulmonary rehabilitation based on FEV_1 or severity of symptoms. To date the majority of studies of home-based pulmonary rehabilitation have been in people with stable COPD; whether it is safe and efficacious in people with other chronic lung diseases, or people with COPD who are recovering from an acute exacerbation, remains to be convincingly demonstrated. There may be some patients in whom direct monitoring and supervision is required, such as those with severe exertional desaturation, pulmonary hypertension or multiple comorbidities. Other patients may require extensive involvement of the multi-disciplinary team, which could be less accessible for home-based patients, depending on the program model. Patients with significant musculoskeletal limitations to exercise may not be suitable for a home program that focuses predominantly on walking. Such issues should be identified in the comprehensive assessment that is conducted prior to commencing any pulmonary rehabilitation program [2]. Some people prefer exercising in a group environment with direct access to clinicians, whilst others will value the opportunity to undertake a program in their home environment [15]. Providing patients with choice regarding the model of pulmonary rehabilitation may assist with uptake, adherence and completion.

22.2.2 Community Pulmonary Rehabilitation

Centre-based programs that are delivered outside the hospital setting may be more accessible for patients and provide greater options for commissioning of programs. Community settings for pulmonary rehabilitation have included primary health care facilities (including general practitioner's clinics) [18, 19], community gymnasiums [20], physiotherapy practices [21] and other community health facilities [22]. A recent systematic review reported wide variability in the way that community pulmonary rehabilitation had been delivered, particularly for the exercise component [5]. Four studies delivered exercise sessions of at least moderate intensity supervised twice weekly [21–24] ($n = 259$), which is consistent with international best practice [2]. These programs resulted in clinically significant improvements in health-related quality of life (St George Respiratory Questionnaire total score improved by −4.2 units, 95% CI −6.5 to −1.9), similar to the improvements reported from hospital-based programs [1]. For other programs where the exercise component was of low intensity or was delivered once weekly [18–20], benefits were less consistently documented. This contributes to the smaller overall effect of community-based pulmonary rehabilitation on exercise capacity that has been demonstrated in clinical trials (Fig. 22.1).

Extending pulmonary rehabilitation into community settings provides an opportunity to engage with patients at a location within their community, and to better integrate care with that delivered by their primary providers. As with any pulmonary rehabilitation program attention must be paid to the exercise prescription, to ensure that an effective exercise dose is delivered, particularly with regard to frequency and intensity of training. To date all studies have enrolled patients with stable COPD; whether community-based pulmonary rehabilitation is suitable for patients who are recovering from an acute exacerbation, or those with other diagnoses, is unknown. Community locations vary widely in the facilities available. For instance, not all may be able to provide supplemental oxygen with training, which may preclude participation by patients with severe exertional desaturation. Similar to home-based programs, a thorough assessment and triage should be undertaken for each individual at entry to the pulmonary rehabilitation program, to ensure that the location of the program is a good fit with the patient's physical and psychosocial needs, pathophysiology, values and preferences.

22.3 Changing the Exercise Modality for Pulmonary Rehabilitation

22.3.1 Water-Based Exercise

People with COPD frequently present with physical comorbidities that may limit their ability to participate in traditional land-based exercise training. These could include musculoskeletal limitations (e.g. pain or reduced range of motion related to osteoarthritis, rheumatoid arthritis, chronic low back pain, previous joint replacement), chronic neurological conditions or obesity. Many people with significant physical comorbidities are frequently not offered referral to pulmonary rehabilitation or may not accept the referral. In addition, experiencing pain during exercise classes contributes to non-completion of pulmonary rehabilitation [25]. Because water-based exercise uses buoyancy to support the body weight and reduce the impact of gravity, it may provide a more comfortable exercise environment whilst facilitating a more effective exercise training dose.

The evidence to support water-based exercise for COPD has been synthesized in a Cochrane review [26]. Five randomized controlled trials were included with 176 participants. The water-based training programs ranged from 4 to 12 weeks in duration with a similar weekly frequency to land-based programs. Most studies recruited people with COPD with a range of disease severity, and one study specifically included those who had one or more physical comorbidities [27]. Compared to no exercise training, water-based training had clinically important effects on exercise capacity and quality of life. The improvements were similar to those seen in traditional land-based exercise training programs, with the exception of endurance exercise time and fatigue, which both improved to a greater extent in the water-based training group. These latter positive results were demonstrated in the one study which included people with physical comorbidities, suggesting that these individuals may have greater gains from a water-based program, possibly because water-based training allows them to exercise at a greater intensity.

Water-based training programs aim to use the unique properties of the aquatic environment (buoyancy, water resistance and turbulence) to deliver exercise training of similar intensity to land-based programs. Typically programs include upper and lower limb aerobics; cycling, jogging or walking in the water, sometimes with flotation devices; strengthening exercises with foam dumbbells using water resistance; stretches for upper limbs and the thoracic cage; and sometimes breathing exercises. Participants are encouraged to exercise at a similar intensity to land-based programs, with Borg dyspnoea score targets of 3–5. Although people with COPD have lower respiratory function when immersed in water compared to land this does not appear to have a significant impact on oxyhaemoglobin saturation in patients who are not hypoxaemic at rest [28]. No adverse events have been reported with water-based training programs in COPD, most of whom had moderate disease [26]. The impact of water-based training on patients with more severe disease has not been documented.

Water-based exercise programs generally take place in community swimming pools or in hydrotherapy pools located at a rehabilitation facility. People with COPD participating in clinical trials have reported high levels of satisfaction with water-based training and the aquatic environment [29]. Whilst a suitable location for water-based training is unlikely to be accessible or necessary for all patients, it is a very promising exercise training modality for those in whom comorbidities limit participation in land-based training programs.

22.3.2 Tai Chi for People with COPD

Tai chi is an ancient form of exercise that originated in China. It is characterized by slow and rhythmic circular motions, moving from one form (or movement) to another. Tai Chi is commonly performed in a semi-squat position and it involves muscle strength, endurance, balance, relaxation and diaphragmatic breathing [30]. Many styles of Tai Chi are practiced including Chen, Yang, Wu and Sun, which are distinguished by the forms or movements that are included. Tai Chi is quick to learn and it does not require specialized exercise equipment, so it is easy to perform at home or in the community. As a result, Tai Chi is increasing in popularity across the world.

A Cochrane review reports the results of 12 randomized controlled trials of Tai Chi in people with COPD [31]. A wide variety of styles were used including Yang, Quigong and Sun styles, and there was also variety in the number of forms included. The duration of exercise ranged from 15 to 60 min per session, on 5–7 days of the week. The most common program length was 12 weeks. Tai Chi resulted in clinically significant gains in 6-min walk distance compared to usual care controls (mean 30 m, 95% confidence interval 11–49 m, 6 studies with 318 participants). Improvements in health-related quality of life were greater in the Tai Chi group but did not reach statistical significance. One study [30] also reported improvements in balance outcomes, which may be highly significant in people with COPD who are known to be at high risk of falls [32].

The effective components of Tai Chi for exercise training are not clearly understood. The physiological load imposed by Tai Chi is of moderate intensity (equivalent to treadmill walking at 60% of maximal workload)[33] and thus it is likely that it delivers similar improvements in cardiopulmonary fitness to standard programs. Inclusion of concentric and eccentric muscle contractions is likely to improve both strength and endurance, whilst squatting and weight shifting will improve balance. Diaphragmatic breathing may also be an important component. It is not yet clear whether one style is most applicable to people with COPD. Some studies used modifications of traditional styles, including a reduced number of forms or addition of hand weights [31]. It seems likely that any style that delivers a moderate intensity training stimulus for a sufficient period will be beneficial.

An advantage of Tai Chi is that it may be more culturally acceptable than gymnasium-based training for some individuals and in some parts of the world. Many people choose to practice Tai Chi in a group in public spaces such as parks, with the added advantages of enhanced social connectedness. Whilst few pulmonary rehabilitation programs currently provide Tai Chi, there are frequently opportunities for older people to participate in community groups.

22.3.3 Nordic Walking

Nordic walking involves walking with a flexible pole held in each hand. The pole compresses when it comes in contact with the ground and springs back at push off, increasing both muscle use and walking speed. It has gained popularity, both in the general population and in people with chronic health conditions, as a form of whole body exercise that increases energy expenditure compared to normal walking without an increase in symptoms. In people with moderate to severe COPD the use of Nordic poles generates higher oxygen uptake than standard walking, but does not increase exertional dyspnoea [34]. A single RCT has examined Nordic walking in 60 people with stable COPD and a wide range of disease severity [35]. Intriguingly, 3 months of supervised Nordic walking training at 75% of maximum heart rate resulted in significant improvements in physical activity (increased standing and walking time, decreased sitting time) that were maintained at 6 months after the supervised training period had ended. The impact of Nordic walking on physical activity in this trial is greater than that reported following a traditional pulmonary rehabilitation program [36]. This large effect size could be a 'first trial' effect, however if it is replicated in other groups this suggests a new, safe and accessible training method that could have long-term benefits for people with COPD.

22.4 Enhancing the Traditional Pulmonary Rehabilitation Model

22.4.1 Combined COPD and Heart Failure Rehabilitation

People with chronic heart failure (CHF) frequently have debilitating dyspnoea and fatigue that limits functional exercise capacity. Frailty, mood disturbance and skeletal muscle dysfunction are also common. Similar to COPD, CHF is characterized by physical inactivity, systemic inflammation, oxidative stress and hypoxia, all of which contribute to poor outcomes [37]. The two conditions frequently coexist; in a recent study 12% of those in COPD outpatient clinics had CHF, and 32% of those in CHF clinics had COPD [38]. Similarly, 15% of those with COPD in pulmonary rehabilitation have co-existing CHF [39]. Although there is strong evidence supporting rehabilitation for CHF [40], program access remains limited, with many cardiac rehabilitation programs focusing on secondary prevention following myocardial infarction and/or surgery.

Acknowledging these similarities and the unmet need for CHF rehabilitation, several groups have reported a new approach to 'breathlessness rehabilitation' [41–43], taking a symptom-focused (rather than disease focused) perspective. In a randomized controlled trial, people with CHF underwent rehabilitation in an existing pulmonary rehabilitation program [41]. Rehabilitation was symptom-focused and all patients undertook twice weekly sessions consisting of endurance training, strength training and education. No adverse events were reported. People with CHF had clinically important improvements in exercise capacity and quality of life, of a similar magnitude to people with COPD who undertook the program concurrently. Other authors have reported a high level of satisfaction when people with COPD and chronic cardiac disease undertook a shared community-based exercise rehabilitation program [43]. A consensus process in the United Kingdom reported that 75% of stakeholders supported this symptom-based approach to rehabilitation for COPD and CHF, whilst 87% thought that COPD exercise training principles could be applied to CHF and vice versa [42]. A number of non-exercise and self management components that could be included in a breathlessness rehabilitation program were identified, including management of dyspnoea, activity pacing, anxiety management, psychosocial support, emergency plans for breathing crises, relaxation, nutrition and hydration advice, medication review and support for carers [42].

Whilst pulmonary rehabilitation appears to be a suitable environment in which to deliver 'breathlessness rehabilitation' to people with CHF and COPD, perhaps improving rehabilitation access and patient outcomes, some modifications may be required. It has been suggested that people with CHF undergo exercise assessment that includes electrocardiogram prior to program entry, to exclude important arrhythmias; that pulmonary rehabilitation practitioners are taught to recognize the signs and symptoms of decompensated heart failure; and that consideration is given to provision of disease specific education for CHF, either within the program or via coordination with existing CHF services [37].

22.4.2 Advance Care Planning in Pulmonary Rehabilitation

Advance care planning (ACP) refers to a process by which an individual prepares for future loss of capacity by making their values and preferences for medical and lifestyle care known to others. Such discussions are particularly relevant for people with chronic respiratory disease who frequently experience distressing symptoms, an uncertain prognosis and unexpected changes in health status. Advance care planning can improve the experience and outcomes of end of life care in older people with chronic disease, increasing the likelihood that end of life care wishes are known and followed, and reducing stress anxiety and depression for family members [44]. Despite this, few people with chronic respiratory disease have the opportunity to discuss end of life care or document their wishes. Only 25% of people entering pulmonary rehabilitation reported having an advance directive [45]. Although 99% of pulmonary rehabilitation participants wanted to discuss advance directives with their physicians, only 19% had previously had such a discussion and only 14% thought their physician understood their wishes for end of life care [46].

Pulmonary rehabilitation may offer unique opportunities to engage participants in advance care planning, in a setting where they have established trusting relationships with health professionals, and at a time when they are willing and able to participate. In a group of 67 people participating in pulmonary rehabilitation or maintenance programs, most of whom had COPD, an education session on advance care planning was well accepted and the information was valued [47]. Participants were happy to receive such information in a group setting, and for some this method of delivery was perceived to have advantages over individual sessions. One-third of participants went on to complete advance directive documentation, and many more reported discussing their wishes for end of life care with their families and friends, which is another important element of advance care planning. People with interstitial lung disease have also reported that they would like to discuss end of life planning in pulmonary rehabilitation, with many seeking information on what would happen at the end of their life and what could be done to manage their symptoms [48]. Participants commented on the importance of a skilled facilitator for such discussions [47] who should be honest, sensitive, compassionate and empathetic [49]. It should be acknowledged that a small number of pulmonary rehabilitation participants would prefer not to participate in advance care planning discussions [47] and this preference should be acknowledged and respected.

Conclusion

Whilst centre-based programs remain the core of pulmonary rehabilitation practice, there is increasing evidence that alternative models may also deliver clinically meaningful benefits. Regardless of the location or modality employed, contemporary programs should ensure that the key components of pulmonary rehabilitation are delivered, which include a thorough patient assessment, exercise training of the appropriate intensity and frequency, education and behaviour change [2]. Expanding the range of options by which patients can engage in pulmonary rehabilitation provides new opportunities for patient-centred care, and may contribute to enhanced uptake of this important treatment.

References

1. McCarthy B, et al. Pulmonary rehabilitation for chronic obstructive pulmonary disease. Cochrane Database Syst Rev. 2015;2:CD003793.
2. Spruit MA, et al. An Official American Thoracic Society/European Respiratory Society statement: key concepts and advances in pulmonary rehabilitation. Am J Respir Crit Care Med. 2013;188(8):e13–64.
3. Rochester CL, et al. An Official American Thoracic Society/European Respiratory Society Policy Statement: enhancing implementation, use, and delivery of pulmonary rehabilitation. Am J Respir Crit Care Med. 2015;192(11):1373–86.
4. Keating A, Lee A, Holland AE. What prevents people with chronic obstructive pulmonary disease from attending pulmonary rehabilitation? A systematic review. Chron Respir Dis. 2011;8(2):89–99.
5. Alison JA, et al. Australian and New Zealand Pulmonary Rehabilitation Guidelines. Respirology. 2017;22(4):800–19.
6. Maltais F, et al. Effects of home-based pulmonary rehabilitation in patients with chronic obstructive pulmonary disease: a randomized trial. Ann Intern Med. 2008;149(12):869–78.
7. Holland AE, et al. Short term improvement in exercise capacity and symptoms following exercise training in interstitial lung disease. Thorax. 2008;63(6):549–54.
8. Strijbos JH, et al. A comparison between an outpatient hospital-based pulmonary rehabilitation program and a home-care pulmonary rehabilitation program in patients with COPD. A follow-up of 18 months. Chest. 1996;109(2):366–72.
9. Wijkstra PJ, et al. Effects of home rehabilitation on physical performance in patients with chronic obstructive pulmonary disease (COPD). Eur Respir J. 1996;9(1):104–10.
10. Wedzicha JA, et al. Randomized controlled trial of pulmonary rehabilitation in severe chronic obstructive pulmonary disease patients, stratified with the MRC dyspnoea scale. Eur Respir J. 1998;12(2):363–9.
11. Spruit MA, et al. Differences in content and organisational aspects of pulmonary rehabilitation programmes. Eur Respir J. 2014;43(5):1326–37.
12. Ghanem M, et al. Home-based pulmonary rehabilitation program: effect on exercise tolerance and quality of life in chronic obstructive pulmonary disease patients. Ann Thorac Med. 2010;5(1):18–25.
13. Dias FD, et al. Home-based pulmonary rehabilitation in patients with chronic obstructive pulmonary disease: a randomized clinical trial. Int J Chron Obstruct Pulmon Dis. 2013;8:537–44.
14. Pradella CO, et al. home-based pulmonary rehabilitation for subjects with COPD: a randomized study. Respir Care. 2015;60(4):526–32.
15. Holland AE, et al. Home-based rehabilitation for COPD using minimal resources: a randomised, controlled equivalence trial. Thorax. 2017;72(1):57–65.

16. Boxall AM, et al. Managing chronic obstructive pulmonary disease in the community. A randomized controlled trial of home-based pulmonary rehabilitation for elderly housebound patients. J Cardiopulm Rehabil. 2005;25(6):378–85.
17. Busch AJ, McClements JD. Effects of a supervised home exercise program on patients with severe chronic obstructive pulmonary disease. Phys Ther. 1988;68(4):469–74.
18. Casey D, et al. The effectiveness of a structured education pulmonary rehabilitation programme for improving the health status of people with moderate and severe chronic obstructive pulmonary disease in primary care: the PRINCE cluster randomised trial. Thorax. 2013;68(10):922–8.
19. Roman M, et al. Efficacy of pulmonary rehabilitation in patients with moderate chronic obstructive pulmonary disease: a randomized controlled trial. BMC Fam Pract. 2013;14:21.
20. Faulkner J, et al. The feasibility of recruiting patients with early COPD to a pilot trial assessing the effects of a physical activity intervention. Prim Care Respir J. 2010;19(2):124–30.
21. Cambach W, et al. The effects of a community-based pulmonary rehabilitation programme on exercise tolerance and quality of life: a randomized controlled trial. Eur Respir J. 1997;10(1):104–13.
22. Gottlieb V, et al. Pulmonary rehabilitation for moderate COPD (GOLD 2)--does it have an effect? COPD. 2011;8(5):380–6.
23. Amin S, et al. A controlled study of community-based exercise training in patients with moderate COPD. BMC Pulm Med. 2014;14:125.
24. van Wetering CR, et al. Short- and long-term efficacy of a community-based COPD management programme in less advanced COPD: a randomised controlled trial. Thorax. 2010;65(1):7–13.
25. Keating A, Lee AL, Holland AE. Lack of perceived benefit and inadequate transport influence uptake and completion of pulmonary rehabilitation in people with chronic obstructive pulmonary disease: a qualitative study. J Physiother. 2011;57(3):183–90.
26. McNamara RJ, et al. Water-based exercise training for chronic obstructive pulmonary disease. Cochrane Database Syst Rev. 2013;12:CD008290.
27. McNamara RJ, et al. Water-based exercise in COPD with physical comorbidities: a randomised controlled trial. Eur Respir J. 2013;41(6):1284–91.
28. Perk J, Perk L, Boden C. Cardiorespiratory adaptation of COPD patients to physical training on land and in water. Eur Respir J. 1996;9(2):248–52.
29. McNamara RJ, et al. Acceptability of the aquatic environment for exercise training by people with chronic obstructive pulmonary disease with physical comorbidities: additional results from a randomised controlled trial. Physiotherapy. 2015;101(2):187–92.
30. Leung RW, et al. Short-form Sun-style t'ai chi as an exercise training modality in people with COPD. Eur Respir J. 2013;41(5):1051–7.
31. Ngai SP, Jones AY, Tam WW. Tai Chi for chronic obstructive pulmonary disease (COPD). Cochrane Database Syst Rev. 2016;6:CD009953.
32. Oliveira CC, et al. Fear of falling in people with chronic obstructive pulmonary disease. Respir Med. 2015;109(4):483–9.
33. Qiu ZH, et al. Physiological responses to Tai Chi in stable patients with COPD. Respir Physiol Neurobiol. 2016;221:30–4.
34. Barberan-Garcia A, et al. Nordic walking enhances oxygen uptake without increasing the rate of perceived exertion in patients with chronic obstructive pulmonary disease. Respiration. 2015;89(3):221–5.
35. Breyer MK, et al. Nordic walking improves daily physical activities in COPD: a randomised controlled trial. Respir Res. 2010;11:112.
36. Cindy Ng LW, et al. Does exercise training change physical activity in people with COPD? A systematic review and meta-analysis. Chron Respir Dis. 2012;9(1):17–26.
37. Evans RA. Developing the model of pulmonary rehabilitation for chronic heart failure. Chron Respir Dis. 2011;8(4):259–69.
38. Griffo R, et al. Frequent coexistence of chronic heart failure and chronic obstructive pulmonary disease in respiratory and cardiac outpatients: evidence from SUSPIRIUM, a multicentre Italian survey. Eur J Prev Cardiol. 2017:2047487316687425.
39. Crisafulli E, et al. Role of comorbidities in a cohort of patients with COPD undergoing pulmonary rehabilitation. Thorax. 2008;63(6):487–92.
40. Taylor RS, et al. Exercise-based rehabilitation for heart failure. Cochrane Database Syst Rev. 2014; 4:CD003331.
41. Evans RA, et al. Generic, symptom based, exercise rehabilitation; integrating patients with COPD and heart failure. Respir Med. 2010;104(10):1473–81.
42. Man WD, et al. Building consensus for provision of breathlessness rehabilitation for patients with chronic obstructive pulmonary disease and chronic heart failure. Chron Respir Dis. 2016;13(3):229–39.
43. McNamara RJ, et al. Community-based exercise training for people with chronic respiratory and chronic cardiac disease: a mixed-methods evaluation. Int J Chron Obstruct Pulmon Dis. 2016;11:2839–50.
44. Detering KM, et al. The impact of advance care planning on end of life care in elderly patients: randomised controlled trial. BMJ. 2010;340:c1345.
45. Gerald LB, et al. Advance directives in cardiac and pulmonary rehabilitation patients. J Cardiopulm Rehabil. 2000;20(6):340–5.
46. Heffner JE, et al. Attitudes regarding advance directives among patients in pulmonary rehabilitation. Am J Respir Crit Care Med. 1996;154(6 Pt 1):1735–40.
47. Burge AT, et al. Advance care planning education in pulmonary rehabilitation: a qualitative study exploring participant perspectives. Palliat Med. 2013;27(6):508–15.
48. Holland AE, et al. Be honest and help me prepare for the future: what people with interstitial lung disease

want from education in pulmonary rehabilitation. Chron Respir Dis. 2015;12(2):93–101.
49. Janssen DJ, et al. Advance care planning for patients with COPD: past, present and future. Patient Educ Couns. 2012;86(1):19–24.
50. Puente-Maestu L, et al. Comparison of effects of supervised versus self-monitored training programmes in patients with chronic obstructive pulmonary disease. Eur Respir J. 2000;15(3):517–25.
51. Murphy N, Bell C, Costello RW. Extending a home from hospital care programme for COPD exacerbations to include pulmonary rehabilitation. Respir Med. 2005;99(10):1297–302.
52. Guell MR, et al. Home vs hospital-based pulmonary rehabilitation for patients with chronic obstructive pulmonary disease: a Spanish multicenter trial. Arch Bronconeumol. 2008;44(10):512–8.
53. Behnke M, et al. Home-based exercise is capable of preserving hospital-based improvements in severe chronic obstructive pulmonary disease. Respir Med. 2000;94(12):1184–91.
54. Fernandez AM, et al. Home-based pulmonary rehabilitation in very severe COPD: is it safe and useful? J Cardiopulm Rehabil Prev. 2009;29(5):325–31.
55. Oh EG. The effects of home-based pulmonary rehabilitation in patients with chronic lung disease. Int J Nurs Stud. 2003;40(8):873–9.
56. Hernandez MT, et al. Results of a home-based training program for patients with COPD. Chest. 2000;118(1):106–14.
57. de Sousa Pinto JM, et al. Clinical benefits of home-based pulmonary rehabilitation in patients with chronic obstructive pulmonary disease. J Cardiopulm Rehabil Prev. 2014;34(5):355–9.
58. Mendes de Oliveira JC, et al. Outpatient vs. home-based pulmonary rehabilitation in COPD: a randomized controlled trial. Multidiscip Respir Med. 2010;5(6):401–8.
59. Xie SL, et al. Influence of home-based training program on patients with COPD. Chin J Clin Rehab. 2003;7(18):2554–5.
60. Singh V, et al. Pulmonary rehabilitation in patients with chronic obstructive pulmonary disease. Indian J Chest Dis Allied Sci. 2003;45(1):13–7.
61. Larson JL, et al. Cycle ergometer and inspiratory muscle training in chronic obstructive pulmonary disease. Am J Respir Crit Care Med. 1999; 160(2):500–7.

23 Telehealth in Pulmonary Rehabilitation

Michele Vitacca and Anne Holland

23.1 Definitions

Telehealth has been defined as the use of information and communication technologies (ICT) to deliver healthcare services and transmit medical data over long and short distances [1]. It encompasses a wide variety of technologies such as videoconferencing, internet platforms, store-and-forward devices, streaming media, and terrestrial and wireless communication. Telehealth may be used for a wide range of purposes, including decreasing demand on existing hospital and healthcare services; reducing the cost of care; measuring treatment adherence; identifying disease worsening; improving accessibility of services; and extending the reach of services to remote locations. Telehealth is therefore a broad concept that could involve diagnosis, treatment, monitoring, education and prevention.

Within telehealth there are a number of domains relevant to pulmonary rehabilitation:

- Telemonitoring—the use of ICT to monitor patients at a distance
- Tele-assistance—the provision of clinical care from a distance using ICT
- Telerehabilitation—the use of ICT to provide clinical rehabilitation services from a distance [2].

23.2 Rationale for TeleHealth in Pulmonary Rehabilitation

23.2.1 Optimizing Care

People with chronic respiratory disease who undertake pulmonary rehabilitation have complex health problems and high numbers of comorbidities. Pulmonary rehabilitation provides an ideal opportunity to enhance disease management via comprehensive patient assessment, applying optimal treatments, improved self-monitoring, better understanding of prescribed treatments, improved adherence and better communication with health professionals [3]. Opportunities to aid these goals using telehealth are growing. A wide range of telehealth interventions could be used to optimize care and patient outcomes, including daily monitoring of physiological signals (e.g. pulse oximetry, home ventilator wave forms) or symptoms (cough, sputum, dyspnoea); early notification of clinical deterioration for both patients and clinicians; telephone

M. Vitacca, M.D., F.E.R.S. (✉)
Respiratory Rehabilitation Division, Istituti Clinici Scientifici Maugeri, IRCSS, Lumezzane, Brescia, Italy
e-mail: michele.vitacca@icsmaugeri.it

A. Holland, B.App.Sci., Ph.D.
Alfred Health and Institute for Breathing and Sleep, La Trobe University, Melbourne, Australia

© Springer International Publishing AG 2018
E. Clini et al. (eds.), *Textbook of Pulmonary Rehabilitation*,
https://doi.org/10.1007/978-3-319-65888-9_23

support; web-based education programmes; and case management via videoconferencing.

23.2.2 Improving Access

Despite compelling evidence for the benefits of pulmonary rehabilitation and unequivocal recommendations in COPD guidelines [4] only 5–10% of those with symptomatic COPD have ever accessed a pulmonary rehabilitation programme [5–7]. Contributors to poor uptake include system-related barriers such as insufficient programmes and inadequate numbers of qualified health professionals, particularly in rural and regional areas [7, 8]. These problems are predicted to worsen in coming years due to population ageing in many developed nations. There are also patient-related barriers to attendance, such as poor physical mobility, distressing symptoms and inability to travel [9]. Using ICT, rehabilitation can be delivered directly to the patient's location, regardless of physical proximity to a rehabilitation centre. This may involve (but is not limited to) assessment of exercise capacity; supervised exercise training; disease-specific education; goal setting and problem solving; health coaching; and peer support. It can also involve training and supervision of health professionals delivering a pulmonary rehabilitation programme in a remote location. Whilst telerehabilitation may be particularly useful to improve pulmonary rehabilitation access for patients located away from major centres, it may also enhance uptake for those in whom ill health precludes travel to centre-based programmes.

23.3 Tele-Assistance

In the last decade, several studies focusing on the effects of various tele-assistance programmes for patients with chronic respiratory insufficiency (with COPD being the main diagnosis) have been published (Table 23.1, chapter 6). Reduction in hospitalization and use of other acute health-care services, improvement in the quality of life and patient satisfaction have been reported in the majority of studies providing at distance chronic home care interventions and patient education. These programmes are based on strict adherence to interventions to enhance symptom self-monitoring by patients and their caregivers; increasing their understanding of drug therapy, symptom and treatment monitoring; and acting as a liaison between primary care providers and hospital services. This involves the delivery of time-intensive education by nurses and other personnel such as respiratory therapists [10–13]. Literature has shown the best telemonitoring success are expected in (1) programmes dedicated to very sick patients with severe symptoms, frequent exacerbations, multi-morbidity, and limited community support; (2) long-term interventions; and (3) programmes using the third-generation telemonitoring systems providing constant analytical and decision-making support, where monitoring centres are led by a physician, staffed by specialist nurses, and have full therapeutic authority 24 h/day, 7 days/week. If an extensive home care package with strong community links exists, telemonitoring may add little additional benefit.

23.4 TeleMonitoring of Signals and Traces

23.4.1 TeleMonitoring of Home Ventilated Patients

An accurate count of the number of patients receiving home mechanical ventilation in the word is unknown. The estimated prevalence of ventilator-dependent individuals in Europe is 6.6 per 100,000 people [38]. Extrapolating the EU prevalence to the United States population in 2010 would suggest that the total American home ventilator population could be estimated to be 20,377 individuals whilst there are roughly 47,981 Medicare patients receiving some form of home ventilation [39]. In Canada 4334 ventilator-assisted individuals have been identified with an estimated prevalence of 12.9/100,000 population [40]. In Australia the estimated prevalence was 9.9 patients per 100,000 population in 2013 [41]. The increasing number and costs of

Table 23.1 Summary of main published studies on tele-assistance (Chapter 6)

Study	Population	Outcomes	Costs
Johnston [14]	102 TM vs 102 controls; CHF, COPD, cerebral vascular accident, cancer, diabetes, anxiety	QOL >	27 % <
Farrero [15]	COPD under LTOT; 46 TM vs 48 controls	H and ER <	Total saving 46.823 dollars
Agha [16]	Mixed; TM vs controls vs on site care	Costs	43% < in TM group
Hernandez [17]	COPD exacerbations at ER; 121 TM vs 101 controls	QOL >; H and ER <	NA
Bourbeau [18]	COPD	QOL >; ER and GP calls <	NA
Pare [19]	COPD; 19 TM vs 10 controls	H <	15% <
Casas [20]	COPD at discharge; 65 TM vs 90 controls	No effect on survival ; H <	NA
Miyasaka [21]	7 paediatric patients for home ventilatory care	GP calls, visits, H <	NA
Vitacca [22]	ALS (*n* = 73: 18 on NIV; 18 on invasive ventilation)	TM timing, TM feasibility, team time consuming, costs	TM costs 105€/pt/month
Vitacca [23]	ALS (*n* = 40: 19 on NIV; 12 on invasive ventilation)	TM use, patient requests for TM , TM staff activities, TM satisfaction	NA
Zamith [24]	Asthma *n* = 21 + CRF *n* = 51, 41 on LTOT ; 32 on NIV	TM use and acceptance; H < and QOL >	NA
Bertini [25]	16 HMV (5 Invasive MV, 11 NIV ; 3 COPD, 4 RTD, 8 NMD, 1 Ondine Syndrome)	TM use and acceptance; ER <; good satisfaction	NA
Vontetsianos [26]	COPD (*n* = 18) + at least 4 H in previous 2 years	H and ER <	NA
Trappenburg [27]	COPD (study *n* = 59; controls *n* = 56)	H and relapses <; QOL =	NA
Segrelles calvo [28]	30 home telehealth, 30 controls; FEV1<50%, age >=50 years, LTOT, non-smokers, with at least one H for respiratory illness in the previous year.	H, H days, need for NIV <; good satisfaction	NA
Jodar sanchez [29]	TM (*n* = 24) control group (*n* = 21) on usual care. Under LTOT and with at least one hospitalization for respiratory illness in the previous year	ER < ; H > ; QOL >; good satisfaction.	NA
Maiolo [30]	20 COPD patients on LTOT+3 RTD	QOL >; H and relapses <	17% <
Moreira [31]	35 patients (OSA 40,0%, COPD 22,8%, NMD 11,4%, TB sequelae 2,9%, Kyphoscoliosis 2,9%; 20,0% other CRF causes	In TM group hours use and % of usage days >	NA
Pinnock [32]	128 patients randomized to TM; 128 to usual care	H, H days, QOL = to controls	NA
Pedone [33]	50 COPD patients in the TM group, 49 controls.	Relapses and H <	NA
Vitacca [34]	CRF patients needing LTOT or HMV+ at least one H for respiratory illness in the previous year. COPD: 56%, RTD: 15%, NMD: 10%, ALS: 9%, other 10%. 46% on NIV, 21.4% IMV, 63% LTOT	No effect on survival ; QOL >; H, ER, GP visits, relapses <	33% <
Lopes de Almeida {Lopes de Almeida, 2012 #3814}	ALS patients; age 18-75 years; 40 patients: 20 TM; 20 controls.	Intention-to-treat analysis considering three different type of costs; costs.	TM of NIV in ALS is cost-effective. 700€ patient/year estimated long-term annual cost-saving.

(continued)

Table 23.1 (continued)

Study	Population	Outcomes	Costs
Cartwright [35]	CHF, COPD or diabetes; 845 were randomized to TM and 728 to controls	cost per quality adjusted life year gained	Quality adjusted life year gain was similar between TM and controls. Costs associated with TM were higher.
Chatwin [36]	1,211 adult and paediatric patients with neuromuscular disease, chronic obstructive pulmonary disease or chest wall disease receiving HMV	TM time consuming: 528 daytime calls/month Home visits from internal staff: < 2/month	NA
Chatwin [37]	68 CRF patients (38 COPD) with or without home mechanical ventilation	No differences for risk of H; H and home visits > in TM group; GP visits unchanged; self-efficacy fell during TM	NA

TM telemonitoring, *CHF* chronic congestive failure, *COPD* chronic obstructive pulmonary disease, *LTOT* long-term oxygen therapy, *ER* emergency room; *ALS* amyotrophic lateral sclerosis, *NIV* non-invasive ventilation, *MV* mechanical ventilation, *RTD* restrictive thoracic disease; *NMD* neuromuscular diseases; *H* hospitalizations; *FEV1* forced expiratory volume at the first second; *CRF* chronic respiratory failure; *OSA* obstructive sleep apnoea; *TB* tuberculosis; *HMV* home mechanical ventilation; *IMV* invasive mechanical ventilation; *QOL* quality of life; *GP* general practitioner; *ABG* arterial blood gases; *NA* not available

these complex patients make present health organizations largely insufficient to face their needs.

In a multicentre quality control survey of home mechanical ventilation (HMV) performed at the home of 300 patients included in the HMV programmes, considerable differences were found between actual, set, and prescribed values of ventilator variables [42]. The study stressed current limitations of the quality control of HMV and suggests that improvements should be made to ensure adequate ventilator settings and correct ventilator performance and ventilator alarm operation. As a consequence, the burden lies mostly with families. The need to reduce healthcare costs and to increase safety has prompted the development of telemonitoring for home ventilatory assistance. Many remote health monitoring systems are available, ensuring safety, feasibility, effectiveness, sustainability and flexibility to meet different patients' needs. The possible use of telemonitoring for HMV patients has been proposed to assist patients to adapt remotely to MV, monitor the side effects and residual apnoeas or desaturations, predict forthcoming relapses, reduce health costs, improve the patient-related outcomes (PRO), improve adherence to HMV, improve lifestyles or improve palliation and meet end of life needs.

Table 23.2 (chapter 6) summarized literature on population and outcomes studied using telemonitoring of HMV patients. The overall body of literature on this topic reveal that the magnitude and significance of effects on patients' conditions and economical organizational expectations are not sufficiently consistent and sometime remain inconclusive.

The 'one glove fits all' approach in offering telemonitoring for chronic respiratory insufficiency seems to be too simplistic for a heterogeneous population such as these patients. Factors that would be important for the successful implementation of telemonitoring are an individually tailored approach, flexibility, and a service that is locally responsive. Chronic diseases increase the burden on healthcare systems. Primary care needs to be sustained in the face of increasing demands: home care and telemonitoring may

Table 23.2 Summary of main published studies on telemonitoring of HMV patients (Chapter 6)

Study	Population	Outcomes
Pinto [43]	ALS ($N = 40$, all ventilated):	Good adaptation to NIV; visits and ER <
Hazenberg [44]	Seventy-seven patients were included, of which 38 patients started HMV at home (neuromuscular or thoracic cage disease)	Home Initiation of HMV with TM improves ABG and QoL not inferior to controls TM is safe, feasible and cheaper.
Janssens JP [45]	Patients treated by non-invasive ventilation (NIV)	Data provided by ventilator software helps by estimating ventilation, tidal volume, leaks, rate of inspiratory or expiratory triggering by the patient. Autonomic markers of sympathetic tone using signals such as pulse wave amplitude of the pulse-oximetry signal can provide reliable information of sleep fragmentation.
Georges M [46]	10 stable subjects with obesity-hypoventilation syndrome	Correlation between AHI-NIV and AHI-PSG was highly significant. Ventilator software had a sensitivity of 90.9%, a specificity and positive predictive value of 100%, and a negative predictive value of 71%.
Pasquina [47]	Data downloaded from home ventilators in 150 clinically stable patients under long-term NIV (mixed diseases)	Built-in software of home ventilators provides the clinician with new parameters (leaks, compliance, triggered ventilators acts, respiratory rate, residual apnoeas and hypopneas) useful to care and better to understand residual hypoventilation and/or desaturations.
Borel [48]	COPD on home NIV	Relapses prediction with TM monitoring of breathing pattern; 21 exacerbations were correctly detected

See Table 23.1 chapter 6; *AHI-NIV* apnoea hypopnea index on NIV, *AHI-PSG* apnoea hypopnea index on polysomnography

help primary care professionals and specialists to reduce the expected burden. Hospitalization of chronically ill patients is a ‘failure’ for healthcare systems and chronic diseases exemplify the case for the large-scale deployment of follow-up programmes. For these reasons, home care programmes and telemonitoring may provide an opportunity for health organizations to develop new strategies and clinical procedures.

23.4.2 Telemonitoring in Sleep-Related Breathing Disorders

Sleep-related breathing disorders (SRD) are characterized by abnormalities of the respiratory pattern during sleep. Continuous positive airway pressure and NIV may benefit these patients. In addition, nocturnal monitoring of SRD is complex and unforeseen problems arise for many reasons, such as (a) physiological variations of different variables, (b) clinical problems (pain and secretions, among others) or (c) sleep disturbances [49, 50]. According to the American Academy of Sleep Medicine recommendations, titration based on polysomnography using conventionally available parameters is an important tool for accurately establishing devices settings, to avoid abnormalities in most of the patients and to achieve optimal treatment and maximal clinical improvement [51].

Self-management should be an essential ingredient in the SRD Chronic Care Model. Tele-assistance and telemonitoring by itself may be one of the tools for improving patient behaviour through direct and timely intervention by a health professional. By combining tele-assistance and telemonitoring with self-management, there should be a boost in patient behaviour encompassing proactivity and willingness to self-monitor symptoms, as well as improving decision-making and providing tools to solve day-to-day problems. In this way, self-management skills can be built on and used at home, as well as in routine healthcare system interactions and the provision of patient support. Tele-assistance and telemonitoring can implement some tasks, such as monitoring, support, education and behavioural changes, with more frequency and lower cost than home intervention programmes conducted face to face [52].

With the aim of improving compliance as well as finding new diagnostic strategies, some studies investigated the role of telemonitoring in SRD [52–57]. However RCTs evaluating the effect on CPAP compliance of additional interventions to standard care, based on telemonitoring, have had contradictory results [52, 58–61]. Differences in the selection of patients, type and intensity of interventions and high CPAP compliance in the control group can explain the discrepancies. The potential of telemonitoring in hypoventilation syndrome has been less studied and no clear recommendations exist in clinical protocols [50–52, 62–66] or procedures [63, 67].

Information communications technology seems to have a great potential in the comprehensive care of SRD. For example, since in many cases one night and follow-up visits in the sleep laboratory are not enough to adequately set the ventilator, ICT can support the home refinement of the titration of these patients [68]. A recent multicentre randomized controlled trial provided evidence that a strategy based on a web platform and tele-consultations, for the CPAP follow-up of OSA patients is as effective as the face-to-face approach at lower costs [52]. However, caution is needed because data transmitted by commercial devices come from different manufacturers with varying data collection strategies. Standardization and homogenization of these data collection and transmission should be regulated by scientific societies [69].

Despite these encouraging results, the penetration of these technological advances in clinical practice is still slow, especially when compared with other chronic respiratory diseases or other pathologies [68, 70]. Furthermore recently published results questioned the validity of this technology as a method to deliver healthcare for all populations [71]. Consequently, it appears crucial to carefully select proper outcomes and target the most receptive patient groups.

23.5 Telerehabilitation

Telerehabilitation affords new opportunities to improve pulmonary rehabilitation access and deliver good clinical outcomes. The components of pulmonary rehabilitation have been defined [3] and emerging evidence suggests that many components, if not all, can be delivered effectively using a variety of ICT approaches. This includes supervised or unsupervised exercise training; monitoring of physiology and symptoms; self-management training; disease education; goal setting; and peer support. Whilst only a few pulmonary rehabilitation programmes worldwide are currently offering telerehabilitation [72], this is likely to grow as telehealth applications become increasingly accessible to patients and clinicians.

To date there have been seven clinical trials testing telerehabilitation in patients with COPD (Table 23.3., chapter 6). No adverse events related to telerehabilitation were reported. A number of models have been used:

23.5.1 Telephone Coaching

Two large trials that delivered PR using weekly telephone calls and unsupervised exercise training reported equivalent benefits to a traditional centre-based pulmonary rehabilitation programme [73, 74]. Telephone calls were delivered by exercise specialists in both cases, but the nature of the calls differed. One study used the telephone calls to reinforce the importance of the exercises and to detect problems [74] and the other used the calls to deliver motivational interviewing, set exercise goals and conduct disease self-management training [73]. Both studies included one home visit from an exercise specialist before the telephone calls were commenced.

23.5.2 Videoconferencing

Videoconferencing was used to link a large expert centre with smaller, regional centres [75]. This allowed experienced pulmonary rehabilitation clinicians to provide support to clinicians, and to deliver education sessions from the multidisciplinary team at the larger centre. Exercise training was not directly supervised via videolink. This controlled trial reported similar outcomes to those who undertook traditional pulmonary rehabilitation at the larger centre. Videoconferencing has also been used to deliver pulmonary rehabilitation directly into the participant's home in a virtual 'group', with up to four participants at a time [76]. Compared to usual care the participants had significant improvements in exercise capacity and mood, although the study was underpowered to detect differences in quality of life.

23.5.3 Internet Platforms and Remote Monitoring

One pilot RCT has illustrated the potential of more complex strategies which integrate remote monitoring, videoconferencing and online diaries [77]. Eighty-four percent of participants were satisfied with the service, with improvements in clinical outcomes that were similar to those in a retrospective control group undergoing centre-based rehabilitation. Other bespoke internet platforms have been tested in single group studies with similar conclusions [78–80].

23.5.4 Smartphone Applications

The 'activity coach' was an accelerometer that connected wirelessly to a smartphone, to register the number of steps taken and provide real time feedback [81]. The smartphone provided graphical feedback, goals and motivational text messages. A web portal provided a symptom diary for self-treatment of exacerbations and an overview of the measured activity levels. Adherence was high, although this small RCT ($n = 30$) was not powered to show differences in clinical outcomes.

Limitations of current studies on telerehabilitation include the wide variety of platforms and equipment used; a plethora of pilot studies describing models that have not been tested in robust trials; few studies powered for equivalence against centre-based pulmonary rehabilitation; a lack of data regarding the cost-effectiveness of different telerehabilitation models; relatively narrow selection criteria which have often excluded patients with severe disease and those with conditions other than COPD; and a lack of robust methods, including random allocation, assessor blinding and intention to treat. Despite this, the body of evidence provides consistent signals suggesting that telerehabilitation may deliver clinically important benefits. Trials are currently underway that will combine a number of telerehabilitation approaches and address the limitations of previous literature [82].

23.5.5 Acceptability of Telerehabilitation

Prior use of the internet does not appear to be required for acceptance of simple telerehabilitation equipment [83] and adherence to sessions is high [76]. However a study that used more complex platform reported that 22% of participants found the technology 'unfriendly' [77]. A study that used videoconferencing for group exercise and education reported that patients valued the supportive social environment, for motivation and sharing of experiences [79]. Participants also valued regular contact with healthcare professionals as it made them feel safe [84]. Experiencing health benefits from telerehabilitation was a powerful motivator to persist with the programme [84]. It is possible that some individuals do not participate in telerehabilitation trials as they are not comfortable with this approach [85]. As a result, these data may not reflect the full range of views of individuals with chronic lung disease who are eligible for pulmonary rehabilitation.

Table 23.3. Controlled trials of telerehabilitation (Chapter 6)

Author	Design	*n*	Telerehabilitation model	Outcomes
Oh 2003 [87]	RCT	23	**Telephone calls** twice weekly from a nurse to discuss problems and concerns; unsupervised exercise training at home	Significant improvement in exercise capacity, dyspnoea and HRQoL compared to control (no PR)
Maltais 2008 [74]	RCT	252	**Telephone calls** weekly from a nurse to reinforce exercises and detect problems; unsupervised exercise training at home	Equivalent improvements in dyspnoea, HRQoL and exercise capacity compared to centre-based PR
Holland 2017 [73]	RCT	166	**Telephone calls** weekly from a physiotherapist using motivational interviewing to set exercise goals; unsupervised exercise training at home	Equivalent improvements in dyspnoea, HRQoL and exercise capacity compared to centre-based PR
Stickland [75]	CCT	409	**Videoconferencing** from major centre to smaller satellite centres; support for remote clinicians and joint education sessions	Similar improvements in HRQoL and exercise capacity compared to centre-based PR
Tsai 2017 [76]	RCT	37	**Videoconferencing** for supervised group exercise training at home	Significant improvement in exercise capacity, self-efficacy and mood compared to control (no PR)
Paneroni 2015 [77]	Pilot CCT	36	**Internet platform** including telemonitoring, tele-prescription, video-assistance and phone-calls	No difference in exercise capacity, symptoms or HRQOL compared to control (retrospectively matched group who had undertaken centre-based PR)
Tabak 2013 [81]	RCT	30	**Smartphone** with wireless accelerometer to measure physical activity; web portal with symptom diary	No difference in physical activity levels compared to control (no PR)

CCT controlled clinical trial, *RCT* randomized controlled trial, *n* number of included participants

There is no single 'optimal' model for telerehabilitation. The following factors could be considered in choosing the best model for a given clinical setting:

- Aims of the telerehabilitation programme—videoconferencing between centres can be used to support and educate clinicians at geographically distant centres [75], whereas in-home telerehabilitation may improve access for debilitated patients [76].
- Patient characteristics—this includes willingness and capacity to use the internet; limitations to sight and vision that might affect the ability to use screen-based applications and videoconferencing; falls risk that may be exacerbated by equipment placed in the home; social situation that may preclude home-based rehabilitation.
- Characteristics of the home environment, including whether there is space for equipment such as exercise bikes [76] or treadmills [86]. Models that have low equipment needs [73] may be more suitable for some.
- Patient preference for setting of care—some patients prefer a centre-based programme [73], usually because it affords greater supervision or greater peer support. However it is possible to achieve these aspects using telerehabilitation with remote monitoring and virtual groups [79].
- Cost of telerehabilitation—telephone-based models are low in cost [73] whilst others require more sophisticated equipment [77]. In many instances funding is required for transport of equipment and an initial home visit. Reimbursement may not be well established for these new models of care.

- Accessibility of ICT equipment—some trials have used bespoke systems [77], whilst others use 'off the shelf' equipment such as tablets, exercise bikes and pulse oximeters [83]. The increasingly widespread use of smartphones may make this an efficient means to deliver telerehabilitation.
- Ability to deliver all components of pulmonary rehabilitation, including disease education and behaviour change.

In conclusion, there is growing evidence that telerehabilitation can achieve clinical benefits that are meaningful for patients. The optimal model has not been identified and may vary across patients and settings. Robust RCTs and cost-effectiveness studies are needed to drive uptake into practice, particularly for more complex telerehabilitation models. Whilst it will not replace the gold standard of centre-based programmes, telerehabilitation has great potential to extend the known benefits of pulmonary rehabilitation to a greater number of people who would benefit.

23.6 Opportunities and Risks

23.6.1 Legal Issues

The legal problems associated with TA and TM are still controversial. Despite many processes of tele-consultation are unique, the legal principles applying to conventional, face-to-face, doctor–patient relationships may be equally as valid in the context of the practice of medicine at a distance [88, 89]. In TA and TM, three roles can be held legally liable for the delivered performance [89]:

(1) *The person who transmits the data.* Any application of TA and TM is considered a medical act. The relationship between the person using the service (especially when he/she is the patient) and other stakeholders, must be governed by 'informed consent'. This preliminary action allows the patient to be adequately informed about the characteristics of the service, the potential risks, the precautions to reduce them and to ensure the confidentiality of the information [88].
(2) *The person who receives data.* The person who conducts the remote health service: he/she is the medical user of the service and the medical consultant [88].
(3) *The service provider(s).* The quality and confidentiality of the transmitted and received data must be ensured by service providers [88].

The use of TA and TM carries several risks distance [88–90]: tele-consultation may fail to reach standard of care; equipment or system may fail; electronic data can be manipulated; the electronic record may be subject to abuse; the network may suffer from poor data protection (poor confidentiality, authenticity, data report, procedure certification, security and privacy); the network may show difficulty to ascertain responsibilities and potential obligations of health professionals.

Important system precautions need to be used by e-Health users [91, 92]:

(a) **Data security and confidentiality**. Suppliers and users must ensure the confidentiality, the authenticity of the data and their report, the authorized certification of procedures with digital signature, the protection of confidentiality, the security and privacy of the assisted persons, the storage and transfer of sensitive data in real time between one unit and the other without manipulation.
(b) **Responsibilities and potential obligations of health professionals**. Three key aspects need to be specified: (a) the responsibility of the physician (tele-consultant) and the patient at distance (tele-consulted); (b) the relationship and co-responsibility between specialist consultant and the requesting physician; (c) the responsibility and the relationship among the applicant, consultant and service supplier or suppliers.
(c) **Interoperability.** Mutual exchange of ICT-enabled solutions and of data is necessary for better coordination and integration across the entire chain of healthcare delivery to offer personalized solutions.

With the increasing diffusion of this technology, case law will be updated and give answers to issues unresolved now. National governments should promote common, ethical, legal, regulatory, technical, administrative standards for remote medicine to assist VDIs and care givers in providing safe and effective services.

23.6.2 Economic Considerations

Tele-assistance and TM can be considered as both a challenge and an opportunity for the Health Services [93]. Home mechanical ventilation requires a large amount of human and financial resources [94]. Some studies have evaluated and compared the costs associated to home and institutional or hospital setting alternative solutions. An early paper from Fields et al. [95] on the cost-effectiveness of home care technology for respiratory technology—dependent children, reports a mean annual home care costs greater than 100,000 US $ for ventilator-dependent children, and greater than 60,000 $ for oxygen-dependent tracheostomized patients, respectively. This corresponds to about 79,000 and 83,000 $ per patient saving, respectively, compared to alternative institutional care. A recent literature review [96] outlines that HMV is a more cost-effective therapy compared to inpatient care in ICUs reporting a cost reduction ranging 62–74% in general. Furthermore, invasive HMV has higher costs compared to home NIV principally due to the care equipment and partially need of 24 care by highly qualified personnel. Available comparisons of institutional and at home solutions in VDI may underestimate the importance of comparing at home alternatives such as:

(a) Telemonitoring *vs* formal caregiver monitoring in VDI's home care, to highlight the savings associated to telemonitoring when compared to high intensity labour home activities;
(b) Quality of life comparison in patients using home and hospital care solutions.

Few studies reporting the cost-effectiveness of remote monitoring in VDIs. For example, the study by Vitacca et al. [34] concluded that telemonitoring was cost-effective in case of severe and frail patients when LTOT and/or either NIV ventilator or invasive mechanical ventilation are needed, considering activation and healthcare service provision costs. Constant costs were mainly based on the number of calls, and savings in healthcare services costs were mainly due to the prevented hospitalizations. Per patient costs were about 33% less than for usual outpatient follow-up, whereas per COPD patients telemonitoring costs were about 50% less than for usual outpatient follow-up. Despite these preliminary studies have shown an advantage in applying telehealth systems, recent research casts some doubts that these systems are more effective and less expensive than usual care [35, 97, 98]. To evaluate the real cost/effectiveness of new methods such as remote monitoring in this population, it is important to understand what do 'standard therapy' and 'usual therapy' mean in the papers published until now. It is clear that the superiority (if any) of this new method of care must be compared to a 'gold standard' of home care that is very variable amongst countries.

On the other side telemonitoring may represent also an opportunity for Health Services. Despite the economic crisis, the potential e-Health market is strong. The global telemedicine market has grown from $ 9.8 billion in 2010 to $ 11.6 billion in 2011, and is expected to continue to grow to $ 27.3 billion in 2016, representing a compound 18.6% annual growth rate [99]. The health market enabled by digital technologies (mobile applications, devices) is rapidly growing. The convergence between wireless communication technologies and healthcare devices and between health and social care is creating new businesses [99].

23.7 Future Directions

23.7.1 Research

The ATS/ERS Statement on Pulmonary Rehabilitation nominates 'defining the role of telehealth and other new technologies' as key to addressing the research priority of 'Increasing the accessibility to pulmonary rehabilitation' (page e45) [3]. Critical future steps towards this would be:

- Achieving consensus on what constitutes 'usual care', such that the additional benefits offered by telehealth can be quantified
- Standardizing models of telehealth in chronic lung disease, to allow consistent implementation and meaningful comparison across studies
- Defining the role of telemonitoring and tele-assistance across the spectrum of chronic lung disease—in which diagnostic groups is it most useful, when should it be offered (including considerations of disease severity and acute vs stable disease) and when should it be stopped
- Conducting robust cost-effectiveness studies to inform health policy.

23.7.2 Clinical Practice

Telehealth can improve access to care, particularly for those living away from major centres. Simple yet innovative telehealth solutions to improve access and uptake are already implemented in clinical practice, with good results [75]. Such programmes, including simple telerehabilitation models and tele-consulting, should be made more widely available. Where high quality clinical care is already available it is less clear that telerehabilitation adds significant benefit. Current data do not yet justify the routine implementation of telehealth in such a setting, although individual patients may benefit.

Conclusions

Home telemonitoring and telerehabilitation of chronic diseases seems to be a promising patient management strategy that could produce accurate and reliable data, empower patients, influence their attitudes and behaviour, and potentially improve their medical conditions. Clinical trials of telerehabilitation have demonstrated meaningful improvements in pulmonary rehabilitation outcomes such as exercise capacity and quality of life. However, systematic reviews of home telemonitoring [100–102] reveal that the magnitude and significance of effects on patients' conditions remain inconclusive. The impact on clinical effectiveness outcomes and economic viability likewise remain unresolved.

In conclusion, at the moment the fundamental pre-requisite for the efficacy of telemonitoring in chronic respiratory insufficiency management is to establish common standardized protocols rather than determine how to deliver the care [103]. The absence of conclusive evidence for the benefit of telemonitoring in chronic respiratory insufficiency should, however, not be taken as evidence of an absence of benefit. It is clear that telemonitoring alone is not sufficient in itself to yield a better outcome; telemonitoring could be a key element in management of chronic respiratory insufficiency patients, but it is difficult to evaluate its benefit without considering the other services received by patients (home care, access to hospital, social care). Considering the overall care 'package' received by the patient, telemonitoring may be included as one of the services offered within the package. But other aspects—quality improvement, integration of programmes and services, increase of collaboration and communication across the different care settings and the development of a shared vision, goals and priorities—are needed to improve the efficiency of the healthcare services provided for chronic patients [103]. The key point in optimizing the use of telemonitoring is to correctly identify who the ideal candidates are, and at what time they should receive it and for how long [103]. In other words, oscillating between expectations and disillusionment, the current dilemma is not 'telemonitoring—yes or no?', but how to use it in a mature and balanced manner in such a way as to enhance the health outcomes for our chronic patients.

References

1. International Organisation for Standardization. ISO Strategy for Services—Case study 1: International SOS (ISO/TS 13131, Telehealth services); 2016.
2. Kairy D, et al. A systematic review of clinical outcomes, clinical process, healthcare utilization and costs associated with telerehabilitation. Disabil Rehabil. 2009;31(6):427–47.
3. Spruit MA, et al. An official American Thoracic Society/European Respiratory Society statement: key concepts and advances in pulmonary rehabilitation. American Journal of Respiratory and Critical Care Medicine. 2013;188(8):e13–64.
4. Global strategy for the diagnosis, management, and prevention of chronic obstructive pulmonary disease. www.goldcopd.org
5. Australian Institute for Health and Welfare. Monitoring pulmonary rehabilitation and long-term oxygen therapy for people with chronic obstructive pulmonary disease (COPD) in Australia: a discussion paper. Canberra: AIHW; 2013.
6. Yohannes AM, Connolly MJ. Pulmonary rehabilitation programmes in the UK: a national representative survey. Clin Rehabil. 2004;18(4):444–9.
7. Brooks D, et al. Characterization of pulmonary rehabilitation programs in Canada in 2005. Can Respir J. 2007;14(2):87–92.
8. Johnston CL, et al. How prepared are rural and remote health care practitioners to provide evidence-based management for people with chronic lung disease? Aust J Rural Health. 2012;20(4):200–7.
9. Keating A, Lee A, Holland AE. What prevents people with chronic obstructive pulmonary disease from attending pulmonary rehabilitation? A systematic review. Chron Respir Dis. 2011;8(2):89–99.
10. Tougaard L, et al. Economic benefits of teaching patients with chronic obstructive pulmonary disease about their illness. The PASTMA Group. Lancet. 1992;339(8808):1517–20.
11. Haggerty MC, Stockdale-Woolley R, Nair S. Respi-Care. An innovative home care program for the patient with chronic obstructive pulmonary disease. Chest. 1991;100(3):607–12.
12. Littlejohns P, et al. Randomised controlled trial of the effectiveness of a respiratory health worker in reducing impairment, disability, and handicap due to chronic airflow limitation. Thorax. 1991;46(8):559–64.
13. Cockcroft A, et al. Controlled trial of respiratory health worker visiting patients with chronic respiratory disability. Br Med J (Clin Res Ed). 1987;294(6566):225–8.
14. Johnston B, et al. Outcomes of the Kaiser Permanente Tele-Home Health Research Project. Arch Fam Med. 2000;9(1):40–5.
15. Farrero E, et al. Impact of a hospital-based home-care program on the management of COPD patients receiving long-term oxygen therapy. Chest. 2001;119(2):364–9.
16. Agha Z, Schapira RM, Maker AH. Cost effectiveness of telemedicine for the delivery of outpatient pulmonary care to a rural population. Telemed J E Health. 2002;8(3):281–91.
17. Hernandez C, et al. Home hospitalisation of exacerbated chronic obstructive pulmonary disease patients. Eur Respir J. 2003;21(1):58–67.
18. Bourbeau J, et al. Reduction of hospital utilization in patients with chronic obstructive pulmonary disease: a disease-specific self-management intervention. Arch Intern Med. 2003;163(5):585–91.
19. Pare G, et al. Cost-minimization analysis of a telehomecare program for patients with chronic obstructive pulmonary disease. Telemed J E Health. 2006;12(2):114–21.
20. Casas A, et al. Integrated care prevents hospitalisations for exacerbations in COPD patients. Eur Respir J. 2006;28(1):123–30.
21. Miyasaka K, et al. Interactive communication in high-technology home care: videophones for pediatric ventilatory care. Pediatrics. 1997;99(1):E1.
22. Vitacca M, et al. Tele-assistance in patients with amyotrophic lateral sclerosis: long term activity and costs. Disabil Rehabil Assist Technol. 2012;7(6):494–500.
23. Vitacca M, et al. A pilot trial of telemedicine-assisted, integrated care for patients with advanced amyotrophic lateral sclerosis and their caregivers. J Telemed Telecare. 2010;16(2):83–8.
24. Zamith M, et al. Home telemonitoring of severe chronic respiratory insufficient and asthmatic patients. Rev Port Pneumol. 2009;15(3):385–417.
25. Bertini S, et al. Telemonitoring in chronic ventilatory failure: a new model of survellaince, a pilot study. Monaldi Arch Chest Dis. 2012;77(2):57–66.
26. Vontetsianos T, et al. Telemedicine-assisted home support for patients with advanced chronic obstructive pulmonary disease: preliminary results after nine-month follow-up. J Telemed Telecare. 2005;11(Suppl 1):86–8.
27. Trappenburg JC, et al. Effects of telemonitoring in patients with chronic obstructive pulmonary disease. Telemed J E Health. 2008;14(2):138–46.
28. Segrelles Calvo G, et al. A home telehealth program for patients with severe COPD: the PROMETE study. Respir Med. 2014;108(3):453–62.
29. Jodar-Sanchez F, et al. Implementation of a telehealth programme for patients with severe chronic obstructive pulmonary disease treated with long-term oxygen therapy. J Telemed Telecare. 2013;19(1):11–7.
30. Maiolo C, et al. Home telemonitoring for patients with severe respiratory illness: the Italian experience. J Telemed Telecare. 2003;9(2):67–71.
31. Moreira J, et al. Compliance with home non-invasive mechanical ventilation in patients with chronic respiratory failure: telemonitoring versus usual care surveillance—a randomized pilot study. Eur Respir J. 2014;44(Suppl 58):447.
32. Pinnock H, et al. Effectiveness of telemonitoring integrated into existing clinical services on hospital admission for exacerbation of chronic obstructive

pulmonary disease: researcher blind, multicentre, randomised controlled trial. BMJ. 2013;347:f6070.
33. Pedone C, et al. Efficacy of multiparametric telemonitoring on respiratory outcomes in elderly people with COPD: a randomized controlled trial. BMC Health Serv Res. 2013;13:82.
34. Vitacca M, et al. Tele-assistance in chronic respiratory failure patients: a randomised clinical trial. Eur Respir J. 2009;33(2):411–8.
35. Cartwright M, et al. Effect of telehealth on quality of life and psychological outcomes over 12 months (Whole Systems Demonstrator telehealth questionnaire study): nested study of patient reported outcomes in a pragmatic, cluster randomised controlled trial. BMJ. 2013;346:f653.
36. Chatwin M, et al. Analysis of home support and ventilator malfunction in 1211 ventilator-dependent patients. Eur Respir J. 2010;35(2):310–6.
37. Chatwin M, et al. Randomised crossover trial of telemonitoring in chronic respiratory patients (TeleCRAFT trial). Thorax. 2016;71(4):305–11.
38. Lloyd-Owen SJ, et al. Patterns of home mechanical ventilation use in Europe: results from the Eurovent survey. Eur Respir J. 2005;25(6):1025–31.
39. King AC. Long-term home mechanical ventilation in the United States. Respir Care. 2012;57(6):921–30. discussion 930-2
40. Rose L, et al. Home mechanical ventilation in Canada: a national survey. Respir Care. 2015;60(5):695–704.
41. Garner DJ, et al. Home mechanical ventilation in Australia and New Zealand. Eur Respir J. 2013;41(1):39–45.
42. Farre R, et al. Performance of mechanical ventilators at the patient's home: a multicentre quality control study. Thorax. 2006;61(5):400–4.
43. Pinto A, et al. Home telemonitoring of non-invasive ventilation decreases healthcare utilisation in a prospective controlled trial of patients with amyotrophic lateral sclerosis. J Neurol Neurosurg Psychiatry. 2010;81(11):1238–42.
44. Hazenberg A, et al. Initiation of home mechanical ventilation at home: a randomised controlled trial of efficacy, feasibility and costs. Respir Med. 2014;108(9):1387–95.
45. Janssens JP, et al. Nocturnal monitoring of home non-invasive ventilation: Contribution of simple tools such as pulse-oximetry, capnography, built-in ventilator software and autonomic markers of sleep fragmentation. Rev Mal Respir. 2014;31(2):107–18.
46. Georges M, et al. Reliability of apnea-hypopnea index measured by a home bi-level pressure support ventilator versus a polysomnographic assessment. Respir Care. 2015;60(7):1051–6.
47. Pasquina P, et al. What does built-in software of home ventilators tell us? An observational study of 150 patients on home ventilation. Respiration. 2012;83(4):293–9.
48. Borel JC, et al. Parameters recorded by software of non-invasive ventilators predict COPD exacerbation: a proof-of-concept study. Thorax. 2015;70(3):284–5.
49. Rabec C, et al. Ventilator modes and settings during non-invasive ventilation: effects on respiratory events and implications for their identification. Thorax. 2011;66(2):170–8.
50. Gonzalez-Bermejo J, et al. Proposal for a systematic analysis of polygraphy or polysomnography for identifying and scoring abnormal events occurring during non-invasive ventilation. Thorax. 2012;67(6):546–52.
51. Berry RB, et al. Rules for scoring respiratory events in sleep: update of the 2007 AASM manual for the scoring of sleep and associated events. Deliberations of the Sleep Apnea Definitions Task Force of the American Academy of Sleep Medicine. J Clin Sleep Med. 2012;8(5):597–619.
52. Isetta V, et al. A Bayesian cost-effectiveness analysis of a telemedicine-based strategy for the management of sleep apnoea: a multicentre randomised controlled trial. Thorax. 2015;70(11):1054–61.
53. Wozniak DR, Lasserson TJ, Smith I. Educational, supportive and behavioural interventions to improve usage of continuous positive airway pressure machines in adults with obstructive sleep apnoea. Cochrane Database Syst Rev. 2014;1:CD007736.
54. Bruyneel M, Ninane V. Unattended home-based polysomnography for sleep disordered breathing: current concepts and perspectives. Sleep Med Rev. 2014;18(4):341–7.
55. Coma-Del-Corral MJ, et al. Reliability of telemedicine in the diagnosis and treatment of sleep apnea syndrome. Telemed J E Health. 2013;19(1):7–12.
56. Isetta V, et al. Telemedicine-based approach for obstructive sleep apnea management: building evidence. Interact J Med Res. 2014;3(1):e6.
57. Dellaca R, et al. Telemetric CPAP titration at home in patients with sleep apnea-hypopnea syndrome. Sleep Med. 2011;12(2):153–7.
58. Taylor Y, et al. The role of telemedicine in CPAP compliance for patients with obstructive sleep apnea syndrome. Sleep Breath. 2006;10(3):132–8.
59. Fox N, et al. The impact of a telemedicine monitoring system on positive airway pressure adherence in patients with obstructive sleep apnea: a randomized controlled trial. Sleep. 2012;35(4):477–81.
60. Sparrow D, et al. A telemedicine intervention to improve adherence to continuous positive airway pressure: a randomised controlled trial. Thorax. 2010;65(12):1061–6.
61. Mendelson M, et al. CPAP treatment supported by telemedicine does not improve blood pressure in high cardiovascular risk OSA patients: a randomized, controlled trial. Sleep. 2014;37(11):1863–70.
62. Fraysse JL, et al. Home telemonitoring of CPAP: a feasibility study. Rev Mal Respir. 2012;29(1):60–3.
63. Mokhlesi B, Tulaimat A. Recent advances in obesity hypoventilation syndrome. Chest. 2007;132(4):1322–36.
64. Benditt JO, Boitano LJ. Pulmonary issues in patients with chronic neuromuscular disease. Am J Respir Crit Care Med. 2013;187(10):1046–55.

65. Hess DR. The growing role of noninvasive ventilation in patients requiring prolonged mechanical ventilation. Respir Care. 2012;57(6):900–18. discussion 918-20
66. Piper AJ. Nocturnal hypoventilation—identifying & treating syndromes. Indian J Med Res. 2010;131:350–65.
67. Piper AJ, Grunstein RR. Big breathing: the complex interaction of obesity, hypoventilation, weight loss, and respiratory function. J Appl Physiol 1985. 2010;108(1):199–205.
68. Kitsiou S, Pare G, Jaana M. Systematic reviews and meta-analyses of home telemonitoring interventions for patients with chronic diseases: a critical assessment of their methodological quality. J Med Internet Res. 2013;15(7):e150.
69. Lujan M, Pomares X. Noninvasive mechanical ventilation. Reflections on home monitoring. Arch Bronconeumol. 2014;50(3):85–6.
70. Wootton R. Twenty years of telemedicine in chronic disease management--an evidence synthesis. J Telemed Telecare. 2012;18(4):211–20.
71. Hall WJ, ACP Journal Club. Telemonitoring did not reduce hospitalizations or ED visits in high-risk elderly patients. Ann Intern Med. 2012;157(6):JC3–8.
72. Spruit MA, et al. Differences in content and organisational aspects of pulmonary rehabilitation programmes. Eur Respir J. 2014;43(5):1326–37.
73. Holland AE, et al. Home-based rehabilitation for COPD using minimal resources: a randomised, controlled equivalence trial. Thorax. 2017;72(1):57–65.
74. Maltais F, et al. Effects of home-based pulmonary rehabilitation in patients with chronic obstructive pulmonary disease: a randomized trial. Ann Intern Med. 2008;149(12):869–78.
75. Stickland M, et al. Using Telehealth technology to deliver pulmonary rehabilitation in chronic obstructive pulmonary disease patients. Canadian Respiratory Journal. 2011;18(4):216–20.
76. Tsai, L.L., et al., Home-based telerehabilitation via real-time videoconferencing improves endurance exercise capacity in patients with COPD: The randomized controlled TeleR Study. Respirology, 2016.
77. Paneroni M, et al. Is telerehabilitation a safe and viable option for patients with COPD? A Feasibility Study. COPD. 2015;12(2):217–25.
78. Tousignant M, et al. In-home telerehabilitation for older persons with chronic obstructive pulmonary disease: a pilot study. International Journal of Telerehabilitation. 2012;4(1):7–13.
79. Burkow TM, et al. Comprehensive pulmonary rehabilitation in home-based online groups: a mixed method pilot study in COPD. BMC Res Notes. 2015;8:766.
80. Marquis N, et al. In-home pulmonary telerehabilitation for patients with chronic obstructive pulmonary disease: a pre-experimental study on effectiveness, satisfaction, and adherence. Telemed J E Health. 2015;21(11):870–9.
81. Tabak M, et al. A telerehabilitation intervention for patients with Chronic Obstructive Pulmonary Disease: a randomized controlled pilot trial. Clinical Rehabilitation. 2013;28(6):582–91.
82. Bernocchi P, et al. A multidisciplinary telehealth program in patients with combined chronic obstructive pulmonary disease and chronic heart failure: study protocol for a randomized controlled trial. Trials. 2016;17(1):462.
83. Holland AE, et al. Telerehabilitation for people with chronic obstructive pulmonary disease: feasibility of a simple, real time model of supervised exercise training. Journal of Telemedicine and Telecare. 2013;19(4):222–6.
84. Hoaas H, et al. Adherence and factors affecting satisfaction in long-term telerehabilitation for patients with chronic obstructive pulmonary disease: a mixed methods study. BMC Med Inform Decis Mak. 2016;16:26.
85. Crotty M, et al. Telerehabilitation for older people using off-the-shelf applications: acceptability and feasibility. J Telemed Telecare. 2014;20(7):370–6.
86. Zanaboni P, et al. Long-term integrated telerehabilitation of COPD Patients: a multicentre randomised controlled trial (iTrain). BMC Pulm Med. 2016;16(1):126.
87. Oh EG. The effects of home-based pulmonary rehabilitation in patients with chronic lung disease. Int J Nurs Stud. 2003;40(8):873–9.
88. Bauer KA. The ethical and social dimensions of home-based telemedicine. Crit Rev Biomed Eng. 2000;28(3–4):541–4.
89. Stanberry B. Legal and ethical aspects of telemedicine. J Telemed Telecare. 2006;12(4):166–75.
90. Brahams D. The medicolegal implications of teleconsulting in the UK. J Telemed Telecare. 1995;1(4):196–201.
91. E-Health and Its Impact on Medical Practice. Position Paper. 2008, Available from American College of Physicians, 190 N. Independence Mall West, Philadelphia, PA 19106.
92. Kaufman DR, et al. Usability in the real world: assessing medical information technologies in patients' homes. J Biomed Inform. 2003;36(1-2):45–60.
93. Doherty ST, Oh P. A multi-sensor monitoring system of human physiology and daily activities. Telemed J E Health. 2012;18(3):185–92.
94. Sevick MA, et al. A confirmatory factor analysis of the Caregiving Appraisal Scale for caregivers of home-based ventilator-assisted individuals. Heart Lung. 1997;26(6):430–8.
95. Fields AI, et al. Home care cost-effectiveness for respiratory technology-dependent children. Am J Dis Child. 1991;145(7):729–33.
96. Geiseler J, et al. Invasive home mechanical ventilation, mainly focused on neuromuscular disorders. GMS Health Technol Assess. 2010;6. Doc08
97. Henderson C, et al. Cost effectiveness of telehealth for patients with long term conditions (Whole

Systems Demonstrator telehealth questionnaire study): nested economic evaluation in a pragmatic, cluster randomised controlled trial. BMJ. 2013;346:f1035.
98. Stoddart A, et al. Telemonitoring for chronic obstructive pulmonary disease: a cost and cost-utility analysis of a randomised controlled trial. J Telemed Telecare. 2015;21(2):108–18.
99. Communication from the commission to the European Parliament, the council, the European economic and social committee and the committee of the regions. eHealth Action Plan. 2012–2020;6(12):2012.
100. Pare G, Jaana M, Sicotte C. Systematic review of home telemonitoring for chronic diseases: the evidence base. J Am Med Inform Assoc. 2007;14(3):269–77.
101. Jaana M, Pare G, Sicotte C. Home telemonitoring for respiratory conditions: a systematic review. Am J Manag Care. 2009;15(5):313–20.
102. Polisena J, et al. Home telehealth for chronic obstructive pulmonary disease: a systematic review and meta-analysis. J Telemed Telecare. 2010;16(3):120–7.
103. Vitacca M. Telemonitoring in patients with chronic respiratory insufficiency: expectations deluded? Thorax. 2016;71(4):299–301.

Part VII

Specific Scenarios

Thoracic Oncology and Surgery 24

Catherine L. Granger and Gill Arbane

24.1 An Overview of Thoracic Oncology

Cancer is a significant contributor to the global burden of disease. It is a disease that results from abnormal cells not being destroyed by normal metabolic processes but instead they proliferate and spread out of control [1]. Thoracic oncology refers to cancers affecting the chest area and includes lung cancer, malignant mesothelioma, mediastinal tumours and carcinoid tumours. This chapter focuses specifically on pulmonary rehabilitation for patients with lung cancer.

Lung cancer is the most common cancer and the leading cause of cancer death worldwide [2]. The most common type of primary lung cancer is non-small cell lung cancer (NSCLC) (88% of cases). This is a carcinoma arising from the epithelial cells of the lung and includes the histological types: adenocarcinoma, squamous cell carcinoma and large cell carcinoma. Small cell lung cancer (SCLC) (12% of cases) is the other more aggressive type of lung cancer [3]. Lung cancer is most commonly caused by smoking (cigarettes, cigars and pipes). Other risk factors include exposure to second-hand smoke; exposure to asbestos, radon, chromium, nickel, arsenic, soot or tar; exposure to air pollution; genetic predisposition; chronic pulmonary inflammation; poor diet; and physical inactivity. The lung carcinogenesis process is likely to result from the interaction of a number of these factors, and if smoking is combined with another risk factor, the risk of lung cancer increases significantly [3]. Due to the poor lifestyle factors (smoking, diet and physical inactivity) associated with the disease aetiology multi-morbidity is common. Approximately 67% of patients with lung cancer have two or more other chronic conditions [4] and COPD is particularly common (40–70%) [5]. Therefore, when delivering pulmonary rehabilitation for patients with lung cancer, assessment and consideration of their past medical history, co-existing chronic diseases, and past and current lifestyle behaviours is important.

C.L. Granger (✉)
Department of Physiotherapy, University of Melbourne, Melbourne, Australia
e-mail: catherine.granger@unimelb.edu.au

G. Arbane
Department PCCP, Guy's and St Thomas' NHS Foundation Trust, London, UK

24.1.1 Medical Treatment of Lung Cancer and Side-Effects

Treatment options for lung cancer include thoracic surgery, chemotherapy, radiotherapy or targeted therapy [3, 6]. The type of treatment combination depends on a number of factors including the tumour(s) location, stage of disease (size and spread), and the patient's degree of frailty which influences their ability to tolerate the treatment(s). Each treatment is associated with side-effects which add to the overall disease burden and impacts on the patient's ability to be

© Springer International Publishing AG 2018
E. Clini et al. (eds.), *Textbook of Pulmonary Rehabilitation*,
https://doi.org/10.1007/978-3-319-65888-9_24

Table 24.1 Treatment side-effects

Treatment	Side-effects
Surgery	Pain Reduced mobility Cough Dyspnoea Fatigue
Chemotherapy	Fatigue Nausea Infection (immunosuppression) Anaemia Vomiting Diarrhoea Constipation Loss of appetite Hair loss Mouth ulcers Weight gain or weight loss
Radiotherapy	Fatigue Cough Rigours Skin erythema Oesophagitis Nausea Vomiting Diarrhoea Loss of appetite Hair loss Flu-like symptoms
Molecular targeted therapies	Fatigue Nausea Vomiting Loss of appetite Diarrhoea Constipation Skin and hair changes

physically active. These are outlined briefly below and summarised in Table 24.1.

24.1.1.1 Surgery

Surgery is the preferred treatment for patients with early stage NSCLC (stage I, II and IIIA) [3, 6] and is associated with the best chance of cure. After surgery, depending on the stage of disease, patients may also receive post-operative chemotherapy or radiotherapy. The thoracic surgery is performed either via a thoracotomy (open chest surgery) or video assisted thoracoscopic surgery (VATS). The following lung resection procedures can be used:

- *Wedge resection*—removal of a small wedge shaped portion of the lung
- *Segment resection*—removal of a larger portion of the lobe than in a wedge resection
- *Lobectomy*—removal of one lobe of the lung
- *Sleeve lobectomy*—removal a cancerous lobe and the bronchus attached to it. The remaining lobe is connected to the remaining bronchus.
- *Pneumonectomy*—removal of one entire lung. This procedure is used if the cancer cannot be removed effectively by removing a wedge, segment or lobe.

To be considered for surgery patients require sufficient cardiopulmonary fitness (to withstand the procedure and loss of lung segments). Generally, patients with peak oxygen consumption (VO_2peak) of less than 10ml/kg/min are considered inoperable and will be offered chemotherapy and or radiotherapy instead of surgery [7]. Small pilot studies suggest pulmonary rehabilitation may be beneficial in improving VO_2peak in these at risk patients in attempt to move them into the fit for surgery category [8]. However, this is not routine clinical practice currently and further definitive research needs to be conducted before this specific indication of pulmonary rehabilitation is understood (see Sect. 24.4.2).

Prevention of post-operative pulmonary complications (PPCs) after thoracic surgery is important. These occur in approximately 4–15% of patients following a thoracotomy and approximately 2% in patients following VATS [9–12]. Complications include respiratory failure (such as prolonged mechanical ventilation, re-intubation or acute respiratory distress syndrome), pneumonia, atelectasis requiring bronchoscopy, myocardial infarction and arrhythmias [13]. The independent risk factors for PPCs after thoracic surgery are older age (≥75 years), higher body mass index (>30 kg/m^2), diagnosis of COPD, and being a current smoker [9, 10]. There is evidence to suggest pulmonary rehabilitation before surgery in people scheduled for surgery can reduce their risk of PPCs [8] (see Sect. 24.4.2).

Lung resection results in an immediate reduction in VO_2peak by 12% following a lobectomy and 18% following pneumonectomy [14]. In most patients following a lobectomy exercise capacity recovers to baseline by 6 months [15, 16], but this is not the case following a pneumonectomy with 20% loss still evident 6 months post-op [15]. Pulmonary function is not a good predictor of changes in post-operative exercise capacity [15]. Reduction in physical activity levels post-surgery is also common and sustained at 6 months [16]. Other common side-effects include post-operative pain and reduced shoulder range of motion (Table 24.1). These impairments can be targeted with post-operative pulmonary rehabilitation (see Sect. 24.4.3).

24.1.1.2 Chemotherapy

Chemotherapy, also known as adjuvant therapy, uses anti-cancer (cytotoxic) drugs to destroy cancer cells by disrupting their growth. This is delivered to the patient via an injection into a vein, through a drip, or via a tablet. Commonly used chemotherapeutic agents for NSCLC are alkylating agents' cisplatin and carboplatin. Chemotherapy is usually delivered with four to six treatments, separated by 3–4 weeks, over a period of 3–6 months. Chemotherapy is commonly used in the following circumstances:

- Post-surgery in stage IB-IIIA NSCLC (with or without concurrent radiotherapy) [6]. In this case chemotherapy is usually started within 8 weeks of surgery.
- Locally advanced NSCLC (i.e. the cancer has spread beyond the lung into lymph nodes or tissues surrounding the lung). In this case chemotherapy can slow the growth and/or shrink the metastatic NSCLC.
- Small cell lung cancer

Cytotoxic drugs result in side-effects from the damage caused to normal cells (Table 24.1). Two important side-effects to screen for and consider in pulmonary rehabilitation are immunosuppression (increased infection risk) and anaemia. Immunosuppression occurs due to bone marrow suppression where the white blood cell count is lowest about 2 weeks following treatment. Therefore, infection control measures are especially important for patients participating in pulmonary rehabilitation during or up to a month following chemotherapy. Anaemia is another important side-effect to screen for in patient assessment. The reduced haemoglobin levels impair the body's oxygen delivering capacity and consequently the patient may experience increased levels of fatigue and poorer exercise tolerance. Exercise should be avoided if the haemoglobin levels are <80 grams/litre (Table 24.2).

24.1.1.3 Radiotherapy

Radiotherapy uses high energy rays to kill cancerous cells. There are two main types of radiotherapy: internal and external radiotherapy. Internal radiotherapy (known as brachytherapy or endobronchial therapy) is given to the patient during a bronchoscopy and is used to shrink a tumour that may be blocking airways. External radiotherapy, the more common form, is a treatment given where radiation is aimed at the tumour in the lung from an external machine. The treatment dosage depends on the intent of the therapy and stage of disease:

- Radical therapy (for curative intent): 20–36 treatments in total, 5 days per week, for 4–7 weeks
- Continuous hyperfractionated accelerated radiotherapy (CHART): three treatments per day for 12 days
- Palliation (for symptom control): one or two treatments a week apart, or daily for up to 3 weeks

A number of side-effects occur due to the damage of surrounding normal tissue. Areas with normal rapidly dividing cells, such as the oesophageal mucosa, are particularly susceptible. The widespread inflammatory response and release of cytokines also cause systemic side-effects (Table 24.1) which typically last for 4–6 weeks.

In 2009 the European Respiratory Society set up a task force to create guidelines for fitness for radical therapy in patients with lung cancer. They identified the need for patients to be fit enough to undertake radiotherapy or chemotherapy; however, they were unable to recommend any specific test, cut-off value, or algorithm before radio-chemotherapy due to the lack of data. They recommended management of these patients in specialised settings by multidisciplinary teams.

Table 24.2 Contraindications and precautions to pulmonary rehabilitation in lung cancer. Adapted from [8]

Exercise	Condition	Action
All	Extreme fatigue	Avoid exercise
	Severe nausea	Avoid exercise
	Temperature > 38 °C	Avoid exercise
	Haemoglobin level < 80 g/L	Avoid exercise
	Platelet count < 50 × 10^9/μL	Avoid exercise
	Neutrophil count ≤0.5 × 10^9/μL	Avoid exercise
	Lymphedema (upper or lower limb)	Wear compression garment during exercise
Aerobic	Severe cancer cachexia or muscle atrophy	Commence with resistance training and then progress to incorporate aerobic training once muscle bulk and strength is improved
Resistance	Known or high risk for bone metastases	Prescribe with caution (recommend medical clearance before commencement particularly for unstable bone or spinal metastases/fractures)
	High risk for osteoporosis	Prescribe with caution
	High risk for bone fracture	Prescribe with caution
	Cardiorespiratory limitation such as chemotherapy-induced left ventricular dysfunction or severe anaemia	Generally contra-indicated (recommend medical clearance before commencement)
	Post-operative patients	Care with wound healing—often require 6–8 weeks post-operatively for healing prior to commencement of resistance exercises (recommend medical clearance before commencement post-operative)
Stretches	Post-operative patients	Avoid upper-limb stretches until removal of inter-costal catheter (chest drain)

24.1.2 Symptoms

Symptoms vary over the disease trajectory in lung cancer. In early stage disease the most common symptoms are fatigue, pain, cough, loss of appetite and insomnia; and in advanced disease the most common symptoms are pain, dyspnoea and anorexia [17]. The symptom profile is often unique to the individual patient depending on the timing relative to their diagnosis/treatments and other multimorbidities [17, 18]. The most frequent 'cluster' of symptom combinations is fatigue, dyspnoea and cough [18]. However, the symptoms which cause the highest patient distress and interference with activities of daily living are fatigue, pain and dyspnoea [19–21]. Physical activity is often viewed by patients as a trigger for their symptoms and avoidance of physical activity promotes a vicious cycle of lack of activity and deconditioning [22]. An important part of patient education in pulmonary rehabilitation is the message that exercise will not make symptoms worse but in fact the evidence shows that exercise is often associated with a reduction in cancer symptoms including fatigue [23, 24].

24.1.3 Physical and Physiological Impairments

Patients with lung cancer can have a number of physical and psychological impairments. These include:

- Poor exercise capacity
- Peripheral muscle weakness
- Poor respiratory function
- Reduced shoulder range of motion (post-surgery)
- Low physical activity levels
- Poor nutrition
- Anxiety
- Depression
- Distress
- Poor health-related quality of life

Many of these impairments are already present at the time of diagnosis and continue to worsen over the trajectory of the disease. Patients with lung cancer are particularly at risk for low physical activity levels. At time of diagnosis less than 40% of patients meet the physical activity guidelines for older adults [22, 25, 26] and following diagnosis and treatment, activity levels reduce further [22, 26]. Preventing the cycle of avoidance of physical activity after diagnosis and empowering the patient to lead an active lifestyle are important targets of pulmonary rehabilitation. Functional decline after diagnosis is also rapid and patients can lose up to 20% of their baseline exercise capacity (6-min walk test at diagnosis) over the first 6 months from diagnosis especially in those with inoperable disease [16, 22]. Assessment of the patient's impairments and individualised exercise prescription to target these is important, because many of these impairments are responsive to pulmonary rehabilitation [27–30].

Cancer cachexia is "a multi-factorial syndrome defined by an ongoing loss of skeletal muscle mass (with or without loss of fat mass) that cannot be fully reversed by conventional nutritional support and leads to progressive functional impairment" [31]. This is common in lung cancer and contributes to the clinical pattern of malnutrition, muscle wasting, weight loss and decline in muscle strength. Exercise limitation is commonly due to skeletal muscle dysfunction in lung cancer [32, 33] and declining muscle strength is problematic.

24.2 The Role of Physical Activity in Cancer

24.2.1 Cancer Prevention

For cancer prevention, the American Cancer Society [34] recommend adults:

- Maintain a physically active lifestyle (≥150 min of moderate intensity or 75 min of vigorous intensity physical activity per week)
- Avoid smoking and second-hand smoke exposure
- Maintain a healthy weight
- Consume a healthy diet

These recommendations are supported by evidence demonstrating that physical activity is an independent risk factor for the development of colon, pancreatic, endometrial and prostate cancer [35]. There is up to a 40-50% risk reduction for colorectal cancer and 30-40% risk reduction for breast cancer with increased physical activity [36]. Increased sedentary time is also an independent risk factor for cancer (independent to moderate and vigorous physical activity) [37]. For lung cancer prevention there is a small amount of evidence linking increased physical activity with reduced risk but study results are conflicting.

24.2.1.1 Cancer Management

There is a vast body of evidence demonstrating the powerful effects of physical activity and exercise training to prevent and treat cancer morbidity [23, 24]. The American Cancer Society recommend adults with cancer undertake:

- ≥150 min of moderate intensity physical activity per week
- Two to three resistance training sessions per week
- Avoid sedentary time [23, 24]

Historically the advice provided to patients with cancer was to 'rest' and avoid physical activity; however this advice is no longer appropriate due to the compelling evidence supporting the safety and efficacy of physical activity and exercise training in cancer. Expected outcomes include improved exercise capacity, cancer symptoms (including fatigue) and health-related quality of life [23, 24]. The majority of evidence comes from trials in breast, colon or prostate cancer. Fewer trials have been conducted in lung cancer, yet the findings are similar (see Sect. 24.4). Exercise after cancer diagnosis (breast, colon and prostrate) may also be associated with reduced cancer-specific and all-cause mortality [38, 39]. Despite the evidence supporting physical activity and exercise training for people with cancer, evidence has not translated effectively into practice, and there has not been routine integration of exercise/cancer rehabilitation programmes for patients in most parts of the world.

The evidence supporting the safety, feasibility and efficacy of exercise training for patients with lung cancer is much newer, but has developed rapidly [8, 29, 30, 40]. The role of pulmonary rehabilitation is to prevent deterioration and to maximise or restore physical status prior to, during and following lung cancer treatment. The majority of research has been focused on operable NSCLC (pre or post-surgery), but there is growing evidence focused on exercise during chemotherapy or radiotherapy and for patients with advanced/palliative disease [8, 30]. The timing of exercise delivery relative to treatment is discussed in Sect. 24.4.

24.3 Patient Assessment in Pulmonary Rehabilitation

Patients with lung cancer should receive the usual pulmonary rehabilitation patient assessment (as described in Part 3 of this Textbook). The same physical tests can be used as in other respiratory diseases, and many of these are specifically validated for use in lung cancer [41]. For questionnaire-based assessment there are a number of cancer-specific questionnaires which can be used instead of other generic or respiratory questionnaires. These include the European Organisation for the Research and Treatment of Cancer core questionnaire and lung cancer ((EORTC-QLQ-C30 and LC13) supplementary module, and the Functional Assessment of Cancer Therapy core questionnaire and lung cancer supplementary module (FACT); both assess HRQoL and lung cancer symptoms and have been used to evaluate efficacy of exercise programmes in lung cancer [30].

In addition to the usual patient assessment, there are a number of additional aspects to include in the assessment of a patient with lung cancer before commencing pulmonary rehabilitation. These include:

- Type and severity of cancer symptoms (see Table 24.2)
- Type of medical treatment(s) planned and or received
- Treatment side-effects or complications (see Table 24.2)
- Wound healing (surgical patients)
- Shoulder range of motion on operated side (surgical patients)
- Presence of cancer metastases (see Table 24.2)
- Patient goals—this is especially important if prognosis is poor such as in stage IV disease
- Psychological distress (can use the Distress Thermometer for assessment)
- Screening for other exercise precautions or contraindications (Table 24.2).

Patients who have undergone chemotherapy or radiotherapy, or have advanced disease, should be screened for peripheral neuropathies, cardiac conditions, bone fractures, muscle atrophy and severe cancer cachexia; and the identification of any of these conditions warrants medical clearance prior to commencing exercise (Table 24.2). Before each training session patients should be briefly assessed for symptom severity as this can fluctuate on a daily basis. In the presence of extreme fatigue exercise should be delayed (Table 24.2).

24.4 Pulmonary Rehabilitation in Lung Cancer

24.4.1 Exercise Prescription

The prescription of exercise in pulmonary rehabilitation for patients with lung cancer is the same as for other respiratory populations receiving pulmonary rehabilitation such as COPD. The programmes tested in the studies to date predominately involve aerobic and resistance exercises and are delivered as a supervised outpatient training programme [27–30]. Given the paucity of research published comparing different exercise prescription or training modalities in lung cancer, at present the usual pulmonary rehabilitation programme is recommended in lung cancer:

- 30 min of moderate intensity aerobic exercise, can be made up of bouts of 10 min, use of the BORG scale to determine and monitor intensity, exercises include: treadmill, stationary cycle, walking, climbing stairs or stepping machine
- Upper and lower limb resistance exercises, can be performed using body weight, free weights, elastic-bands or weight machines
- Whole body stretches following exercise, especially upper body

However, individualisation of prescription is important and programmes can be adapted as needed based on the patients' baseline level of fitness, contraindications to exercises, current symptoms, and goals/preference. Due to symptoms, the incorporation of a rest day is important, particularly between days of resistance training. Educating patients about rest and energy conservation is also important in those experiencing fatigue.

To date the pulmonary rehabilitation programmes have been tested in three stages: before surgery, after surgery, and advanced disease (+/- during chemotherapy or radiotherapy) (Fig. 24.1). The delivery of pulmonary rehabilitation during these discrete time points is discussed in the following sections.

24.4.2 Prehabilitation

Prehabilitation in lung cancer refers to the delivery of exercise training prior to thoracic surgery (Fig. 24.1) [27]. Prehabilitation is not part of usual care in most hospitals, however it is a rapidly developing area of research. Prehabilitation can be used for patients scheduled for surgery to maximise their fitness before going through surgery, or for patients deemed inoperable (due to insufficient cardiorespiratory fitness) in attempt to increase their fitness levels to become eligible for surgery. Given surgery is the best chance for cure in lung cancer, the later indication may have potential survival benefits although research in this area is minimal (the current RCTs do not have long-term outcomes) and such outcomes are yet to be shown [8].

There is growing evidence from randomised controlled trials which have tested prehabilitation compared to usual care (no exercise programme before surgery) for patients scheduled to undergo lung resection. Despite the number of randomised controlled trials being small, the results to date are promising. Results suggest that prehabilitation is associated with reduced PPCs, reduced duration of chest tube post-operatively, reduced hospital length of stay, and improved exercise capacity immediately following prehabilitation [8]. There is currently minimal or no evidence to suggest prehabilitation improves lung function, fatigue or dyspnoea compared to usual care from randomised controlled trials [8]. Studies lack longer term follow-up measures and therefore the impact on long-term outcomes including survival is unknown.

The exercise programmes delivered as part of prehabilitation are short (1–4 weeks) to fit within the time between diagnosis and surgery. It is currently not recommended to delay surgery in order to be able to deliver prehabilitation in someone already fit for surgery. The programmes tested generally run five times per week in a supervised outpatient setting [8]. All studies conducted to date include aerobic training and over half of the studies also include resistance training. Whilst prehabilitation is safe and beneficial, in some countries and settings it may not be feasible due to the short time frame available before surgery. This issue may challenge the adoption of prehabilitation into routine clinical practice.

24.4.3 Pulmonary Rehabilitation After Curative Intent Treatment

Pulmonary rehabilitation delivered after curative intent treatment (surgery, chemotherapy and or radiotherapy) (Fig. 24.1) aims to improve or restore impairments associated with the disease and treatment, in particular exercise capacity and muscle strength which are markedly reduced in the short term [22]. Pulmonary rehabilitation at this time point also aims to promote a healthy lifestyle as the patient emerges into the survivorship phase by maximising their physical function, reducing symptoms and improving HRQoL. There are a number of systematic reviews and a Cochrane review summarising evidence in this area [29, 30, 40]. Overall exercise post-surgery, chemotherapy and or radiotherapy with curative intent is effective at improving exercise capacity, muscle strength (if resistance exercise is undertaken), muscle mass, and reducing symptoms including anxiety and depression. However, there is conflicting evidence as to whether exercise at this time point improves HRQoL or lung function.

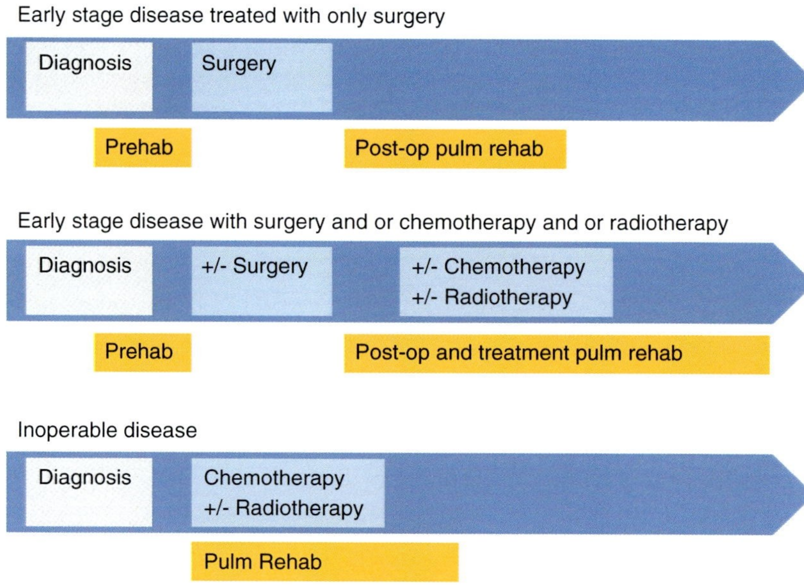

Fig. 24.1 Timing options of pulmonary rehabilitation relative to treatment in lung cancer. Abbreviations: *op* operation, *prehab* prehabilitation, *pulm* pulmonary, *rehab* rehabilitation

The exercise programmes utilised in the studies to date are longer in duration (3–20 weeks) (more similar to traditional pulmonary rehabilitation programmes in COPD), given they are not confined by the time pre-treatment. The timing of commencement of exercise varies. Some programmes start on the first day after surgery whilst the patient is still hospitalised and then continue once they discharge home [42, 43] whereas other programmes wait 1–3 months (whilst the patient recovers naturally) before commencing [30]. There is no clear evidence to suggest when is the best time to start exercise, although delaying exercise commencement much beyond 3 months risks a prolonged time in which the patient may be sedentary (and deconditioning) after the insult of treatment. There have been a number of different exercise programmes used with good effect and the most common being combined moderate intensity aerobic exercise with or without resistance training. High-intensity endurance training is also an option and has been shown in a recent randomised controlled trial to be safe and effective when commenced 5–7 weeks post-surgery [44]. Whilst the majority of RCTs have implemented outpatient exercise programmes, there are a number of earlier single group studies which successfully testing inpatient rehabilitation programmes [45, 46], however, the reality of an 8-week inpatient programme may not be feasible with many health care providers. It is unknown if inpatient pulmonary rehabilitation is more or less effective than outpatient rehabilitation in lung cancer at present, and therefore the recommendation is for patients to access pulmonary rehabilitation in any form and time that is available.

24.4.4 Exercise in Advanced Disease

Pulmonary rehabilitation for patients during treatment and or with advanced disease aims to minimise physical deterioration and maximise functional independence and HRQoL (Fig. 24.1). There is less relative research conducted in this area compared to patients with early stage disease; however it is an area being actively investigated at present with many randomised controlled trials in progress. It appears pulmonary rehabilitation at this time point is associated with either improved or maintained exercise capacity, physical function, muscle strength, symptoms and HRQoL [47–52]. Given functional decline is rapid and problematic in advanced disease, maintenance of patient outcomes is a positive outcome. The studies conducted to date include patients with advanced lung cancer undergoing treatment (chemotherapy, radiotherapy and or targeted therapy) and have found exercise to be safe.

Similar to the other time points, the exercise programmes tested to date are combined aerobic and resistance exercise delivered in either outpatient [48, 51, 52], inpatient [47, 53], or both in- and outpatient settings [49, 50]. One issue with pulmonary rehabilitation in the setting of advanced lung cancer is the poorer adherence and completion rates of programmes. It is important to consider that patients with stage IV disease have poor prognosis (17% and 22% 1-year survival in males and females, respectively) [54] and therefore where pulmonary rehabilitation fits within the patient's priorities is an important consideration. Whilst there is growing evidence supporting the efficacy of pulmonary rehabilitation to improve many patient outcomes, whether or not it improves survival in lung cancer (at any stage) is currently unknown. The majority of the studies conducted to date do not have long-term follow-up and until further research is conducting it is unclear if pulmonary rehabilitation has a survival benefit in lung cancer. The studies incorporating supervised hospital (in or outpatient) training report the highest adherence rates in this patient group [49–52] compared to unsupervised home training [50]. The feasibility and efficacy of home-based training and the potential use of telerehabilitation warrants further investigation and may be a great asset to delivery of pulmonary rehabilitation for this patient group.

Conclusion

Pulmonary rehabilitation is an important aspect in the management of lung cancer. Preventing or minimising the cycle of inactivity and functional decline after lung cancer diagnosis with pulmonary rehabilitation is important. Patients with lung cancer experience symptoms and physical and psychological impairments such as fatigue, exercise intolerance, muscle weakness and inactivity, which are responsive to pulmonary rehabilitation. Pulmonary rehabilitation can be safely and effectively delivered before surgery, during treatment (chemotherapy, radiotherapy or targeted therapy) or after treatment. Patients with lung cancer have a number of specific precautions and contraindications to exercise which should be screened for in the patient assessment before commencing. Pulmonary rehabilitation in lung cancer is a rapidly evolving area of research and hopefully with the generation of further research in the next decade access to pulmonary rehabilitation will become more routine practice.

References

1. Australian Institute of Health and Welfare & Australasian Association of Cancer Registries. (2012). Cancer in Australia: an overview 2012. Cancer series no. 74. Cat. no. CAN 70. Canberra: AIHW.
2. Ervik, M., Lam, F., Ferlay, J., Mery, L., Soerjomataram, I., & Bray, F. (2016). Cancer today. Lyon, France: International Agency for Research on Cancer. Cancer Today. Available from: http://gco.iarc.fr/today, accessed [27/09/2016].
3. NICE. (2011). National Institute for Health and Clinical Excellence Clinical Guidelines, CG 121 Lung cancer: The diagnosis and treatment of lung cancer.
4. Smith A, Reeve B, Bellizzi K, Harlan L, Klabunde C, Amsellem M, et al. Cancer, comorbidities, and health-related quality of life of older adults. Health Care Financ Rev. 2008;24(9):41–56.
5. Dela Cruz C, Tanoue L, Matthay R. Lung cancer: epidemiology, etiology, and prevention. Clin Chest Med. 2011;32(4):605–44.
6. NCCN. (2012). NCCN Clinical Practice Guidelines in Oncology (NCCN Guidelines): Non-small Cell Lung Cancer. National Comprehensive Cancer Network, Version 3; 2012.
7. Loewen G, Watson D, Kohman L, Herndon J, Shennib H, Kernstine K, et al. Preoperative exercise Vo2 measurement for lung resection candidates: results of cancer and leukemia group B protocol 9238. J Thorac Oncol. 2007;2(7):619–25.
8. Granger C. Physiotherapy management of lung cancer. J Physiother. 2016;62(2):60–7.
9. Agostini P, Cieslik H, Rathinam S, Bishay E, Kalkat M, Rajesh P, et al. Postoperative pulmonary complications following thoracic surgery: are there any modifiable risk factors? Thorax. 2010;65:815–8.
10. Lugg S, Agostini P, Tikka T, Kerr A, Adams K, Bishay E, et al. Long-term impact of developing a postoperative pulmonary complication after lung surgery. Thorax. 2016;71(2):171–6.
11. McKenna R, Houck W, Fuller C. Video-assisted thoracic surgery lobectomy: experience with 1100 cases. Ann Thorac Surg. 2006;81(2):425–6.

12. Reeve J, Nicol K, Stiller K, McPherson K, Birch P, Gordon I, Denehy L. Does physiotherapy reduce the incidence of postoperative pulmonary complications following pulmonary resection via open thoracotomy? A preliminary randomised single-blind clinical trial. Eur J Cardiothorac Surg. 2010;37(5):1158–66.
13. Benzo R, Kelley G, Recchi L, Hofman A, Sciurba F. Complications of lung resection and exercise capacity: a meta-analysis. Respir Med. 2007;101(8):1790–77.
14. Brunelli A, Belardinelli R, Refai M, Salati M, Socci L, Pompili C, Sabbatini A. Peak oxygen consumption during cardiopulmonary exercise test improves risk stratification in candidates to major lung resection. Chest. 2009;135(5):1260–7.
15. Bolliger C, Jordan P, Soler M, Stulz P, Tamm C, Wyser M, et al. Pulmonary function and exercise capacity after lung resection. Eur Respir J. 1996;9:415–21.
16. Granger C, Parry S, Edbrooke L, Denehy L. Deterioration in physical activity and function differs according to treatment type in non-small cell lung cancer - future directions for physiotherapy management. Physiotherapy. 2016;102(3):256–63.
17. Cooley M. Symptoms in adults with lung cancer. A systematic research review. J Pain Symptom Manage. 2000;19(2):137–53.
18. Cheville A, Novotny P, Sloan J, Basford J, Wampfler J, Garces Y, et al. The value of a symptom cluster of fatigue, dyspnea, and cough in predicting clinical outcomes in lung cancer survivors. J Pain Symptom Manage. 2011;42(2):213–21.
19. Degner L, Sloan J. Symptom distress in newly diagnosed ambulatory care patients and as a predictor of survival in lung cancer. J Pain Symptom Manage. 1995;10(6):423–31.
20. Tanaka K, Akechi T, Okuyama T, Nishiwaki Y, Uchitomi Y. Impact of dyspnea, pain, and fatigue on daily life activities in ambulatory patients with advanced lung cancer. J Pain Symptom Manage. 2002;23(5):417–23.
21. Tishelman C, Petersson LM, Degner LF, Sprangers MA. Symptom prevalence, intensity, and distress in patients with inoperable lung cancer in relation to time of death. J Clin Oncol. 2007;25(34):5281–9.
22. Granger C, McDonald C, Irving L, Clark R, Gough K, Murnane A, et al. Low physical activity levels and functional decline in individuals with lung cancer. Lung Cancer. 2014;83(2):292–9.
23. Rock C, Doyle C, Demark-Wahnefried W, Meyerhardt J, Courneya K, Schwartz A, et al. Nutrition and physical activity guidelines for cancer survivors. CA: Cancer J Clin. 2013;62(4):242–74.
24. Schmitz K, Courneya K, Matthews C, Demark-Wahnefried W, Galvao D, Pinto B, et al. ACSM roundtable on exercise guidelines for cancer survivors. Med Sci Sports Exerc. 2010;42(7):1409–26.
25. Coups E, Park B, Feinstein M, Steingart R, Egleston B, Wilson D, Ostroff J. Physical activity among lung cancer survivors: changes across the cancer trajectory and associations with quality of life. Cancer Epidemiol Biomarkers Prev. 2009;18(2):664–72.
26. Novoa N, Varela G, Jimenez M, Aranda J. Influence of major pulmonary resection on postoperative daily ambulatory activity of the patients. Interact Cardiovasc Thorac Surg. 2009;9(6):934–8.
27. Cavalheri, V., & Granger, C. (2015). Preoperative exercise training for patients with non-small cell lung cancer. Cochrane Database Syst Rev (7).
28. Cavalheri, V., Tahirah, F., Nonoyama, M., Sue Jenkins, S., & Hill, K. (2013). Exercise training for people following lung resection for non-small cell lung cancer. Cochrane Database Syst Rev (7), Art. No.: CD009955.
29. Crandall K, Roma Maguire R, Campbell A, Kearney N. Exercise intervention for patients surgically treated for Non-Small Cell Lung Cancer (NSCLC): a systematic review. Surg Oncol. 2014;23(1):17–30.
30. Granger C, McDonald C, Berney S, Chao C, Denehy L. Exercise intervention to improve exercise capacity and health related quality of life for patients with Non-small cell lung cancer: a systematic review. Lung Cancer. 2011;72(2):139–53.
31. Blum D, Omlin A, Baracos V, Solheim T, Tan B, Stone P, et al. Cancer cachexia: a systematic literature review of items and domains associated with involuntary weight loss in cancer. Crit Rev Oncol Hematol. 2011;80(1):114–44.
32. Morice R, Peters E, Ryan M, Putnam J, Ali M, Roth J. Exercise testing in the evaluation of patients at high risk for complications from lung resection. Chest. 1992;101(2):356–61.
33. Nezu K, Kushibe K, Tojo T, Takahama M, Kitamura S. Recovery and limitation of exercise capacity after lung resection for lung cancer. Chest. 1998;113(6):1511–6.
34. American Cancer Society. Cancer prevention & early detection facts & figures 2012. Atlanta: American Cancer Society Website; 2012.
35. World Health Organization. Global recommendations on physical activity for health. Geneva: World Health Organization; 2010. p. 1–58. ISBN: 9789241599979
36. Friedenreich C. Physical activity and cancer prevention: from observational to intervention research. Cancer Epidemiol Biomarkers Prev. 2001;10(4):287–301.
37. Biswas A, Oh P, Faulkner G, Bajaj R, Silver M, Mitchell M, Alter D. Sedentary time and its association with risk for disease incidence, mortality, and hospitalization in adults: a systematic review and meta-analysis. Ann Intern Med. 2015;162(2):123–32.
38. Ballard-Barbash R, Friedenreich C, Courneya K, Siddiqi S, McTiernan A, Alfano C. Physical activity, biomarkers, and disease outcomes in cancer survivors: a systematic review. J Natl Cancer Inst. 2012;104(11):815–40.
39. Lee I, Wolin K, Freeman S, Sattlemair J, Sesso H. Physical activity and survival after cancer diagnosis in men. J Phys Act Health. 2014;11(1):85–90.
40. Cavalheri V, Tahirah F, Nonoyama M, Jenkins S, Hill K. Exercise training undertaken by people within

12 months of lung resection for non-small cell lung cancer. Cochrane Database Syst Rev. 2015;7
41. Granger C, Denehy L, Parry S, Oliveira C, McDonald C. Functional capacity, physical activity and muscle strength of individuals with non-small cell lung cancer: a systematic review of outcome measures and their measurement properties. BMC Cancer. 2012;13(135)
42. Arbane G, Tropman D, Jackson D, Garrod R. Evaluation of an early exercise intervention after thoracotomy for non-small cell lung cancer: effects on quality of life, muscle strength and exercise tolerance: Randomised controlled trial. Lung Cancer. 2011;71(2):229–34.
43. Granger C, Chao C, McDonald C, Berney S, Denehy L. Safety and feasibility of an exercise intervention for patients following lung resection: a pilot randomized controlled trial. Integr Cancer Ther. 2013;12(3):213–24.
44. Edvardsen E, Skjonsberg O, Holme I, Nordsletten L, Borchsenius F, Anderssen S. High-intensity training following lung cancer surgery: a randomised controlled trial. Thorax. 2015;70(3):244–50.
45. Cesario A, Ferri L, Galetta D, Pasqua F, Bonassi S, Clini E, et al. Post-operative respiratory rehabilitation after lung resection for non-small cell lung cancer. Lung Cancer. 2007;57(2):175–80.
46. Spruit M, Janssen P, Willemsen S, Hochstenbag M, Wouters E. Exercise capacity before and after an 8-week multidisciplinary inpatient rehabilitation program in lung cancer patients: a pilot study. Lung Cancer. 2006;52(2):257–60.
47. Henke C, Cabri J, Fricke L, Pankow W, Kandilakis G, Feyer P, de Wit M. Strength and endurance training in the treatment of lung cancer patients in stages IIIA/IIIB/IV. Support Care Cancer. 2014;22(1):95–101.
48. Hwang C, Yu C, Shih J, Yang P, Wu Y. Effects of exercise training on exercise capacity in patients with non-small cell lung cancer receiving targeted therapy. Support Care Cancer. 2012;20(12):3169–77.
49. Kuehr L, Wiskemann J, Abel U, Ulrich C, Hummler S, Thomas M. Exercise in patients with non-small cell lung cancer. Med Sci Sports Exerc. 2014;46(4):656–63.
50. Quist M, Rorth M, Langer S, Jones LW, Laursen JH, Pappot H, et al. Safety and feasibility of a combined exercise intervention for inoperable lung cancer patients undergoing chemotherapy: A pilot study. Lung Cancer. 2012;75(2):203–8.
51. Quist M, Adamsen L, Rorth M, Laursen J, Christensen K, Langer S. The impact of a multidimensional exercise intervention on physical and functional capacity, anxiety, and depression in patients with advanced-stage lung cancer undergoing chemotherapy. Integr Cancer Ther. 2015;14(4):341–9.
52. Temel J, Greer J, Goldberg S, Vogel P, Sullivan M, Pirl W, et al. A structured exercise program for patients with advanced non-small cell lung cancer. J Thorac Oncol. 2009;4(5):595–601.
53. Jastrzębski D, Maksymiak M, Kostorz S, Bezubka B, Osmanska I, Młynczak T, et al. Pulmonary rehabilitation in advanced lung cancer patients during chemotherapy. Adv Exp Med Biol. 2015;861:57–64.
54. National Cancer Intelligence Network. Cancer survival in England by stage 2012. London: NCIN; 2014.

25 Transplantation

Rainer Gloeckl, Tessa Schneeberger, Inga Jarosch, and Klaus Kenn

25.1 Pulmonary Rehabilitation Prior to Lung Transplantation (LTx)

Pulmonary rehabilitation (PR) plays a key role in disease management of patients before and following LTx and is recommended as a component of care in the current statement on PR by the *American Thoracic Society/European Respiratory Society* (ATS/ERS) [1]. PR is recognized to improve exercise tolerance, symptoms, and health-related quality of life in patients with chronic obstructive pulmonary disease (COPD) and also other forms of severe chronic respiratory diseases such as interstitial lung disease, cystic fibrosis, and pulmonary hypertension. Beside these aims of general PR programs, pre-LTx PR is meant to additionally prepare patients for surgery, to give information about risks after LTx and to identify patients who may be poor candidates for LTx [2]. The benefit of PR in LTx candidates was observed to be independent of the kind of chronic respiratory disease, age, sex, body mass index, 6-min walk distance (6MWD), and health-related quality of life level [3]. Thus, this treatment option should be considered for all patients with chronic respiratory diseases who are on the waiting list for LTx or in evaluation for LTx.

A multidisciplinary pre LTx PR program should focus on optimizing or maintaining the functional status until the time of surgery. Following components are necessary to meet the multidimensional needs of lung transplant candidates.

25.1.1 Exercise Training

Exercise training is declared as the cornerstone of PR to improve muscle function in patients with chronic respiratory diseases. Despite more adverse events reported during training compared to other high-risk populations, patients prior to heart or lung transplantation have generally been shown to tolerate exercise training very well [4]. Even patients with severe physical impairments are able to sustain necessary training intensities and durations to adapt in skeletal muscle [1] in order to improve exercise capacity despite the absence of improvements in lung function [5]. As a consequence of an increased oxidative capacity in skeletal muscle, delayed lactic acidosis leads to a decreased ventilatory drive and thus dynamic hyperinflation might be reduced at a given submaximal workrate [6]. This phenomenon helps to reduce perceived dyspnea during exercise training.

R. Gloeckl, Ph.D. (✉) • T. Schneeberger
I. Jarosch • K. Kenn, M.D.
Department of Respiratory Medicine & Pulmonary Rehabilitation, Schoen Klinik Berchtesgadener Land, Malterhoeh 1, 83471 Schoenau am Koenigssee, Germany
e-mail: rgloeckl@schoen-kliniken.de

© Springer International Publishing AG 2018
E. Clini et al. (eds.), *Textbook of Pulmonary Rehabilitation*,
https://doi.org/10.1007/978-3-319-65888-9_25

There are no formal guidelines available which are specialized on exercise training for patients in preparation for LTx. Most programs use the general exercise training recommendations stated in the ATS/ERS guidelines of pulmonary rehabilitation [1]. Basically, patients with chronic respiratory diseases need training intensities and durations targeted to the individual requirements to be effective in improving endurance capacity and muscle strength. Modalities need to be adapted in order to give an adequate training stimulus and to further improve exercise capacity.

Exercise training commonly consists of endurance and strength training. Furthermore, flexibility training, neuromuscular electrical stimulation (NMES), or inspiratory muscle training (IMT) in selected patients with substantial inspiratory muscle weakness may be complementary exercise modalities.

25.1.1.1 Endurance Training

To maximize physiological benefits, endurance training is recommended three to five times a week with an intensity of ≥60% of the individual maximal workload for 20–60 min per session. Values of perceived dyspnea or fatigue on a 10-point Borg scale can be used to target the training intensity (between four [moderate] to six [(very) severe]) [7]. The most common modality applying endurance training is walking or cycling. Walking is a very functional training modality to improve walking capacity and thus is important for activities of daily life. Training on a bicycle often leads to less exercise-induced desaturation as well as lower dyspnea levels and applies a greater stimulus on M.quadriceps compared to walking. Gloeckl et al. [8] investigated the effect of an interval compared to continuous training in a randomized controlled trial including COPD patients prior to LTx. Patients in the interval group were instructed to cycle for 30 s at a training intensity of 100% of the maximal workload that was followed by 30 s of resting. The continuous training group cycled at 60% of maximal workload. Interval training resulted in lower dyspnea levels rated on the Borg scale and fewer unintended breaks during the training by inducing the same level of improvement in the 6-min walk test (6MWT) compared to the continuous training group. Also one-legged training on a bicycle resulting in lower levels of dyspnea was suggested as an appropriate alternative for symptom-limited patients [9].

During exercise training, hemodynamic parameters should be monitored closely and supplemental oxygen should be available. For selected patients with exercise-induced hypercapnia, a noninvasive ventilation can be applied during exercise training to enable patients to perform an effective endurance training program with an adequate intensity and duration. However, this treatment needs close supervision by a health care professional with special qualification to adjust in- and expiratory pressures as well as breathing frequency promptly.

25.1.1.2 Strength Training

Strength training mainly addresses the increase in muscle mass and muscle strength, which is only modestly caused by endurance training. It has been proven that strength training in patients with chronic respiratory diseases is very effective and safe [10]. Recommendations for strength training in adults from the *American College of Sports Medicine* are also often used in patients with respiratory disorders [11]. One to three sets of 8–12 repetitions on 2–3 days per week are recommended. The load should be equivalent to 60–70% of the one repetition maximum or has to evoke fatigue after 8–12 repetitions. Exercise dosage has to be increased over time to induce skeletal muscle adaptations continuously.

Beside exercises for the lower limb to preserve or improve patients' mobility, also exercises for the upper limb are of interest in order to facilitate daily activities involving the upper extremities such as dressing, bathing, and household tasks [12]. Aerobic exercises (e.g., arm ergometer training) or strength exercise (e.g., free weights, elastic bands) can be used to improve upper limb capacity.

25.1.1.3 NMES

Especially in patients who are unable to participate in a regular exercise training program during PR (e.g., due to exacerbation), transcutaneous NMES might be a feasible and effective component. This technique elicits muscle contractions and thus trains selected muscle groups of the lower limbs without causing dyspnea. NMES has been shown to improve exercise capacity, muscle strength and to reduce dyspnea levels in stable COPD patients with poor exercise performance [13]. The effect of NMES remains unclear in patients with preserved exercise capacity levels. Frequencies should be adapted for each training session to individuals' highest tolerable frequency to optimize the effect on skeletal muscle. Attention should be paid for individuals with implanted electrical devices (pacemakers, implanted defibrillators), patients with seizure disorders, uncontrolled cardiac arrhythmias, unstable angina, recent myocardial infarction, intracranial clips, and/or total knee or hip replacement.

25.1.2 Physical and Breathing Therapy

Physical therapy is applied to reduce dynamic hyperinflation and dyspnea in patients with chronic respiratory disorders. According to the main functional disorder of the individual patient, different techniques such as thoracic mobilization, mucociliary clearance (e.g., cough techniques), or special breathing strategies are available to improve patients' symptoms and to reduce the risk for infections. Breathing strategies are aimed to slow down and to deepen the breathing frequency in order to reduce dynamic hyperinflation and dyspnea. Pursed-lips breathing, computer-supported breathing feedback, and yoga-breathing have been shown to be effective tools in reducing dyspnea or dynamic hyperinflation.

Due to the loss of cough reflex following LTx, it is of special importance for patients to learn adequate techniques for airway clearance such as autogenous drainage combined with "huffing" technique prior to LTx in order to be able to use them directly following LTx.

25.1.3 Education

Education prior to LTx can provide patients with a comprehensive knowledge addressing benefits and the importance of pre- and postoperative exercise training to optimize outcomes of the surgery. Energy conservating strategies, nutritional counseling, the management of anxiety and depression and understanding the disease are of special interest for the time bridging to transplant. To enhance compliance and adherence to the medical treatment, also the benefits and possible adverse effects of current medications and those given after LTx, such as immunosuppressants can be discussed. Patients also need to learn the effective use of their respiratory devices. In preparation of the surgery, patients should be familiarized with the LTx procedure including the potential benefits, expected outcomes as well as perioperative and postoperative risks. Supplying background information is essential for each patient to give informed consent for LTx. For the perioperative time period, patients have to consider special manners such as controlled cough, incentive spirometries, pain management, and the importance of early mobilization [3, 14]. A multidisciplinary PR is an ideal setting to address these issues to the patients.

25.1.4 Psychological Support

Patients on the waiting list for LTx have been shown to suffer from very poor quality of life. The implementation of quality of life interventions is important to cope successfully with the decline in physical performance and physical health, and to manage the stressful waiting time up to surgery. Also anxiety and depression symptoms are common in patients prior to LTx and together with the reduced quality of life, outcome of LTx can be affected [15]. Anxiety and panic can also negatively influence breathing pattern that often induce severe dynamic hyperinflation. PR programs including psychological support, breathing training, and coping strategies are of particular interest to reduce anxiety and depression symptoms in these patients. PR is suggested with evidence grade A as a treatment option [16].

25.1.5 Physical Activity

The level of physical activity (PA) is markedly reduced in patients listed for LTx. Also in comparison to COPD patients not listed for LTx, pretransplant COPD patients demonstrated a significantly more inactive lifestyle. Beside the influence of seasonal variation and the use of long-term oxygen therapy, exercise capacity (6MWD) was observed to have the strongest impact on PA level [17]. By reducing sedentary behavior, the risk of developing comorbidities can be reduced. This might be of particular interest because especially pretransplant patients have a high prevalence of comorbidities that might worsen in the time course after LTx as a side effect of pharmacological therapy (corticosteroids, immunosuppressive). Therefore, enhancing PA in LTx candidates is an important goal during PR to reduce the risk of exacerbating comorbidities. Studies with COPD patients showed that a behavioral change is necessary to motivate patients in favor of a more active lifestyle. Several methods such as activity measurements with activity monitors or simple pedometers and education sessions are available to help patients with this difficult task [18].

25.1.6 Maintenance Programs

Individuals are encouraged to continue exercise training to a feasible amount at home to maintain functional capacity achieved during PR up to the time of surgery [1]. Also activities of daily living might sustain physical performance and thus is highly recommended. Due to the progression of the underlying diseases, frequent visits with diagnostics and reassessments are necessary [19]. The regular contact with health care professionals can be used to adapt home exercise training program to patients' recent condition.

25.2 Lung Transplantation

The International Society for Heart and Lung Transplantation (ISHLT) administrates a worldwide registry that contains data from more than 50.000 adult lung transplants performed since 1985 with continuously increasing numbers every year. In 2013 a total of 3.893 lung transplants with a ratio of 1:4 concerning single and double LTx were registered. The most common indications were emphysema (~30%), idiopathic pulmonary fibrosis (~30%), and cystic fibrosis (~15%).

25.2.1 Candidate Identification

The pretransplant evaluation is recommended for clinically stable patients and not as a rescue strategy for critically ill patients. The decision to refer a patient for LTx particularly the timing of the decision is difficult (Table 25.1, according to [20]). A patient should not be exposed to the risk of the transplant surgery until all other viable treatment options were considered. Listing a patient for LTx requires the explicit knowledge that a patient has a limited life expectancy without LTx and that the risk-to-benefit ratio favors LTx over conventional medical treatment. Patients who have already been fully evaluated by the transplant team and all medical and psychosocial risk factors identified before, bridging strategies, as mechanical ventilation or extracorporeal life support can be applied in selected cases [20].

25.2.2 Disease-Specific Candidate Selection

25.2.2.1 COPD

Apart from survival an improvement in quality of life is the most important clinical benefit in patients with COPD. Considering the prevalence of end-stage COPD and the continuing shortage of donor organs it remains a challenging task to determine the optimal time point of LTx listing in COPD and whether quality of life issues should also be taken into account when making that decision. The median survival in patients with emphysema after LTx is 6.0 years [21]. A specific issue to the COPD population is the option for interventions like lung volume reduction surgery, endobronchial valves or coils. According to strict in- and exclusion criteria these procedures may be offered first to improve functional status.

25.2.2.2 Interstitial Lung Disease

Interstitial lung disease (ILD) and in particular idiopathic pulmonary fibrosis (IPF) carries the worst prognosis among the common disease indications for LTx. Retrospective cohort studies indicate a median survival of 2–3 years from diagnosis and only 20–30% patients survive >5 years after diagnosis resulting in a high waiting list mortality [22].

Beside the very limited drug treatment options, supplemental oxygen and LTx are the only treatments for IPF patients that were strongly recommended by ATS consensus documents [23, 24]. Especially in IPF patients it is also recommended to start a transplant discussion already at the time of diagnosis. The median survival in IPF patients after LTx is 4.7 years [21].

25.2.2.3 Cystic Fibrosis

LTx should be considered for suitable patients with cystic fibrosis (CF) who have a 2-year predicted survival of <50% and who have functional limitations classified as New York Heart Association Class III or IV. A routinely measurement of lung function has been shown to be the most useful predictor of disease progression [25]. The FEV1 has been the most frequently used parameter in CF patients to predict mortality. A FEV1 <30% of predicted is associated with a 2-year mortality rate of approximately 40% in men and 55% in women [26, 27]. Other preoperative parameters that have been shown to affect survival after LTx are a 6MWD <400 m and the presence of pulmonary hypertension [28, 29]. Due to the younger age of CF patients the median survival in these patients after LTx is longer (8.6 years) compared to other indications [21].

Table 25.1 General candidate considerations for lung transplantation

LTx should be considered for patients with a chronic, end-stage lung disease who meet the following general criteria:
1. High (>50%) risk of death from lung disease within 2 years if LTx is not performed
2. High (>80%) likelihood of surviving at least 90 days after LTx
3. High (>80%) likelihood of 5-year post LTx survival from a general medical perspective provided that there is adequate graft function

25.2.3 Allocation

Allocation systems vary around the world and depend on geographical conditions, urgency criteria, or accumulated waiting time. Center-based regional distribution is common in some European countries while others place emphasis on waiting period, urgency, or prospective transplant benefit [30].

In 2005 the United Network for Organ Sharing (UNOS) implemented the Lung Allocation Score (LAS) in the United States (US). The Eurotransplant Foundation® adopted the LAS for the allocation of donor lungs in some European countries in 2011.

The LAS is used to prioritize waiting list candidates based on a combination of waiting list urgency and estimated posttransplant survival to assess the prospective survival benefit [31]. Consequently, a drop in waiting list mortality has been reported [30]. The implementation of the LAS resulted in an increased number of patients with idiopathic pulmonary disease (IPF) receiving LTx making IPF one of the most common indications for LTx [30].

25.2.4 Single Versus Double Lung Transplantation

Single (SLTx) and double (DLTx) lung transplantation represent therapeutic options in patients with advanced lung disease without any further medical management options [32]. Some centers provide SLTX to older patients or patients with comorbidities to reduce the risk of short-term mortality. In contrast, although younger patients might benefit from larger lung volumes they might be less affected by problems arising from the remaining native lung. Hence, it is not clear whether SLTx or DLTx provides the best outcome. An analysis of the ISHLT registry has shown that survival is better in DLTx than SLTx recipients (median survival, 6.7 vs 4.6 years;

$p < 0.001$) [33]. However, this finding is confounded by the large differences between the various disease populations. A more recent study reviewed data after the LAS was implemented from 7308 LTx surgeries on disease-specific outcomes after SLTx and DLTx. It was found that in patients with IPF DLTx was associated with better survival compared to SLTx. In COPD patients there was no significant survival difference between SLTx and DLTx at 5 years [34].

In general, a decision on the type of procedure must be made on an individual case-by-case basis supported by a multidisciplinary approach. Disease severity, existing comorbidities, recipient age, nutritional and functional status, presence of pulmonary hypertension, and center experience have to be taken into account. Also waiting time on the transplant list is generally longer in DLTx recipients generating a greater risk of dying while waiting for a suitable donor organ [35]. Furthermore, shortage of donor organs is a problem all over the world. Accordingly, the decision to give DLTx to a single patient rather than to give SLTx to two patients must be considered carefully.

25.3 Pulmonary Rehabilitation After Lung Transplantation

Despite near normal pulmonary function and gas exchange, exercise intolerance, decreased PA, and reductions in health-related quality of life are not uncommon in LTx recipients, and often last up to years after surgery [36]. Therefore, extrapulmonary factors like skeletal muscle dysfunction, or inactivity should be improved. Existing preoperative muscle weakness can even worsen in the early period after LTx. Consequently LTx recipients report leg fatigue as the major symptom limiting exercise capacity, instead of the ventilator limiting mechanisms prior to LTx [37].

It has been shown that reduced skeletal muscle mass and limitations in quadriceps strength lingered up to 3 years after LTx surgery [38]. Structural alterations, like decreased muscle mass, reductions in type I fiber proportion and altered oxidative enzymes, favoring anaerobic metabolism of the peripheral muscles, are similar to those in COPD patients [39]. Additionally, the skeletal muscle function can be negatively impacted by postoperative factors, like prolonged hospitalization and side effects of immunosuppressive drugs.

Considering the fact of persisting impairments and limitations in the skeletal muscle function, exercise training in PR could be a key item to help this special group of patients to regain the best possible level of exercise capacity and health-related quality of life. Furthermore, a specific and multimodal PR program seems to be very important to help LTx recipients to deal with relevant topics like hygiene or nutrition in their daily life.

Although most individuals enrolled in PR are COPD patients, the current ATS/ERS statement contains a recommendation for including non-COPD individuals due to the increasing evidence of similar effects [1].

There is some evidence that PR after LTx increases muscle strength, physical exercise capacity, and health-related quality of life in [1]. However, the number of studies in the LTx population is still very low [1, 40]. Findings from cohort studies in the early phase after LTx must be interpreted with caution. Due to the lack of a control group, it is not possible to differentiate between the effects of an intervention and spontaneous improvements due to the natural recovery.

25.3.1 Components of a Pulmonary Rehabilitation After Lung Transplantation

PR begins within the first 48 h after surgeries without any major complications and is focused on optimizing lung expansion, secretion clearance, breathing pattern efficiency, range of motion of upper and lower extremities, strength, basic transfers, and gait stabilization [1]. Alterations in muscle mass and muscle strength can occur early after admission to the intensive care unit and are associated with functional disability and increased mortality. Even when there is a lack of evidence concerning the rehabilitation of LTx patients during hospitalization in the early postoperative period, an early active muscle training is seen as an important intervention to minimize further reductions in muscle function [41].

A first small pilot study [42] investigated the feasibility of WBVT in LTx patients directly after ICU discharge (13 ± 10 days post-LTx). The WBVT protocol (body starting position: standing or sitting; frequency: up to 10 Hz; 5 d/week for 10 min) was found to be a safe and feasible treatment option. For patients who are not able to participate in any active exercise treatment, neuromuscular electrical stimulation could also be a supportive treatment modality [43].

However, in the early postoperative phase, it is very important to increase training progression slowly concerning the range of motion of upper extremities to ensure the patient's safety [1]. Precautions in treatment recommendations depend on the used surgical method (minimally invasive LTx or transverse thoracosternotomy/"clamshell incision"), as well as on the reference given by the operating surgeon, which can sometimes differentiate, depending on the transplant center. Therefore, special considerations must be made concerning further interventions like exercise training or physical therapy incl. breathing therapy. Some examples of postoperative care limitations are given in Tables 25.2 and 25.3.

After discharge from the transplantation center, patients should participate in an outpatient or inpatient PR program in a specialized center. An indication to PR is not limited to the early period after LTx, it can also be indicated in the further course if there are signs of chronic rejection (bronchiolitis obliterans syndrome), or other comorbidities which lead to relevant restrictions in quality of life or physical performance [44].

A comprehensive, PR following LTx markedly differs from standard care in complexity and care intensity. Conventional multimodal aspects like exercise training, breathing therapy, psychological support, and structured education sessions are focusing on LTx-specific topics like proper use of medication, nutritional recommendations, and hygiene management. A benefit of an inpatient program is the additional consistent medical care, including clinical diagnostics throughout the whole course of the PR. Besides fundamental medical diagnostics, like pulmonary function, blood gas analyses and functional tests, imaging and endoscopic procedures can be promptly done. Therefore, it is possible to detect any impairments due to infection, rejection, respiratory insufficiency, or anastomotic problems at an early stage. Continuous monitoring of blood samples concerning infection screening, CMV titer, controlling immunosuppressives, and its adverse reactions is essential. In the early postoperative period, in some cases, an indication for a continuation of ambulatory oxygen or noninvasive ventilation could be given, because of severe complications, or a notable ventilatory insufficiency.

25.3.2 Exercise Training After Lung Transplantation

Despite the well-investigated phenomenon of persisting muscle dysfunction and the general belief that LTx recipients benefit from an exercise training program, there is only one randomized controlled trial that investigated the effects in this LTx recipients [45]. Langer et al. showed that a supervised exercise training following hospital discharge improves the functional recovery in LTx subjects. On top of the natural recovery clinically relevant improvements were observed in the amount of daily PA, quadriceps force, functional exercise capacity, and quality of life. However, optimal exercise training recommendations have not yet been described [36]. Therefore, it is advisable to follow general recommendations for frequency, intensity, and timing concerning exercise training interventions as suggested for patients with chronic respiratory diseases [7, 41]. Principles of an adequate muscle stimulus and progression of intensity should also be considered [1, 46]. In the beginning of a PR program, different assessments should be performed to evaluate the current status of functional exercise capacity (e.g., using 6MWT, shuttle-walk tests, cardiopulmonary exercise testing) and measurements of muscle strength [41].

Exercise training usually consists of a combination of endurance training and strength training. LTx recipients are no longer limited by ventilatory symptoms. Therefore, exercise training should be progressed to a higher intensity and longer duration over time. Contrary to the pre-LTx period, exertional dyspnea usually is no longer a major limitation. Therefore, a continuous endurance training at moderate intensities on either bicycle or treadmill can be performed. Interval training modalities could also be seen as a good opportunity in LTx recipients who still suffer from ventilatory impairments.

Strength training can be performed by using various exercises for major muscle groups of the lower (and upper) limbs, 1–3 sets of 8–12 repetitions each at 60–70% of the maximum tolerated load, with a progressive increase of resistance, as tolerated [41]. Special attention must be paid to strength exercises of the upper limbs in the early period according to post surgery limitations listed in Tables 25.2 and 25.3. Furthermore, some LTx recipients also suffer from tendinopathies [41]. Therefore, symptoms should be monitored and overloading tendons by repetitive, demanding exercises combined with high resistances should be avoided.

A WBVT on top of conventional endurance and strength training seems to be promising and may even enhance the benefits of a comprehensive PR concerning exercise capacity. Improvements in 6MWD and peak work rate were significantly ($p < 0.05$) higher in the WBVT group (83.5 m and 16.8 W) compared to the control group (55.2 m and 12.6 W). The complementary WBVT was performed on 3 days per week and LTx recipients were instructed to do 4 × 2 min of bilateral dynamic squat exercises, on a side-alternating vibration platform at 24–26 Hz [39]. No adverse events related to the WBVT were observed.

To prevent infections and reduce the risk of acute rejections, hygiene issues must also be taken into consideration during training sessions. LTx recipients should wear face masks during exercise training and disinfect their hands, as well as the handles of their training equipment, before and after each exercise [41].

Table 25.2 Postoperative limitations following minimal invasive LTx surgery

Postoperative progress	Limitations
1–2 weeks post LTx	– No stretch or traction to the scar tissue, m. pectoralis major, m. serratus anterior and carry loads < 5 kg
3–6 weeks post LTx	Glenohumeral joint: flexion and abduction maximally 90°
After 6 weeks post LTx	Carry loads > 5 kg
After 3 month post LTx	Range of motion of the upper body and load capacity should be fully given

Table 25.3 Postoperative limitations following transverse thoracosternotomy LTx surgery ("clamshell incision")

Postoperative progress	Limitations
1–8 weeks post LTx	Sternum protection: change of body position only with patient's arms crossed before breast; fix the sternum while coughing; Patients should not:—brace their body with arms—elevate arms over 90°—lie on the side—pull or push heavy objects—carry items which weigh more than 1.5 kg—rotate their upper body
After 9 weeks post LTx	Carry loads < 5 kg; bilateral distribution of load
After 3 month post LTx	Working on full range of movement of the upper body and load capacity; Carry loads > 5 kg; overhead loads possible

25.3.3 Physical and Breathing Therapy

Preexisting respiratory deficits often deteriorate immediately after LTx surgery due to operation induced pain, pleural effusion, or diaphragm paresis. Furthermore, the mucociliary clearance (MCC) is affected and decreased because of the denervation of the transplanted lung and the loss of the cough reflex [47]. Due to less effective coughing, the risk of an infection can be increased. Therefore, aim of the breathing therapy is to improve ventilation and airway clearance.

Viable options are: to enhance vital capacity, scar tissue treatment, performing breathing exercises, or mobilizing thorax structures. Dyspnea induced breathing patterns (high breathing frequency) must be retrained with some LTx recipients. Furthermore, special cough techniques (Huffing, autogenic drainage) that improve airway clearance should be taught [48]. The cough reflex probably recovers within the first year after surgery [49]. However, the MCC stays abnormal [50]. Therefore, it is necessary to take special care of the MCC (e.g., inhalation of isotonic Ems salt via jet nebulizer) and instruct the patients to prevent infections. The usage of assistive breathing devices, e.g., oscillating devices to improve airway clearance, has to be given special attention. Only devices that can be sterilized accordingly should be used to ensure hygiene management. Physical therapy should also train activities of daily life (e.g., step training, gait training, balance or coordination exercises), in order to prepare the patients for daily challenges and reintegration. The treatment approach depends on the functional and structural problems of the single patient.

However, there are no studies available concerning the effects of breathing therapy in patients after LTx.

25.3.4 Education

The educational component of PR after LTx is essential. It is important to promote adaptive behavior changes and especially collaborative self-management skills [1]. Relevant post LTx topics include the proper use of medication, nutrition, and hygiene management. The risk of infection is increased due to the medical suppression of the immune defense. For an early medical treatment it is important that patients are aware of the early signs of an acute infection. In context with infection prevention, LTx recipients must be strictly adhered to hygiene rules. Hygiene management has to be educated and the transmission to the daily life of organ recipients must be clear (e.g., intensive body/dental hygiene, routine hand disinfection, wearing face masks in public, contact avoidance with adults or children with the cold, no contact with pets or flower soil). Possible side effects of immunosuppressive drugs should also be discussed. Considering the fact that essential drugs can increase the incidence of diabetes, osteoporosis, obesity, hypertension, hyperlipidemia and hyperkalemia, a healthy and preventive diet is important from the beginning, but especially for the long-time course [51]. The right nutrition therapy for LTx recipients is aimed at minimizing these medication-induced side effects of immunosuppressives, high-dose corticosteroids and calcineurin inhibitors [51]. The intake of pathogenic substances by food, or possible interactions between food and medications (e.g., grapefruit/immunosuppressive) make nutrition a very important component of everyday care for each LTx recipient. An additional bioelectrical impedance analyses could be helpful to measure exactly the changes in body composition and might therefore be another external motivation for the patient.

25.3.5 Psychological Support

Psychologists are an important professional group that should not be missing in the team of a multidisciplinary PR program. Despite the LTx, patients experience the remaining physical impairments as frustrating and limiting concerning their quality of life. Issues like the fear of organ rejection and making plans for the future or including the patients' return to work are of great importance. The probability in LTx recipients to return to work is increased for patients with a younger age and a good quality of life before LTx [52]. In the long-term course, after 1 year 28.7% and after 5 years 7.4% of LTx recipients, have a part- or full time job [53].

A regular exchange with other LTx recipients can also be of great relevance. In the long-term progress, a psychological support is especially useful, when LTx recipients suffer from beginning impairments due to chronic organ failure.

25.3.6 Physical Activity

Physical functioning is a main component of health-related quality of life. It affects the ability to perform activities of the daily life including the return to work and participation in social life. In patients with COPD, PA has been identified as an important predictor of mortality [54]. Persisting limitations in exercise capacity and repeated episodes of infection and rejection, the use of immunosuppressives and a sedentary lifestyle could also have a negative influence on PA in the daily life of LTx recipients [55].

A randomized controlled trial showed that daily activity is substantially reduced after LTx and most patients do not return to a normal, active lifestyle. Daily steps, standing time, and moderate-intense activity of LTx recipients were shown to be reduced by 42%, 29%, and 66%, respectively, relative to health controls 1 year after LTx [55]. Wickerson et al. showed that 3 months after LTx the largest improvement in PA had occurred. However, the level of daily steps reached only 55% of the general population. The fact that daily steps correlated with self-reported physical functioning (r = 0.81), 6MWD (r = 0.63), quadriceps force (r = 0.66), and maximum workload (r = 0.63) suggested that PR, and in particular exercise training, could also be applied to increase PA [55]. Higher PA levels were related to higher leg muscle strength and exercise capacity [55].

Since LTx recipients are at risk to develop hypertension, diabetes, etc., PA may play a relevant role in the long-term management of common comorbidities that could positively influence posttransplant outcomes.

25.3.7 Maintenance Programs

Use it or lose it—abandoning training for a longer period decreases physical fitness not only for healthy people or athletes. This will also be the case in LTx-recipients that quit exercise training after a successful PR participation. Therefore, one of the main goals of PR must be the maintenance of exercise training and the motivation to aim for higher levels of PA. Improvements developed through PR must be transferred into everyday lives of patients by means of PA and self-management skills.

Currently, there is a lack of studies investigating the long-term effects of exercise training or PA interventions on muscle dysfunction, health-related quality of life, survival, risk of rejection, or infections and the development of comorbidities [41]. For patients who do have the ability to perform an exercise training autonomously, a supervised exercise training might not be mandatory. A home-based exercise program, or a pedometer-based walking intervention could also be interesting in the long-term post LTx course [41].

References

1. Spruit MA, Singh SJ, Garvey C, et al. An official American Thoracic Society/European Respiratory Society statement: key concepts and advances in pulmonary rehabilitation. Am J Respir Crit Care Med. 2013;188:e13–64.
2. Rochester CL. Pulmonary rehabilitation for patients who undergo lung-volume-reduction surgery or lung transplantation. Respir Care. 2008;53:1196–202.
3. Kenn K, Gloeckl R, Soennichsen A, et al. Predictors of success for pulmonary rehabilitation in patients awaiting lung transplantation. Transplantation. 2015;99(5):1072–7.
4. Wallen MP, Skinner TL, Pavey TG et al (2016) Safety, adherence and efficacy of exercise training in solid-organ transplant candidates: a systematic review. Transplant Rev
5. Franssen FM, Broekhuizen R, Janssen PP, et al. Effects of whole-body exercise training on body composition and functional capacity in normal-weight patients with COPD. Chest. 2004;125:2021–8.
6. Porszasz J, Emtner M, Goto S, et al. Exercise training decreases ventilatory requirements and exercise-induced hyperinflation at submaximal intensities in patients with COPD. Chest. 2005;128:2025–34.
7. Gloeckl R, Marinov B, Pitta F. Practical recommendations for exercise training in patients with COPD. Eur Respir Rev. 2013;22:178–86.
8. Gloeckl R, Halle M, Kenn K. Interval versus continuous training in lung transplant candidates: a randomized trial. J Heart Lung Transplant. 2012;31:934–41.
9. Dolmage TE, Goldstein RS. Effects of one-legged exercise training of patients with COPD. Chest. 2008;133:370–6.
10. O'Shea SD, Taylor NF, Paratz JD. Progressive resistance exercise improves muscle strength and may improve elements of performance of daily activities for people with COPD: a systematic review. Chest. 2009;136:1269–83.
11. American College of Sports Medicine. American College of Sports Medicine position stand. Progression

models in resistance training for healthy adults. Med Sci Sports Exerc. 2009;41:687–708.
12. Annegarn J, Meijer K, Passos VL, et al. Problematic activities of daily life are weakly associated with clinical characteristics in COPD. J Am Med Dir Assoc. 2012;13:284–90.
13. Sillen MJ, Speksnijder CM, Eterman RM, et al. Effects of neuromuscular electrical stimulation of muscles of ambulation in patients with chronic heart failure or COPD: a systematic review of the English-language literature. Chest. 2009;136:44–61.
14. Langer D. Rehabilitation in patients before and after lung transplantation. Respiration. 2015;89:353–62.
15. Singer HK, Ruchinskas RA, Riley KC, et al. The psychological impact of end-stage lung disease. Chest. 2001;120:1246–52.
16. Cafarella PA, Effing TW, Usmani ZA, et al. Treatments for anxiety and depression in patients with chronic obstructive pulmonary disease: a literature review. Respirology. 2012;17:627–38.
17. Langer D, Cebria i Iranzo MA, Burtin C, et al. Determinants of physical activity in daily life in candidates for lung transplantation. Respir Med. 2012;106:747–54.
18. Mantoani LC, Rubio N, McKinstry B, et al. Interventions to modify physical activity in patients with COPD: a systematic review. Eur Respir J. 2016;48:69–81.
19. Rochester CL, Fairburn C, Crouch RH. Pulmonary rehabilitation for respiratory disorders other than chronic obstructive pulmonary disease. Clin Chest Med. 2014;35:369–89.
20. Weill D, Benden C, Corris PA, et al. A consensus document for the selection of lung transplant candidates: 2014—an update from the Pulmonary Transplantation Council of the International Society for Heart and Lung Transplantation. J Heart Lung Transplant. 2015;34:1–15.
21. Yusen RD, Edwards LB, Kucheryavaya AY, et al. The Registry of the International Society for Heart and Lung Transplantation: Thirty-second Official Adult Lung and Heart-Lung Transplantation Report--2015; Focus Theme: Early Graft Failure. J Heart Lung Transplant. 2015;34:1264–77.
22. Brown AW, Shlobin OA, Weir N, et al. Dynamic patient counseling: a novel concept in idiopathic pulmonary fibrosis. Chest. 2012;142:1005–10.
23. Raghu G, Collard HR, Egan JJ, et al. An official ATS/ERS/JRS/ALAT statement: idiopathic pulmonary fibrosis: evidence-based guidelines for diagnosis and management. Am J Respir Crit Care Med. 2011;183:788–824.
24. Raghu G, Rochwerg B, Zhang Y, et al. An Official ATS/ERS/JRS/ALAT Clinical Practice Guideline: treatment of idiopathic pulmonary fibrosis. an update of the 2011 Clinical Practice Guideline. Am J Respir Crit Care Med. 2015;192:e3–e19.
25. Rosenbluth DB, Wilson K, Ferkol T, et al. Lung function decline in cystic fibrosis patients and timing for lung transplantation referral. Chest. 2004;126:412–9.
26. Kerem E, Reisman J, Corey M, et al. Prediction of mortality in patients with cystic fibrosis. N Engl J Med. 1992;326:1187–91.
27. Mayer-Hamblett N, Rosenfeld M, Emerson J, et al. Developing cystic fibrosis lung transplant referral criteria using predictors of 2-year mortality. Am J Respir Crit Care Med. 2002;166:1550–5.
28. Tuppin MP, Paratz JD, Chang AT, et al. Predictive utility of the 6-minute walk distance on survival in patients awaiting lung transplantation. J Heart Lung Transplant. 2008;27:729–34.
29. Venuta F, Tonelli AR, Anile M, et al. Pulmonary hypertension is associated with higher mortality in cystic fibrosis patients awaiting lung transplantation. J Cardiovasc Surg (Torino). 2012;53:817–20.
30. Gottlieb J, Greer M, Sommerwerck U, et al. Introduction of the lung allocation score in Germany. Am J Transplant. 2014;14:1318–27.
31. Egan TM, Murray S, Bustami RT, et al. Development of the new lung allocation system in the United States. Am J Transplant. 2006;6:1212–27.
32. Kotloff RM, Thabut G. Lung transplantation. Am J Respir Crit Care Med. 2011;184:159–71.
33. Christie JD, Edwards LB, Kucheryavaya AY, et al. The Registry of the International Society for Heart and Lung Transplantation: 29th adult lung and heart-lung transplant report-2012. J Heart Lung Transplant. 2012;31:1073–86.
34. Schaffer JM, Singh SK, Reitz BA, et al. Single- vs double-lung transplantation in patients with chronic obstructive pulmonary disease and idiopathic pulmonary fibrosis since the implementation of lung allocation based on medical need. JAMA. 2015;313:936–48.
35. Nathan SD, Shlobin OA, Ahmad S, et al. Comparison of wait times and mortality for idiopathic pulmonary fibrosis patients listed for single or bilateral lung transplantation. J Heart Lung Transplant. 2010;29:1165–71.
36. Wickerson L, Mathur S, Brooks D. Exercise training after lung transplantation: a systematic review. J Heart Lung Transplant. 2010;29:497–503.
37. Chhajed PN, Plit ML, Hopkins PM, et al. Achilles tendon disease in lung transplant recipients: association with ciprofloxacin. Eur Respir J. 2002;19:469–71.
38. Rozenberg D, Wickerson L, Singer LG, et al. Sarcopenia in lung transplantation: a systematic review. J Heart Lung Transplant. 2014;33:1203–12.
39. Gloeckl R, Heinzelmann I, Seeberg S, et al. Effects of complementary whole-body vibration training in patients after lung transplantation: A randomized, controlled trial. J Heart Lung Transplant. 2015;34(11):1455–61.
40. Puri V, Patterson GA, Meyers BF. Single versus bilateral lung transplantation: do guidelines exist? Thorac Surg Clin. 2015;25:47–54.
41. Langer D. Rehabilitation in patients before and after lung transplantation respiration. Int Rev Thorac Dis. 2015;89:353–62.

42. Brunner S, Brunner D, Winter H, et al. Feasibility of whole-body vibration as an early inpatient rehabilitation tool after lung transplantation--a pilot study. Clin Transplant. 2016;30:93–8.
43. Segers J, Hermans G, Bruyninckx F, et al. Feasibility of neuromuscular electrical stimulation in critically ill patients. J Crit Care. 2014;29:1082–8.
44. van Den BJ, Geertsma A, van Der BW, et al. Bronchiolitis obliterans syndrome after lung transplantation and health-related quality of life. Am J Respir Crit Care Med. 2000;161:1937–41.
45. Langer D, Burtin C, Schepers L, et al. Exercise training after lung transplantation improves participation in daily activity: a randomized controlled trial. Am J Transplant. 2012;12:1584–92.
46. Osadnik CR, Rodrigues FM, Camillo CA, et al. Principles of rehabilitation and reactivation. Respir Int Rev Thorac Dis. 2015;89:2–11.
47. Dolovich M, Rossmann C, Chambers C. Mucociliary function in patients following single lung or lung/heart transplantation. Am Rev Respir Dis. 1987;135:336.
48. Downs AM. Physical therapy in lung transplantation. Phys Ther. 1996;76:626–42.
49. Duarte AG, Terminella L, Smith JT, et al. Restoration of cough reflex in lung transplant recipients. Chest. 2008;134:310–6.
50. Herve P, Silbert D, Cerrina J, et al. Impairment of bronchial mucociliary clearance in long-term survivors of heart/lung and double-lung transplantation. The Paris-Sud Lung Transplant Group Chest. 1993;103:59–63.
51. Tynan C, Hasse JM. Current nutrition practices in adult lung transplantation. Nutr Clin Pract. 2004;19:587–96.
52. Petrucci L, Ricotti S, Michelini I, et al. Return to work after thoracic organ transplantation in a clinically-stable population. Eur J Heart Fail. 2007;9:1112–9.
53. Kugler C, Tegtbur U, Gottlieb J, et al. Health-related quality of life in long-term survivors after heart and lung transplantation: a prospective cohort study. Transplantation. 2010;90:451–7.
54. Waschki B, Kirsten A, Holz O, et al. Physical activity is the strongest predictor of all-cause mortality in patients with COPD: a prospective cohort study. Chest. 2011;140:331–42.
55. Langer D, Gosselink R, Pitta F, et al. Physical activity in daily life 1 year after lung transplantation. J Heart Lung Transplant. 2009;28:572–8.

26 Rehabilitation in Intensive Care

Rik Gosselink and Enrico Clini

26.1 Background and Rationale

The progress of intensive care medicine has dramatically improved survival of patients, especially those with acute respiratory distress syndrome (ARDS) and sepsis [1–3]. This improved survival is, however, often associated with general deconditioning, muscle weakness, prolonged mechanical ventilation, dyspnoea, depression and anxiety, reduced health-related quality of life following discharge from an intensive care unit (ICU) [4, 5]. Deconditioning and specifically muscle weakness have a key role in impaired functional status after ICU stay [6, 7].

Optimal physiological functioning depends on the upright position [8–10], so bed rest and limited mobility during critical illness result in profound physical deconditioning and dysfunction of the respiratory, cardiovascular, musculoskeletal, neurological, renal and endocrine systems [11]. These effects can be exacerbated by inflammation and pharmacological agents, such as corticosteroids, neuromuscular blockers and antibiotics. The prevalence of skeletal muscle weakness in the intensive care unit (ICU-acquired weakness-ICUAW) varies up to 50%. Muscle wasting appears to be the highest during the first 2–3 weeks of stay [12–15]. In addition, muscle weakness may already be present before ICU admission in patients with underlying chronic disease. Development of this neuropathy or myopathy also contributes to weaning failure [16]. Although most patients under mechanical ventilation are extubated in less than 3 days, approximately 20% of them still requires prolonged ventilatory support. Chronic ventilator dependence is a major medical problem, but it is also an extremely uncomfortable state for a patient, leading to important physical and psychosocial implications. Indeed, muscle weakness has been linked with ICU and hospital length of stay and increased 1-year mortality [6, 17, 18].

The above-mentioned changes in functional performance and limb and/or respiratory muscle function indicate the need for rehabilitation *after* ICU stay [19–21], but also underscores the need for assessment and measures to prevent deconditioning and loss of physical function *during* ICU stay. The amount of rehabilitation performed in ICUs is often inad-

R. Gosselink (✉)
Department Rehabilitation Sciences, Faculty of Kinesiology and Rehabilitation Sciences-KU Leuven, Cardiovascular and Respiratory Research Unit, University Hospitals Leuven, Leuven, Belgium
e-mail: rik.gosselink@uz.kuleuven.ac.be

E. Clini
Department of Medical and Surgical Sciences, University of Modena, Azienda Ospedaliero Universitaria di Modena Policlinico, Modena, Italy

© Springer International Publishing AG 2018
E. Clini et al. (eds.), *Textbook of Pulmonary Rehabilitation*,
https://doi.org/10.1007/978-3-319-65888-9_26

equate [22–24] due to lack of knowledge and barriers [25–27]. As a rule, rehabilitation is better organized in weaning centres or respiratory ICUs (RICUs) [28–30]. The major reason is that the approach in rehabilitation is less driven by medical diagnosis; instead rehabilitation is focusing on deficiencies in the broader scope of health problems as defined in the International Classification of Functioning, Disability and Health. This leads to identification of problems and the prescription of one or more interventions at a level of *body structure and function* as well as *activities* and *participation*.

Therefore, members of the rehabilitation team in the ICU (doctors, physiotherapists, nurses and occupational therapists) should be able to prioritize, and identify aims and parameters of treatments, ensuring that these are both therapeutic and safe by appropriate monitoring of vital functions [31]. This team approach has been shown effective [28, 32–35].

Exercise and muscle training can improve muscle force and functionality in stable critically ill patients admitted to a RICU because of weaning failure [30, 36, 37]. Indeed, it is important to prevent or attenuate muscle deconditioning as early as possible in patients with expected prolonged bed rest. To quote the 1944 paper 'The evil sequelae of complete bed rest' [38]: 'The physician must always consider complete bed rest as a highly *unphysiologic* and definitely *hazardous* form of therapy, to be ordered only for *specific indications* and *discontinued as early as possible*'. Mobilization has been part of the physiotherapy management of acutely ill patients for several decades [39] and the recommendation document of European Respiratory Society (ERS)/European Society of Intensive Care Medicine advices to start early with active and passive exercise in critically ill patients [40]. Over the last decade increasing scientific and clinical interest and evidence have given support for a safe and early physical activity and mobilization approach towards the critically ill patient by ICU team members [41, 42].

26.2 Safety Assessment and Efficacy

The detrimental physiological effects of recumbency and restricted mobility on all systems, and the benefits of being upright and moving have been widely reported. However, issues related to early physical activity and mobilization of patients in the ICU as a therapeutic option including *safety*, *dose* and *implementation* have only recently been a shared focus of interest to interdisciplinary teams practising in the ICU [28, 32, 34, 43]. Accurate assessment of cardiorespiratory reserve and rigorous screening for other factors that could preclude early mobilization is of paramount importance [31].

In addition to assessment of the safety and readiness of the patient for exercise and spontaneous physical activity, specific measures of function (e.g. muscle strength, joint mobility), functional status (e.g. outcomes for functional performance such as the Functional Independence Measure, Berg Balance scale, Functional Ambulation Categories, Physical Function ICU Test (PFIT), Chelsea Critical Care Physical Assessment (CPAx) and quality of life (e.g. Medical Outcome Survey Short Form 36 [SF-36], disease-specific questionnaires) must be considered [44] (see in Box 26.1).

26.3 Cooperation

In addition to the Glasgow Coma Scale, the Confusion Assessment for the ICU (CAM ICU), and the Richmond Agitation and Sedation Scale (RASS), the Standardized 5 Questions (see in Box 26.2) are oftentimes used to assess the level of cooperation and adequacy in clinical practice.

26.3.1 Joint Mobility

Knowledge on the epidemiology of major joint contractures is limited. A systematic review reported a high prevalence in patient population frequently admitted to ICU (spinal cord injuries, burns, brain injuries and stroke) [45]. Functional

Box 26.1: Assessment of critically patient

Cooperation—level of confusion, agitation, sedation and consciousness

- Glasgow Coma Scale
- Confusion Assessment for the ICU (CAM ICU)
- Richmond Agitation and Sedation Scale (RASS)
- Standardized 5 Questions

Joint mobility

- Active and passive range of motion

Muscle function

- Medical Research Council 0–5 scale/ Medical Research Council sum score
- Handheld dynamometry
- Muscle twitch stimulation force
- Muscle thickness with ultrasonography

Overall functional status

- Barthel Index
- Functional Independence Measure
- Katz ADL Scale
- Berg Balance Scale
- Functional Ambulation Categories
- 4 Meter Gait speed test
- Physical Function ICU Test (PFIT)
- Chelsea Critical Care Physical Assessment (CPAx)

Well-being and quality of life

- Short-Form Health Survey
- Nottingham Health Profile
- Chronic Respiratory Disease Questionnaire

Box 26.2: Five standardized questions (S5Q) to assess the level of cooperation and adequacy

- Open and close your eyes
- Look at me
- Open your mouth and put out your tongue
- Nod your head
- Raise your eyebrows after I have counted up to five

significant contracture of major joints occurred in more than 30% of patients with prolonged ICU stay [46]. Elbow and ankle were the mostly affected joints both at ICU discharge and hospital discharge. This underlines the need for both assessment and treatment of (passive) range of motion in ICU patients. Frequent assessment of joint mobility and causes of limitation of range of motion (muscle tone, muscle length, capsule, skin and oedema) is requested. Detailed assessment of joint mobility by physiotherapists can reveal undetected injuries.

26.4 Limb Muscle Strength Testing

Muscle strength, or more precisely the maximum muscle force or tension generated by a muscle or (more commonly) a group of muscles, can be measured in several ways and with a range of different equipments. Manual muscle testing with the 0–5 Medical Research Council (MRC) scale is very often used in clinical practice. Good reliability of the MRC sum score has been shown in critically ill patients [47]. This MRC sum score comprehends both upper limb (arm abductors, forearm flexors and wrist extensors) and lower limb (leg flexors, knee extensors and dorsal flexors of the foot) muscles. De Jonghe et al. have proposed that a sum score less than 48 reflects significant ICU-acquired weakness [48]. Recently, the American Thoracic Society has published a statement on the diagnosis of ICUAW and concluded that there is lack of a *gold standard*. All available tests have their limitations, but until more data emerge, manual muscle testing is the preferred evaluation method [49]. However, manual muscle testing seems to be less sensitive to assess differences in muscle strength of values above grade 3 (active movement against gravity over the full range of motion) [50].

Therefore, several tools have been developed to measure muscle strength more accurately.

Dynamometry with mechanical or electrical equipment is used to measure isometric muscle force. Handgrip dynamometry has been shown to be reliable, and reference values are available

[47, 51]. For other upper and lower extremity muscle groups, handheld electrical devices have been developed. Two methods of isometric testing have been described: the make-test and the break-test. In the make-test, the maximal force the subject can exert is equal to the force of the assessor. In the break-test, the force of the assessor exceeds the force of the patient slightly. The test is reproducible in critically ill patients [52]. Handheld dynamometry is a viable alternative to costlier modes of isometric strength measurements, provided the assessor's strength is greater than that of the specific muscle group being measured. References values are available, also for elderly healthy subjects [53]. The limitation of the use of maximal voluntary contractions is the potential to observe submaximal contractions due to submaximal effort and cortical drive [54]. The use of superimposed electric or magnetic twitch contractions anticipates this potential variation in voluntary activation [54]. Moreover, it is less painful than electrical stimulation, and the 'twitch' stimulations are relatively reproducible, but only clinically tested on the adductor pollicis. Ultrasound measurement of muscle thickness of the quadriceps was introduced and validated against MRI, the gold standard for muscle cross-sectional area and has recently been validated in ICU patients [13, 14]. This allows non-invasive and accurate assessment of muscle size in uncooperative critically ill patients.

26.4.1 Respiratory Muscle Testing

In clinical practice, respiratory muscle strength is measured as maximal inspiratory and expiratory mouth pressures (P_{Imax} and P_{Emax}, respectively). These pressure measurements are made via a small cylinder attached to the mouth with a circular mouthpiece. The American Thoracic Society (ATS)/European Respiratory Society (ERS) statement describes respiratory muscle testing in more detail [55]. In ventilated patients inspiratory muscle strength is estimated from temporary occlusion of the airway. The procedure involves a unidirectional expiratory valve to allow the patient to expire while inspiration is occluded. Optimal length of occlusion time is considered 25–30 s in adults [56]. Several groups have developed normal values, however, regardless of which set of normal values is used, the standard deviation is large. The presence of inspiratory weakness is accepted when P_{Imax} is lower than 50% of the predicted value.

Goligher and colleagues assessed diaphragm thickness and documented that a lower contractile activity of the diaphragm during mechanical ventilation was associated with further reduction of diaphragm thickness [57]. Very recently, the ultrasound assessment of the diaphragm has been proposed as a reliable and useful method to assess muscular dysfunction, which in turn is associated with a worse prognosis in ventilated patients suffering from acute on chronic obstruction of the airways [58]. This might reflect the ability to be weaned from mechanical ventilation is such population.

More invasive techniques such as electric or magnetic diaphragm stimulation provide more accurate information on diaphragm function and are useful in the diagnosis of diaphragmatic paresis and weakness [15].

26.4.2 Functional Status

The assessment of functional status may seem to be inapplicable for acutely ill ICU patients, but can be implemented in long-term weaning facilities and after discharge. Functional assessment tools are also successfully used to monitor progress of patients in several studies [29, 33, 35, 44, 59]. Furthermore, several of these tools are helpful reconstructing the patient's functionality before ICU admission.

The Barthel Index, Functional Independence Measure (FIM), Katz ADL Scale and Timed Up and Go test are commonly used and valid tools to score the patient's ability to independently perform a range of activities, mostly related to mobility (e.g. transfers from bed to chair, walking, stair climbing) and self-care (e.g. bathing, grooming, toileting, dressing, feeding). The Berg Balance Scale quantifies impairment in balance function by scoring the performance of simple functional tasks (e.g. sitting, standing, transfers, reaching forward, turning). Walking ability can also be simply assessed using the Functional Ambulation Categories. In patients who are able to walk, the Shuttle walk test, 6-min walking test or the 4 m gait speed test can be used to evaluate functional exercise capacity [60, 61].

26.4.3 Quality of Life

As health-related quality of life is often reduced after prolonged ICU stay [7, 62], appropriate evaluation of physical and mental health components is mandatory. The SF-36 is a widely used generic quality of life questionnaire which includes 8 multiple-item scales that assess physical functioning, social functioning, physical role, emotional role, mental health, pain, vitality and general health. As an alternative tool the Nottingham Health Profile covers six different quality of life areas: pain, energy, physical mobility, sleep, social isolation and emotional interaction. Both questionnaires have been used frequently in post-ICU quality of life studies. In patients with underlying chronic respiratory diseases, disease-specific questionnaires such as the Chronic Respiratory Disease Questionnaire (CRDQ) or the St George's Respiratory Questionnaire (SGRQ) can provide more specific information on the impact of the ICU stay on the disease perception.

26.5 Physiotherapy in the Prevention and Treatment of Deconditioning

Exercise training is a cornerstone component of each rehabilitation programme, in addition to psychosocial interventions. Avoiding or minimizing physical deconditioning and other complications, and shortening of duration of mechanical ventilation with early extubation are prime goals of the critical care team.

Early mobilization was shown to reduce the time to wean from mechanical ventilation 30 years ago and more recently proven evidence based [33]. It is the basis for long-term functional recovery. Evidence for the benefits of body positioning, mobilization, exercise and muscle training, on the prevention and treatment of deconditioning in other patient groups as well as in healthy subjects, was confirmed in the management of critically ill patients [41]. In addition to safety issues, exercise should also be targeted at the appropriate intensity and exercise modality. These will be dependent on the stability and cooperation of the patient.

Acutely ill, uncooperative patients are treated with modalities that will not need cooperation and will not put stress on the cardiorespiratory system, such as passive range of motion, muscle stretching, splinting, body positioning, passive cycling with a bed cycle or electrical muscle stimulation. On the other hand, the stable cooperative patient, beyond the acute illness phase but still on mechanical ventilation, will be able to be mobilized on the edge of the bed, transfer to a chair, perform resistance muscle training or active cycling with a bed cycle or chair cycle and walk with or without assistance. The flow diagram developed by Gosselink et al. [63] and based upon the scheme of Morris et al. [34]. Fig. 26.1 is an example of such step-up approach.

The paragraphs as illustrated in the Fig. 26.1 deal with modalities of exercise training with progressive intensity and increasing need of cooperation of the patient. The risk of moving a critically ill patient is weighed against the risk of immobility and recumbency and when employed requires stringent monitoring to ensure that mobilization is instituted appropriately and safely [31].

26.5.1 Uncooperative Critically Ill Patient

The importance of body positioning ('stirring up' patients) was reported as early as the 1940s [39]. Since that time, positioning has been used prescriptively to remediate oxygen transport deficits such as impaired gas exchange by altering the distribution of ventilation (V) and perfusion (Q),

UZ LEUVEN 'START TO MOVE' ASAP *(from day 2 with an expected prolonged MICU stay of 5 more days)*

MULTIDISCIPLINARY APPROACH

	LEVEL 0	LEVEL 1	LEVEL 2	LEVEL 3	LEVEL 4	LEVEL 5
CLINICAL INVESTIGATION	**NO COOPERATION** **S5Q[1] = 0** **FAILS BASIC ASSESSMENT[2]**	**VARIABLE COOP.** **S5Q[1] = 0-5** **PASSES BASIC ASSESSMENT[3]** TRANSFER to chair **not allowed** because of neurological or surgical or trauma condition	**VARIABLE COOP.** **S5Q[1] = 0-5** **PASSES BASIC ASSESSMENT[3]** ACTIVE TRANSFER to chair **not allowed** because of obesity or neurological or surgical or trauma condition	**CLOSE-FULL COOP.** **S5Q[1] ≥ 4/5** **PASSES BASIC ASSESSMENT[3]** MRCsum ≥ 36 ($MRCsum_{LL}$ ≥ 36) BBS Sit to stand = 0 BBS Standing = 0 BBS Sitting ≥ 1	**FULL COOP.** **S5Q[1] = 5** **PASSES BASIC ASSESSMENT[3]** MRCsum ≥ 48 ($MRCsum_{LL}$ ≥ 24) BBS Sit to stand ≥ 0 BBS Standing ≥ 0 BBS Sitting ≥ 2	**FULL COOP.** **S5Q[1] = 5** **PASSES BASIC ASSESSMENT[3]** MRCsum ≥ 48 BBS Sit to stand ≥ 1 BBS Standing ≥ 2 BBS Sitting ≥ 3
REHABILITATION	**BODY POSITIONING[4]** °2h turning °Splinting °Positioning	**BODY POSITIONING[4]** °2h turning °Splinting °Fowler's position	**BODY POSITIONING[4]** °2h turning °Splinting °Upright sitting position in bed °**Passive** transfer bed to chair	**BODY POSITIONING[4]** °2h turning °**Passive** transfer bed to chair °Sitting out of bed °Standing with assist (≥ 2 pers)	**BODY POSITIONING[4]** °**Active** transfer bed to chair °Sitting out of bed °Standing with assist (≥ 1 pers)	**BODY POSITIONING[4]** °**Active** transfer bed to chair °Sitting out of bed °Standing
	PHYSIOTHERAPY °No treatment	**PHYSIOTHERAPY[4]** °Passive/active ROM °Passive/active leg and/or arm cycling in bed °NMES	**PHYSIOTHERAPY[4]** °Passive/active ROM °Resistance training arms and legs °Passive/active leg and/or arm cycling in bed or chair °NMES	**PHYSIOTHERAPY[4]** °Passive/active ROM °Resistance training arms and legs °Active leg and/or arm cycling in bed or chair °Standing (with assistance/frame) °NMES °ADL	**PHYSIOTHERAPY[4]** °Passive/active ROM °Resistance training arms and legs °Active leg and/or arm cycling in bed or chair °Walking (with assistance/frame) °NMES °ADL	**PHYSIOTHERAPY[4]** °Passive/active ROM °Resistance training arms and legs °Active leg and/or arm cycling in chair °Walking (with assistance) °NMES °ADL

UZ LEUVEN INTENSIEVE GENEESKUNDE

[1]: score 5 questions: adequate response to 5 standardized orders
[2]: FAILS = at least 1 risk factor present
[3]: if basic assessment failed, decrease to level 0
[4]: safety and feasibility: each activity should be deferred if severe adverse events (cv., resp., internal and subject. intolerance) occur during the intervention

ADEQUACY SCORE
A. Open and close your eyes
B. Loo at me
C. Open your mouth and put out your tongue
D. Nod your head
E. Raise your eyebrows when I have counted up to five

BASIC ASSESSMENT =
-Cardiorespiratory unstable
 * MAP < 60mmHg or
 * FiO_2 > 60% or
 * PaO_2/FiO_2 < 200 or
 * RR > 30 bpm
-Neurological unstable
-Acute surgery
-Temp > 40°C

BERG BALANCE SCORE

SITTING TO STANDING
4 able to stand without using hands and stabilize independently
3 able to stand independently using hands
2 able to stand using hands after several tries
1 needs minimal aid to stand or stabilize
0 needs moderate or maximal assist to stand

STANDING UNSUPPORTED
4 able to stand safely for 2 minutes
3 able to stand 2 minutes with supervision
2 able to stand 30 seconds unsupported
1 needs several tries to stand 30 seconds unsupported
0 unable to stand 30 seconds unsupported

SITTING WITH BACK UNSUPPORTED BUT FEET SUPPORTED ON FLOOR OR ON A STOOL
4 able to sit safely and securely 2 minutes
3 able to sit 2 minutes under supervision
2 able to sit 30 seconds
1 able to sit 10 seconds
0 unable to sit 10 seconds unsupported

MRC-SUMSCORE Pre-existing NMD: ☐ **No** ☐ **Yes** ___________

	Right	Reason	EP	Left	Reason	EP	
MS: Abduction of the arm							
MS: Flexion of the forearm							
MS: Extension of the wrist							
MS: Flexion of the leg							
MS: Extension of the knee							
MS: Dorsal flexion of the foot							
STRENGTH SUBTOTAL VALUE						STRENGTH TOTAL=	
EP SUBTOTAL VALUE						EP TOTAL =	
MRC TOTAL SUMSCORE							

MRC-SCALE
0 = no visible contraction
1 = visible contraction without movements of the limbs
2 = movements of the limbs but not against gravity
3 = movement against gravity over (almost) the full range
4 = movement against gravity and resistance
5 = normal

Dominance:

Fig. 26.1 'Start to move'—protocol University Hospital Leuven: step-up approach of progressive mobilization and physical activity programme (adapted from [63]). *NMES* neuromuscular electrical stimulation, *ADL* activities of daily living, *MRC* (Medical Research Council) muscle strength sum scale(0–60), *BBS* Berg Balance score

V/Q matching, airway closure, work of breathing, and work of the heart, as well as mucociliary transport (postural drainage). Recumbency during bed rest in patients who are critically ill exposes them to risk because the vertical gravitational gradient is eliminated, and exercise stress is restricted. To simulate the normal perturbations that the human body experiences in health, the patient who is critically ill needs to be positioned upright (well supported), and rotated when recumbent. These perturbations need to be scheduled frequently to avoid the adverse effects of prolonged static positioning on respiratory, cardiac, and circulatory function. The potent and direct physiological effects of changing body position on oxygen transport and oxygenation are exploited when mobilization is contraindicated. This evidence comes primarily from the space science literature in which bed rest has been used as a model of weightlessness. The prone position has been of particular interest in the management of the critically ill patient, but is underused. Knowledge of the physiologic effects of body position enables the physiotherapist to prescribe a positioning regimen to exploit its beneficial effects as well as minimize the effects of deleterious body positions. Other indications for active and passive positioning include the management of soft tissue contracture, protection of flaccid limbs and lax joints, nerve impingement and skin breakdown.

Although a specific body position may be indicated for a patient, varied positions and frequent body position changes, particularly extreme body positions, are based on the assessment findings. The efficacy of 2-h patient rotation, which is common in clinical practice, has not been verified scientifically. A rotation schedule that is more frequent and promotes turning from one extreme position to another approximates more normal heart-lung function than a standardized 2-hourly turning regimen. Medically unstable patients who require a rotating or kinetic bed, benefit from continuous side-to-side perturbation, which supports the hypothesis that patients may benefit from frequent and extreme position changes rather than fixed, prolonged periods in given positions [64].

Bed design features in critical care should include hip and knee breaks so the patient can approximate upright sitting as much as can be tolerated. Heavy care patients such as those who are sedated, heavy or overweight may need chairs with greater support such as stretcher chairs. Lifts may be needed to change a patient's position safely.

Passive stretching or range of motion exercise may have a particularly important role in the management of patients who are unable to move spontaneously. In healthy subjects passive stretching decreases stiffness and increases extensibility of the muscle. Evidence for using continuous dynamic stretching (and counter balancing the 'silencing' of the muscle in critically ill patients [65]) is based on the observation in patients with critical illness subjected to prolonged inactivity. Nine hours of continuous passive motion per day reduced the loss of muscle strength, muscle atrophy and protein loss, compared with passive stretching for 5 min, twice daily [66, 67].

For patients who cannot be actively mobilized and have high risk on soft tissue contracture, such as following severe burns, trauma, and some neurological conditions, splinting may be indicated. Splinting of the periarticular structures in the stretched position for more than half an hour per day was shown to have a beneficial effect on the range of motion (ROM) in an animal model [68]. In burns patients, fixing the position of joints reduced muscle and skin contraction [69]. In patients with neurological dysfunction, splinting may reduce muscle tone [70].

Finally, the application of exercise training in the early phase of ICU admission is often more complicated due to lack of cooperation and the clinical status of the patient. Although early active training at the very beginning of patient's cooperation is feasible and effective even with low-cost devices [71], technological development resulted in a bedside cycle ergometer for (active or passive) leg cycling during bed rest (Fig. 26.2). The application of this training modality has been shown to be a safe and feasible exercise tool in (neuro) ICU patients [35, 72, 73]. The bedside cycle ergometer can perform a

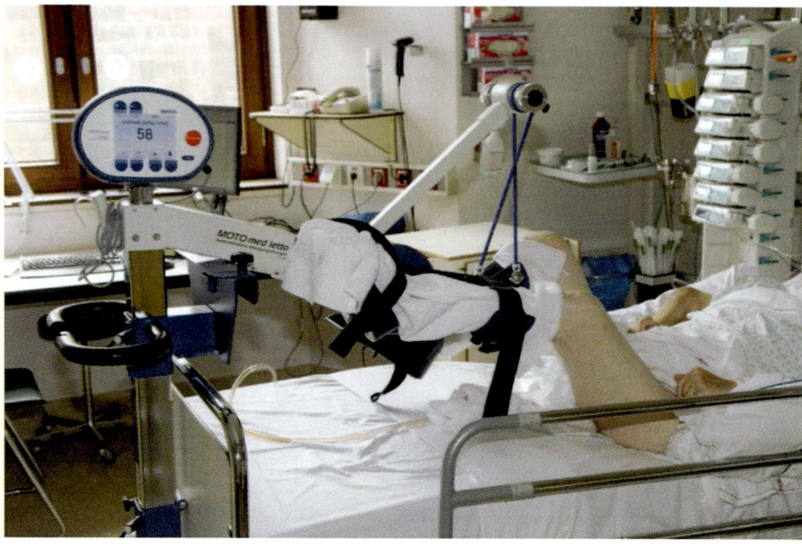

Fig. 26.2 Device for active and passive cycling in a bedridden patient in the intensive care

prolonged continuous mobilization allowing rigorous control of exercise intensity and duration. A randomized controlled trial of early application of daily bedside leg cycling in critically ill patients showed improved functional status, muscle function and exercise performance at hospital discharge compared with patients receiving standard physiotherapy without leg cycling [35].

In patients unable to perform voluntary muscle contractions, neuromuscular electrical stimulation (NMES) has been used to prevent disuse muscle atrophy. Daily NMES for at least 1-h during an immobilization period reduced in patients with lower limb fractures and cast immobilization the decrease in cross-sectional area of the quadriceps and enhanced normal muscle protein synthesis [74]. A slower muscle protein catabolism and increase in total RNA content were also seen after NMES in patients with major abdominal surgery [75]. In patients in the ICU not able to move actively, NMES was also introduced to preserve muscle strength and muscle mass in critically ill patients. Although the trend of the effectiveness is positive, results of the studies are conflicting [76, 77]. Several reasons may account for these findings, such as patient characteristics (sepsis, oedema, use of vasopressives [78]), timing of NMES related to ICU admission, protocol for stimulation (devices, stimulation duration and frequency), and also methodology for assessment of muscle function (muscle mass, strength) varied substantially. NMES of the quadriceps, in addition to active limb mobilization, enhanced muscle strength and hastened independent transfer from bed to chair in patients with prolonged critical illness [79].

26.5.2 Cooperative Critically Ill Patient

Mobilization and ambulation has been part of the physiotherapy management of acutely ill patients for several decades [39]. Mobilization refers to physical activity sufficient to elicit acute physiological effects that enhance ventilation, central and peripheral perfusion, circulation, muscle metabolism and alertness. Strategies—in order of intensity—include sitting over the edge of the bed, standing, stepping in place, transferring in bed and from bed to chair, and walking with or without support. Although the approach of early mobilization has face validity, its effectiveness was evaluated in only three (randomized) controlled trials [3, 19, 33, 34]. Two studies [3, 34] demonstrated that patients receiving early mobility therapy had reduced ICU stay and hospital stay with no differences in weaning time. No differences were observed in discharge location or in hospital costs of the usual care and early mobility patients. Schweickert et al. observed that early physical and occupational therapy improved functional status at hospital discharge, shortened duration of delirium and increased ventilator-free days. These findings did not result in differences in length of ICU or hospital stay [33].

The team approach (doctor, nurse, physiotherapist and occupational therapist) is an important and strong point in establishing an early ambulation programme [80]. The early intervention approach is, although not easily, specifically delivered in patients still in need of supportive devices (mechanical ventilation, cardiac assists) or unable to stand without support of personnel or standing aids, a worthwhile experience for the patient [34, 81]. This difference in the mentality of the team was elegantly demonstrated by Thomsen et al. [28] in a study including 104 respiratory failure patients who required mechanical ventilation for more than 4 days. After correction for confounders, transferring a patient from the acute intensive care to the RICU substantially increased the number of patients ambulating threefold compared with pre-transfer rates. Improvements in ambulation with transfer to the RICU were allocated to the differences in the team approach towards ambulating the patients [28].

Standing and walking frames enable the patient to mobilize safely with attachments for bags, lines and leads that cannot be disconnected. The arm support on a frame or rollator has been shown to increase ventilatory capacity in patients with severe chronic obstructive pulmonary disease [82]. The frame either needs to be able to accommodate a portable oxygen tank, or a portable mechanical ventilator and seat, or a suitable trolley for equipment can be used.

Walking and standing aids, and tilt tables, enhance physiological responses [83] and enable early mobilization of critically ill patients. The tilt table may be used when the patient is unable to move the legs to counter dependent fluid displacement, and may be at risk of orthostatic intolerance. Abdominal belts need to be carefully positioned to support, not restrict, respiration during mobilization. In patients with spinal cord injury this improves vital capacity [84]. Transfer belts facilitate heavy lifts and protect both the patient and the physiotherapist or nurse. Non-invasive ventilation (NIV) during mobilization might improve exercise tolerance for non-intubated patients, similar to that demonstrated in patients with stable chronic obstructive pulmonary disease [85]. Accordingly, the ventilator settings may require adjustment to the patient's needs (i.e. increased minute ventilation).

Aerobic training and muscle strengthening, in addition to routine mobilization, improved walking distance more than mobilization alone in patients on long-term mechanical ventilation and chronic critical illness [30, 36]. A randomized controlled trial showed that a 6-week upper and lower limb training programme improved limb muscle strength, ventilator-free time and functional outcomes in patients requiring long-term mechanical ventilation compared to a control group [36]. These results are in line with a retrospective analysis of patients on long-term mechanical ventilation who participated in a whole-body and respiratory muscle training [29]. In patients recently weaned from mechanical ventilation, the addition of upper-limb exercise enhanced the effects of general mobilization on exercise endurance performance and dyspnoea [86].

Low-resistance multiple repetitions of resistive muscle training can augment muscle mass, force generation, and oxidative enzymes. Sets of repetitions (three sets of 8–10 repetitions at 50–70% of one repetition maximum [1RM]) within the patient's tolerance can be scheduled daily, commensurate with their goals. Resistive muscle training can include the use of pulleys, elastic bands and weight belts.

The chair cycle and the earlier mentioned bed cycle allow patients to perform an individualized exercise training programme. The intensity of cycling can be adjusted to the individual and progressive patient's capacity (i.e. from passive cycling, via assisted cycling, to cycling against resistance). The prescription of exercise intensity, duration and frequency is response-dependent rather than time-dependent and is based on clinical challenge tests, such as the response to a nursing or investigative procedure, or to a specific mobilization challenge. Exercise should be safely tolerated in any treatment session and if the patient responds positively, greater intensity and duration can be applied. For acutely ill patients, frequent short sessions (analogous to interval training) allow for greater recovery than the less frequent, longer sessions prescribed for patients with chronic stable conditions [87]. Patients with haemodynamic instability, or with little to no oxygen transport reserve capacity (e.g. those on high concentrations of oxygen and high levels of ventilatory support, or those with anaemia or cardiovascular instability), are not candidates for aggressive mobilization. The risk of moving a critically ill patient should be weighed against the risk of immobility and requires stringent monitoring to ensure effectiveness and safety [31].

26.6 Physiotherapy in the Treatment of Respiratory Conditions

The aims of physiotherapy in respiratory dysfunction are to improve lung inflation, clear airway secretions, reduce the work of breathing, and enhance inspiratory muscle function thus promoting recovery of spontaneous breathing [40]. In a recent systematic review Stiller concluded that the evidence from randomized controlled trials evaluating the effectiveness of routine multimodality respiratory physiotherapy is still conflicting [88]. In the following paragraphs the physiotherapy treatment will be discussed in different clinical conditions.

26.6.1 Prevention of Post-Operative Pulmonary Complications

The majority of patients undergoing major thoracic or abdominal surgery recover without complications. Preoperative physiotherapy, including inspiratory muscle training, in cardiac surgery patients with an increased risk profile reduced the development of post-operative pulmonary complications [89]. After routine cardiac surgery, optimal post-operative management includes early mobilization and body positioning [90].

Further prophylactic physiotherapy interventions are not required in uncomplicated patients [91] or during (short time) intubation and mechanical ventilation [41, 92] . Early mobilization and upright body positioning after major surgery is of primary importance to increase lung volume and to prevent pulmonary complications. Routine breathing exercises should not be used following uncomplicated coronary artery bypass surgery. Perioperative physiotherapy should be instituted if warranted, e.g. in high risk patients, rather than administered routinely. Two randomized controlled studies have provided strong evidence that supports the role of prophylactic physiotherapy in preventing pulmonary complications after upper abdominal surgery [93, 94]. However, a meta-analysis showed no added value of physiotherapy to the effectiveness of early mobilization in high risk patients after abdominal surgery [95].

Incentive spirometry (IS) and non-invasive ventilation (NIV) are frequently used in the post-operative setting. IS is used in the management of non-intubated patients to encourage lung volume recruitment, but has not been shown to be of added benefit (beyond physiotherapy, early mobilization and body position) in the routine management of post-operative patients [96, 97]. NIV has been used successfully to support patients following thoracotomy [98]. Continuous Positive Airway Pressure (CPAP) is effective in the treatment of atelectasis, since it increases FRC and improves compliance, minimizing post-operative airways collapse. NIV has been shown superior to CPAP in the treatment of atelectasis in patients after cardiac surgery [99].

26.6.2 Retained Airway Secretions and Atelectasis

Figure 26.3 provides an overview of pathways and treatment modalities for increasing airway clearance. Interventions aimed at increasing inspiratory volume (deep breathing exercises, mobilization and body positioning) may affect lung expansion, increase regional ventilation, reduce airway resistance and optimize pulmonary

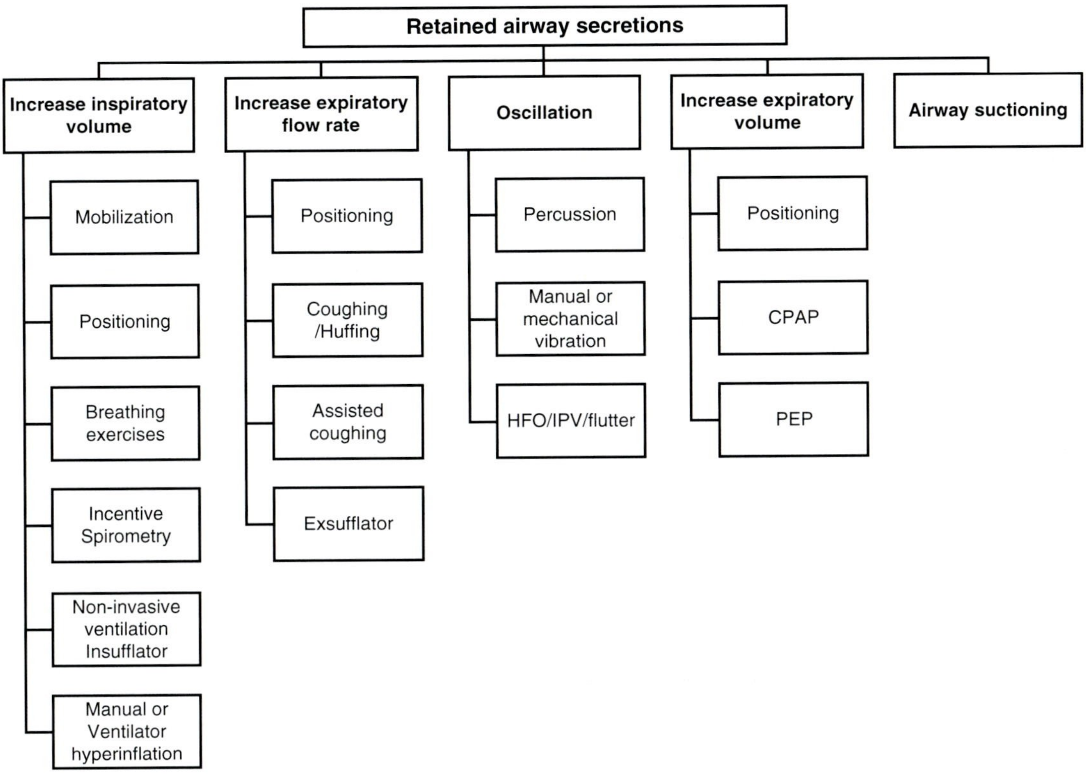

Fig. 26.3 Pathways and treatment modalities for enhancing airway clearance. *PEP* positive expiratory pressure, *CPAP* continuous positive airway pressure; *HFO* high frequency oscillation, *IPV* intrapulmonary percussive ventilation, *NIV* non-invasive ventilation, *IPPB* intermittent positive pressure breathing

compliance. Interventions aimed at increasing expiratory flow include forced expirations (huffing and coughing). Manually assisted cough, using thoracic or abdominal compression may be indicated for patients with expiratory muscle weakness or fatigue [48].

The mechanical in- and exsufflator can be used to deliver an inspiratory pressure followed by a high negative expiratory force, via a mouthpiece or facemask. It has been applied in the management of neuromuscular patients with retained secretions secondary to respiratory muscle weakness with variable success [100], but was successful in difficult to wean neuromuscular patients undergoing NIV [101]. Airway suctioning is used solely to clear central secretions that are considered a primary problem when other techniques are ineffective. Treatment of acute lobar atelectasis and airway clearance should incorporate body positioning and techniques to increase inspiratory volume and enhance forced expiration [40]. Chest wall vibration provided no additional benefit in these conditions. Low quality research has shown CPAP to be effective in the treatment of atelectasis [102].

26.6.3 Mechanically Ventilated Patients

In intubated and ventilated patients manual hyperinflation (MHI) or ventilator hyperinflation, by positive end-expiratory pressure ventilation, postural drainage, chest wall compression and airway suctioning may assist in secretion clearance. The aims of MHI are to prevent pulmonary atelectasis, re-expand collapsed alveola [103], improve oxygenation [104] and lung compliance [103], and facilitate movement of airway secretions towards the central airways [105].

MHI involves a slow deep inspiration with manual resuscitator bag, an inspiratory hold of 2–3 s [106], followed by a quick release of the bag to enhance expiratory flow and mimic a forced expiration. However, MHI might also have important negative side effects. First, MHI can precipitate marked hemodynamic changes associated with a decreased cardiac output, which result from large fluctuations in intra-thoracic pressure [107]. Second, MHI can also increase intracranial pressure, which might have implications for patients with brain injury. This increase is, however, usually limited such that cerebral perfusion pressure remains stable [57]; a pressure of 40 cmH_2O has been recommended as an upper limit.

Two studies in ventilated patients reported that bronchoscopy offered no additional benefit over physiotherapy (postural drainage, percussion, manual hyperinflation and suctioning) in the management of acute lobar atelectasis [58, 59].

Airway suctioning may have detrimental side effects (bronchial lesions, hypoxaemia), but reassurance, sedation, and pre-oxygenation of the patient may minimize these consequences [60]. Suctioning can be performed via an in-line closed system or an open system. The in-line system increased the costs, but did not decrease the incidence of ventilator-associated pneumonia (VAP) nor the duration of mechanical ventilation, and length of ICU stay or mortality [61]. Closed suctioning may be less effective than open suctioning for secretion clearance during pressure support ventilation [62]. The routine instillation of normal saline during airway suctioning has potential adverse effects on oxygen saturation and cardiovascular stability, and variable results in terms of increasing sputum yield [63]. Chest wall compression prior to endotracheal suctioning did not improve airway secretion removal, oxygenation, or ventilation after endotracheal suctioning in an unselected population of mechanically ventilated patients [64].

VAP is a common complication in mechanically ventilated patients and is associated with higher mortality rates, prolonged hospitalization, and high medical costs [65]. Studies have shown that avoidance of intubation with NIV reduces the incidence of nosocomial pneumonia in a subgroup of patients [66, 67]. Physiotherapy including manual hyperinflation, positioning plus suctioning, showed contrasting results in the incidence of VAP compared with no treatment [68–70].

26.6.4 Weaning and Respiratory Muscle Training

Fifteen to 20% of patients fails liberation from mechanical ventilation, but they require a disproportionate amount of resources. A spontaneous breathing trial can be used to assess readiness for extubation with the performance of serial measurements [108]. Early detection of worsening clinical signs such as distress, airway obstruction, and paradoxical chest wall motion, ensures that serious problems are prevented.

Airway patency and protection (i.e. an effective cough mechanism) should be assessed prior to commencement of weaning. Peak cough flow is a useful parameter to predict successful weaning in patients with neuromuscular disease or spinal cord injury when extubation is anticipated [109]. An 'airway care score' has been developed based on quality of the patient's cough during airway suctioning, the absence of 'excessive' secretions, and the frequency of airway suctioning [110].

Weaning failure has been extensively studied in the clinical literature and, several factors are likely to contribute to this. These factors include inadequate ventilatory drive, respiratory muscle weakness, respiratory muscle fatigue, increased work of breathing or cardiac failure [111]. The inability to breathe spontaneously relates to an imbalance between *load on* the respiratory muscles and the *capacity of* the respiratory muscles [112]. Respiratory muscle dysfunction in mechanically ventilated patients is observed in 80% of patients with ICUAW [113], showing a decline in transdiaphragmatic pressure by approximately 2–4% per day in the first weeks of ICU stay [15]. A rapid decline in diaphragm muscle strength is associated with sepsis [16].

There is accumulating evidence that weaning problems are associated with failure of the respiratory muscles to resume ventilation [114]. Indeed, high rates of respiratory muscle effort (ratio of workload and muscle capacity (P_I/P_{Imax})) are major cause of ventilator dependency and predict the outcome of successful weaning [114]. Since *in*activity contributes considerably to muscle atrophy: 'mechanical silencing' has been identified as an important contributor to the loss of contractile properties [66]. A lower contractile activity of the diaphragm during mechanical ventilation was associated with further reduction of diaphragm thickness [57]. This observation supports the idea that well-balanced intermittent loading of the respiratory muscles during the process of mechanical ventilation might be beneficial to prevent or ameliorate muscle atrophy. Indeed, modalities inducing (intermittent) loading of the respiratory muscles such as spontaneous breathing trials and early mobilization have been shown to increase muscle strength [115] and to shorten the duration of mechanical ventilation [33], respectively.

In patients at risk for failing the weaning process, *unloading* of the respiratory muscles with non-invasive ventilation has been shown successful [116]. Surprisingly, little attention has been given to specific interventions to enhance strength and endurance of the respiratory muscles [117]. Indeed, daily intermittent inspiratory loading with 6–8 contractions repeated in 3–4 series at moderate to high intensity was safe, improved inspiratory muscle strength and success in patients with difficult weaning [118]. One of the challenges of these studies is that patients who might benefit from the intervention are oftentimes not sufficiently capable to collaborate during the training sessions. Biofeedback to display the breathing pattern has been shown to enhance weaning [119]. Voice and touch may be used to augment weaning success either by stimulation to improve ventilatory drive, or by reducing anxiety [120]. Environmental influences, such as ambulating with a portable ventilator have been shown to benefit attitudes and outlooks in long-term ventilator-dependent patients [121]. Alternatively in patients unable to cooperate with respiratory muscle training, intermittent electrical stimulation of the diaphragm through phrenic nerve pacing might be applied [122]. So far only studies in patients with spinal cord injury have been reported to support this concept [123].

References

1. Eisner MD, Thompson T, Hudson LD, Luce JM, Hayden D, Schoenfeld D, et al. Efficacy of low tidal volume ventilation in patients with different clinical risk factors for acute lung injury and the acute respiratory distress syndrome. Am J Respir Crit Care Med. 2001;164(2):231–6.
2. Kaukonen KM, Bailey M, Suzuki S, Pilcher D, Bellomo R. Mortality related to severe sepsis and septic shock among critically ill patients in Australia and New Zealand, 2000–2012. JAMA. 2014;311(13):1308–16.
3. Schaller SJ, Anstey M, Blobner M, Edrich T, Grabitz SD, Gradwohl-Matis I, et al. Early, goal-directed mobilisation in the surgical intensive care unit: a randomised controlled trial. Lancet. 2016;388(10052):1377–88.
4. Herridge MS. Recovery and long-term outcome in acute respiratory distress syndrome. Crit Care Clin. 2011;27(3):685–704.
5. Borges RC, Carvalho CR, Colombo AS, da Silva Borges MP, Soriano FG. Physical activity, muscle strength, and exercise capacity 3 months after severe sepsis and septic shock. Intensive Care Med. 2015;41(8):1433–44.
6. Hermans G, Van Mechelen H, Clerckx B, Vanhullebusch T, Mesotten D, Wilmer A, et al. Acute outcomes and 1-year mortality of intensive care unit-acquired weakness. A cohort study and propensity-matched analysis. Am J Respir Crit Care Med. 2014;190(4):410–20.
7. Wieske L, Dettling-Ihnenfeldt DS, Verhamme C, Nollet F, van Schaik IN, Schultz MJ, et al. Impact of ICU-acquired weakness on post-ICU physical functioning: a follow-up study. Crit Care. 2015;19:196.
8. Convertino VA. Value of orthostatic stress in maintaining functional status soon after myocardial infarction or cardiac artery bypass grafting. J Cardiovasc Nurs. 2003;18(2):124–30.
9. Dittmer DK, Teasell R. Complications of immobilization and bed rest. Part 1: Musculoskeletal and cardiovascular complications. Can Fam Physician. 1993;39:1428–32. 35-7
10. Teasell R, Dittmer DK. Complications of immobilization and bed rest. Part 2: other complications. Can Fam Physician. 1993;39:1440–2. 5-6
11. Parry SM, Puthucheary ZA. The impact of extended bed rest on the musculoskeletal system in the critical care environment. Extrem Physiol Med. 2015;4:16.

12. Gruther W, Benesch T, Zorn C, Paternostro-Sluga T, Quittan M, Fialka-Moser V, et al. Muscle wasting in intensive care patients: ultrasound observation of the M. Quadriceps femoris muscle layer. J Rehabil Med. 2008;40(3):185–9.
13. Puthucheary ZA, Rawal J, McPhail M, Connolly B, Ratnayake G, Chan P, et al. Acute skeletal muscle wasting in critical illness. JAMA. 2013;310(15):1591–600.
14. Segers J, Hermans G, Charususin N, Fivez T, Vanhorebeek I, Van den Berghe G, et al. Assessment of quadriceps muscle mass with ultrasound in critically ill patients: intra- and inter-observer agreement and sensitivity. Intensive Care Med. 2015;41(3):562–3.
15. Hermans G, Agten A, Testelmans D, Decramer M, Gayan-Ramirez G. Increased duration of mechanical ventilation is associated with decreased diaphragmatic force: a prospective observational study. Crit Care. 2010;14(4):R127.
16. De Jonghe B, Bastuji-Garin S, Durand MC, Malissin I, Rodrigues P, Cerf C, et al. Respiratory weakness is associated with limb weakness and delayed weaning in critical illness. Crit Care Med. 2007;35(9):2007–15.
17. Ali NA, O'Brien JM Jr, Hoffmann SP, Phillips G, Garland A, Finley JC, et al. Acquired weakness, handgrip strength, and mortality in critically ill patients. Am J Respir Crit Care Med. 2008;178(3): 261–8.
18. Marchioni A, Fantini R, Antenora F, Clini E, Fabbri L. Chronic critical illness: the price of survival. Eur J Clin Invest. 2015;45(12):1341–9.
19. Rehabilitation After Critical Illness. National Institute for Health and Clinical Excellence: Guidance. London: Rehabilitation After Critical Illness; 2009.
20. Major ME, Kwakman R, Kho ME, Connolly B, McWilliams D, Denehy L, et al. Surviving critical illness: what is next? An expert consensus statement on physical rehabilitation after hospital discharge. Crit Care. 2016;20(1):354.
21. Hodgson CL, Turnbull AE, Iwashyna TJ, Parker A, Davis W, Bingham CO 3rd, et al. Core domains in evaluating patient outcomes after acute respiratory failure: international multidisciplinary clinician consultation. Phys Ther. 2017;97(2):168–74.
22. Corrado A, Roussos C, Ambrosino N, Confalonieri M, Cuvelier A, Elliott M, et al. Respiratory intermediate care units: a European survey. Eur Respir J. 2002;20(5):1343–50.
23. Jolley SE, Moss M, Needham DM, Caldwell E, Morris PE, Miller RR, et al. Point prevalence study of mobilization practices for acute respiratory failure patients in the United States. Crit Care Med. 2017;45(2):205–15.
24. Bakhru RN, Wiebe DJ, McWilliams DJ, Spuhler VJ, Schweickert WD. An environmental scan for early mobilization practices in U.S. ICUs. Crit Care Med. 2015;43(11):2360–9.
25. Koo KK, Choong K, Cook DJ, Herridge M, Newman A, Lo V, et al. Early mobilization of critically ill adults: a survey of knowledge, perceptions and practices of Canadian physicians and physiotherapists. CMAJ Open. 2016;4(3):E448–54.
26. Harrold ME, Salisbury LG, Webb SA, Allison GT, Australia, Scotland ICUPC. Early mobilisation in intensive care units in Australia and Scotland: a prospective, observational cohort study examining mobilisation practises and barriers. Crit Care. 2015;19:336.
27. Bourdin G, Barbier J, Burle JF, Durante G, Passant S, Vincent B, et al. The feasibility of early physical activity in intensive care unit patients: a prospective observational one-center study. Respir Care. 2010;55(4):400–7.
28. Thomsen GE, Snow GL, Rodriguez L, Hopkins RO. Patients with respiratory failure increase ambulation after transfer to an intensive care unit where early activity is a priority. Crit Care Med. 2008;36(4):1119–24.
29. Martin UJ, Hincapie L, Nimchuk M, Gaughan J, Criner GJ. Impact of whole-body rehabilitation in patients receiving chronic mechanical ventilation. Crit Care Med. 2005;33(10):2259–65.
30. Nava S. Rehabilitation of patients admitted to a respiratory intensive care unit. Arch Phys Med Rehabil. 1998;79(7):849–54.
31. Hodgson CL, Stiller K, Needham DM, Tipping CJ, Harrold M, Baldwin CE, et al. Expert consensus and recommendations on safety criteria for active mobilization of mechanically ventilated critically ill adults. Crit Care. 2014;18(6):658.
32. Bailey P, Thomsen GE, Spuhler VJ, Blair R, Jewkes J, Bezdjian L, et al. Early activity is feasible and safe in respiratory failure patients. Crit Care Med. 2007;35(1):139–45.
33. Schweickert WD, Pohlman MC, Pohlman AS, Nigos C, Pawlik AJ, Esbrook CL, et al. Early physical and occupational therapy in mechanically ventilated, critically ill patients: a randomised controlled trial. Lancet. 2009;373(9678):1874–82.
34. Morris PE, Goad A, Thompson C, Taylor K, Harry B, Passmore L, et al. Early intensive care unit mobility therapy in the treatment of acute respiratory failure. Crit Care Med. 2008;36(8):2238–43.
35. Burtin C, Clerckx B, Robbeets C, Ferdinande P, Langer D, Troosters T, et al. Early exercise in critically ill patients enhances short-term functional recovery. Crit Care Med. 2009;37(9):2499–505.
36. Chiang LL, Wang LY, Wu CP, Wu HD, Wu YT. Effects of physical training on functional status in patients with prolonged mechanical ventilation. Phys Ther. 2006;86(9):1271–81.
37. Ambrosino N, Venturelli E, Vagheggini G, Clini E. Rehabilitation, weaning and physical therapy strategies in chronic critically ill patients. Eur Respir J. 2012;39(2):487–92.
38. Dock W. The evil sequelae of complete bed rest. JAMA. 1944;125:5.

39. Dripps RWW, R.M. Nursing care of surgical patients. Am J Nurs. 1941;41:4.
40. Gosselink R, Bott J, Johnson M, Dean E, Nava S, Norrenberg M, et al. Physiotherapy for adult patients with critical illness: recommendations of the European Respiratory Society and European Society of Intensive Care Medicine Task Force on Physiotherapy For Critically Ill Patients. Intensive Care Med. 2008;34(7):1188–99.
41. Castro-Avila AC, Seron P, Fan E, Gaete M, Mickan S. Effect of early rehabilitation during intensive care unit stay on functional status: systematic review and meta-analysis. PLoS One. 2015;10(7):e0130722.
42. Connolly B, O'Neill B, Salisbury L, Blackwood B. Enhanced recovery after critical illness Programme G. Physical rehabilitation interventions for adult patients during critical illness: an overview of systematic reviews. Thorax. 2016;71(10):881–90.
43. Stiller K. Safety issues that should be considered when mobilizing critically ill patients. Crit Care Clin. 2007;23(1):35–53.
44. Parry SM, Granger CL, Berney S, Jones J, Beach L, El-Ansary D, et al. Assessment of impairment and activity limitations in the critically ill: a systematic review of measurement instruments and their clinimetric properties. Intensive Care Med. 2015;41(5):744–62.
45. Fergusson D, Hutton B, Drodge A. The epidemiology of major joint contractures: a systematic review of the literature. Clin Orthop Relat Res. 2007;456:22–9.
46. Clavet H, Hebert PC, Fergusson D, Doucette S, Trudel G. Joint contracture following prolonged stay in the intensive care unit. CMAJ. 2008;178(6):691–7.
47. Hermans G, Clerckx B, Vanhullebusch T, Segers J, Vanpee G, Robbeets C, et al. Interobserver agreement of Medical Research Council sum-score and handgrip strength in the intensive care unit. Muscle Nerve. 2012;45(1):18–25.
48. De Jonghe B, Sharshar T, Lefaucheur JP, Authier FJ, Durand-Zaleski I, Boussarsar M, et al. Paresis acquired in the intensive care unit: a prospective multicenter study. JAMA. 2002;288(22):2859–67.
49. Fan E, Cheek F, Chlan L, Gosselink R, Hart N, Herridge MS, et al. An official American Thoracic Society Clinical Practice Guideline: the diagnosis of intensive care unit-acquired weakness in adults. Am J Respir Crit Care Med. 2014;190(12):1437–46.
50. Bohannon RW. Norm references are essential if therapists are to correctly identify individuals who have physical limitations. J Orthop Sports Phys Ther. 2005;35(6):388.
51. Mathiowetz V, Kashman N, Volland G, Weber K, Dowe M, Rogers S. Grip and pinch strength: normative data for adults. Arch Phys Med Rehabil. 1985;66(2):69–74.
52. Vanpee G, Segers J, Van Mechelen H, Wouters P, Van den Berghe G, Hermans G, et al. The interobserver agreement of handheld dynamometry for muscle strength assessment in critically ill patients. Crit Care Med. 2011;39(8):1929–34.
53. Bohannon RW. Reference values for extremity muscle strength obtained by hand-held dynamometry from adults aged 20–79 years. Arch Phys Med Rehabil. 1997;78(1):26–32.
54. Allen GM, Gandevia SC, McKenzie DK. Reliability of measurements of muscle strength and voluntary activation using twitch interpolation. Muscle Nerve. 1995;18(6):593–600.
55. American Thoracic Society/European Respiratory Society. ATS/ERS Statement on respiratory muscle testing. Am J Respir Crit Care Med. 2002;166(4):518–624.
56. Marini JJ, Smith TC, Lamb V. Estimation of inspiratory muscle strength in mechanically ventilated patients: the measurement of maximal inspiratory pressure. J Crit Care. 1986;1:6.
57. Goligher EC, Fan E, Herridge MS, Murray A, Vorona S, Brace D, et al. Evolution of diaphragm thickness during mechanical ventilation. Impact of inspiratory effort. Am J Respir Crit Care Med. 2015;192(9):1080–8.
58. Fantini R, Mandrioli J, Zona S, Antenora F, Iattoni A, Monelli M, et al. Ultrasound assessment of diaphragmatic function in patients with amyotrophic lateral sclerosis. Respirology. 2016;21(5):932–8.
59. Parry SM, Denehy L, Beach LJ, Berney S, Williamson HC, Granger CL. Functional outcomes in ICU—what should we be using? An observational study. Crit Care. 2015;19:127.
60. Chan KS, Aronson Friedman L, Dinglas VD, Hough CL, Morris PE, Mendez-Tellez PA, et al. Evaluating physical outcomes in acute respiratory distress syndrome survivors: validity, responsiveness, and minimal important difference of 4-meter gait speed test. Crit Care Med. 2016;44(5):859–68.
61. Singh SJ, Puhan MA, Andrianopoulos V, Hernandes NA, Mitchell KE, Hill CJ, et al. An official systematic review of the European Respiratory Society/American Thoracic Society: measurement properties of field walking tests in chronic respiratory disease. Eur Respir J. 2014;44(6):1447–78.
62. Herridge MS, Tansey CM, Matte A, Tomlinson G, Diaz-Granados N, Cooper A, et al. Functional disability 5 years after acute respiratory distress syndrome. N Engl J Med. 2011;364(14):1293–304.
63. Gosselink R, Clerckx B, Robbeets C, Vanhullenbusch T, Vanpee G, Segers J. Physiotherapy in the intensive care unit. Neth J Int Care. 2011;15:9.
64. Fink MP, Helsmoortel CM, Stein KL, Lee PC, Cohn SM. The efficacy of an oscillating bed in the prevention of lower respiratory tract infection in critically ill victims of blunt trauma. A prospective study. Chest. 1990;97(1):132–7.
65. Friedrich O, Reid MB, Van den Berghe G, Vanhorebeek I, Hermans G, Rich MM, et al. The sick and the weak: neuropathies/myopathies in the critically ill. Physiol Rev. 2015;95(3):1025–109.

66. Llano-Diez M, Renaud G, Andersson M, Marrero HG, Cacciani N, Engquist H, et al. Mechanisms underlying ICU muscle wasting and effects of passive mechanical loading. Crit Care. 2012;16(1):R209.
67. Griffiths RD, Palmer TE, Helliwell T, MacLennan P, MacMillan RR. Effect of passive stretching on the wasting of muscle in the critically ill. Nutrition. 1995;11(5):428–32.
68. Williams PE. Use of intermittent stretch in the prevention of serial sarcomere loss in immobilised muscle. Ann Rheum Dis. 1990;49(5):316–7.
69. Kwan MW, Ha KW. Splinting programme for patients with burnt hand. Hand Surg. 2002;7(2):231–41.
70. Hinderer SR, Dixon K. Physiologic and clinical monitoring of spastic hypertonia. Phys Med Rehabil Clin N Am. 2001;12(4):733–46.
71. Clini EM, Crisafulli E, Antoni FD, Beneventi C, Trianni L, Costi S, et al. Functional recovery following physical training in tracheotomized and chronically ventilated patients. Respir Care. 2011;56(3):306–13.
72. Camargo Pires-Neto R, Fogaca Kawaguchi YM, Sayuri Hirota A, Fu C, Tanaka C, Caruso P, et al. Very early passive cycling exercise in mechanically ventilated critically ill patients: physiological and safety aspects--a case series. PLoS One. 2013;8(9):e74182.
73. Thelandersson A, Nellgard B, Ricksten SE, Cider A. Effects of early bedside cycle exercise on intracranial pressure and systemic hemodynamics in critically Ill patients in a neurointensive care unit. Neurocrit Care. 2016;25(3):434–9.
74. Gibson JN, Smith K, Rennie MJ. Prevention of disuse muscle atrophy by means of electrical stimulation: maintenance of protein synthesis. Lancet. 1988;2(8614):767–70.
75. Strasser EM, Stattner S, Karner J, Klimpfinger M, Freynhofer M, Zaller V, et al. Neuromuscular electrical stimulation reduces skeletal muscle protein degradation and stimulates insulin-like growth factors in an age- and current-dependent manner: a randomized, controlled clinical trial in major abdominal surgical patients. Ann Surg. 2009;249(5):738–43.
76. Williams N, Flynn M. A review of the efficacy of neuromuscular electrical stimulation in critically ill patients. Physiother Theory Pract. 2014;30(1):6–11.
77. Maffiuletti NA, Roig M, Karatzanos E, Nanas S. Neuromuscular electrical stimulation for preventing skeletal-muscle weakness and wasting in critically ill patients: a systematic review. BMC Med. 2013;11:137.
78. Segers J, Hermans G, Bruyninckx F, Meyfroidt G, Langer D, Gosselink R. Feasibility of neuromuscular electrical stimulation in critically ill patients. J Crit Care. 2014;29(6):1082–8.
79. Zanotti E, Felicetti G, Maini M, Fracchia C. Peripheral muscle strength training in bed-bound patients with COPD receiving mechanical ventilation: effect of electrical stimulation. Chest. 2003;124(1):292–6.
80. Perme C, Chandrashekar R. Early mobility and walking program for patients in intensive care units: creating a standard of care. Am J Crit Care. 2009;18(3):212–21.
81. Needham DM. Mobilizing patients in the intensive care unit: improving neuromuscular weakness and physical function. JAMA. 2008;300(14):1685–90.
82. Probst VS, Troosters T, Coosemans I, Spruit MA, Pitta Fde O, Decramer M, et al. Mechanisms of improvement in exercise capacity using a rollator in patients with COPD. Chest. 2004;126(4):1102–7.
83. Chang AT, Boots R, Hodges PW, Paratz J. Standing with assistance of a tilt table in intensive care: a survey of Australian physiotherapy practice. Aust J Physiother. 2004;50(1):51–4.
84. Goldman JM, Rose LS, Williams SJ, Silver JR, Denison DM. Effect of abdominal binders on breathing in tetraplegic patients. Thorax. 1986;41(12):940–5.
85. van 't Hul A, Gosselink R, Hollander P, Postmus P, Kwakkel G. Acute effects of inspiratory pressure support during exercise in patients with COPD. Eur Respir J. 2004;23(1):34–40.
86. Porta R, Vitacca M, Gile LS, Clini E, Bianchi L, Zanotti E, et al. Supported arm training in patients recently weaned from mechanical ventilation. Chest. 2005;128(4):2511–20.
87. Vogiatzis I, Nanas S, Roussos C. Interval training as an alternative modality to continuous exercise in patients with COPD. Eur Respir J. 2002;20(1):12–9.
88. Stiller K. Physiotherapy in intensive care: an updated systematic review. Chest. 2013;144(3):825–47.
89. Hulzebos EH, Helders PJ, Favie NJ, De Bie RA, Brutel de la Riviere A, van Meeteren NL. Preoperative intensive inspiratory muscle training to prevent postoperative pulmonary complications in high-risk patients undergoing CABG surgery: a randomized clinical trial. JAMA. 2006;296(15):1851–7.
90. Jenkins SC, Soutar SA, Loukota JM, Johnson LC, Moxham J. Physiotherapy after coronary artery surgery: are breathing exercises necessary? Thorax. 1989;44(8):634–9.
91. Pasquina P, Tramer MR, Walder B. Prophylactic respiratory physiotherapy after cardiac surgery: systematic review. BMJ. 2003;327(7428):1379.
92. Patman S, Sanderson D, Blackmore M. Physiotherapy following cardiac surgery: is it necessary during the intubation period? Aust J Physiother. 2001;47(1):7–16.
93. Celli BR, Rodriguez KS, Snider GL. A controlled trial of intermittent positive pressure breathing, incentive spirometry, and deep breathing exercises in preventing pulmonary complications after abdominal surgery. Am Rev Respir Dis. 1984;130(1):12–5.
94. Roukema JA, Carol EJ, Prins JG. The prevention of pulmonary complications after upper abdominal surgery in patients with noncompromised pulmonary status. Arch Surg. 1988;123(1):30–4.
95. Pasquina P, Tramer MR, Granier JM, Walder B. Respiratory physiotherapy to prevent pulmonary

complications after abdominal surgery: a systematic review. Chest. 2006;130(6):1887–99.
96. Overend TJ, Anderson CM, Lucy SD, Bhatia C, Jonsson BI, Timmermans C. The effect of incentive spirometry on postoperative pulmonary complications: a systematic review. Chest. 2001;120(3):971–8.
97. Gosselink R, Schrever K, Cops P, Witvrouwen H, De Leyn P, Troosters T, et al. Incentive spirometry does not enhance recovery after thoracic surgery. Crit Care Med. 2000;28(3):679–83.
98. Aguilo R, Togores B, Pons S, Rubi M, Barbe F, Agusti AG. Noninvasive ventilatory support after lung resectional surgery. Chest. 1997;112(1):117–21.
99. Pasquina P, Merlani P, Granier JM, Ricou B. Continuous positive airway pressure versus noninvasive pressure support ventilation to treat atelectasis after cardiac surgery. Anesth Analg. 2004;99(4):1001–8.
100. Morrow B, Zampoli M, van Aswegen H, Argent A. Mechanical insufflation-exsufflation for people with neuromuscular disorders. Cochrane Database Syst Rev. 2013;12:CD010044.
101. Bach JR, Sinquee DM, Saporito LR, Botticello AL. Efficacy of mechanical insufflation-exsufflation in extubating unweanable subjects with restrictive pulmonary disorders. Respir Care. 2015;60(4):477–83.
102. Ireland CJ, Chapman TM, Mathew SF, Herbison GP, Zacharias M. Continuous positive airway pressure (CPAP) during the postoperative period for prevention of postoperative morbidity and mortality following major abdominal surgery. Cochrane Database Syst Rev. 2014;8:CD008930.
103. Hodgson C, Denehy L, Ntoumenopoulos G, Santamaria J, Carroll S. An investigation of the early effects of manual lung hyperinflation in critically ill patients. Anaesth Intensive Care. 2000;28(3):255–61.
104. Patman S, Jenkins S, Stiller K. Manual hyperinflation—effects on respiratory parameters. Physiother Res Int. 2000;5(3):157–71.
105. Hodgson C, Ntoumenopoulos G, Dawson H, Paratz J. The Mapleson C circuit clears more secretions than the Laerdal circuit during manual hyperinflation in mechanically-ventilated patients: a randomised cross-over trial. Aust J Physiother. 2007;53(1):33–8.
106. Albert SP, DiRocco J, Allen GB, Bates JH, Lafollette R, Kubiak BD, et al. The role of time and pressure on alveolar recruitment. J Appl Physiol (1985). 2009;106(3):757–65.
107. Singer M, Vermaat J, Hall G, Latter G, Patel M. Hemodynamic effects of manual hyperinflation in critically ill mechanically ventilated patients. Chest. 1994;106(4):1182–7.
108. Yang KL, Tobin MJ. A prospective study of indexes predicting the outcome of trials of weaning from mechanical ventilation. N Engl J Med. 1991;324(21):1445–50.
109. Bach JR, Saporito LR. Criteria for extubation and tracheostomy tube removal for patients with ventilatory failure. A different approach to weaning. Chest. 1996;110(6):1566–71.
110. Ely EW, Baker AM, Dunagan DP, Burke HL, Smith AC, Kelly PT, et al. Effect on the duration of mechanical ventilation of identifying patients capable of breathing spontaneously. N Engl J Med. 1996;335(25):1864–9.
111. Penuelas O, Frutos-Vivar F, Fernandez C, Anzueto A, Epstein SK, Apezteguia C, et al. Characteristics and outcomes of ventilated patients according to time to liberation from mechanical ventilation. Am J Respir Crit Care Med. 2011;184(4):430–7.
112. Goldstone J, Moxham J. Assisted ventilation. 4. Weaning from mechanical ventilation. Thorax. 1991;46(1):56–62.
113. Jung B, Moury PH, Mahul M, de Jong A, Galia F, Prades A, et al. Diaphragmatic dysfunction in patients with ICU-acquired weakness and its impact on extubation failure. Intensive Care Med. 2016;42(5):853–61.
114. Vassilakopoulos T, Zakynthinos S, Roussos C. The tension-time index and the frequency/tidal volume ratio are the major pathophysiologic determinants of weaning failure and success. Am J Respir Crit Care Med. 1998;158(2):378–85.
115. Gayan-Ramirez G, Testelmans D, Maes K, Racz GZ, Cadot P, Zador E, et al. Intermittent spontaneous breathing protects the rat diaphragm from mechanical ventilation effects. Crit Care Med. 2005;33(12):2804–9.
116. Nava S, Gregoretti C, Fanfulla F, Squadrone E, Grassi M, Carlucci A, et al. Noninvasive ventilation to prevent respiratory failure after extubation in high-risk patients. Crit Care Med. 2005;33(11):2465–70.
117. Gosselink R, Langer D. Recovery from ICU-acquired weakness; do not forget the respiratory muscles! Thorax. 2016;71(9):779–80.
118. Elkins M, Dentice R. Inspiratory muscle training facilitates weaning from mechanical ventilation among patients in the intensive care unit: a systematic review. J Physiother. 2015;61(3):125–34.
119. Holliday JE, Hyers TM. The reduction of weaning time from mechanical ventilation using tidal volume and relaxation biofeedback. Am Rev Respir Dis. 1990;141(5 Pt 1):1214–20.
120. Hall JB, Wood LD. Liberation of the patient from mechanical ventilation. JAMA. 1987;257(12):1621–8.
121. Esteban A, Alia I, Ibanez J, Benito S, Tobin MJ. Modes of mechanical ventilation and weaning. A national survey of Spanish hospitals. The Spanish Lung Failure Collaborative Group. Chest. 1994;106(4):1188–93.
122. Pavlovic D, Wendt M. Diaphragm pacing during prolonged mechanical ventilation of the lungs could prevent from respiratory muscle fatigue. Med Hypotheses. 2003;60(3):398–403.
123. DiMarco AF, Onders RP, Ignagni A, Kowalski KE. Inspiratory muscle pacing in spinal cord injury: case report and clinical commentary. J Spinal Cord Med. 2006;29(2):95–108.

27 Cystic Fibrosis

Thomas Radtke, Susi Kriemler,
and Helge Hebestreit

27.1 Settings of Pulmonary Rehabilitation

In general, pulmonary rehabilitation in CF is offered for inpatients and outpatients. The inpatient setting includes acute care hospitals and rehabilitation hospitals. The latter are more common in some countries than in others and provide a 3–4 weeks multicomponent rehabilitation program consisting of medical support, nutritional and psychological counseling, and exercise training. While pulmonary rehabilitation during acute hospital stays is usually done on an individual basis allowing for targeted therapy and optimal infection control, rehabilitation hospitals can often provide a more intense rehabilitation for selected groups of patients at a very high level of expertise. Furthermore, specific climatic conditions such as warm and dry weather in winter and/or high barometric pressure with increased salt content may support the success of the rehabilitation. One challenge in this setting is to select the patients based on the pathogens present in their airways. Despite sputum examinations and stringent selection criteria prior to the rehabilitation, some patients are tested positive for a pathogen at the beginning of the rehabilitation, which has not been identified in this patient before. In such a case, the patient cannot be included in the planned rehabilitation program. And even with all these measures in place, patient-to-patient transmission of pathogens cannot be completely excluded but can be minimized with proper infection control measures [1].

Pulmonary rehabilitation in an outpatient setting is usually conducted near home on an individual basis and includes physical therapy with focus on airway clearance and thorax mobilization, and an exercise program.

Although discouraged by the Infection Prevention and Control Guideline for CF [2], some patient organizations still provide settings which combine some aspects of a structured rehabilitation program as in specialized hospitals and an outpatient setting by organized trips for people with CF, for example, to the Canary Islands. The patients are accommodated in individual apartments or hotel rooms and participate in both group sessions and individual therapies.

T. Radtke • S. Kriemler
Epidemiology, Biostatistics and Prevention Institute, University of Zürich, Zurich, Switzerland

H. Hebestreit (✉)
Paediatric Department, Julius-Maximilians University Würzburg, Wuerzburg, Germany

© Springer International Publishing AG 2018
E. Clini et al. (eds.), *Textbook of Pulmonary Rehabilitation*,
https://doi.org/10.1007/978-3-319-65888-9_27

27.2 Infection Control

Several reports highlight the importance of infection control during pulmonary rehabilitation in CF [3, 4]. The Infection Prevention and Control guideline of the Cystic Fibrosis Foundation [2] contains many recommendations which apply to pulmonary rehabilitation such as education of all health care professionals and people with CF about infection control, hand hygiene for both groups, face masks for all patients in the health care setting, a 6 foot (2 m) distance between patients, proper disinfection of testing and rehabilitation equipment, etc. With respect to some rehabilitation settings, the statements are even more restrictive: "The CF Foundation recommends against CF-specific camps or CF-specific educational retreats for groups of people with CF. In other words, only one individual with CF should attend any camp or educational retreat unless they live in the same household" [2]. However, recent studies indicate that educational programs in a hospital setting with repeated group sessions among children and adolescents with CF may not be associated with transmission of bacteria [5], and the benefits of educational and rehabilitation programs are documented in the literature [6–8]. This ambiguous situation requires a careful benefit-harm assessment.

27.3 Components of Pulmonary Rehabilitation

27.3.1 Nutrition

Pulmonary rehabilitation is often used for nutritional counseling. In general, people with CF are slim or even suffer from underweight. A better nutritional status has long been associated with a better pulmonary condition [9] and aerobic fitness [10]. Thus, a nutrition rich in fat and calories combined with adequate supplementation of pancreatic enzymes and fat-soluble vitamins is generally recommended. However, an increasing number of patients are overweight or even obese [11, 12] who require different advice.

27.3.2 Airway Clearance

Several airway clearance techniques have been established for people with CF such as—for example—the active cycle of breathing technique, autogenic drainage, huffing, positive expiratory pressure therapy, and breathing with oscillating positive end-expiratory pressure devices like the Flutter®, Cornet®, or Acapella®. In general, there is no evidence to prefer one technique over the other [13]. However, compared to positive expiratory pressure therapy, high frequency chest wall oscillation appears to be less effective with respect to pulmonary exacerbation rates [14]. For an individual patient, the technique(s) selected depend on the actual pulmonary condition, individual experiences and preferences, and the experience of the therapist administering/teaching the technique.

In clinical practice, many patients—especially those with advanced lung disease and/or bronchial secretions—perform airway clearance before exercise. They claim that their performance is improved and dyspnea is reduced. However, others use airway clearance techniques after an exercise session to expectorate the secretions, which have been mobilized during the exercise session [15].

27.3.3 Psychosocial Support

Stress, anxiety, and depression are quite prevalent in CF [16] and can influence treatment adherence and health-related quality of life (HRQoL). Especially depression may interfere with the self-management in CF and can, thus, jeopardize the effects of a pulmonary rehabilitation program. On the other hand, pulmonary rehabilitation involving a group of patients may have psychosocial benefits. Although—to these authors' knowledge—no systematic study has been performed on this topic, patients report a boost of motivation from rehabilitation. Furthermore, using a tailored family oriented program, rehabilitation may also positively affect HRQoL of parents [17].

27.3.4 Exercise

27.3.4.1 Importance of Physical Activity and Fitness in CF

Physical activity and exercise training are accepted and integral components of CF health care. High levels of physical activity have been related to a better HRQoL [18], bone health [19], reduced hospital admissions and hospital days [20] and a slower pulmonary function decline over time [20, 21]. Furthermore, patients with higher physical activity levels have higher levels of aerobic exercise capacity [20, 22]. A high aerobic exercise capacity in CF is associated with a higher HRQoL [18], muscle strength [22], and a higher life expectancy [23–25]. Figure 27.1 shows the association between peak oxygen uptake (VO_2peak), a measure of aerobic fitness, and two selected HRQoL domains.

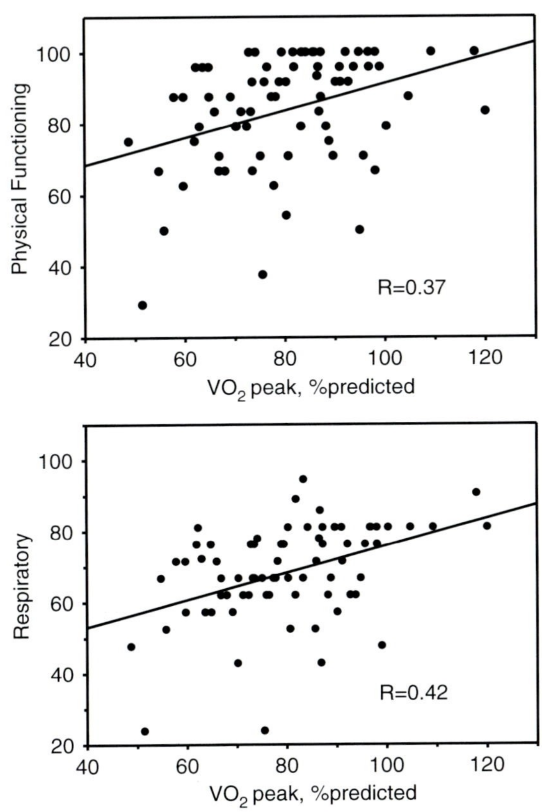

Fig. 27.1 Relationship between VO_2peak and the health-related quality of life domains "Physical Functioning" (**a**) and "Respiratory" (**b**) of the CFQ-R questionnaire. Data are from Hebestreit et al. [18]

27.3.4.2 Assessing Exercise Capacity

Prior to initiation of any exercise training, exercise testing is recommended to assess the physiological health of a patient, screen for exercise-related risks, and provide exercise training recommendations [26]. A statement on exercise testing including recommendations on the choice of exercise test, testing protocols, and interpretation has been recently published [26]. Exercise capacity can be assessed by simple field tests such as walking, step or shuttle tests or preferably a cardiopulmonary exercise test with analysis of expired gases using a cycle ergometer or treadmill. All tests have their advantages and disadvantages and the choice of the test should be clearly driven by the question and the aim of the test. The European Cystic Fibrosis Society Exercise Working Group recommends the Godfrey cycle ergometer protocol [27] with measurement of expired gases and monitoring of oxygen saturation in patients 10 years and older. Alternative tests include a cycle ergometer test using the Godfrey protocol with pulse oximetry but without measurements of gas exchange or a treadmill exercise test with gas exchange analysis and pulse oximetry [26].

27.3.4.3 Improving Physical Fitness

Much of the knowledge on the effects of exercise training on aerobic and anaerobic exercise capacity, muscle strength, and patient reported outcomes such as HRQoL has been derived from predominantly small observational and non-controlled studies. A Cochrane Database Systematic Review summarized findings from 13 randomized controlled trials including 402 patients on exercise capacity, lung function (forced expiratory volume in 1 s), and HRQoL. Although there was large heterogeneity among studies with respect to study duration (<1 months up to 3 years), disease severity, training modalities (aerobic, anaerobic, and combinations of both vs no training), and levels of supervision (fully supervised, partially supervised, and non-supervised training), the majority of longer-term training studies (≥1 month) showed improvements in aerobic exercise capacity (see Fig. 27.2) with unclear effects on FEV_1 and HRQoL.

Specific to the pulmonary rehabilitation setting, Gruber et al. [29] investigated an interval exercise-training program as part of a 6-week inpatient rehabilitation program. In this study, patients with CF and severe pulmonary function impairment ($FEV_1 \leq 40\%$ predicted) and unable to take part in the standard exercise training program received an individually adapted treadmill interval training (1:2 work-recovery ratio). After 6 weeks, submaximal and maximal exercise capacity improved significantly demonstrating that even patients with severe pulmonary function impairment can benefit from structured interval exercise training.

In some CF centers, structured exercise training is performed during hospitalization. In a study by Selvadurai et al. [30] children and adolescents (8–16 years) referred to the hospital for treatment of an infectious pulmonary exacerbation were randomized into an aerobic-training group, a resistance-training group or a control group. Children in the training groups received supervised training five times per week and the control group received standard treatment including chest physiotherapy and nutritional counseling. After hospital discharge, FEV_1 and body mass was improved in all three groups, the aerobic training group increased their VO_2peak (~22%) and HRQoL (~14%), and the resistance-training group improved their leg muscle strength (~18%). The effects were sustained 1 month after discharge.

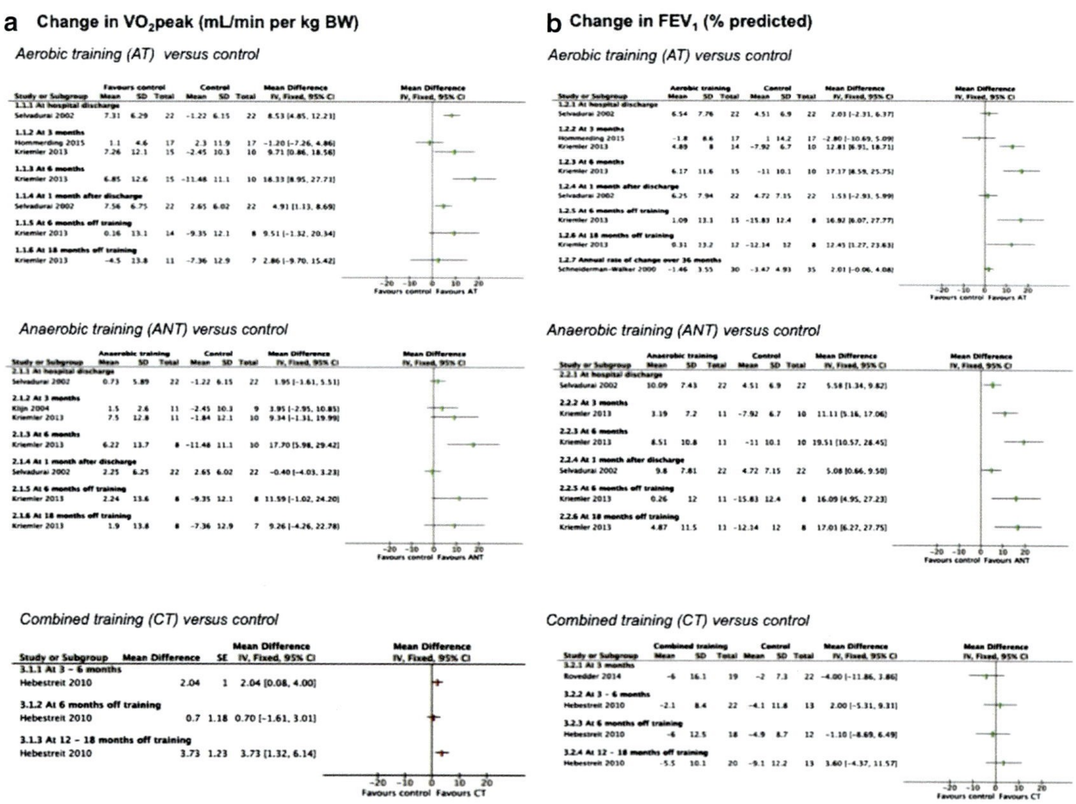

Fig 27.2 Comparison of aerobic training (*AT*) versus no physical training; anaerobic training (*ANT*) versus no physical training and combined training (*CT*) versus no physical training on peak oxygen uptake (VO_2 peak in mL/min per kg BW). *BW* body weight. Data are from Radtke et al. [28]

27.4 Special Considerations

27.4.1 Lung Transplantation

According to registry data of the International Society for Heart and Lung Transplantation (ISHLT), CF is the third most common indication for lung transplantation (LTx) and most effective in improving survival and HRQoL in end-stage lung disease. Lung transplant recipients with CF have reduced exercise capacity and habitual physical activity levels, a low lactate threshold, reduced systemic oxygen extraction and substantially impaired peripheral muscle strength [31–33]. In lung transplant recipients, several factors contribute to the impairment in muscle strength, for example, muscle fiber atrophy, changes in muscle fiber proportion from type I to type II due to long periods of immobilization, the use of immunosuppressives and corticosteroids and others [33, 34]. Peripheral muscle weakness, however, appears to be the major determinant for the reduced aerobic exercise capacity after LTx in CF [31]. A systematic review provided some evidence that structured exercise training has the potential to improve exercise capacity and muscle strength in lung transplant recipients including CF [35]. Exercise training, ideally a combination of endurance and resistance exercises, should be performed at least three times per week and should be tailored to the individual's exercise capacity. A 3-months structured exercise training program (3 times weekly for about 90 min) consisting of endurance and strengthening exercises has been shown to improve daily physical activity, 6-min walk test distance, muscle strength, and self-reported physical functioning [36]. In patients with severe pulmonary function impairment and substantial muscle deconditioning interval training is a feasible training modality. In contrast to continuous exercise training, interval training elicits less dyspnea and muscle fatigue in patients with chronic obstructive pulmonary disease and can be sustained for longer periods [37–39]. Ideally, exercise training should be started in a preoperative rehabilitation setting aiming to improve (or maintain) muscle strength, aerobic exercise capacity, and mobility to achieve a better starting point for LTx and to achieve a better postoperative outcome [40]. The training must be adapted to the individual's exercise capacity and adequate resting periods should be implemented to allow sufficient recovery between training stimuli. After LTx, early mobilization, physiotherapy, and individualized exercise training are essential. The long-term effects of exercise training programs on exercise capacity and patient-reported outcomes in lung transplant recipients require further studies.

27.4.2 Supplemental Oxygen/ Noninvasive Ventilation

Patients with moderate-to-severe CF may experience oxygen desaturation during exercise. The risk of oxygen desaturation, defined as oxygen saturation (SpO_2) below 90% may increase with increasing disease severity [41–43]. SpO_2 at peak exercise and during a formal hypoxic challenge is related to pulmonary function (e.g., FEV_1, forced vital capacity (FVC), the diffusion capacity of the lung for nitric oxide and carbon monoxide), body mass index, clinical and radiological scores, and resting SpO_2 [41–46]. However, none of the aforementioned studies could reliably predict oxygen desaturation during exercise from data collected at rest, and others have shown that even patients with an FEV_1 between 70 and 90% of the FVC demonstrate oxygen desaturation during cardiopulmonary exercise testing [43]. Consequently, patients should undergo (cardiopulmonary) exercise testing with pulse oximetry monitoring to accurately identify those with exercise induced oxygen desaturation [26].

Exercise-induced hypoxemia is associated with cardiac arrhythmias and it has been recommended that SpO_2 shall not drop below 90% during exercise in people with CF [47, 48]. In people who desaturate only at peak exercise intensities, a limitation of exercise intensity based on target heart rate, or interval training with sufficient recovery periods may be sufficient to prevent hypoxemia while still allowing for effective training stimuli [49].

Supplemental oxygen during exercise can also be useful in patients with oxygen desaturation and has been shown to prolong exercise duration during submaximal [50] and maximal exercise [51] and to minimize oxygen desaturation in moderate-to-severe CF lung disease [50–52]. A Cochrane Database Systematic Review concluded that there is limited evidence for additional oxygen supplementation during exercise in chronic obstructive pulmonary disease [53], in particular for patient-reported outcomes such as HRQoL and symptoms. However, it may be useful for the patient to achieve a sufficient training stimulus due to longer exercise durations with oxygen supplementation compared to no supplementation [53] and may therefore optimize the training benefit in the rehabilitation setting. During pulmonary rehabilitation, the physiotherapist or exercise therapist may instruct the patient to self-monitor SpO_2 during exercise and adapt the exercise intensity if SpO_2 drops below 90%. Furthermore, heart rate limits may help to guide training intensities (see Fig. 27.3). In addition, interval training (in combination with additional oxygen supplementation) maybe preferred to avoid oxygen desaturation for patients with severe lung disease and significant peripheral muscle dysfunction. Interval compared to continuous exercise appears to induce less metabolic stress and dynamic hyperinflation [54], which is quite common in CF lung disease and associated with lower exercise performance and higher exertional dyspnea [55].

In addition to supplemental oxygen, noninvasive ventilation (NIV), for example, continuous positive airway pressure (CPAP), inspiratory pressure support (IPS), or proportional assist ventilation (PAV) has been studied during exercise in patients with chronic lung disease [56–58]. During exercise, dynamic hyperinflation occurs as a result of increased end-expiratory lung volumes due to expiratory flow limitation and high respiratory frequencies. Consequently, the work of breathing substantially increases and causes the patient to stop exercise due to shortness of breath. NIV has been used to unload respiratory muscles and to minimize symptoms of breathlessness in obstructive lung disease. Studies in children and adults with CF reported improvements in exercise tolerance, lung function, and oxygen saturation during submaximal exercise with ventilatory support, with controversial effects on patient's sensations of dyspnea [57, 58]. The beneficial effects of CPAP during submaximal exercise in adults with CF (i.e., reduced oxygen consumption, transdiaphragmatic pressure, and dyspnea, and improved oxygen saturation) appear to be related to lung disease severity with greater effects in patients with severe lung disease [57]. A randomized crossover trial with young patients with CF (7–16 years) measured chest wall volume changes using optoelectronic plethysmography before and after a 6-min treadmill walking test with and without NIV. In the experiment with NIV, walking distance and SpO_2 was significantly higher compared to the experiment without ventilatory support [58]. Moreover, the authors observed changes in thoracoabdominal kinematics, i.e., increased pulmonary ribcage volumes and decreased abdominal volumes of the chest wall due to higher tidal volumes after exercise with ventilatory support. These data suggest beneficial effects of NIV during exercise in the acute setting, but further studies are needed to evaluate long-term effects of NIV in combination with exercise on (functional) exercise capacity and patient-reported outcomes following pulmonary rehabilitation in CF.

Figure 27.3 shows data from two male patients with CF who performed cardiopulmonary exercise testing (gas exchange data not shown) using the Godfrey Cycle Protocol. The first patient (case 1) showed oxygen desaturation ($SpO_2 < 90\%$) at an exercise intensity of 180 W and a heart rate of 151 beats min^{-1}. The work rate at desaturation was very close to that at gas exchange threshold (GET). During counseling, this patient would be advised not to exceed a heart rate limit of 150 beats min^{-1} during continuous exercise training to prevent long periods of oxygen desaturation. Case 2 showed substantial oxygen desaturation and his SpO_2 levels dropped below 90% early during the exercise test and long before the GET. Massive oxygen desaturation during exercise is long known in this patient and

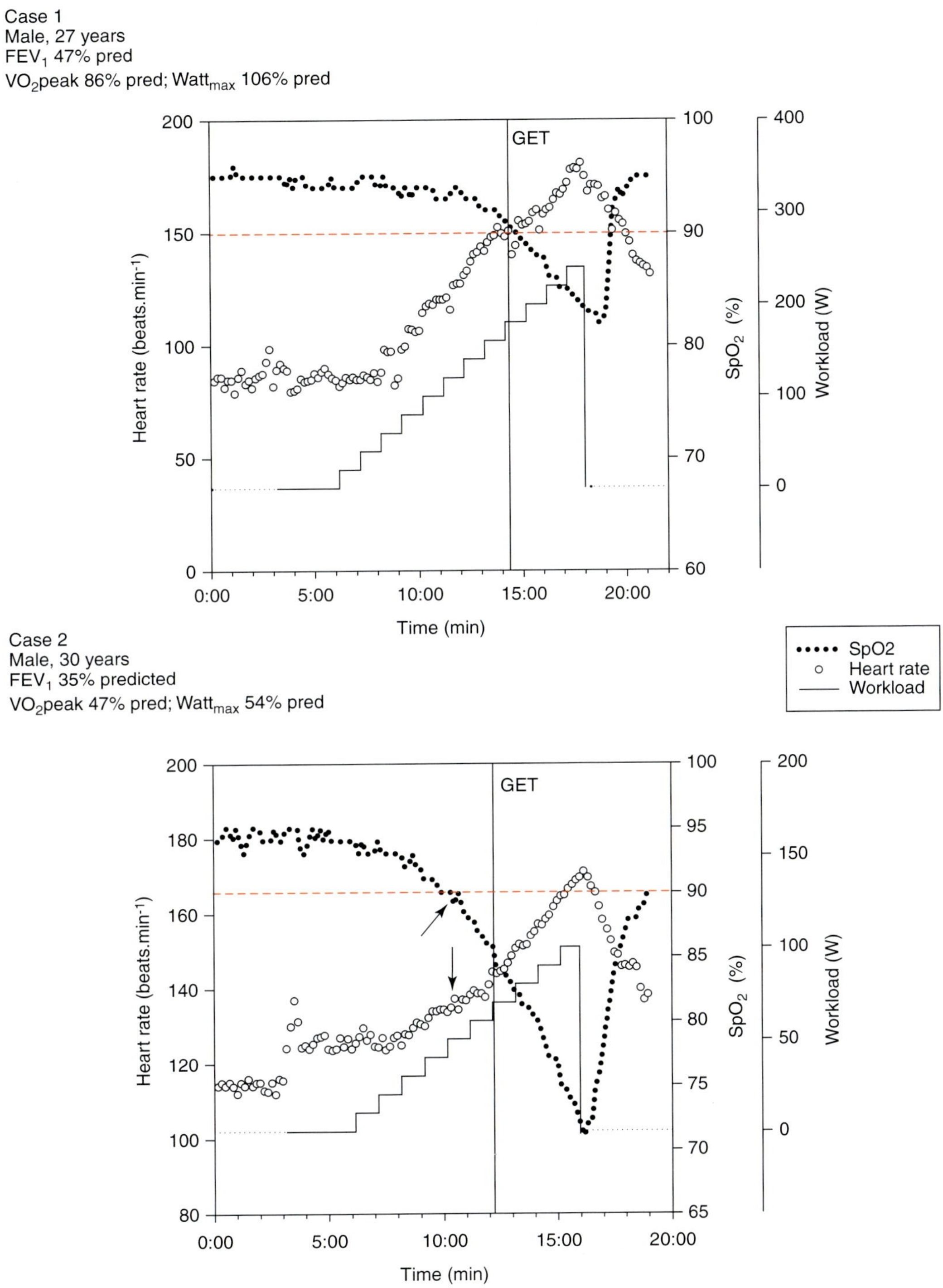

Fig. 27.3 Exercise test in a 27-year-old (case 1) and a 30-year-old (case 2) male patient with cystic fibrosis using the Godfrey Cycle Protocol. In both cases, the test started with a 3-min resting period (*dotted lines*) followed by 3-min's of unloaded pedaling with subsequent increases in workload (20 W and 10 W increments per minute for case 1 and 2, respectively) and followed by a 3-min resting period (*dotted lines*). The *red dashed horizontal line* represents an oxygen saturation (SpO_2) of 90% and the *black vertical line* represents the gas exchange threshold (GET) determined by the V-slope method. Both cases showed oxygen desaturation (case 1 at a workload of 180 W and a heart rate of 151 beats min^{-1}; case 2 at a workload of 50 W and a heart rate of 137 beats min^{-1})

he often exercises at very high intensities without supplemental oxygen. Thus, the test was performed until voluntary exhaustion despite deep desaturation to evaluate the occurrence of cardiac arrhythmias, which were not detected. In this case, we would recommend interval training with supplemental oxygen to allow the patient to achieve sufficient training stimuli and to prevent oxygen desaturation and early muscle fatigue.

27.4.3 Diabetes

Cystic fibrosis related diabetes (CFRD) is the most common comorbidity in CF occurring in about 40–50% of adults [59, 60]. CFRD shares features of both type I and II diabetes [60] and might be associated with exercise intolerance [61]. The diagnosis of CFRD impacts negatively on pulmonary function and is associated with poorer prognosis [60]. Most of the knowledge on the beneficial effects of regular physical activity and structured exercise training on glycemic control has been derived from studies in type II diabetes [62]. With respect to chronic effects, both aerobic and resistance training can improve insulin action, blood glucose levels, fat oxidation and storage in skeletal muscles [62]. Due to the numerous cardiovascular health benefits of regular exercise, the American Diabetes Association [59] recommends patients with CFRD to engage in moderately intense aerobic exercises 150 min per week, consistent with physical activity recommendations for the general population. Specific to CF lung disease, limited data exists to provide sufficient evidence on the benefits of regular physical activity and exercise training for prevention and management of CFRD. Some preliminary data from a small randomized controlled study ($N = 14$) suggest that in adult patients with abnormal glucose tolerance, a combined aerobic and resistance training may improve glycemic control after 12 weeks [63]. These data, however, need to be confirmed by future studies. Acute complications of CFRD include hypoglycemia that can be caused by vigorous or prolonged exercise and in combination with insufficient caloric intake prior to and during exercise. Non-severe hyperglycemia can even occur in patients without CFRD. Patients with CF have a fast catecholamine response to hypoglycemia and a normal hypoglycemia awareness, but their glucagon response to hypoglycemia is insufficient [64]. Therefore, appropriate hypoglycemia education for patients and their families is important. Patients should be instructed to measure blood glucose levels prior to vigorous physical activities and plan their food and drink intake carefully depending on the duration and intensity of the planned activities or exercises [59].

27.4.4 Intravenous Access Devices

In some people with CF, an intravenous antibiotic treatment is necessary during a pulmonary rehabilitation program. In other cases, in-hospital stays for intravenous therapy are used for an intense pulmonary rehabilitation program [30].

In general, four types of devices are employed in such situations: peripheral venous catheters, midline catheters usually inserted in the cubital vein and reaching up to the shoulders, peripherally inserted central catheters (PICC), and implantable devices like the port-a-cath system which can be accessed by a transcutaneous needle when needed.

Although there are no systematic studies on adverse events related to intravenous access devices with exercise, common sense and case reports [65] have guided some recommendations relevant for pulmonary rehabilitation. Swimming is strongly discouraged with all devices except the port-a-cath system when not in use. Furthermore, expert consensus strongly discourages contact sports or activities where trauma to the site of the device might occur [48, 66]. People with CF and a PICC are advised not to perform strenuous exercises with the arm such as weight lifting or tennis. In one case, spring expander exercises with expander elongations before and behind the trunk were associated with a fracture of a port-a-cath catheter and embolization of a fragment into the right pulmonary artery [65]. Thus, the recommendations outlined above might be extended to port-a-cath systems.

27.4.5 Hemoptysis and Pneumothorax

In CF, exercise testing under controlled conditions is safe and severe adverse events for in-hospital exercise training as well as during daily life are low [67]. Yet, as CF-related airways disease worsens, there is an increased likelihood of respiratory complications, such as hemoptysis and pneumothorax that may be serious. Three to 4% of all patients with CF will suffer from a spontaneous pneumothorax during lifetime [67, 68] with an average annual incidence of 1 in 167 [68], a recurrence rate within a week in about 50–90% [69] and a subsequent occurrence on the contralateral side of about 46% [68]. Incidence rates of pneumothoraces during exercise are low with 0.15% per 1000 patient years. These events can occur at any severity of lung disease, but occurred predominantly after a period of infection and were, in at least 50% related to coughing that may or may not be exercise induced [67]. Hemoptysis was reported by 9.1% of patients over a 5-year period [70]. The bleeding is mostly scant to modest, but massive, life-threatening bleeding occurs in about 4% of all patients with CF during their lifetime, and the average annual incidence is 0.87%, or 1 in 115 patients per year [71]. Hemoptysis related to exercise was reported by 3% of patients in a retrospective survey with an incidence rate of 0.12% per 1000 patient years. There were no risk constellations found, and there was no report of how serious the bleeding was. For both events when severe, it is recommended to abstain from airway clearance techniques [72]. Although only recommended in case of a pneumothorax (for the period up to 2 weeks after resolution) it may be wise to abstain from more intense aerobic exercise and weight lifting in both conditions, especially when the exercise induces coughing or higher intrathoracic pressures [72].

27.5 Summary

Pulmonary rehabilitation in CF is multidisciplinary and includes medical support, nutritional and psychological counseling and chest physiotherapy and exercise training, but structured programs as available for COPD patients do not exist. The major difference of pulmonary rehabilitation in CF compared to other lung diseases is due to the nature of the disease and the potential risk of transmission of pathogens between patients. For these reasons, group sessions (i.e., education or exercise) are often avoided in CF care. The evidence for beneficial effects of pulmonary rehabilitation components such as exercise training and chest physiotherapy is predominantly based on studies that have not been performed in the traditional pulmonary rehabilitation setting. Nevertheless, CF patients can benefit in many ways from multicomponent treatment as, for example, a better nutritional status and a higher exercise capacity are associated with improved survival in CF.

References

1. Saiman L. Update on infection prevention and control guidelines. Pediatr Pulmonol. 2013;48(Suppl 36):185–7.
2. Saiman L, Siegel JD, LiPuma JJ, Brown RF, Bryson EA, Chambers MJ, Downer VS, Fliege J, Hazle LA, Jain M, Marshall BC, O'Malley C, Pattee SR, Potter-Bynoe G, Reid S, Robinson KA, Sabadosa KA, Schmidt HJ, Tullis E, Webber J, Weber DJ. Infection prevention and control guideline for cystic fibrosis: 2013 update. Infect Control Hosp Epidemiol. 2014;35(S1):S1–S67
3. Pegues DA, Carson LA, Tablan OC, Fitzsimmons SC, Roman SB, Miller JM, Jarvis WR, Spohn W, Diakew D, Mccoy K, Johnson T, Wilmott RW, Kociela VL, Bivens K, Kanga JF, Christenson J, Woods C, Reisman J, Ciccaletaylor L, Wilson WM, Hennessey R, Eccelstone ER, Hunter E, Keely K. Acquisition of pseudomonas-cepacia at summer camps for patients with cystic-fibrosis. J Pediatr. 1994;124:694–702.
4. Tummler B, Koopmann U, Grothues D, Weissbrodt H, Steinkamp G, Vonderhardt H. Nosocomial acquisition of pseudomonas-aeruginosa by cystic-fibrosis patients. J Clin Microbiol. 1991;29:1265–7.
5. Ridderberg W, Andersen C, Vaeth M, Bregnballe V, Norskov-Lauritsen N, Schiotz PO. Lack of evidence of increased risk of bacterial transmission during cystic fibrosis educational programmes. J Cyst Fibros. 2016;15:109–15.
6. Christian BJ, D'auria JP. Building life skills for children with cystic fibrosis - Effectiveness of an intervention. Nurs Res. 2006;55:300–7.
7. Greenberg D, Yagupsky P, Peled N, Goldbart A, Porat N, Tal A. Lack of evidence of transmission

of Pseudomonas aeruginosa among cystic fibrosis patients attending health camps at the Dead Sea, Israel. Isr Med Assoc J. 2004;6:531–4.

8. Griese M, Busch P, Caroli D, Mertens B, Eismann C, Harari M, Staudter H, Kappler M. Rehabilitation programs for cystic fibrosis—view from a CF center. Open Respir Med J. 2010;4:1–8.
9. Steinkamp G, Wiedemann B. Relationship between nutritional status and lung function in cystic fibrosis: cross sectional and longitudinal analyses from the German CF quality assurance (CFQA) project. Thorax. 2002;57:596–601.
10. Klijn PH, Van Der Net J, Kimpen JL, Helders PJ, Van Der Ent CK. Longitudinal determinants of peak aerobic performance in children with cystic fibrosis. Chest. 2003;124:2215–9.
11. Hanna RM, Weiner DJ. Overweight and obesity in patients with cystic fibrosis: a center-based analysis. Pediatr Pulmonol. 2015;50:35–41.
12. Stephenson AL, Mannik LA, Walsh S, Brotherwood M, Robert R, Darling PB, Nisenbaum R, Moerman J, Stanojevic S. Longitudinal trends in nutritional status and the relation between lung function and BMI in cystic fibrosis: a population-based cohort study. Am J Clin Nutr. 2013;97:872–7.
13. Mckoy NA, Wilson LM, Saldanha IJ, Odelola OA, Robinson KA. Active cycle of breathing technique for cystic fibrosis. Cochrane Database Syst Rev. 2016;7:CD007862.
14. McIlwaine M, Button B, Dwan K. Positive expiratory pressure physiotherapy for airway clearance in people with cystic fibrosis. Cochrane Database Syst Rev. 2015;6:CD003147.
15. Radtke T, Nolan SJ, Hebestreit H, Kriemler S. Physical exercise training for cystic fibrosis. Cochrane Database Syst Rev. 2015; doi:10.1002/14651858.CD002768.pub3CD002768.
16. Quittner AL, Barker DH, Snell C, Grimley ME, Marciel K, Cruz I. Prevalence and impact of depression in cystic fibrosis. Curr Opin Pulm Med. 2008;14:582–8.
17. West CA, Besier T, Borth-Bruhns T, Goldbeck L. Effectiveness of a family-oriented rehabilitation program on the quality of life of parents of chronically ill children. Klin Padiatr. 2009;221:241–6.
18. Hebestreit H, Schmid K, Kieser S, Junge S, Ballmann M, Roth K, Hebestreit A, Schenk T, Schindler C, Posselt H-G, Kriemler S. Quality of life is associated with physical activity and fitness in cystic fibrosis. BMC Pulm Med. 2014;14:26.
19. Tejero Garcia S, Giraldez Sanchez MA, Cejudo P, Quintana Gallego E, Dapena J, Garcia Jimenez R, Cano Luis P, Gomez De Terreros I. Bone health, daily physical activity, and exercise tolerance in patients with cystic fibrosis. Chest. 2011;140:475–81.
20. Cox NS, Alison JA, Button BM, Wilson JW, Morton JM, Holland AE. Physical activity participation by adults with cystic fibrosis: an observational study. Respirology. 2016;21:511–8.
21. Schneiderman JE, Wilkes DL, Atenafu EG, Nguyen T, Wells GD, Alarie N, Tullis E, Lands LC, Coates AL, Corey M, Ratjen F. Longitudinal relationship between physical activity and lung health in patients with cystic fibrosis. Eur Respir J. 2014;43:817–23.
22. Hebestreit H, Kieser S, Rudiger S, Schenk T, Junge S, Hebestreit A, Ballmann M, Posselt HG, Kriemler S. Physical activity is independently related to aerobic capacity in cystic fibrosis. Eur Respir J. 2006;28:734–9.
23. Moorcroft AJ, Dodd ME, Webb AK. Exercise testing and prognosis in adult cystic fibrosis. Thorax. 1994;49:1075–1076P.
24. Nixon PA, Orenstein DM, Kelsey SF, Doershuk CF. The prognostic value of exercise testing in patients with cystic fibrosis. New Engl J Med. 1992;327:1785–8.
25. Pianosi P, Leblanc J, Almudevar A. Peak oxygen uptake and mortality in children with cystic fibrosis. Thorax. 2005;60:50–4.
26. Hebestreit H, Arets HG, Aurora P, Boas S, Cerny F, Hulzebos EH, Karila C, Lands LC, Lowman JD, Swisher A, Urquhart DS, European Cystic Fibrosis Exercise Working Group. Statement on exercise testing in cystic fibrosis. Respiration. 2015;90:332–51.
27. Godfrey S, Davies CT, Wozniak E, Barnes CA. Cardio-respiratory response to exercise in normal children. Clin Sci. 1971;40:419–31.
28. Radtke T, Nolan SJ, Hebestreit H, Kriemler S. Physical exercise training for cystic fibrosis. Paediatr Respir Rev. 2016b;19:42–5.
29. Gruber W, Orenstein DM, Braumann KM, Beneke R. Interval exercise training in cystic fibrosis—effects on exercise capacity in severely affected adults. J Cyst Fibros. 2014;13:86–91.
30. Selvadurai HC, Blimkie CJ, Meyers N, Mellis CM, Cooper PJ, Van Asperen PP. Randomized controlled study of in-hospital exercise training programs in children with cystic fibrosis. Pediatr Pulmonol. 2002;33:194–200.
31. Lands LC, Smountas AA, Mesiano G, Brosseau L, Shennib H, Charbonneau M, Gauthier R. Maximal exercise capacity and peripheral skeletal muscle function following lung transplantation. J Heart Lung Transplant. 1999;18:113–20.
32. Langer D, Gosselink R, Pitta F, Burtin C, Verleden G, Dupont L, Decramer M, Troosters T. Physical activity in daily life 1 year after lung transplantation. J Heart Lung Transplant. 2009;28:572–8.
33. Williams TJ, Mckenna MJ. Exercise limitation following transplantation. Compr Physiol. 2012;2:1937–79.
34. Radtke T, Benden C, Kriemler S. Physical activity and exercise training in lung transplant recipients with cystic fibrosis: 'what we know, what we don't know and where to go'. Lung. 2016a;194:177–8.
35. Wickerson L, Mathur S, Brooks D. Exercise training after lung transplantation: a systematic review. J Heart Lung Transplant. 2010;29:497–503.
36. Langer D, Burtin C, Schepers L, Ivanova A, Verleden G, Decramer M, Troosters T, Gosselink R. Exercise

training after lung transplantation improves participation in daily activity: a randomized controlled trial. Am J Transplant. 2012;12:1584–92.
37. Coppoolse R, Schols AMWJ, Baarends EM, Mostert R, Akkermans MA, Janssen PP, Wouters EFM. Interval versus continuous training in patients with severe COPD: a randomized clinical trial. Eur Respir J. 1999;14:258–63.
38. Vogiatzis I, Nanas S, Roussos C. Interval training as an alternative modality to continuous exercise in patients with COPD. Eur Respir J. 2002;20:12–9.
39. Vogiatzis I, Terzis G, Nanas S, Stratakos G, Simoes DCM, Georgiadou O, Zakynthinos S, Roussos C. Skeletal muscle adaptations to interval training in patients with advanced COPD. Chest. 2005;128:3838–45.
40. Mathur S, Hornblower E, Levy RD. Exercise training before and after lung transplantation. Physician Sports Med. 2009;37:78–87.
41. Henke KG, Orenstein DM. Oxygen saturation during exercise in cystic fibrosis. Am Rev Respir Dis. 1984;129:708–11.
42. Lebecque P, Lapierre JG, Lamarre A, Coates AL. Diffusion capacity and oxygen desaturation effects on exercise in patients with cystic fibrosis. Chest. 1987;91:693–7.
43. Ruf K, Hebestreit H. Exercise-induced hypoxemia and cardiac arrhythmia in cystic fibrosis. J Cyst Fibros. 2009;8:83–90.
44. Marcotte JE, Grisdale RK, Levison H, Coates AL, Canny GJ. Multiple factors limit exercise capacity in cystic fibrosis. Pediatr Pulmonol. 1986;2:274–81.
45. Peckham D, Watson A, Pollard K, Etherington C, Conway SP. Predictors of desaturation during formal hypoxic challenge in adult patients with cystic fibrosis. J Cyst Fibros. 2002;1:281–6.
46. Wheatley CM, Foxx-Lupo WT, Cassuto NA, Wong EC, Daines CL, Morgan WJ, Snyder EM. Impaired lung diffusing capacity for nitric oxide and alveolar-capillary membrane conductance results in oxygen desaturation during exercise in patients with cystic fibrosis. J Cyst Fibros. 2011;10:45–53.
47. Boas SR. Exercise recommendations for individuals with cystic fibrosis. Sports Med. 1997;24:17–37.
48. Swisher AK, Hebestreit H, Meija-Downs A, Lowman JD, Gruber W, Nippins M, Alison J. Exercise and habitual physical activity for people with cystic fibrosis: expert consensus, evidence-based guide for advising patients. Cardiopulm Phys Ther J. 2015;26:85–98.
49. Burtin C, Hebestreit H. Rehabilitation in patients with chronic respiratory disease other than chronic obstructive pulmonary disease: exercise and physical activity interventions in cystic fibrosis and non-cystic fibrosis bronchiectasis. Respiration. 2015;89:181–9.
50. McKone EF, Barry SC, FitzGerald MX, Gallagher CG. The role of supplemental oxygen during submaximal exercise in patients with cystic fibrosis. Eur Respir J. 2002;20:134–42.
51. Marcus CL, Bader D, Stabile MW, Wang CI, Osher AB, Keens TG. Supplemental oxygen and exercise performance in patients with cystic fibrosis with severe pulmonary disease. Chest. 1992;101:52–7.
52. Nixon PA, Orenstein DM, Curtis SE, Ross EA. Oxygen supplementation during exercise in cystic fibrosis. Am Rev Respir Dis. 1990;142:807–11.
53. Nonoyama ML, Brooks D, Lacasse Y, Guyatt GH, Goldstein RS. Oxygen therapy during exercise training in chronic obstructive pulmonary disease. Cochrane Database Syst Rev. 2007; Issue 2:CD005372.
54. Sabapathy S, Kingsley RA, Schneider DA, Adams L, Morris NR. Continuous and intermittent exercise responses in individuals with chronic obstructive pulmonary disease. Thorax. 2004;59:1026–31.
55. Stevens D, Stephenson A, Faughnan ME, Leek E, Tullis E. Prognostic relevance of dynamic hyperinflation during cardiopulmonary exercise testing in adult patients with cystic fibrosis. J Cyst Fibros. 2013;12:655–61.
56. Ambrosino N, Cigni P. Non invasive ventilation as an additional tool for exercise training. Multidiscip Respir Med. 2015;10:14.
57. Henke KG, Regnis JA, Bye PT. Benefits of continuous positive airway pressure during exercise in cystic fibrosis and relationship to disease severity. Am Rev Respir Dis. 1993;148:1272–6.
58. Lima CA, Andrade Ade F, Campos SL, Brandao DC, Fregonezi G, Mourato IP, Aliverti A, Britto MC. Effects of noninvasive ventilation on treadmill 6-min walk distance and regional chest wall volumes in cystic fibrosis: randomized controlled trial. Respir Med. 2014;108:1460–8.
59. Moran A, Brunzell C, Cohen RC, Katz M, Marshall BC, Onady G, Robinson KA, Sabadosa KA, Stecenko A, Slovis B. Clinical care guidelines for cystic fibrosis-related diabetes: a position statement of the American diabetes association and a clinical practice guideline of the cystic fibrosis foundation, endorsed by the pediatric endocrine society. Diabetes Care. 2010;33:2697–708.
60. Moran A, Dunitz J, Nathan B, Saeed A, Holme B, Thomas W. Cystic fibrosis-related diabetes: current trends in prevalence, incidence, and mortality. Diabetes Care. 2009;32:1626–31.
61. Ziegler B, Oliveira CL, Rovedder PM, Schuh SJ, Abreu ESFA, Dalcin Pde T. Glucose intolerance in patients with cystic fibrosis: sex-based differences in clinical score, pulmonary function, radiograph score, and 6-minute walk test. Respir Care. 2011;56:290–7.
62. Colberg SR, Sigal RJ, Fernhall B, Regensteiner JG, Blissmer BJ, Rubin RR, Chasan-Taber L, Albright AL, Braun B, American College of Sports Medicine, American Diabetes Association. Exercise and type 2 diabetes: the American college of sports medicine and the American diabetes association: joint position statement. Diabetes Care. 2010;33:e147–67.
63. Beaudoin N, Bouvet GF, Coriati A, Rabasa-Lhoret R, Berthiaume Y. Combined exercise training improves glycemic control in adults with cystic fibrosis. Med Sci Sports Exerc. 2017;49:231–7.

64. Moran A, Diem P, Klein DJ, Levitt MD, Robertson RP. Pancreatic endocrine function in cystic fibrosis. J Pediatr. 1991;118:715–23.
65. Roggla G, Linkesch M, Roggla M, Wagner A, Haber P, Linkesch W. A rare complication of a central venous catheter system (Port-a-Cath). A case report of a catheter embolization after catheter fracture during power training. Int J Sports Med. 1993;14:345–6.
66. Cystic Fibrosis Foundation. https://www.cff.org/Living-with-CF/Treatments-and-Therapies/Medications/Vascular-Access-Devices-PICCs-and-Ports/; 2017. Accessed 1 Jan 2017.
67. Ruf K, Winkler B, Hebestreit A, Gruber W, Hebestreit H. Risks associated with exercise testing and sports participation in cystic fibrosis. J Cyst Fibros. 2010;9:339–45.
68. Flume PA, Strange C, Ye X, Ebeling M, Hulsey T, Clark LL. Pneumothorax in cystic fibrosis. Chest. 2005a;128:720–8.
69. Flume PA. Pneumothorax in cystic fibrosis. Chest. 2003;123:217–21.
70. Flume PA. Pneumothorax in cystic fibrosis. Curr Opin Pulm Med. 2011;17:220–5.
71. Flume PA, Yankaskas JR, Ebeling M, Hulsey T, Clark LL. Massive hemoptysis in cystic fibrosis. Chest. 2005;128:729–38.
72. Flume PA, Mogayzel PJ Jr, Robinson KA, Rosenblatt RL, Quittell L, Marshall BC, Clinical Practice Guidelines for Pulmonary Therapies Committee, Cystic Fibrosis Foundation Pulmonary Therapies Committee. Cystic fibrosis pulmonary guidelines: pulmonary complications: hemoptysis and pneumothorax. Am J Respir Crit Care Med. 2010;182:298–306.

28 Pulmonary Rehabilitation in Restrictive Thoracic Disorders

Anne Holland and Nicolino Ambrosino

28.1 The Interstitial Lung Diseases

The interstitial lung diseases (ILDs) are a group of over 200 debilitating conditions characterised by lung inflammation and/or fibrosis. Idiopathic pulmonary fibrosis (IPF), the most common and lethal of the ILDs, accounts for approximately one-third of the ILDs and has a median survival of 3 years from diagnosis [1]. However, the clinical course varies widely and some patients with IPF will experience long periods of stability, whilst others will have frequent exacerbations or a rapid decline [2]. Interstitial lung disease may also occur due to an underlying systemic disease process, such as connective tissue disease or sarcoidosis, or an occupational exposure, such as asbestosis or silicosis. The incidence of ILD is increasing globally, largely due to a rise in the number of people who are diagnosed with IPF. Idiopathic pulmonary fibrosis is a disease of older people, with an estimated prevalence of 19 per 100,000 in those aged 55–64 years, rising to 88 per 100,000 in those 75 and over [3]. Consequently there will be more people living with IPF as the population ages in developed nations.

A. Holland
Alfred Health and Institute for Breathing and Sleep, La Trobe University, Melbourne, Australia

N. Ambrosino (✉)
Research Consultant, Pulmonary and Respiratory Medicine Department, Faculty of Medicine, Universitas Sebelas Maret, Surakarta, Indonesia

Istituti Clinici Scientifici Maugeri, Scientific Institute of Montescano, Montescano, Italy
e-mail: nico.ambrosino@gmail.com

28.1.1 Pathophysiology of ILD

The interstitium is the lung tissue between the alveolar epithelium and capillary endothelium. Thickening or inflammation of the interstitium leads to a restrictive ventilatory pattern and impairment of gas exchange, documented by impairments in spirometry and diffusing capacity for carbon monoxide, respectively. Destruction of the pulmonary capillary bed may also occur, contributing to ventilation-perfusion mismatch and oxygen diffusion limitation [4]. As a result, exertional desaturation is a key feature of the ILDs. Circulatory limitation results from pulmonary capillary destruction and vasoconstriction, leading to pulmonary hypertension and cardiac dysfunction in some patients [5]. A high resolution CT scan is required to make a diagnosis of ILD [1]. In some cases a lung biopsy is required to confirm the diagnosis.

28.1.2 Clinical Features

The ILDs are characterised by dyspnoea on exertion, reduced exercise capacity and poor health-related quality of life (HRQoL). In many patients

© Springer International Publishing AG 2018
E. Clini et al. (eds.), *Textbook of Pulmonary Rehabilitation*, https://doi.org/10.1007/978-3-319-65888-9_28

dyspnoea is severe and distressing, particularly in those with rapidly progressive disease. Fatigue and exhaustion are even more bothersome than breathlessness for many patients [6]. Reduction in exercise capacity is clinically important as it is associated with worse HRQoL and poor prognosis. Persistent cough is a characteristic feature of the ILDs and can be difficult to control. Auscultation may reveal bilateral 'velcro' crackles throughout inspiration, particularly in IPF, although they may also be heard in other ILDs such as asbestosis and sarcoidosis [7].

28.1.3 Extrapulmonary Manifestations of ILD

Peripheral muscle dysfunction is increasingly recognised as an important contributor to exercise dysfunction in ILD. Quadriceps force is reduced in people with fibrotic ILDs [8], sarcoidosis [9, 10] and rheumatoid arthritis [11], with average values that are 20 to 35% lower than healthy controls. Those who have worse quadriceps strength have reduced functional exercise capacity [8–10, 12, 13]. Lower peripheral muscle strength is also associated with worse lower quality of life [9, 10] and higher levels of fatigue [9, 10]. The causes of peripheral muscle dysfunction in ILD are not well understood and may relate to the type of underlying ILD. For instance in rheumatoid arthritis, reduced quadriceps force has been associated with longer disease duration, a greater number of joints affected and current use of corticosteroids [14]. In systemic sclerosis (SSc), skeletal muscle dysfunction is also associated with longer disease duration, and is worse in those with diffuse cutaneous SSc compared to limited cutaneous SSc [15]. It is likely that physical inactivity also makes a significant contribution to peripheral muscle dysfunction. People with ILD take 65% fewer daily steps compared to healthy age matched peers [16] and those with the lowest levels of physical activity have the worst HRQoL, independent of respiratory function [17]. There is a threefold increase in the hazard of death for patients with ILD who are highly sedentary (walk less than 3300 steps per day) [16].

Other important comorbidities that are prevalent and known to impact on outcome (particularly in IPF) include gastro-oesophageal reflux, cardiovascular disease, sleep disordered breathing and mood disorders [18]. Although some of these share common risk factors with IPF (e.g. smoking) they are still more prevalent than expected. Coronary artery disease may occur in up to one-third of patients [19] and gastro-oesophageal reflux in up to 94% [20]. Anxiety is present in up to one-third of individuals with ILD, especially in those with higher levels of dyspnoea [21]. Depression occurs in approximately 25%, more often in those with higher levels of dyspnoea and a greater number of comorbidities [21]. Depression does not resolve without treatment [22]. A study including 272 patients with IPF reported that 58% of patients had one to three comorbid conditions, 30% had four to seven comorbid conditions, and only 12% had no comorbidities [23]. This reinforces the importance of comprehensive treatment for people with ILD.

28.1.4 Clinical Management of ILD

Recent years have seen major advances in the treatment of IPF. Two anti-fibrotic agents have been shown to reduce disease progression [24, 25], demonstrating for the first time that IPF is a treatable disease. However there are no curative treatments and patients continue to experience a significant disease burden including reduced functional capacity, dyspnoea on exertion and reduced HRQoL. New treatments are likely to emerge in the future. Currently supportive care has an important role in IPF management, including referral for pulmonary rehabilitation, oxygen therapy, and lung transplantation [1, 26]. For patients with hypersensitivity pneumonitis (e.g. 'bird fancier's lung'), treatment focuses on removal of the antigen and prednisolone may be prescribed in some cases. Prednisolone may also be used to treat sarcoidosis if there is evidence of progressive disease or extra-pulmonary involvement. Immunosuppressive therapy may be used in connective tissue disease and scleroderma lung. In some ILDs there may be no pharmacological management available [27]. Most people with ILD will continue to experience symptoms despite best available medical care, illustrating the importance of treatments such as pulmonary rehabilitation that assist patients to live well with a chronic lung disease.

28.2 Evidence for the Role of Pulmonary Rehabilitation in ILD

Pulmonary rehabilitation is designed to '... *improve the physical and psychological condition of people with chronic respiratory disease and to promote the long-term adherence to health-enhancing behaviours*' [28]. Whilst evidence for its considerable benefits has been predominantly gathered in COPD, a disease with differing pathophysiology, the symptoms and impairments experienced by people with ILD are frequently similar, including dyspnoea, fatigue, reduced exercise capacity and impaired HRQoL. A number of randomised controlled trials have evaluated the efficacy of pulmonary rehabilitation on these outcomes and results have been summarised in a Cochrane review [29]. Nine studies were identified, most of which included a range of ILD diagnoses. There was a total of 386 participants, including 153 with IPF. Programmes typically used aerobic exercise training or a combination of aerobic and resistance training, whilst some also included education, nutritional advice, stress management and psychosocial support. Programmes ranged from 5 to 12 weeks, with all programmes offering two or more supervised sessions each week. Quality of the evidence was rated as low to moderate as only one study used a blinded assessor and one used intention to treat analysis, with numbers of dropouts poorly reported. This may be important for external validity, particularly in IPF where progressive disease may affect a patient's ability to complete the programme.

Clinically meaningful benefits from pulmonary rehabilitation were reported for 6-min walk distance (weighted mean difference 44 m, 95% confidence interval 26–64 m, 4 studies), dyspnoea (standardised mean difference −0.66, −1.05 to −0.28, 3 studies) and HRQoL (standardised mean difference 0.59, 95% confidence interval 0.2–0.98, 3 studies). Findings were similar when only people with IPF were considered, which means pulmonary rehabilitation is one of the only treatments to improve patient-centred outcomes in this group. The average changes are similar to those documented following pulmonary rehabilitation in COPD [30], although certainty about the size of the effect is lower because there are fewer studies. As a result the confidence intervals do not exclude changes that are less than the minimal important difference (Fig. 28.1). Only two studies have evaluated longer-term outcomes of pulmonary rehabilitation and both suggest that the benefits are diminished by 6 months, particularly in those with progressive disease [31, 32]. As a result, the National Institute for Clinical Excellence guidelines (UK) recommend that patients with IPF are reassessed for rehabilitation every 6–12 months [1].

Gaps remain in our knowledge of pulmonary rehabilitation for people with ILD, particularly with regard to the duration of benefit, the mechanisms underlying these changes, the optimal programme components and when in the disease course it should be offered. However the convincing impact of pulmonary rehabilitation on patient-important outcomes, in a disease group with few therapeutic options, has driven its adoption into clinical practice in many countries. A global survey reported that 74% of pulmonary rehabilitation programmes accepted people with ILD [33]. The American Thoracic Society guidelines for IPF management make a weak recommendation for pulmonary rehabilitation and the American Thoracic Society/European Respiratory Society statement on pulmonary rehabilitation also supports its use [28]. A notable exception is the British Thoracic Society guideline on pulmonary rehabilitation which made no recommendation, largely due to the absence of trials of comprehensive pulmonary rehabilitation programmes (many studies have been exercise only) and variability in the clinical course of the

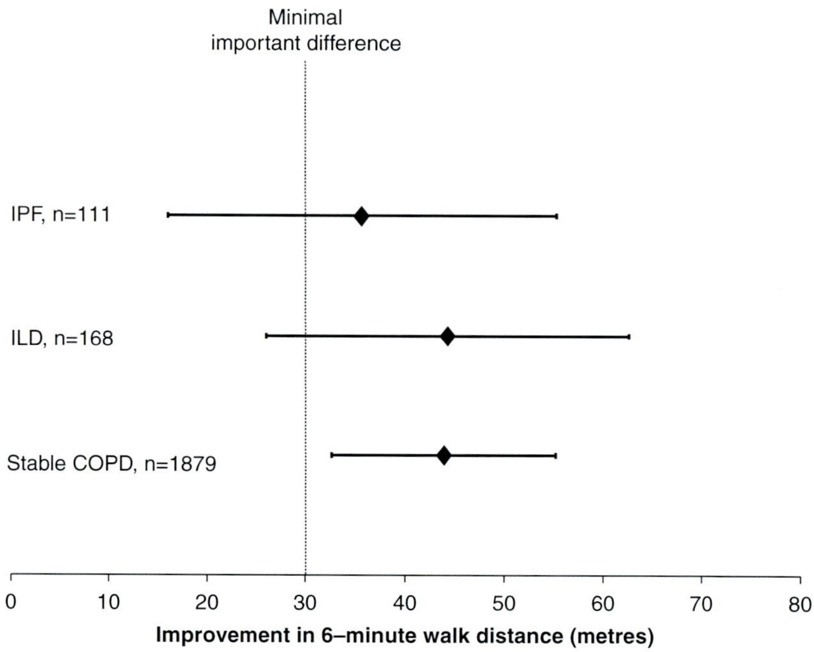

Fig. 28.1 Change in 6-min walk distance following pulmonary rehabilitation. *COPD* chronic obstructive pulmonary disease, *ILD* interstitial lung disease, *IPF* idiopathic pulmonary fibrosis. Data are means and 95% confidence intervals from Cochrane reviews [29, 30]. Dotted line is minimal important difference for 6-min walk test of 30 m [40]

different ILDs [34]. This reflects the remaining uncertainties regarding programme content and timing. Despite these deficiencies, existing studies offer convincing data to suggest that many individuals with ILD will experience meaningful benefits from pulmonary rehabilitation that includes whole body exercise training.

28.2.1 Components of Exercise Training for ILD

Most reports of exercise training for ILD have used a similar programme format to that used in patients with COPD [33]. The training components are outlined in Table 28.1. Aerobic exercise training is conducted on an exercise bike and/or a treadmill, with the goal of at least 30 min per session. Training intensity commences at 60–80% of baseline exercise capacity, measured either on a cardiopulmonary exercise test (CPET) or walking test, with regular progression of workload over the course of the programme. Resistance training is a feature of most programmes and has been delivered in a variety of formats, including free weights, elastic bands and functional activities such as stair training and sit-to-stand. Similar to aerobic training, progression of the workload over the course of the programme is a key feature. Monitoring consists of pulse oximetry to measure oxyhaemoglobin saturation during exercise, as well as symptom monitoring ensure that exercise is of moderate intensity (3–5 on the Borg CR scale [35]). Some programmes also include a flexibility component, consisting of stretches for the upper and lower body that are held for 15–30 s each.

28.2.2 Special Considerations for Exercise Training in ILD

Exertional desaturation is a key feature of the ILDs and is often more severe than that seen in other pulmonary rehabilitation participants [36]. Pulmonary hypertension is also present in many patients and may worsen with exercise [37]. As a result pulmonary rehabilitation programmes for ILD should take place where supplemental oxygen is available and staff are experienced in its use. Whilst it is not certain that supplemental oxygen can prevent exercise-induced elevation of pulmonary pressures [38], it may result in better oxygen delivery to the tissue and enhance both tolerability of training and exercise outcomes. Most programmes report delivering supplemental oxygen during training to maintain oxyhaemoglobin saturation above thresholds ranging from 85 to 90%. These strategies appear safe, with no adverse events reported [29].

A unique challenge of rehabilitation for ILD is that some patients may have rapidly progressive disease, particularly in IPF. This has led to concerns that some patients may be too unwell to achieve benefits [34]. To date no studies have identified a 'threshold' beyond which patients are unlikely to improve with rehabilitation. Conversely a number of studies suggest that those with a lower 6-min walk distance at the beginning of rehabilitation may achieve greater improvements in exercise capacity, suggesting those with the greatest functional impairment may have the most to gain. However other authors have shown that those with higher forced vital capacity and less exertional desaturation are more likely to benefit. Referral early in the disease course is recommended, especially in patients with IPF, to ensure that patients have the best opportunity to participate and attain the benefits of pulmonary rehabilitation. However there is currently no evidence supporting exclusion of those with more severe disease. Health professionals should assist patients with severe or progressive disease to make an informed choice about the costs and benefits of participation in pulmonary rehabilitation.

People with connective tissue related ILD frequently have musculoskeletal limitations that may require modification of the standard exercise prescription (Table 28.1). Arthropathy is common and may particularly affect weightbearing exercise such as walking, stair climbing and chair stands. Alternative training strategies may be required, including aerobic activities that minimise lower limb weightbearing (e.g. cycling or water-based exercise training). Range of motion limitations and pain of the upper and lower limbs should also be carefully assessed at programme entry. Modifications may be required to resistance training regimens, particularly avoidance of loaded upper limb movements that may exacer-

Table 28.1 Programme components and outcome measures for pulmonary rehabilitation in ILD

Programme components	Details
Aerobic exercise training	Exercise bike AND/OR treadmill walking
	Duration 30–40 min per session
	Continuous or interval training
	Starting intensity 60–80% of maximum heart rate OR 80% of peak power on CPET OR 80% of walking speed on 6MWT
	Progressed weekly
Resistance training	Free weights, 2 sets of 10–12 repetitions, major muscle groups of upper and lower limbs
	OR elastic bands
	AND/OR functional tasks/body weight – Sit to stand, stair climbing, squats, wall push ups
Supplemental oxygen during exercise training	To maintain $SpO_2 > 85\%$ OR 88% OR 90%
Monitoring	Pulse oximetry, symptom scores (dyspnoea and fatigue) During exercise and at end-exercise
Other interventions	Flexibility training
	Nutritional advice
	Stress management
	Education
	Psychosocial support
Programme format	5–12 weeks, with 2–5 supervised sessions each week
Outcome measures	Exercise capacity—6MWT, 12MWT CPET, 30 s sit to stand test
	Strength—Quadriceps force
	Dyspnoea—MMRC, BDI/TDI
	Health related quality of life—SGRQ, SGRQ-I, CRQ, WHO Physical activity (self-report)—IPAQ

From randomised controlled trials of pulmonary rehabilitation in ILD [29]

6MWT 6-min walk test, *BDI/TDI* Baseline Dyspnoea Index/Transitional Dyspnoea Index, *CPET* cardiopulmonary exercise test, *CRQ* Chronic Respiratory Questionnaire, *IPAQ* international physical activity questionnaire, *MMRC* Modified Medical Research Council scale, *SGRQ* St George's Respiratory Questionnaire, *SGRQ-I* St George's Respiratory Questionnaire idiopathic pulmonary fibrosis version, SpO_2 oxygen saturation measured by pulse oximetry, *WHO* World Health Organisation questionnaire

bate shoulder pain. Participants should be encouraged to report any pain and discomfort to the supervising therapist immediately, to ensure that appropriate modifications can be made and to maximise adherence.

28.2.3 Non-exercise Components

Pulmonary rehabilitation provides an ideal opportunity to optimise disease management in ILD. People with ILD have expressed their desire for disease-specific education in pulmonary rehabilitation, including information about the expected disease course and how they can prepare for the future [39]. Topics of specific interest to people with ILD include management of dyspnoea and cough, managing medications and their side effects, and strategies to limit disease progression [39]. Although there may be insufficient evidence to provide definitive management strategies in some of these areas, it is likely that patients will benefit from the opportunity to share their experiences. Information about use of supplemental oxygen and lung transplantation may be relevant for some people. Most people with ILD will undertake pulmonary rehabilitation in groups that include people with other lung diseases including COPD; they report that this is acceptable as long as clinicians include some ILD-specific educational content where it is relevant [39]. Because anxiety and depression are very common in ILD, pulmonary rehabilitation may provide an opportunity to optimise management of mood. The inclusion of a psychologist in the multidisciplinary team is highly desirable. Other components that have been included in pulmonary rehabilitation for ILD are in Table 28.1. Individualised patient assessment and goal setting can be used to identify those components that are most likely to be of benefit.

28.3 The Neuromuscular Diseases

Respiratory failure is the most common cause of mortality in patients with rapidly progressive neuromuscular diseases (NMD). Most NMD are associated to peripheral, inspiratory, and expiratory muscle weakness with difficulty to loss of ambulation, and swallowing disorders. Inspiratory muscle weakness reduces alveolar ventilation, whereas expiratory muscle weakness affects cough capacity and airway secretions clearance, both contributing to chronic respiratory insufficiency, as well as to life-threatening conditions, and in most severe cases, death due to acute on chronic respiratory failure [41]. Alterations in lung function may be present earlier than symptoms: a screening study reveals that at first evaluation, about two-third of NMD patients may be candidate for home mechanical ventilation (HMV) [42] (Table 28.2).

Recent advances in respiratory care and comprehensive management of these patients have improved their prognosis and expectations, leading to a more aggressive, supportive approach [43, 44]. Despite this more positive attitude a recent survey found that 24% of all patients suffering from Duchenne muscular dystrophy (DMD) received no regular physiotherapy, 22% of them did not receive serial echocardiograms, and lung function was not regularly assessed in 71% of non-ambulatory patients [45]. In comprehensive management of these patients rehabilitation has an increasingly relevant role. This chapter deals only with the pulmonary rehabilitation approaches to the patients with NMD, without any specific mention to other essential components of their

Table 28.2 Symptoms, signs and laboratory markers of respiratory involvement in NMD

Symptoms
Generalised weakness; dysphagia; dysphonia; exercise and rest dyspnoea; fatigue; sleepiness
Clinical signs
Rapid shallow breathing; tachycardia; weak cough; staccato speech; accessory muscle use; abdominal paradox; orthopnoea; weakness of trapezius and neck muscles; cough after swallowing
Laboratory data
VC <15 mL kg^{-1}, VC <1 L or 50% reduction from stable state, or >20% reduction from sitting to supine position
Maximum inspiratory pressure < 30 cmH_2O
Maximum expiratory pressure < 40 cmH_2O
Nocturnal desaturation
$PaCO_2$ > 45 mmHg

VC vital capacity, *$PaCO_2$* arterial carbon dioxide tension

comprehensive management such as mechanical ventilation (MV), nutritional therapy, general physiotherapy.

28.4 Glossopharyngeal Breathing

Two-thirds of patients with preserved bulbar innervated musculature can use glossopharyngeal breathing (GPB) to increase their tidal volumes. With GPB the glottis takes boluses of air and pushes them into the lungs (gulp). One breath may consist of six to nine gulps of 40–60 to 100–200 mL each. It has been suggested that GPB allows daytime MV free hours, also in patients with inspiratory muscle weakness and that this strategy may delay or avoid tracheostomy or allow the switch from tracheostomy to non-invasive ventilation (NIV) [46]. Manuals and videos are available for training [47, 48].

28.5 Clearing Airways

Spontaneous cough requires functioning inspiratory, expiratory and bulbar-innervated muscles. Optimal airway secretion clearance is crucial to avoid atelectasis, airways infections, pneumonia, and related danger of acute respiratory failure. Bronchial hygiene by means of airway clearance techniques (ACT), including manually and/or mechanically assisted coughing, and secretion mobilisation techniques, are recommended in the management of these patients [49]. Many of such techniques have been described in another chapter of this Textbook (Table 28.3).

Table 28.3 Airway clearance techniques

Postural drainage
Chest percussions and vibrations
Lung volume recruitment
Manually assisted coughing
Mechanically assisted coughing
Bronchoscopy
New devices

28.5.1 Postural Drainage

The physiopathological rationale of postural drainage is that gravity increases mobilisation of airway secretions according to the patient's position. More recently proposed ACT are based on the ability to ventilate behind obstructed lung regions and on the capacity to achieve the minimum expiratory airflow able to move secretions, following the interdependence during deep inspiration and collateral ventilation principles [50].

28.5.2 Chest Percussions and Vibrations

Chet percussions and vibrations can help to move peripheral airway secretions but cannot substitute coughing and have been shown to decrease pulmonary morbidity and mortality [51].

28.5.3 Lung Volume Recruitment

In addition to expiratory muscle weakness, ineffective cough may be also due to low lung volumes, a common condition in NMD. Lung volumes can be increased by lung volume recruitment (LVR) manoeuvres. 'Air stacking' can be delivered through oral, nasal, or oronasal interfaces by means of manual resuscitators such as the AMBU BAG or volume-preset ventilators [52]. An active LVR involves the glottis holding consecutively delivered volumes of air to a 'maximum insufflation capacity' (MIC), a function of pulmonary compliance and strength of glottis closure. Exhalation is passive [53].

28.5.4 Manually Assisted Coughing

Manually Assisted Coughing consists of deep lung insufflation and pushing on the upper abdomen (i.e. abdominal thrust) or chest wall (i.e. anterior chest compression) applied as the glottis opens in synchrony with the subject's own cough effort. Preserved bulbar-innervated muscle function, a co-operative patient and good coordination between the patient and physiotherapist are required for assisted coughing.

28.5.5 Mechanically Assisted Coughing

When manually assisted coughing is not enough, an effective alternative may be the addition of *Mechanical In-Exsufflation* (MI-E) [41]. Positive and negative pressures delivered through an oronasal mask or a tracheostomy with the cuff inflated are usually effective to inflate and deflate the lungs [41]. Indications to MI-E are patients with respiratory muscle weakness and *adequate bulbar function* but insufficient function for air stacking to get an appropriate cough capacity as assessed by a CPF > 5 L s^{-1}. This approach is not usually necessary for patients with intact bulbar-innervated muscle function able to air stack with an abdominal thrust to get a CPF > 6 L s^{-1}. Pneumothorax has been reported with MI-E [54]. More recently, a new mechanical device has been proposed to enhance airway clearance, nevertheless its effectiveness in NMD patients is still to be evaluated [55].

28.5.6 Others

Bronchoscopy should only be considered in cases of persistent atelectasis after all noninvasive airway clearance techniques have been proven to be unsuccessful [56].

Aerosolised medications are used with ACT in some diseases although recent guidelines underline the lack of clear evidence for bronchodilators, mucolytics, mucokinetics, to promote airway clearance in these NMD patients [57].

28.5.7 Clinical Results in Clearing Airways

A study suggests that active LVR may help to maintain vital capacity (VC) in DMD patients [53]. With LVR, the respiratory system compliance remained stable, despite a loss in VC. Decline in VC was slow, and cough peak flow (CPF), a measure of cough capacity, was maintained in an effective range [58]. Manually and mechanically assisted coughing were shown to be effective and safe methods for facilitating airway secretion clearance for NMD under MV who would otherwise be managed by endotracheal suctioning [59]. Mechanical in-exsufflation and standard chest physiotherapy improved the management of airway obstruction in NMD patients with airway infections [60]. In a retrospective study ACT were used to reduce the perioperative risks of NMD patients with low VC [61]. During NIV assisted weaning from MV, MI-E reduced the reintubation rates with consequent reduction in postextubation ICU length of stay [62]. Continuous volume-cycled NIV through oral interfaces and masks and MI-E with oximetry feedback in ambient air allowed safe extubation of unweanable patients with NMD [63]. Although a recent systematic review [64] concludes that the scientific evidence does not support the use of MI-E for cough augmentation in patients with NMD, most guidelines recommend the use of mechanically assisted coughing [49, 65, 66].

28.5.8 Respiratory Muscle Training

There is a paucity of literature of respiratory muscle training in NMD. A study suggests that inspiratory and expiratory muscle strength can be increased in these patients by inspiratory and expiratory muscle training without any improvement in spirometry [67]. There is limited evidence that inspiratory muscle training leads to strengthening of inspiratory muscles in amyotrophic lateral sclerosis (ALS) [68]. The weakness of respiratory muscles in these patients is related to the disease itself, therefore we should be cautious in proposing such approach, until a clearer evidence of effectiveness and lack of harmfulness is available.

28.5.9 Tele-rehabilitation

The feasibility of tele-rehabilitation for NMD patients with impaired cough capacity was assessed in a pilot study. Home chest physiotherapy prescribed according to daily registration and transmission of respiratory signs and symptoms to a remote control centre was associated with reduction in hospitalisations and emergency room admissions [69]. Tele-rehabilitation systems may be useful for those NMD ventilator-dependent patients [70] and those living in remote areas with difficult care access [71].

28.5.10 Rehabilitation in Palliative Care and End of Life

There is great variability between countries and within the same country in the availability of home care at the end of life for patients with ALS or other NMD. Several issues such as health resources, physician attitudes, patient/relatives preferences and support resources, including physiotherapy influence the choice [72]. The prevalence of NMD patients needing HMV as well as the related problems are growing [73]. The main concerning of these patients and their families is the control of symptoms especially dyspnoea [74], and the need of strict supervision to avoid complications of HMV, including unexpected death [75]. Alternative locations are not easy. The rehabilitation programmes to be implemented in specialised inpatient facilities are ill defined and there is a clear need to establish guidelines to define the optimal rehabilitation programmes in these settings [76]. Rehabilitative services are underutilised in the palliative care setting and we need more research to evaluate how patients may benefit from these resources at the end of their lives [77].

Conclusion

Restrictive disorders are common in respiratory medicine with patients developing progressive deterioration in function thus leading to several consequences at the pulmonary and extra-pulmonary level. Overall, rehabilitation is becoming an important component in the long-term management of these individuals, although programmes are still far from being homogenised as well as results are not consistent. Notwithstanding, the advances in caring respiratory problems in patients with NMD, in particular, resulted in longer survival and better quality of life as a major progress.

References

1. NICE. The diagnosis and management of suspected idiopathic pulmonary fibrosis: NICE clinical guideline, vol. 163. United Kingdom: National Institute for Health and Care Excellence; 2013.
2. Ley B, Collard HR, King TE Jr. Clinical course and prediction of survival in idiopathic pulmonary fibrosis. Am J Respir Crit Care Med. 2011;183(4):431–40.
3. Raghu G, Weycker D, Edelsberg J, Bradford WZ, Oster G. Incidence and prevalence of idiopathic pulmonary fibrosis. Am J Respir Crit Care Med. 2006;174(7):810–6.
4. Agusti AG, Roca J, Gea J, Wagner PD, Xaubet A, Rodriguez-Roisin R. Mechanisms of gas-exchange impairment in idiopathic pulmonary fibrosis. Am Rev Respir Dis. 1991;143(2):219–25.
5. Hansen JE, Wasserman K. Pathophysiology of activity limitation in patients with interstitial lung disease. Chest. 1996;109(6):1566–76.
6. Swigris JJ, Stewart AL, Gould MK, Wilson SR. Patients' perspectives on how idiopathic pulmonary fibrosis affects the quality of their lives. Health Qual Life Outcomes. 2005;3:61.
7. Cottin V, Cordier JF. Velcro crackles: the key for early diagnosis of idiopathic pulmonary fibrosis? Eur Respir J. 2012;40(3):519–21.
8. Mendoza L, Gogali A, Shrikrishna D, Cavada G, Kemp SV, Natanek SA, Jackson AS, Polkey MI, Wells AU, Hopkinson NS. Quadriceps strength and endurance in fibrotic idiopathic interstitial pneumonia. Respirology. 2014;19(1):138–43.
9. Spruit MA, Thomeer MJ, Gosselink R, Troosters T, Kasran A, Debrock AJ, Demedts MG, Decramer M. Skeletal muscle weakness in patients with sarcoidosis and its relationship with exercise intolerance and reduced health status. Thorax. 2005;60(1):32–8.
10. Marcellis RG, Lenssen AF, Elfferich MD, De Vries J, Kassim S, Foerster K, Drent M. Exercise capacity, muscle strength and fatigue in sarcoidosis. Eur Respir J. 2011;38(3):628–34.
11. Madsen OR, Egsmose C, Hansen B, Sorensen OH. Soft tissue composition, quadriceps strength, bone quality and bone mass in rheumatoid arthritis. Clin Exp Rheumatol. 1998;16(1):27–32.
12. Watanabe, F., H. Taniguchi, K. Sakamoto, Y. Kondoh, T. Kimura, K. Kataoka, T. Ogawa, S. Arizono, O. Nishiyama, and Y. Hasegawa, Quadriceps weakness contributes to exercise capacity in nonspecific interstitial pneumonia.. Respir Med, 2013;107(4):622-628.
13. Mengshoel AM, Jokstad K, Bjerkhoel F. Associations between walking time, quadriceps muscle strength and cardiovascular capacity in patients with rheumatoid

arthritis and ankylosing spondylitis. Clin Rheumatol. 2004;23(4):299–305.

14. Kramer HR, Fontaine KR, Bathon JM, Giles JT. Muscle density in rheumatoid arthritis: associations with disease features and functional outcomes. Arthritis Rheum. 2012;64(8):2438–50.
15. Marighela TF, Genaro Pde S, Pinheiro MM, Szejnfeld VL, Kayser C. Risk factors for body composition abnormalities in systemic sclerosis. Clin Rheumatol. 2013;32(7):1037–44.
16. Wallaert B, Monge E, Le Rouzic O, Wemeau-Stervinou L, Salleron J, Grosbois JM. Physical activity in daily life of patients with fibrotic idiopathic interstitial pneumonia. Chest. 2013;144(5):1652–8.
17. Bahmer T, Kirsten AM, Waschki B, Rabe KF, Magnussen H, Kirsten D, Gramm M, Hummler S, Brunnemer E, Kreuter M, Watz H. Clinical correlates of reduced physical activity in idiopathic pulmonary fibrosis. Respiration. 2016;91(6):497–502.
18. Collard HR, Ward AJ, Lanes S, Cortney Hayflinger D, Rosenberg DM, Hunsche E. Burden of illness in idiopathic pulmonary fibrosis. J Med Econ. 2012;15(5):829–35.
19. King C, Nathan SD. Identification and treatment of comorbidities in idiopathic pulmonary fibrosis and other fibrotic lung diseases. Curr Opin Pulm Med. 2013;19(5):466–73.
20. King CS, Nathan SD. Idiopathic pulmonary fibrosis: effects and optimal management of comorbidities. Lancet Respir Med. 2017;5(1):72–84.
21. Holland AE, Fiore JF Jr, Bell EC, Goh N, Westall G, Symons K, Dowman L, Glaspole I. Dyspnoea and comorbidity contribute to anxiety and depression in interstitial lung disease. Respirology. 2014;19(8):1215–21.
22. Ryerson CJ, Arean PA, Berkeley J, Carrieri-Kohlman VL, Pantilat SZ, Landefeld CS, Collard HR. Depression is a common and chronic comorbidity in patients with interstitial lung disease. Respirology. 2012;17(3):525–32.
23. Kreuter M, Ehlers-Tenenbaum S, Palmowski K, Bruhwyler J, Oltmanns U, Muley T, Heussel CP, Warth A, Kolb M, Herth FJ. Impact of comorbidities on mortality in patients with idiopathic pulmonary fibrosis. PLoS One. 2016;11(3):e0151425.
24. King TE Jr, Bradford WZ, Castro-Bernardini S, Fagan EA, Glaspole I, Glassberg MK, Gorina E, Hopkins PM, Kardatzke D, Lancaster L, Lederer DJ, Nathan SD, Pereira CA, Sahn SA, Sussman R, Swigris JJ, Noble PW, A.S. Group. A phase 3 trial of pirfenidone in patients with idiopathic pulmonary fibrosis. N Engl J Med. 2014;370(22):2083–92.
25. Richeldi L, du Bois RM, Raghu G, Azuma A, Brown KK, Costabel U, Cottin V, Flaherty KR, Hansell DM, Inoue Y, Kim DS, Kolb M, Nicholson AG, Noble PW, Selman M, Taniguchi H, Brun M, Le Maulf F, Girard M, Stowasser S, Schlenker-Herceg R, Disse B, Collard HR, Investigators IT. Efficacy and safety of nintedanib in idiopathic pulmonary fibrosis. N Engl J Med. 2014;370(22):2071–82.
26. Raghu G, Collard HR, Egan JJ, Martinez FJ, Behr J, Brown KK, Colby TV, Cordier JF, Flaherty KR, Lasky JA, Lynch DA, Ryu JH, Swigris JJ, Wells AU, Ancochea J, Bouros D, Carvalho C, Costabel U, Ebina M, Hansell DM, Johkoh T, Kim DS, King TE Jr, Kondoh Y, Myers J, Muller NL, Nicholson AG, Richeldi L, Selman M, Dudden RF, Griss BS, Protzko SL, Schunemann HJ. An Official ATS/ERS/JRS/ALAT Statement: idiopathic pulmonary fibrosis: evidence-based guidelines for diagnosis and management. Am J Respir Crit Care Med. 2011;183(6):788–824.
27. Bradley B, Branley HM, Egan JJ, Greaves MS, Hansell DM, Harrison NK, Hirani N, Hubbard R, Lake F, Millar AB, Wallace WA, Wells AU, Whyte MK, Wilsher ML. Interstitial lung disease guideline: the British Thoracic Society in collaboration with the Thoracic Society of Australia and New Zealand and the Irish Thoracic Society. Thorax. 2008;63(Suppl 5):v1–58.
28. Spruit MA, Singh SJ, Garvey C, ZuWallack R, Nici L, Rochester C, Hill K, Holland AE, Lareau SC, Man WD, Pitta F, Sewell L, Raskin J, Bourbeau J, Crouch R, Franssen FM, Casaburi R, Vercoulen JH, Vogiatzis I, Gosselink R, Clini EM, Effing TW, Maltais F, van der Palen J, Troosters T, Janssen DJ, Collins E, Garcia-Aymerich J, Brooks D, Fahy BF, Puhan MA, Hoogendoorn M, Garrod R, Schols AM, Carlin B, Benzo R, Meek P, Morgan M, Rutten-van Molken MP, Ries AL, Make B, Goldstein RS, Dowson CA, Brozek JL, Donner CF, Wouters EF. An official American Thoracic Society/European Respiratory Society statement: key concepts and advances in pulmonary rehabilitation. Am J Respir Crit Care Med. 2013;188(8):e13–64.
29. Dowman L, Hill CJ, Holland AE. Pulmonary rehabilitation for interstitial lung disease. Cochrane Database Syst Rev. 2014;10:CD006322.
30. McCarthy B, Casey D, Devane D, Murphy K, Murphy E, Lacasse Y. Pulmonary rehabilitation for chronic obstructive pulmonary disease. Cochrane Database Syst Rev. 2015;2:CD003793.
31. Holland AE, Hill CJ, Conron M, Munro P, McDonald CF. Short term improvement in exercise capacity and symptoms following exercise training in interstitial lung disease. Thorax. 2008;63(6):549–54.
32. Vainshelboim B, Oliveira J, Fox BD, Soreck Y, Fruchter O, Kramer MR. Long-term effects of a 12-week exercise training program on clinical outcomes in idiopathic pulmonary fibrosis. Lung. 2015;193(3):345–54.
33. Spruit MA, Pitta F, Garvey C, ZuWallack RL, Roberts CM, Collins EG, Goldstein R, McNamara R, Surpas P, Atsuyoshi K, Lopez-Campos JL, Vogiatzis I, Williams JE, Lareau S, Brooks D, Troosters T, Singh SJ, Hartl S, Clini EM, Wouters EF, E.R.S. Rehabilitation, C. Chronic, G. Physiotherapists Scientific, C. American Association of, R. Pulmonary, A.T.S.P.R. Assembly, and E.R.S. C.OPD Audit team. Differences in content and organisational aspects of pulmonary rehabilitation programmes. Eur Respir J. 2014;43(5):1326–37.

34. Bolton CE, Bevan-Smith EF, Blakey JD, Crowe P, Elkin SL, Garrod R, Greening NJ, Heslop K, Hull JH, Man WD, Morgan MD, Proud D, Roberts CM, Sewell L, Singh SJ, Walker PP, Walmsley S, G. British Thoracic Society Pulmonary Rehabilitation Guideline Development, and C. British Thoracic Society Standards of Care. British Thoracic Society guideline on pulmonary rehabilitation in adults. Thorax. 2013;68(Suppl 2):ii1–30.
35. Borg G. Psycho physical bases of perceived exertion. Med Sci Sports Exerc. 1982;14(5):377–81.
36. Jenkins S, Cecins N. Six-minute walk test: observed adverse events and oxygen desaturation in a large cohort of patients with chronic lung disease. Intern Med J. 2011;41(5):416–22.
37. Glaser S, Noga O, Koch B, Opitz CF, Schmidt B, Temmesfeld B, Dorr M, Ewert R, Schaper C. Impact of pulmonary hypertension on gas exchange and exercise capacity in patients with pulmonary fibrosis. Respir Med. 2009;103(2):317–24.
38. Pouwels-Fry S, Pouwels S, Fournier C, Duchemin A, Tillie-Leblond I, Le Tourneau T, Wallaert B. Effects of oxygen on exercise-induced increase of pulmonary arterial pressure in idiopathic pulmonary fibrosis. Sarcoidosis Vasc Diffuse Lung Dis. 2008;25(2):133–9.
39. Holland AE, Fiore JF Jr, Goh N, Symons K, Dowman L, Westall G, Hazard A, Glaspole I. Be honest and help me prepare for the future: what people with interstitial lung disease want from education in pulmonary rehabilitation. Chron Respir Dis. 2015;12(2):93–101.
40. Holland AE, Spruit MA, Troosters T, Puhan MA, Pepin V, Saey D, McCormack MC, Carlin BW, Sciurba FC, Pitta F, Wanger J, MacIntyre N, Kaminsky DA, Culver BH, Revill SM, Hernandes NA, Andrianopoulos V, Camillo CA, Mitchell KE, Lee AL, Hill CJ, Singh SJ. An official European Respiratory Society/American Thoracic Society Technical Standard: field walking tests in chronic respiratory disease. Eur Respir J. 2014;44(6):1428–46.
41. Ambrosino N, Carpenè N, Gherardi M. Chronic respiratory care in neuromuscular diseases for adults. Eur Respir J. 2009;34(2):444–51.
42. Fiorenza D, Vitacca M, Bianchi L, Gabbrielli L, Ambrosino N. Lung function and disability in neuromuscular patients at first admission to a respiratory clinic. Respir Med. 2011;105(1):151–8.
43. Bushby K, Finkel R, Birnkrant DJ, Case LE, Clemens PR, Cripe L, Kaul A, Kinnett K, McDonald C, Pandya S, Poysky J, Shapiro F, Tomezsko J, Constantin C, DMD Care Considerations Working Group. Diagnosis and management of Duchenne muscular dystrophy. Part 2: Implementation of multidisciplinary care. Lancet Neurol. 2010;9(2):177–89.
44. Ambrosino N, Confalonieri M, Crescimanno G, Vianello A, Vitacca M. The role of respiratory Management of Pompe disease. Respir Med. 2013;107(8):1124–32.
45. Vry J, Gramsch K, Rodger S, Thompson R, Steffensen BF, Rahbek J, Doerken S, Tassoni A, Beytía ML, Guergueltcheva V, Chamova T, Tournev I, Kostera-Pruszczyk A, Kaminska A, Lusakowska A, Mrazova L, Pavlovska L, Strenkova J, Vondráček P, Garami M, Karcagi V, Herczegfalvi Á, Bushby K, Lochmüller H, Kirschner J. European cross-sectional survey of current care practices for Duchenne Muscular Dystrophy reveals regional and age-dependent differences. J Neuromuscul Dis. 2016;3(4):517–27.
46. Bach JR. Noninvasive respiratory management of high level spinal cord injury. J Spinal Cord Med. 2012;35(2):72–80.
47. Dail C, Rodgers M, Guess V, Adkins HV. Glossopharyngeal breathing. Downey, CA: Rancho Los Amigos Department of Physical Therapy; 1979.
48. Webber B, Higgens J. Glossopharyngeal breathing: what, when and how? [video]. West Sussex, England: Aslan Studios Ltd., Holbrook, Horsham; 1999.
49. Strickland SL, Rubin BK, Drescher GS, Haas CF, O'Malley CA, Volsko TA, Branson RD, Hess DR, American Association for Respiratory Care, Irving, Texas. AARC Clinical Practice Guideline: effectiveness of nonpharmacologic airway clearance therapies in hospitalized patients. Respir Care. 2013;58(12):2187–93.
50. McIlwaine M, Bradley J, Elborn JS, Moran F. Personalising airway clearance in chronic lung disease. Eur Respir Rev. 2017;26(143) doi:10.1183/16000617.0086-2016.
51. Gosselink R. Respiratory physiotherapy. In: Donner CF, Ambrosino N, Goldstein RS, editors. Pulmonary rehabilitation. London: Hodder Arnold; 2005. p. 186–94.
52. Kang SW, Bach JR. Maximum insufflation capacity: vital capacity and cough flows in neuromuscular disease. Am J Phys Med Rehabil. 2000;79(3):222–7.
53. Chiou M, Bach JR, Jethani L, Gallagher MF. Active lung volume recruitment to preserve vital capacity in Duchenne Muscular Distrophy. J Rehabil Med. 2017;49(1):49–53.
54. Suri P, Burns SP, Bach JR. Pneumothorax associated with mechanical insufflation-exsufflation and related factors. Am J Phys Med Rehabil. 2008;87(11):951–5.
55. Venturelli E, Crisafulli E, DeBiase A, Righi D, Berrighi D, Cavicchioli PP, Vagheggini G, Dabrosca F, Balbi B, Paneroni M, Bianchi L, Vitacca M, Galimberti V, Zaurino M, Schiavoni G, Iattoni A, Ambrosino N, Clini EM. Efficacy of temporary positive expiratory pressure (TPEP) in patients with lung diseases and chronic mucus hypersecretion. The UNIKO® project. Clin Rehabil. 2013;27(4):336–46.
56. Guarracino F, Bertini P, Bortolotti U, Stefani M, Ambrosino N. Flexible bronchoscopy during mechanical ventilation in the prone position to treat acute lung injury. Rev Port Pneumol. 2013;19(1):42–4.
57. Strickland SL, Rubin BK, Haas CF, Volsko TA, Drescher GS, O'Malley CA. AARC Clinical Practice Guideline: effectiveness of pharmacologic airway clearance therapies in hospitalized patients. Respir Care. 2015;60(7):1071–7.
58. Katz SL, Barrowman N, Monsour A, Su S, Hoey L, McKim D. Long-term effects of lung volume recruitment on maximal inspiratory capacity and vital capac-

ity in Duchenne muscular dystrophy. Ann Am Thorac Soc. 2016;13(2):217–22.
59. Bach JR. Mechanical insufflation-exsufflation. Comparison of peak expiratory flows with manually assisted and unassisted coughing techniques. Chest. 1993;104(5):1553–62.
60. Vianello A, Corrado A, Arcaro G, Gallan F, Ori C, Minuzzo M, Bevilacqua M. Mechanical insufflation exsufflation improves outcomes for neuromuscular disease patients with respiratory tract infections. Am J Phys Med Rehabil. 2005;84(2):83–8.
61. Lee JW, Won YH, Kim DH, Choi WA, Bach JR, Kim DJ, Kang SW. Pulmonary rehabilitation to decrease perioperative risks of spinal fusion for patients with neuromuscular scoliosis and low vital capacity. Eur J Phys Rehabil Med. 2016;52(1):28–35.
62. Goncalves MR, Honrado T, Winck JC, Paiva JA. Effects of mechanical insufflation-exsufflation in preventing respiratory failure after extubation: a randomized controlled trial. Crit Care. 2012;16(2):R48.
63. Bach JR, Goncalves MR, Hamdani I, Winck JC. Extubation of patients with neuromuscular weakness: a new management paradigm. Chest. 2010;137(5):1033–9.
64. Auger C, Hernando V, Galmiche H. Use of mechanical insufflation-exsufflation devices for airway clearance in subjects with neuromuscular disease. Respir Care. 2017;62(2):236–45.
65. Narayanaswami P, Weiss M, Selcen D, David W, Raynor E, Carter G, Wicklund M, Barohn RJ, Ensrud E, Griggs RC, Gronseth G, Amato AA. Evidence-based guideline summary: diagnosis and treatment of limb-girdle and distal dystrophies: report of the guideline development subcommittee of the American Academy of Neurology and the practice issues review panel of the American Association of Neuromuscular & Electrodiagnostic Medicine. Neurology. 2014;83(16):1453–63.
66. Boentert M, Prigent H, Várdi K, Jones HN, Mellies U, Simonds AK, Wenninger S, Barrot Cortés E, Confalonieri M. Practical recommendations for diagnosis and management of respiratory muscle weakness in late-onset Pompe Disease. Int J Mol Sci. 2016;17(10.) pii: E1735
67. Aslan GK, Gurses HN, Issever H, Kiyan E. Effects of respiratory muscle training on pulmonary functions in patients with slowly progressive neuromuscular disease: a randomized controlled trial. Clin Rehabil. 2014;28(6):573–81.
68. Eidenberger M, Nowotny S. Inspiratory muscle training in patients with amyotrophic lateral sclerosis: a systematic review. NeuroRehabilitation. 2014;35(3):349–61.
69. Garuti G, Bagatti S, Verucchi E, Massobrio M, Spagnolatti L, Vezzani G, Lusuardi M. Pulmonary rehabilitation at home guided by telemonitoring and access to healthcare facilities for respiratory complications in patients with neuromuscular disease. Eur J Phys Rehabil Med. 2013;49(1):51–7.
70. Ambrosino N, Vitacca M, Dreher M, Isetta V, Montserrat JM, Tonia T, Turchetti G, Winck JC, Burgos F, Kampelmacher M, Vagheggini G, ERS Tele-Monitoring of Ventilator-Dependent Patients Task Force. Tele-monitoring of ventilator-dependent patients: a European Respiratory Society Statement. Eur Respir J. 2016;48(3):648–63.
71. Ambrosino N, Makhabah DN. Tele-medicine: a new promised land, just to save resources? Eur Respir J. 2017;49:1700410.
72. Escarrabil J, Vianello A, Farrero E, Ambrosino N, Martínez LJ, Vitacca M. Place of death in patients with amyotrophic lateral sclerosis. Rev Port Pneumol. 2014;20(4):188–93.
73. Lloyd-Owen SJ, Donaldson GC, Ambrosino N, Escarabill J, Farre R, Fauroux B, Robert D, Schoenhofer B, Simonds AK, Wedzicha JA. Patterns of home mechanical ventilation use in Europe: results from the Eurovent survey. Eur Respir J. 2005;25(6):1025–31.
74. Vitacca M, Grassi M, Barbano L, Galavotti G, Sturani C, Vianello A, Zanotti E, Ballerin L, Potena A, Scala R, Peratoner A, Ceriana P, Di Buono L, Clini E, Ambrosino N, Hill N, Nava S. Last 3 months of life in home-ventilated patients: the family perception. Eur Respir J. 2010;35(5):1064–71.
75. Di Paolo M, Evangelisti L, Ambrosino N. Unexpected death of a ventilator-dependent ALS patient. Rev Port Pneumol. 2013;19(4):175–8.
76. Winck J, Camacho R, Ambrosino N. Multidisciplinary rehabilitation in ventilator-dependent patients: call for action in specialized inpatients facilities. Rev Port Pneumol (2006). 2015; doi:10.1016/j.rppnen.2015.03.005.
77. Barawid E, Covarrubias N, Tribuzio B, Liao S. The benefits of rehabilitation for palliative care patients. Am J Hosp Palliat Care. 2015;32(1):34–43.

29 Conclusions: Perspectives in Pulmonary Rehabilitation

Enrico Clini, Anne E. Holland, Fabio Pitta, and Thierry Troosters

By assembling 29 chapters comprehensively written by a great number of authors from all over the world, this book updates previous knowledge in the field and hopefully provides a considerable amount of information concerning the pulmonary rehabilitation process regarding delivery, characteristics, and effectiveness, discussing both strengths and limitations. It was considered essential to review new concepts dealing with this clinical process, i.e., settings and patient's conditions which actually are going to be also considered for appropriate selection and referral.

Overall, emerging from this textbook (and therefore from the current literature in which it is based), a few key concepts can be emphasized, such as:

E. Clini (✉)
Department of Medical and Surgical Sciences, University of Modena, Azienda Ospedaliero Universitaria di Modena Policlinico, Modena, Italy
e-mail: enrico.clini@unimore.it

A.E. Holland
Alfred Health and Institute for Breathing and Sleep, La Trobe University, Melbourne, VIC, Australia
e-mail: A.Holland@alfred.org.au

F. Pitta
Departamento de Fisioterapia, State University of Londrina, Londrina, Paranà, Brazil
e-mail: fabiopitta@uol.com.br

T. Troosters
Department of Rehabilitation Sciences, KU Leuven, Respiratory Division and Rehabilitation, University Hospital Leuven, Leuven, Belgium
e-mail: thierry.troosters@med.kuleuven.ac.be

- Comprehensive, regular, and multidisciplinary assessment, including key outcomes for each specific patient, is necessary to provide a good basis for applying the most adequate interventions in pulmonary rehabilitation and to monitor the patient's progression.
- There is clear role for a variety of forms of exercise training that can be used on an individual basis in order to generate benefits in exercise capacity, muscle function, dyspnea, quality of life, and functional status.
- Interventions related to nutrition, physiotherapy, behavior change, occupational therapy, psychology, pharmacotherapy, education, physical activity coaching, nursing, among the others, also have an important role, so that patients may benefit from the multifaceted care which should be ideally embedded in rehabilitation programs.
- Pulmonary rehabilitation greatly benefits not only patients with COPD but also individuals with chronic respiratory diseases other than COPD. Different options of long-term interventions aiming at maintaining the benefits are available, and new ones are certainly welcome.
- Rehabilitation is an important part of the management of exacerbations, since it is known to impact patient's recovery. A specific emphasis should be given to the acute and post-acute care in COPD patients at risk for recurrent exacerbations.

© Springer International Publishing AG 2018
E. Clini et al. (eds.), *Textbook of Pulmonary Rehabilitation*,
https://doi.org/10.1007/978-3-319-65888-9_29

There is a variety of settings and regimens that can be applied in the context of pulmonary rehabilitation, with varying degrees of scientific basis and cost-effectiveness. Surgery, including lung transplantation, e-health modalities, and intensive care area are those settings where promising results are accumulating and research groups are working to fulfill gaps.

Furthermore, a few points still deserve careful consideration as future perspectives in the field of pulmonary rehabilitation. Indeed, the list below underlines some points which may be the subject to special attention from all those professionals and stakeholders involved:

* There is need to increase the applicability, scope, and accessibility to pulmonary rehabilitation programs. Higher number of programs, developed not only in large centers but also in more remote areas, should reach a higher number of patients. Those affected by milder disease, comorbidities, exacerbations, critical illness, and other "non-COPD" chronic respiratory diseases should be targeted. Barriers should be identified and overcome, as well as patient and clinician awareness may be increased. E-health and new technologies emerge more and more as a viable possibility to help with this goal.

* Since current evidence from pulmonary rehabilitation studies do not show consistent results in modifying physical activity, specific interventions for behavior change (e.g., self-management strategies) may pose as interesting options when targeting to impact on physical activity levels, provided the patient has acquired the physiological capacity to be more active.

* Despite the complexity of treating patients with chronic respiratory disorders, the advance in defining phenotypes and better understanding the diseases' characteristics and heterogeneities has the potential to foster knowledge and practice on the rehabilitative possibilities for these populations.

In summary, assessment tools and interventions linked to pulmonary rehabilitation have the possibility to provide our patients with a much better care, meeting their potential needs and expectations.

Erratum to: The Physical Activity Coach in Pulmonary Rehabilitation

Fabio Pitta and Chris Burtin

Erratum to:
Chapter 15 in: E. Clini et al. (eds.), *Textbook of Pulmonary Rehabilitation*, https://doi.org/10.1007/978-3-319-65888-9

The original version of Chapter 15, was inadvertently published with one author name "C. Burtin" instead of two author names "F. Pitta and C. Burtin" and the running head should read as F. Pitta and C. Burtin. The chapter has been updated.

The updated original online version of the chapter can be found at https://doi.org/10.1007/978-3-319-65888-9_15

F. Pitta (✉) • C. Burtin
Faculty of Medicine and Life Sciences, Rehabilitation Research Centre, Biomedical Research Institute, Hasselt University, Diepenbeek, Belgium

© Springer International Publishing AG 2018
E. Clini et al. (eds.), *Textbook of Pulmonary Rehabilitation*,
https://doi.org/10.1007/978-3-319-65888-9_30